CLINICAL DIAGNOSIS

THE HIPPOCRATIC OATH

*I swear by Apollo, the Physician, by As-
clepius, by Hygeia, by Panacea, and by
all the gods and goddesses, making
them my witnesses, that I will carry out,
according to my ability and judgement,
this oath and this indenture. To hold my
teacher in this art equal to my own parents, to make him partner in my liveli-
hood; when he is in need of money to
share mine with him; to consider his
family as my own brothers, and to
teach them this art, if they want to learn
it, without fee or indenture. I will use
treatment to help the sick according to
my ability and judgement, but never
with a view to injury or wrong-doing. I
will keep pure and holy both my life
and my art. In whatsoever houses I
enter I will enter to help the sick, and I
will abstain from all intentional wrong-
doing and harm. And whatsoever I shall
see or hear in the course of my profession in my intercourse with men, if it be
what should not be published abroad, I
will never divulge, holding such things
to be holy secrets. Now if I carry out this
oath, and break it not, may I gain forever reputation among all men for my
life and for my art; but if I transgress it
and forswear myself, may the opposite
befall me.*

Translation by
WILLIAM HENRY RICH JONES
(1817–1885)

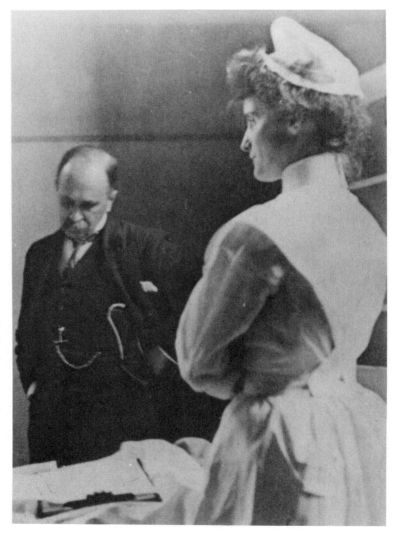

Osler   From the Alan Mason Chesney Medical Archives of The Johns Hopkins Medical Institutions

CLINICAL DIAGNOSIS

A PHYSIOLOGIC APPROACH

FIFTH EDITION

EDITED BY

Richard D. Judge, M.D.

Clinical Professor of Internal Medicine and Assistant Dean
for Student Affairs, University of Michigan Medical School,
Ann Arbor

George D. Zuidema, M.D.

Professor of Surgery and Vice Provost for Medical Affairs,
University of Michigan Medical School; Professor of
Surgery, The University of Michigan Hospitals, Ann Arbor

Faith T. Fitzgerald, M.D.

Professor of Internal Medicine, Vice Chairman, Department
of Medicine, University of California, Davis, School of
Medicine, Davis

With illustrations by
Mary Ann Olson and Leslie H. Arwin, M.D.

*We must turn to nature itself,
to the observations of the
body in health and disease to
learn the truth.*
HIPPOCRATES OF COS
(460?–377? B.C.)

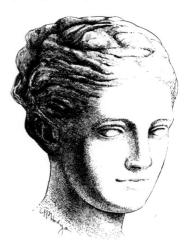

HYGEIA

Little, Brown and Company
Boston/Toronto

The head of Hygeia, Greek goddess of health, on the title page was originally part of a statue that stood outside the Temple of Athena in Tegea, Peloponnesus, Greece, in the fourth century B.C. Its style suggests the influence of the sculptor Praxiteles. The drawing was made by *Gerald P. Hodge,* Professor of Medical and Biological Illustration, The University of Michigan, Ann Arbor.

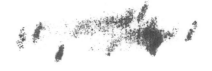

CONTENTS

Contributing Authors   vii

Preface   ix

Section I. INTRODUCTION TO THE HISTORY AND PHYSICAL   1
    1. Introduction   3
    2. Structure and Recording of the Clinical Examination   21
    3. The Patient's History   35

Section II. GENERAL EXAMINATIONS   55
    4. General Appearance   57
    5. Vital Signs   71
    6. Skin   81
    7. Hematopoietic System   101

Section III. HEAD AND NECK   113
    8. Eye   115
    9. Head   153
    10. Neck   185

Section IV. CHEST   195
    11. Respiratory System   197
    12. Cardiovascular System   241
    13. Breast   311

Section V. ABDOMEN AND PELVIS   329
    14. Gastrointestinal System   331
    15. Male Genitourinary System and Hernia   363
    16. Female Genitourinary System   389

Section VI. NEUROMUSCULAR SYSTEM   413
    17. Musculoskeletal System   415
    18. Nervous System   455

Section VII. SPECIAL EXAMINATIONS   503
    19. Pediatric Examination   505
    20. Geriatric Examination   533
    21. Injured Patient   541

Section VIII. THE ART AND SCIENCE OF MEDICINE   573

22. Clinical Problem Solving   575
23. Use of the Clinical Laboratory   585
24. Practical Points for the Wards   589
   History and Physical—Example of the Write-up   589
   Standard Orders   595
   Common Abbreviations   596
   Commonly Used Laboratory Values   612
   Common Drugs, With Brand Names and Uses   613

Index   621

CONTRIBUTING AUTHORS

Terry J. Bergstrom, M.D.
Associate Professor, Department of Ophthalmology, University of Michigan Medical School; Attending Physician, The University of Michigan Hospitals, Ann Arbor

Alan D. Campbell, M.D.
Assistant Professor of Internal Medicine, University of Michigan Medical School; Attending Physician, Division of Hematology/Oncology, Veterans Administration Hospital, Ann Arbor

Eric J. Cassell, M.D.
Clinical Professor of Public Health, Cornell University Medical College; Attending Physician, The New York Hospital, New York

James K. Cooper, M.D.
Associate Professor of Internal Medicine, Director of Geriatrics, Department of Medicine, University of California, Davis, School of Medicine, Davis

Faith T. Fitzgerald, M.D.
Professor of Internal Medicine, Vice Chairman, Department of Medicine, University of California, Davis, School of Medicine, Davis

John C. Floyd, Jr., M.D.
Professor of Internal Medicine, University of Michigan Medical School; Attending Physician, Internal Medicine, The University of Michigan Hospitals, Ann Arbor

Bruce J. Genovese, M.D.
Clinical Instructor of Medicine (Cardiology), University of Michigan Medical School; Director, Coronary Care Unit, St. Joseph Mercy Hospital, Ann Arbor

Sid Gilman, M.D.
Professor and Chairman, Department of Neurology, University of Michigan Medical School; Chief of Service, Department of Neurology, The University of Michigan Hospitals, Ann Arbor

Richard D. Judge, M.D.
Clinical Professor of Internal Medicine and Assistant Dean for Student Affairs, University of Michigan Medical School, Ann Arbor

Theodore M. King, M.D., Ph.D.
Professor, Department of Gynecology and Obstetrics, Johns Hopkins University School of Medicine; Attending Physician, Johns Hopkins Hospital, Baltimore

George H. Lowrey, M.D.
Professor Emeritus of Pediatrics, University of California, Davis, School of Medicine, Davis

Peter J. Lynch, M.D.
Professor and Head, Department of Dermatology, University of Minnesota Medical School—Minneapolis; Attending Staff, Department of Dermatology, University of Minnesota Hospitals and Clinics of the University of Minnesota Health Sciences Center, Minneapolis

Edward J. McGuire, M.D.
Section Head, Urology, University of Michigan Medical School, Ann Arbor

William W. Montgomery, M.D.
Professor, Department of Otolaryngology, Harvard Medical School; Senior Surgeon in Otolaryngology, Massachusetts Eye and Ear Infirmary, Boston

Patricia O'Connor, M.D.
Associate Professor of Pediatrics, University of Michigan Medical School; Attending Physician, Department of Pediatrics, The University of Michigan Hospitals, Ann Arbor

Lee H. Riley, Jr., M.D.
Robinson Professor and Director, Department of Orthopedic Surgery, Johns Hopkins University School of Medicine; Orthopedic Surgeon and Chief, Department of Orthopedic Surgery, Johns Hopkins Hospital, Baltimore

Gerhard Schmeisser, M.D.
Professor, Department of Orthopedic Surgery, Johns Hopkins University School of Medicine, Baltimore

Thomas L. Schwenk, M.D.
Associate Professor and Chairman, Department of Family Practice, University of Michigan Medical School; Attending Physician, The University of Michigan Hospitals, Ann Arbor

Gilbert S. Small, D.D.S.
Clinical Associate Professor of Oral and Maxillofacial Surgery, University of Michigan School of Dentistry; Active Staff, Section of Oral Surgery, Department of General Surgery, St. Joseph Mercy Hospital, Ann Arbor

Ron J. Vanden Belt, M.D.
Clinical Assistant Professor of Internal Medicine, University of Michigan Medical School; Head, Department of Internal Medicine, Catherine MacAuley Health Center, Ann Arbor

John G. Weg, M.D.
Professor of Internal Medicine, University of Michigan Medical School; Attending Physician, Pulmonary Division, The University of Michigan Hospitals, Ann Arbor

Max S. Wicha, M.D.
Professor of Internal Medicine, University of Michigan Medical School; Director, University of Michigan Cancer Center, Ann Arbor

George D. Zuidema, M.D.
Professor of Surgery and Vice Provost for Medical Affairs, University of Michigan Medical School; Professor of Surgery, The University of Michigan Hospitals, Ann Arbor

PREFACE

Why a fifth edition of a textbook on physical diagnosis when there are so many excellent volumes on the market already? And why emphasize *physical* diagnosis at all in an age of medicine in which sophisticated chemical analyzers, Coulter counters, radioisotopes, sonography, radiologic studies, and magnetic resonance imaging have revolutionized laboratory diagnosis?

The first question is easily answered. The authors and editors of this edition, all experienced clinicians, have been impressed by the frequency with which many textbooks of physical diagnosis separate this skill from the rest of medicine, as if it were a technique or set of techniques to be mastered in the first and second years of medical school, then not specifically studied again for the remainder of one's career. We believe, in contrast, that the experienced physician is continually expanding his or her diagnostic skills throughout the years of graduate training and of practice. We have emphasized, therefore, the integration of physical diagnostic techniques with the clinical thought process, problem solving, newer diagnostic laboratory methods, and physician-patient interactions in such a way that we hope the student using this textbook will carry it onto the wards in the clinical clerkships, during house officership, and beyond.

The second question—whether physical diagnosis should be emphasized in an age of technologic medicine—has a somewhat more philosophic answer as well as a pragmatic one. Clinical diagnosis—talking to the patient, touching the patient—has a greater purpose than simply making diagnoses. It is a therapeutic tool as well and is the method by which clinicians bring enrichment and comfort into the lives of their patients, and into their own lives. Heart murmurs are no doubt better "heard" by Doppler ultrasonography than by auscultation with a stethoscope, but the sense of care the patient receives from the physician and the overall understanding of the patient that the physician possesses is probably greater with auscultation than with ultrasonography, if only because the human touch is warmer than that of the machine.

Laboratory technology, in addition, is becoming fearfully expensive and has its dangers. It cannot be done every time a patient is seen: It would be prohibitive both in dollars and, with certain invasive studies, in risk to the patient. As costs rise, the physician of the future will be called on more and more to use his or her clinical diagnostic art *before,* and instead of, the laboratory.

From what we know about the medical marketplace, it is the doctor with good interpersonal skills who will succeed in attracting and keeping patients in the face of a predicted surplus of physicians. It is to this clinician also that the extra time made available by the use of judiciously chosen laboratory and invasive diagnostic tests will be seen as a gift he or she can use to spend in discussion, explanation, and empathy with patients.

This edition has a major contribution from Eric J. Cassell, two of whose works,

The Healer's Art and *Talking with Patients,* have achieved widespread recognition as classics in the field of clinical practice. For those students interested in pursuing these topics in greater depth there are paperback editions available from MIT Press.

R. D. J.
G. D. Z.
F. T. F.

CLINICAL DIAGNOSIS

SECTION I

INTRODUCTION TO THE HISTORY AND PHYSICAL

1. INTRODUCTION
   Eric J. Cassell
2. STRUCTURE AND RECORDING OF THE CLINICAL EXAMINATION
   Faith T. Fitzgerald
   Richard D. Judge
3. THE PATIENT'S HISTORY
   Eric J. Cassell

If you would learn to do a thing, you go to one who does it well; you watch, you listen and your first attempts are made under supervision. The teaching of medical practice began and has continued until recent times under such a simple system of apprenticeship.

SIR THOMAS LEWIS
(1881–1945)

CHAPTER 1

INTRODUCTION

Clinical judgment depends not on knowledge of causes, mechanisms or names of disease but on a knowledge of patients. The background of clinical judgment is clinical experience: the things that clinicians have learned at the bedside in the care of sick people.

ALVAN R. FEINSTEIN
(1925–   )

THE TOOLS OF THE CLINICIAN

To be able to carry out our responsibilities as clinicians, we employ two very different tools, our knowledge of medical science and ourselves. Not only does the faculty (correctly) never lose an opportunity to tell you how vital medical science is, but, if you are like most physicians, you have been pounding scientific knowledge into yourself morning, noon, and night for years. You may not know, however, that the person who is the doctor (you), is equally important. The reason is that doctors treat *individual* patients, while medical science is always about *generalities*—the theory of science will have it no other way. Another way of saying this is that medical science can tell us about pneumonia or liver disease—their causes and treatment—but only a doctor can treat this individual patient with one of those diseases. *Science and technology do not treat patients—doctors do.*

Judgment is the name most often given to the essential quality of physicians that individualizes medical science for individual patients, but we think that the word *judgment* does not cover enough ground. So when we say that this text has but one purpose—to start you on your way to becoming a clinician, we mean that our goal is to start you on your way to acquiring and perfecting your best and most effective diagnostic and therapeutic instrument—*yourself.* A solid foundation of medical science in a doctor who cares about patients and is observant, thorough, disciplined, thoughtful, and self-reflective defines a good clinician.

We would be leaving out perhaps the best part, however, if we stopped there in telling you what we want you to learn. The knowledge of science that you have acquired is necessarily about parts of people—e.g., subcellular, cellular, or organs—but patients always come in wholes, not parts. Clinicians learn to translate what they know about, for example, the molecular biology of the immune system and the physiology of neuromuscular transmission into knowledge about patients with myesthenia gravis. To do this they have to learn how each element in pathophysiology expresses itself in patients who are walking, talking, working, and getting on with their lives. Consequently, clinicians have to learn a whole lot about people and how to help them participate in their own diagnosis and treatment. It takes knowledge about human nature in addition to a bit of Sherlock Holmes and touch of Houdini to make the science of medicine work for sick persons.

THE DOCTOR, THE PATIENT, AND THE RELATIONSHIP

Every history and physical examination, whether it is the full-fledged formal affair that takes place on admission to the hospital, or the less formal questioning and examination that are done in follow-up visits or over the telephone (yes, one can do some physical examination over the telephone!) has a cast of at least three characters: the doctor, the patient, and their relationship. One of the most rewarding and pleasurable aspects of being a clinician comes from the fact that because each patient is different, each relationship varies, and consequently the doctor must change somewhat to meet these differences. When students begin learning how to take a history and examine a patient, they are trying so hard to feel what is in the abdomen or to hear the heart murmur that they overlook the miraculous thing that happened during their introduction to the patient and those few moments of polite conversation in which they tried to put the patient at ease, or vice versa. In what must be one of the oddest phenomena of humankind, a student or a doctor approaches someone who is a total stranger, and within a few minutes is asking the most intimate questions and poking fingers into the most private places. And this complete stranger (the patient) not only lets them do these things, but says thank you when it is over!

There must be something special about being a patient that changes the strictest social rules of behavior in such a short space of time. There must also be something special about the relationship between patient and caregiver that allows the patient to feel safe enough to make such changes in behavior because a physician or a medical student is present. It is not only the patient that changes from everyday social behavior, the medical student (and physician) also shift away from the everyday.

The usual answer to the question of why sick persons allow students (and doctors) to ask all those questions and permit themselves to be undressed and examined is that they are ill and require help. But that cannot be the entire reason because except for the most dire emergencies, sick persons do not allow even the best-meaning friends similar access to their bodies. Neither is it simply medical knowledge that gains entry to the person's confidence. Rather, the answer is that when persons become patients, by beginning a therapeutic relationship with a doctor, they allow doctors entrance to their most private selves. The circularity of the preceding sentence is eliminated by the fact that becoming a patient is a social change that necessarily entails the existence of special persons called doctors and a special relationship. This social change of state (sociologists refer to such transformations as *status passages*) alters the rules of behavior and expectations of all the actors in the drama of medical care. In other words, there would not be patients as we know them, if there were not doctors (as we know them) and if the relationship between the two did not have the unique set of rules that guides it. Just as you have become very sophisticated about human biology, you must leave behind the simplistic notion that the necessary conditions for medical care are merely sick persons and doctors with the knowledge to treat them. When you understand what it is about doctors, patients and their relationship that makes it possible for the professional care of the sick to exist, it will be much easier to do the work for which this text prepares you.

THE PHYSICIAN

The essential human qualities required of candidates seeking ABIM certification are integrity, respect, and compassion . . . . moral behavior is an overriding professional consideration in caring for patients.

AMERICAN BOARD OF INTERNAL MEDICINE
1985

A physician is at the same time an individual private person and someone who inhabits the role known as physician. The same is true of a medical student. When it comes to patient contact, the roles of the two are similar except for the differences imposed by differing responsibility and knowledge. The rules, rewards, and constraints associated with many roles are powerful determinants of behavior. All roles have ideal representatives—in this case, what people believe doctors should be like and how they should behave. Roles also consist of entitlements and limitations—what doctors may do and what they are either not permitted or not required to perform. So that, as mentioned above, you are entitled to handle a woman's breasts or a man's penis, but it is a *serious* breach of the limitations contained in physician's role to make a sexual overture to a patient. Similarly, you are entitled to respect and admiration as a medical student but there are limits to what you can do within that role and still keep the respect.

It is important to keep this idea in mind that you are both the you that you know and also an inhabitant of a role, because it will provide you with important information about patients and protect you from some painful experiences and errors. Doctors are sometimes hurt because a patient becomes angry with them without reason. The physician takes it personally. In fact, the patient was angry, not with Bill Osler, but with Doctor (or medical student) Osler. Realizing the difference, and reflecting on why the patient might be angry with a doctor, the physician now has access to information that may be important in taking care of the patient.

Similarly it is the constraints of the role that sometimes lead to complaints about student dress. It is one thing for Wild Bill Osler to dress like a mountain man, but patients have expectations about medical students that require Bill Osler to rein in that aspect of his personality without feeling personally criticized. It would be all right for students to override the limitations on their dress and personal behavior as long as they are equally willing to give up the respect and admiration usually accorded to medical students—a role is an all-or-none package. As you work with patients over the coming years, you will be learning more about the role called *physician*. As with taking histories and doing physical examinations, you will end up knowing much more if you are self-reflective in the process, learning both the thing itself and the how and the why of learning it.

There is something special about being a doctor, so special that in virtually every culture, in good times and bad, when the profession as a whole is in favor or out of favor, people treat doctors with singular respect and hold them in high esteem. We know that fact, which is why all of us, at certain stages in our training, nonchalantly allow our stethoscopes to show, hoping that the allure of medicine will be attached to us by the onlookers. The source of admiration accorded individual doctors lies in the characteristics believed to be true of the ideal representative of the physician's role.

One reason people respect us is that they dread sickness and death, and they know that physicians have learned to work without fear among the sick and the dying. You may be sceptical about laypersons' faith in your bravery, because you are all too aware of your own fears of disease and the idea of the coming responsibility for life and death decisions weighs heavily. But whatever trepidations doctors may have, the patient's worries and uncertainties are much greater. For this reason physicians must learn to keep their qualms from showing. This does not mean that you must pretend to yourself that you are not frightened, quite the contrary, *fear, repulsion, and uncertainty are controlled best when they are acknowledged* because only then can you succeed in actively keeping them from being evident on the surface. As you learn physical diagnosis you will have an opportunity to practice this because at first (if you are like others) you will be afraid to touch the body, palpate masses, smell certain lesions, or even look closely at sexual organs. Gradually, you will come to know how much pressure will not cause pain, when looking is not staring, how to tolerate what was previously nauseating, and how to dissociate the erotic implications from sexual body parts. It is important to realize that you are not merely "getting used to" examining sick people, you are learning something essential to the care of the sick—how to be a bridge between the person and their disease. Patients are also offended by the sight, smell, and feel of their diseased body; because of this they frequently tend to conceive of their sick selves as repellent. When you look and touch each patient as though whatever the body is like it is totally acceptable to you, you make patients acceptable to themselves despite their disease and that actively reduces the burden of their sickness.

Just as it is doctors not science that treat disease, hands alone do not palpate the abdomen, and ears alone do not listen to heart sounds; doctors do these things, employing their hands or their ears. The distinction is important because not only are you training yourself to attend to the faintest variations under your hands in size, texture, or temperature and to remember the sensations—things that laypersons are unable to do—at the same time *you are teaching yourself to be a physician,* someone whose every action has the potential for helping the patient. You will learn this best if you actively remember that *every diagnostic act is a therapeutic act.*

Sometimes students tell us that this is the last thing they want to remember because initially they are so conscious of their own ineptitude. As humbling as it may be, no one, including the patients, expects you to be more expert than is customary at your stage of training. Students and doctors tend to forget how knowledgeable patients are. Patients constantly talk among themselves about the staff, and in university hospitals they are usually able to distinguish students, interns, residents, fellows, and attendings, although they may not know what each is called. When a student tries to pretend to an expertise that he or she does not have, the student generally looks not like an expert, but like someone pretending to be one. Nothing more surely tells of ignorance then pretensions. Perhaps the worst thing about trying to look like someone you are not is that you become more concerned about what the patient will see in you than what you will see in the patient.

People also respect physicians because of their knowledge. They expect us, correctly, to be knowledgeable about the body and its ills, but also to be aware of the latest findings of medical science. Their respect is not only for the corpus of information that we possess, but for the attitude towards learning that is believed to be characteristic of ideal physicians. Doctors, like science itself, are believed to be people who are always probing and searching for the answers to the mysteries of disease. Ours is understood to be a restless intellect. For this reason, patients not only respect us for our knowledge, but, strangely, for our ignorance. Everyone knows both that no doctor can know everything and that only people who know a lot can admit to ignorance. Thus, when a doctor says, "I don't know," the implications are both that he or she has confidence (because of being knowledgeable) and that he or she will try and find out. It is frequently said that good physicians are perpetual students, and this should be understood not only in terms of reading published information, but in terms of being continually a student where *the patient is the teacher.*

This textbook will introduce you to the concepts and methods of clinical diagnosis so that in the future you bring that knowledge with you to every patient, but also so that every time you approach sick persons you are prepared to learn from them. We understand how different are these views of knowledge from the ones you learned in the intensively competitive atmosphere of the premed and preclinical classroom, but those other attitudes that seemed (falsely, we believe) to serve you best in relation to your colleagues are merely another aspect of being a layman that you must learn to change to achieve mastery as a physician.

Many of us presumed early in our careers that patients should trust us because we had the latest in medical training. But patients take it for granted that we are knowledgeable; they trust us because we are trustworthy. There are many characteristics in physicians that make them trustworthy, for example, thoroughness, attention to detail, overriding concern for the patient, being there when needed, maintenance of knowledge, self-discipline, and self-knowledge. Trust, which should never be confused with blind trust, is granted to physicians because of their role and then grows or shrinks as the patient has experience with the individual physician's behavior.

Two important characteristics of the trustworthy physician can be developed from your earliest experiences in physical diagnosis: thoroughness and attention to detail. As you examine even your first patient, pay attention to the small details of the examination, the patient's words, his or her appearance, the appearance of the room, bedside table, and bed. Be thorough as you examine the patient even though it may seem to go on endlessly. Most students are so worried about bothering the patient that they do not spend sufficient time. Although it is not wrong to be considerate of patients' welfare, it is a waste of their time if through inattention to detail or lack of thoroughness you learned little or nothing. We are all aware that in the beginning it is virtually impossible to keep all these requirements in mind, but it is not your beginner's proficiency that is your primary goal—nor the goal of this text—but your ultimate mastery.

Empathy, an essential and highly developed skill in effective clinicians, is difficult to describe despite the fact that the social world could not exist without it. As we drive, walk, talk, and move in our daily world, we give way, make room, wait, and provide help for others almost constantly even when it slows us down or is inconvenient. We do that because we understand and accept their behavior as they do ours. Similarly, we are embarrassed for others when they fall or make a mess in public because we feel what it would be like if it had happened to us. In other words, empathy—knowing, understanding, or feeling the feelings and thoughts of others—is a natural part of the human condition.

The empathy of physicians differs because its goal is different—to help patients. Empathy in physicians also differs in that it seeks to know thoughts and feelings about aspects of the personal life, sickness, and relationships to the body of the patient that are not part of the public experience that trains everyday empathy. Although empathy is a necessary part of the kindness and compassion that doctors should develop, it also serves practical diagnostic and therapeutic ends. For example, we are much better able to evaluate the importance of a symptom if we are aware of the extent of distress it causes the patient. Asking questions (see Chap. 3) will provide some information about this, but language is a poor tool for the expression of feelings. It is our ability to empathize that allows us to extend the information provided by the patient's answers to our questions. Frequently, what we wish to know is intensely private and painful to the patient. Patient's awareness of the physician's understanding and concern (external forms that empathy takes) allows them to overcome their inhibitions, embarrassments, or fears of ridicule sufficiently to tell us. Our empathy is tolerant (another dress of empathy) of their weaknesses, and so their protective shields are lowered sufficiently to let us help. So too is the doctor's empathy patient (yet another guise of empathy) with the time it takes patients to do things; thus, patients whose clumsiness would otherwise inhibit them will make extra efforts at recovery.

All these rewards should spur physicians toward developing empathy, but usually doctors hold back. One reason appears to be that most of the behaviors we try to empathetically accept in patients are behaviors we do not permit in ourselves. Consequently, to become more empathetic towards the sick we must become more accepting of ourselves. This is another example of how medical students and doctors change within themselves as they achieve diagnostic and therapeutic skills. Another impediment to developing empathy is that there are no teaching tools for it that are equivalent to the heart sound recordings. Just as when you listen to heart sounds you should be developing the skill of attending to the sounds coming from the stethoscope (rather than all the other sounds in the room), or when you are palpating you should be attending to the tips of your fingers, empathy requires attending to and concentrating on the patient rather than on his or her words alone. It may be useful to you to know that some clinicians believe that their noses are their primary tool for empathy! We do not want to leave the subject without saying that aside from their enormous diagnostic and therapeutic utility, empathetic

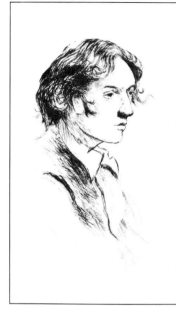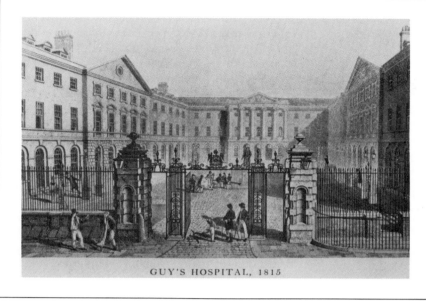

GUY'S HOSPITAL, 1815

FIGURE 1—1
John Keats was only 26 years old when he died of tuberculosis. During his short adult life, he was a medical student at Guy's Hospital for 5 years. He passed his qualifying examinations but never practiced. (Used by permission of the Easton Press, Norwalk, Conn.)

connections with patients provide physicians with much of their pleasure in medicine.

The ideal physician is also believed to be humane, kind, considerate, and caring. Many physicians-in-training think of all the characteristics that are said to exemplify physicians and wonder whether they can ever meet such expectations. Dr. Walsh McDermott, who was one of the most admired physicians of our time, told how when he was a medical student he knew that he personally did not match up to these descriptions of the best physicians. But, he said, he also knew what he had to do and how he had to act in order to fulfill the expectations of others in these regards, and so he did it. That is all any one can ask of you.

THE PATIENT
One who is ill has not only the right but also the duty to seek medical aid.

MAIMONIDES
(1135–1204)

A patient, we stated above, is someone who goes to a doctor. From this one can infer the foremost characteristic of patienthood: *it is a consensual, voluntary state.* If your image of medical care is formed by *M*A*S*H,* with the wounded on stretchers coming in by helicopter, the preceding sentence may seem nonsensical. Medical care, however, is a process not an event. Even those soldiers, when they emerged from the surgical tent, might choose not to follow doctors orders, covertly refuse medications, or exert their independence in any number of ways. One might wonder why they, or any other patient, would want to do that when their doctors are trying to help them get better. The verb, to want, used in this sense also implies that patients have choice. To say that doctors try to help people get better suggests the cooperative nature of caring for the sick. Disregarding these two facts—that patients have choice and that medical care is a cooperative venture—is the major cause of the difficulties that students and physicians have with patients.

Nobody would forget these obvious truths, however, were it not for another essential feature of patienthood. Every person who becomes a patient does so because he or she is sick, believes sickness to be present, fears sickness, is trying to prevent sickness, or is motivated by some aspect of sickness. Patienthood, which is voluntary and consensual, is commonly mistakenly considered to be the equivalent of sickness, which is involuntary and coercive. The world of the sick is different from the world of the well, and the sick have different behaviors. They can be demanding, irritating, clinging, rebellious, forgetful, self-absorbed, self-defeating, self-endangering, self-deluding, angry, seductive, changeable, loving, manipulative, needy, denying, untruthful, worshipful, foolish, and they need the help of others much more than the well. We forgive them all of these traits (when we are able to remember that they are sick) because the sick also die, suffer, choke, become disabled, go blind, have pain, lose everything that counts, and need the help of others much more than the well. Because of all the terrible things that can happen to the sick, compassion forces us to extend ourselves towards them and to help them. In modern medicine, because of the advances of science and technology, our compassion is armed with the knowledge and powerful weapons to make patients better. We physicians believe in our science and in our abilities. Little wonder, in view of all this, that we doctors often act as if patients are passive folks who have been depersonalized by the diseases that carried them to us for our cure.

You may believe that the idea of the voluntary and consensual nature of patienthood has arisen only in the current climate of medical ethics which emphasizes patient autonomy, but that is mistaken. It is true that in our society, the days of "doctor knows best" have disappeared in company with many other evidences of overriding respect for authority. Effective clinicians, however, have always understood the importance of discussions with patients about their disease and its treatment to obtain their cooperation. Even Plato talks about the value of physicians acting as teachers with their patients. What has changed recently is the language that is employed to discuss these issues. You will find it easier to understand if you rid yourself of the words "patient compliance" and use in their stead "patient cooperation" or "patient participation." It was possible to believe in the authoritarian nature of doctors as long as we were able to sustain the odd notion that doctors treat diseases, and that patients and their ideas are inconveniences that get between a doctor and a disease. Diseases, to the contrary, have no free-standing existence—

they can only be found in patients. Doctors do not treat diseases; they treat patients.

If your image of disease is pneumococcal pneumonia, then it seems reasonable to envision treatment as, for example, giving antibiotics. Nowadays most sick patients do not have pneumococcal pneumonia; their illnesses are more complicated and more often chronic. In these instances, patients treat themselves—taking their medications, giving themselves insulin, changing their dressings, following their diets, and doing their exercises—on the basis of what their doctors have taught them and to the degree that their doctors have motivated them. Just as you do not learn just because you should, but more often because you like and respect the teacher, patients act in the same manner.

It follows from what we have said that communication skills are essential for patient care. Actually, students beginning physical diagnosis have already learned one of the basic uses of doctor-patient communication—talking patients into saying yes—otherwise the students would never have gotten to examine even their first patients. Rhetoric, the art of persuasive speaking, which is what this use of language is called, has come to have a bad reputation because of its connection with doubtful causes and inflated language. It is, on the other hand, a required skill in medicine where it is so often necessary to convince patients to take an action (e.g., be operated on or start chemotherapy) they would like to avoid but which we (and parts of them) know to be in their best interests. You will be learning this skill from your first contacts with patients.

Most physicians believe they are immune from the dangers of practicing overly persuasive rhetoric because they only suggest to patients what they know to be in the patient's best interests. This attitude, which is quite common, reflects a confusion. Even the most knowledgeable and experienced physicians among us can know with certainty solely what is best *for the patient's disease;* only the *patient knows what is in the best interest of the patient.* The correct thing to do for the disease is most often the right thing for the patient, but not always. This is especially true in relation to high-risk therapies and in the care of terminally ill patients. Somehow, even in complex and highly technical circumstances, patients must be made sufficiently aware of the facts so that they can balance them against what is important in their lives. You may wonder how you are to meet that requirement in view of all the seemingly irrational behaviors of sick patients that might interfere with clear-headed judgments about the best alternatives. Here is where your empathy and communication skills meet their strictest test. Your task, in diagnosis, is not only to find out what is the patient's disease, but also to discover who the patient is. Both kinds of knowledge are necessary to take care of individual sick patients. The instrument that best serves these demanding aims is yourself, armed with knowledge of medical science and knowledge of persons. If this task was dumped on you all at once, the responsibility would be awesome, which is why the system of medical education increases your responsibility as your competence improves. We want you to be aware that as you approach patients in your physical diagnosis course you are starting to learn how to achieve both of these goals: to know the disease and to know the patient.

THE RELATIONSHIP

The principal objective of the medical profession is to render service to humanity with full respect to the dignity of man . . . . rendering to each a full measure of service and devotion.

AMA ETHICAL CODE
1957

The vehicle that makes your work as a student and a physician possible is the relationship to the patient. Much has been written about the doctor-patient relationship, but aside from the fact that it is universally considered to be benevolent, its true nature remains elusive. It has been compared to the relationship between parent and child, but while similarities are present, the comparison is lacking. Some have applied the concept of business contract, while others have employed the idea of a covenant. Although each concept explains one or another aspect of the relationship, the total continues to be obscure. We believe that it is fundamentally based on two human traits; the power of sickness or its threat to make patients receptive to change at all levels of the human condition, and the power of benevolence to induce persons who care for the sick to extend *themselves* at all levels of the human condition. From this it follows that the relationship exerts an influence on both patients and doctors. If you are like most doctors, you will find yourself going out of your way to be kind and careful when you are with patients. As you develop professionally, you will expect from yourself higher standards of behavior with patients then you use in the usual social interactions. Not only is this a source of gratification to students and doctors, but patients are more responsive to students and physicians whom they perceive as caring. It is also true that students and physicians experience the pain of loss when their patients die. The personal involvement with patients that leads to these observations is not only unavoidable, but there could not be medical care in its absence. Learning how much of yourself to give to your patients and how to manage the emotional strains produced by caring for the sick and dying will occupy you for virtually *all* of your professional life. The fact that you are in a relationship with patients that is different from others in your experience will probably be apparent to you with your first patient contacts.

Students frequently express their discomfort at inconveniencing patients. Because they are not equipped to diagnose or treat, they tend to feel that the intrusions made upon patients' time and person are unjustified. Students interrupt naptimes or meals, ask embarrassing questions for hours on end, and awkwardly poke away at them. And from all of this, there is no concrete benefit to the patient. If, as is the case, the ruling moral dictum of medicine is "Above all, do no harm," how is all this inconvenience justified?

Medical training is an apprenticeship. There is no better way to learn than at the bedside, and there are no better teachers than our patients. For each of us there is always a first patient, one to whom little advantage is returned for the discomforts. The skill necessary to give benefit, however, is only acquired through multiple contacts with many patients. Yet the patients may benefit. Many will delight in students visits; they are frequently happy to participate in your training, and being an active part of your teaching enhances their sense of self-worth and allows them to take pride in their students. Sickness and hospitalization are lonely conditions. The student visit may be the high point of the patient's week. Although students lack skill, they have one thing to offer which patients often find lacking in other staff: time. If you demonstrate your interest, your patients will recount their experiences and tell you their troubles. They need a listener who is not, as visitors so often do, trying to top them or responding with platitudes or moral judgments. It is a therapeutic act to allow someone to tell his or her story without interruption. Students are frequently afraid that once the patients starts, the narrative will go on forever. It is more usual for them to be afraid of wasting *your* time. Be patient and you will both help the patient and learn much about the experience of illness, medical care, and hospitalization.

THE GOALS OF HISTORY TAKING AND PHYSICAL DIAGNOSIS

The Physician must be able to tell the antecedents, know the present, and foretell the future—must meditate these things and have two special objects in view with regard to diseases, namely, to do good or to do no harm. The art consists in three things—the disease, the patient, and the physician. The physician is the servant of the art, and the patient must combat the disease along with the physician.

HIPPOCRATES
460?–377? B.C.

Doctors who are directly involved in the care of patients have four fundamental tasks:

1. Making a diagnosis.
2. Discovering the cause of the problem.
3. Determining treatment.
4. Establishing a prognosis.

Everything that we clinicians do to and for our patients—for example, well-baby examinations, preventive medicine, nutritional guidance, family counseling, treating the very sick, emergency medicine, surgical procedures, and the care of the dying—includes one or another of these basic jobs.

MAKING A DIAGNOSIS

As you can see, each one of the succeeding tasks depends on the first, the diagnosis of the patient's sickness. The techniques described in this text are employed by all physicians in discovering the patient's disease. *This is the central methodology of medicine.* No matter how experienced or sophisticated you become, you will be employing these diagnostic procedures all of your professional life. The generation of physicians who preceded you would never have doubted that fact, but because of current diagnostic technologies, the centrality of taking histories and doing physical examinations has been questioned by some medical students and doctors. The capability of computed tomographic (CT) scans, the potential of magnetic resonance imaging, immunologic testing based on monoclonal antibodies, and the host of other techniques for visualizing or revealing disease seem to cast doubt on what one doctor can do by merely asking questions or feeling for lumps.

Progress in diagnostic capabilities has not diminished the importance of taking a good history and doing a careful physical examination. The reasons for this come from the fact that the name of the disease is only one part of a description of the patient's problem. At first glance it would appear that to make a diagnosis is to discover the patient's disease. Pneumococcal pneumonia, lupus erythematosis, adenocarcinoma of the lung, and acute myocardial infarction are typical disease diagnoses. If we were to say to a clinician that we have a patient with pneumococcal pneumonia and ask how to treat, we might be told to give penicillin. But you already know that allergy to penicillin would require modification of the treatment as would concurrent diseases such as sickle cell anemia or some immune disorder. For the patient with lupus, your consultant needs to know whether the patient has already been treated and how, how long the disease has been present, and what the complications are—whether, in fact, the patient is ill at the present time. For the patient with adenocarcinoma of the lung, an immediate question would be where in the lung the tumor is situated and whether metastatic disease is present. Where the patient lives, the availability of medical services, the presence or absence of family, and other seemingly nonmedical issues all have a bearing on treatment. For the patient with a myocardial infarction, the doctor's actions will be influenced by how recent the episode is, the patient's age, the presence of other diseases, and associated risk factors.

All of these other factors are not strictly part of a diagnosis, but for clinicians they are equally important because no effective action can be taken in the absence of such knowledge. Clinicians, then, are seeking to discover: (1) the disease; (2) the factors that modify it within or external to the patient; (3) at what point in the overall course of the disease is the patient at this moment; and (4) what is there about *this* sick person that modifies the presentation, course, treatment, or outcome of the disease. The information that provides the answers to these questions comes from taking a history, the physical examination, laboratory and other diagnostic technologies, and the observation over time of the patient's illness. No one source can be used to the exclusion of others.

FINDING A CAUSE

The term scientific cannot be denied to an accurate observation at the bedside, if it is conceded to a similarly accurate observation made by means of the microscope; nor can it be denied to a correct description of a process observed in a patient, while conceded to the correct description of a process observed in a rabbit or guinea pig. The clinic is scientific, not merely in so far as it utilizes chemical or physical methods and technique, but primarily because it represents a determined, fearless, and painstaking effort to observe, to explore, to interpret, to unravel.

ABRAHAM FLEXNER
(1866–1959)

The cause we are seeking is not merely the immediate cause (the pneumococcus in pneumococcal pneumonia or human immunodeficiency virus (HIV) infection in acquired immunodeficiency syndrome), but rather the chain of events by which the patient moved from a healthy person to a sick person. Thus, in persons with chronic obstructive pulmonary disease, we are interested not only in whether they smoked cigarettes, but whether their occupation or other environmental exposures may have contributed to the illness, whether they have obtained adequate medical care, whether they understand their medications, or whether alpha$_1$-trypsonase deficiency is present. In persons with recurrent urinary tract infections, we might look for anatomical abnormalities that may be promoting infection (for example, bladder stones, cystocele, or urethral stricture), the nature of the infecting organism, personal habits that may promote recurrence, and inadequate understanding by the patient of the nature of the illness and its treatment so that medication was not correctly used. The clinical diagnosis of coronary heart disease based on a history of angina pectoris prompts the search for known risk factors, including dietary habits and level of physical activity, in addition to being alert to other diseases or factors that might have precipitated the angina in this patient at this time. Another example is discovering that a patient's hip fracture is a result of alcoholism.

TREATMENT

A proper understanding of cause leads to the concept that all diseases are processes that involve a chain of events taking place over time. Treatment is the activity that interrupts the chain in order to change the outcome. Modern medicine is at its most effective when a knowledge of the pathophysiology of a disease leads to a treatment that stops the disease. The interruption of the metabolism of uric acid by allopurinol is an example, as is the use of vasodilators to reduce the afterload of a failing heart. However, *any intervention* that interferes with the disease process, inside or outside of the patient, is equally acceptable. Changing diet, promoting exercise, stopping smoking, and educating patients in the proper use of insulin can be more effective therapy, ultimately, than more direct interventions such as antibiotics. The knowledge on which treatment is based is equally knowledge of medical science, knowledge of patients and their diseases, and the knowledge of how to elicit the participation of patients in their own care. Although this is not a textbook on therapeutics, it should be apparent that learning the necessary information about patients and their diseases starts with taking a good history and doing a careful physical examination.

PROGNOSIS

Hippocrates knew, and all doctors learn, the importance of predicting the course and outcome of their patients' illnesses. Doctors are not magicians or fortune tellers. Their ability to predict the future comes from a knowledge of the behavior of specific diseases, knowledge of the factors in *this* patient that might modify the course of the disease, and an ability to learn the tempo of the disease by watching its progress over time. For this reason, as well as to determine the effects of treatment or the occurence of complications, physicians carefully reexamine and question patients daily while they are in the hospital. Accurate prognostication protects physicians against surprise happenings, allows the early detection of deviations from the predicted course, and keeps patients abreast of their circumstances. In addition, patients who understand what is most likely to happen can prepare in advance for the best and the worst rather than depending only on their fears or the gossip of their friends.

As you examine patients, now and in the future, learn the skill of making small predictions about what you expect to see in your next encounter with the patient: how will the wound appear, what will the chest sound like, what will the patient's face look like. Make these prognostic statements aloud to *yourself* (not to the patient); then check on their accuracy when you next meet the patient. Learn what supported and what defeated your predictions. Just as continued examination of patients will sharpen your diagnostic skills, so actively making and checking your predictions will hone your prognostic abilities.

INFORMATION

This entire book is concerned with methods for obtaining information. Your professional life will be spent gathering information about patients based on their statements, your examination of them, and your inspection of diagnostic studies. In these activities, *it is vital to learn, and never forget, the difference between information and the conclusions drawn from it.* This failure to distinguish the interpretation from the observation is the basis for many diagnostic errors. In the discussion of heart murmurs (pp. 289-302), for example, you will find a language and a simple system for describing the sounds you hear when listening to the heart. Given the information about the heart that these sounds provide, you may draw conclusions about disturbances in its anatomy or physiology. For example, based primarily upon its location and the timing in systole you may believe that a particular murmur is produced by aortic stenosis. If you record the description of the findings (the information), it is always open for possible reinterpretation in the light of other information. If you fall into the common error of writing that the patient has "the murmur of aortic stenosis," this statement, which is a conclusion, closes the door to further interpretation. In addition such assertions make it impossible for others to know what the patient's heart sounded like at your examination.

In similar fashion, one sees admitting notes that state that a patient has a "hot joint," a "lipoma," a "basal cell," or a "parkinsonian gait." These diagnostic conclusions may be correct, but they contain very little information from which others can draw conclusions. Perhaps worse, physicians who get into the habit of recording such interpretations lose their observational skills. These doctors become pattern recognizers, fitting everything into known categories rather than training themselves to be consciously aware of what is presented to their senses and only then drawing inferences. Developing excellent observational skills requires discipline and plenty of practice. Pattern recognizers see only what they know, whereas good observers can continue to learn new things. The mind cannot be prevented from jumping to conclusions; it takes discipline to train yourself to go back and actively and consciously note all the details even when you believe the immediate interpretation to be correct. The key is consciously recording what your senses report; some diagnosticians suggest that in your early training you say everything aloud to yourself. We cannot stress too strongly that if you spend the time to develop observational skills now, they will continue to serve you. It is very difficult to undo bad habits learned early in training.

Well-developed observational skills will give you the confidence to stand by your findings. Too often when there is a conflict between a finding on physical examination and the results of a test or an x-ray film, physicians will conclude that their observation was incorrect. If you felt a mass in the abdomen, then there is something in the abdomen that felt like a mass. If a sonogram or CT scan fails to reveal it, then you must explain what it was that you felt. Perhaps it was feces in the bowel; if so, on reexamining the abdomen the mass should be gone. If it is still present, perhaps the imaging study is incorrect—it is of another patient or has been incorrectly interpreted. If there is a large mass in the left upper quadrant of the abdomen where you expect to palpate the spleen, perhaps it is the spleen or perhaps the kidney, but it *is* something, and it should not be dismissed until it has been explained.

All information is true only between confidence limits. The clinician's task is to narrow the confidence limits, that is, increase the accuracy of information to the degree possible. Whenever inferences are drawn, the probability that the information on which they are based is correct must always be kept actively in mind. To do this, you should get into the habit of assessing probabilities. Perhaps, on the basis of a chest roentgenogram, you believe a hilar mass is present; tell yourself *in numbers* what you believe to be the probability that your conclusion is correct. Gradually you will acquire the ability to think in terms of competing probabilities. In another instance, perhaps the evidence suggests that a patient has an intraabdominal abscess. But the white blood count is normal and there is no fever. Both fever and leukocytosis are reliable indicators of infection (fever and leukocytosis commonly accompany infection) and the tests for both are quite accurate (confidence limits are narrow). The probability is that no abscess is present, and an alternative explanation for the other findings must be sought. Everyday thinking is not carried out with probabilities, reliability, accuracy, and precision in mind. Learning to do this, however, and making it a habit will greatly increase your diagnostic effectiveness. You may observe fine clinicians who seem to be pattern recognizers and who do not appear to think in these terms. We believe that excellent, experienced clinicians do think in the manner we have described, although they may use other words for what they do and be so proficient and fast that their thought processes are not apparent.

The Goal

You should have actively in your mind what you are trying to find out when you take a history and examine a patient. Conceptualizing this is easier if you realize that medicine has become a profession of action. Whatever you discover in the diagnostic process will serve as a basis for action. Because our acts are so powerful (and expensive), they need to be thought out in advance to ensure that they are appropriate to the primary goal of helping the patient, while not wasting time or money or placing the patient at undue risk. It might seem that the most desirable diagnostic result is the name of the disease, but, as we have pointed out repeatedly, this is not sufficient. Knowing that the patient has, for example, acute cholecystitis leads to an immediate therapeutic plan. But rarely do we know that a patient has acute cholecystitis; rather, based on the reliability of the information that has been gathered, we suspect it with some level of probability. It is the suspicion that leads us to our next diagnostic and therapeutic actions, and those acts are conditioned by the information that tells how sick or threatened the patient is.

So it is with the vast majority of diagnoses, even those that appear the most straightforward. If examination of the breast reveals what seems most surely to be carcinoma of the breast, the diagnostic process has probably revealed the name of the disease. But that diagnosis alone will not permit action, because the next act is telling the patient something that will convince her of the need for biopsy (because "probably" is insufficiently accurate where malignancy is suspected). Therefore something must be known about the patient because if the suspected diagnosis is presented incorrectly, she may, for example, delay surgery, flee in panic, or develop disabling emotional symptoms. In addition, the extent of her disease and much other information about the patient and her tumor must be discovered before definitive plans can be made. Each step in that process will be dependent on diagnostic information obtained in the preceding steps. Even when no disease name is forthcoming, diagnostic efforts are successful if they tell you clearly what to do next. The knowledge that a patient has rectal bleeding where the blood is intermixed with the stool is sufficient to determine that endoscopy is necessary even though you cannot know the source of the bleeding. The "diagnosis" is that the patient requires endoscopy because of the real possibility that a tumor or inflammatory disease is present.

When the diagnostic process is understood in these terms, then it must be true that all diagnostic methodologies, from asking questions to angiography, are in pursuit of a basis for the actions that will most benefit this individual patient. For an action to benefit the patient, the patient must be either sick and at risk, or only at risk. For the patient to cooperate in diagnostic or therapeutic actions, the patient must comprehend the sickness and the risk. Patients should not merely fear the threat, because fear is a short-lived motivator; they must be helped to understanding in their own terms. In saying that diagnostic activities are meant not only to explain the sickness but estimate the threat to the patient, we provide the focus for the questions clinicians must always ask themselves whenever they see a patient. All diagnostic activities are attempting to answer three questions in the service of the fourth: *What is the pathophysiologic process? What is the threat? Who is this patient? What should be done at this time?* Earlier we showed the necessity for clinicians to know the context of the illness and the patient in whom it occurs and pointed out that the name of a disease is only part of a diagnosis. In going further, we are emphasizing the importance of remaining focused on the threat to the patient. This will prevent you from merely finding and diagnosing diseases just because they are present. In the care of elderly this is particularly important because they frequently have many diseases, but they may be threatened by something that is not literally a disease process. For example, because of weakness in the quadriceps, it is not uncommon for the aged to be unable to rise, unassisted, from a chair. This disability, which is not a disease, usually results from simple inactivity, yet it may seriously threaten their function and independence.

We recognize what a difficult and burdensome responsibility the diagnostic process would be were it to suddenly fall on your shoulders. It is in the nature of the educational process that you are introduced to the ideas and methods of clinical diagnosis well before full clinical responsibility is yours. Take advantage of the opportunity. Take the time necessary to develop your skills; learn to focus your entire attention on the information coming from your senses; now and always seek help when you are in doubt. We hope you will view this volume as the entrance to one of medicine's most exciting pursuits, whose mastery will occupy your entire life in clinical medicine.

CHAPTER 2

STRUCTURE AND RECORDING OF THE CLINICAL EXAMINATION

The best history taker is he who can best interpret the answer to a leading question.

PAUL H. WOOD
(1907–1962)

THE HISTORY

When taking or recording a medical history (and doing a physical exam), a reproducible, orderly approach is best. It ensures completeness and provides a structure on which to display the infinitely variable histories that patients may give.

The physician's most effective tool for controlling the interview process is the way in which he frames his questions. The experienced physician uses all types of questions to gather information. In evaluating the responses, he is conscious of the possible introduction of bias into the interview by the question itself. Certain types of general questions are neutral and virtually free of biasing effects. Others may be strongly weighted in one direction or another. It is only when the physician is unaware of the potential distorting influence of this or that type of question that he is likely to get into trouble. Let us consider several basic types of questions.

The *neutral question* should be used whenever possible. It is structured so that it does not suggest that any particular response is more acceptable to the physician or more beneficial to the patient than another. A neutral question can be open or closed. The open neutral question simply establishes a topic: "Tell me more about your headaches." The closed neutral question incorporates several alternative answers in the question: "Are your headaches more likely to occur in the morning, afternoon, or evening?"

The *simple direct question* is always closed because it requires simply a yes or no answer: "Do your headaches upset your stomach?" Direct questions may or may not be neutral, depending on such factors as voice inflection, context, and previous questions. Although direct questions will speed the interview, too many of them tend to overwhelm the patient and put words into his mouth. They are indispensable but require moderation.

The *leading question* is one that tempts the patient to give one answer rather than another. Although it automatically introduces bias, it may yield special information unobtainable by any other means. This technique is particularly useful in testing the reliability of a series of questions by loading the final query: "Would you say that your headaches come on only when you are feeling very tired?" Most physicians occasionally use leading questions.

The *loaded question* is usually interjected to study the reaction of the patient, since it is so heavily biased that the answer itself is unimportant: "Do you ever think you might be better off dead?" Such a question rarely if ever is needed under ordinary circumstances. It would be directed to a depressed patient only after laying considerable groundwork. This shock technique would be used primarily to assess his response to the suggestion of suicide.

Supplementary remarks are brief comments that are intended to stimulate the patient to proceed. They tell the patient that he is doing well and should continue. They may consist of a simple assertion such as "I see" or "Umm." A simple pause is sometimes an effective way of encouraging the patient to go ahead. Certain neutral remarks such as "Anything else?" "How do you mean?" and "Tell me more about that" have the same positive effect.

By using these different techniques selectively, you will gradually set a pattern that becomes intelligible to the patient. A head nod or an encouraging murmur is a reward that tells him that the topic is relevant and that he should continue. When the response is inadequate, you probe with a direct question. If the patient wanders too far afield, you may have to interrupt and change the subject. Interruption should be used only as a last resort, for if the patient's feelings are hurt, he will surely retreat. This must be avoided if possible. By carefully observing the effect of your remarks on the patient, your questions should improve as you proceed.

As you elicit your information, you simultaneously estimate its significance. You probe for precise temporal relationships and try to determine the relative severity of the various complaints. Certain symptoms considered extremely important by the patient may be discarded as irrelevant in the light of your insight and experience, while other symptoms that might be considered trivial by the patient are retained by you as significant. The interrelationships between symptoms must be determined as the interview proceeds, and you must decide whether any single complaint has more than one cause. This process of probing and measuring continues throughout the interview.

How to Record the History
It is often harder to boil down than to write.

Sir William Osler
(1849–1919)

During the interview, no attempt should be made to record the complete history in final form. There are several good reasons for this. First, it is literally impossible to do so; it distracts the patient and disrupts the procedure. Jotting down reminders, dates, ages, and numbers, however, is not only acceptable but indispensable. Second, the medical record is not meant to be a repository for raw data. The information must be suitably condensed, logically sequenced, and converted (as far as possible) into crisp, pertinent medical terminology before it is recorded. The procedure requires time and thought.

The classic approach to the history is outlined below. (A pocket copy for your reference is provided in the pocket inside the back cover of this book.)

OUTLINE OF THE HISTORY

1. **Biographical data.** Use the patient's stamp or clinic card if possible, including name and number. Add the date of admission or interview and the time at which you took the history. (The time of the history is important if clinical events change. It can be used as a baseline with more meaning if the reader knows when it was taken. This is particularly true in patients with rapidly changing clinical events, such as cardiac or neurologic disease.)

2. **Source of history and estimate of reliability.** The source should be very brief and might contain no more than "the patient," "old records," "the patient's wife," or whatever. If the source is unreliable (e.g., because of confusion), say so here.

3. **Chief complaint.** Statement of the chief complaint can be given in the patient's own words (using quotation marks liberally). Or you may with justice restructure what the patient has said to make it clearer, but without altering the basic meaning. Beware of inserting a premature diagnosis in the chief complaint, as it may lead you astray: Use symptoms rather than someone's opinion of what is wrong. The chief complaint should include age, race, sex, the complaint, and duration of the complaint. For example: "This 63-year-old man presents with 'headache' for 3 days." There may be multiple chief complaints. For example: "This 34-year-old woman has had nausea, vomiting, abdominal pain, and a rash for a week." Include in the chief complaint any major underlying illness of which you are aware, that is of such importance as to lead to immediate understanding of the chief complaint. For example, if the woman mentioned above has known diabetes, the sentence would be restructured to read "This 34-year-old woman with known diabetes has had nausea, vomiting. . . ." Adults should be referred to as men and women, not males and females (the latter is dehumanizing, not being species-specific).

4. **History of present illness (HPI).** The history of present illness (HPI) is the most challenging part of the clinical examination and requires more skill than the physical examination. It should be recorded as a paragraphic, orderly, logical, and grammatically correct description of the features of the chief complaint(s), written in full sentences. Think of it rather as a short story or a mystery story in which positive and negative clues contribute to a total understanding of the sequential events that have led to the patient's coming to you. The HPI should include *all* information referable to the system(s) involved in each major complaint. For example, for a cardiovascular complaint (angina), a *past history* of rheumatic fever belongs in the HPI, as do a *family history* of heart disease, a *social history* of severe work stress, and the entire cardiovascular *review of systems,* including all negatives.

   In recording the present illness, you are more than a scribe, more than a simple recorder of information. It is your job to take the patient's story, examine it, probe it, and order and clarify it to the point where it most clearly describes the most likely illness or illnesses involved. This requires an ever-increasing familiarity on your part with the classic presentations of disease. Early on (and even later) in your career, it would be wise for you to take an initial history, do a physical, and then go immediately to a major textbook to read about the pathophysiology and clinical presentation of the disorder you suspect. Then go back to the patient to ask the additional questions and do the points of physical examination that you had, through ignorance, not known to ask and do before.

   At the end of the HPI, the reader or listener should have a very good idea of the patient's status. Often the diagnosis will be quite clear at this point; sometimes it will be apparent that you do not know the diagnosis, but you will have explored many alternative possibilities in your mind.

The difficulty for the beginner is in eliminating irrelevant material, condensing and concentrating relevant findings into usable forms, and systematically arranging these findings into logical clusters or patterns. As you become more knowledgeable about disease, what to keep and what to throw away in the HPI becomes easier to determine. *All* abnormalities may *not* be related to the patient's current illness and thus are recorded in the past history or review of systems.

The HPI may be long or short, depending on the nature of the illness, and it should be carefully scrutinized for excess verbiage, which should then be removed. Trivial pieces of information that have no bearing on the real complaint can be culled from the HPI. For example: "The patient was well until April 1982, when, while walking down the street on a sunny day, with the birds singing overhead, she experienced pain in her chest." Write instead, "This woman was well until April 1982, when, while walking easily, she had chest pain."

You will save both time and trouble by leaving out the stultified English so characteristic of medical workups. You may omit such statements as "The patient noted," or "The patient states that he was . . . at that time." It will be assumed, unless otherwise specified, that what is in the history is what the patient stated or noted. Similarly, "at that time" can usually be omitted and the history still will make sense. If not, use "then," which is shorter. "The patient" is more readily (and more humanely) referred to as "he," "she," or "Mr."

Minimize abbreviations; they tend to be unintelligible. Because they are impossible to avoid altogether, however, we have listed some of the more common ones in Chapter 23.

If the patient has multiple problems, you might wish to describe them in paragraphs under separate problem headings, such as

a. **Heart disease** (and then fully describe that chronologically)

b. **Renal failure** (and then fully describe that chronologically)

This is generally easier than trying to write them all up together.

With the exception of the HPI, the remainder of the history and the physical may be written in truncated, staccato, incomplete sentences. The same caution about abbreviations should stand throughout, however.

5. **Past history (PH)**

a. **Childhood illnesses** (e.g., measles, mumps, chickenpox, rheumatic fever, scarlet fever).

b. **Adult illnesses.** Generally, record any for which the patient was hospitalized. Append dates if possible.

c. **Trauma.** Major trauma (e.g., fractures) should be listed with dates and sequelae, if any.

d. **Surgery.** Operations, with dates and, if known, the hospitals in which each procedure was done.

e. **Allergies.** Describe not only what the patient is allergic to, but also the manifestations of that allergy. Drug allergies are especially important.

f. **Medications.** Even if these have been included in the HPI, they should be listed, using both generic and brand names, with dose and frequency. If the indication for the medication is neither obvious nor stated elsewhere, include that here as well.

g. **Travel.** Especially outside the continental United States.

h. **Habits.** This generally refers most prominently to smoking, drinking, the use of illicit drugs, and bizarre diets.

i. **Immunizations.** Particularly important in pediatric patients. Include measles, mumps, DPT, polio. Influenza, tetanus, and pneumococcal vaccination histories are more important in older patients.

6. **Family history (FH).** You may do this by outlining a family tree or by simply listing blood kin, either living or dead, giving their ages and any health problems they may have had. Look especially for possible genetic disease if your patient's history of present illness is suggestive (certain forms of arthritis, kidney disease, and endocrine disease run in families.) In blacks, seek specifically a history of sickle cell anemia. In all patients, ask about heart disease, hypertension, diabetes, and cancer.

7. **Social history (SH).** What you really want to know here is "who is this person who is sick?" Illness is really a limitation of function rather than the histopathologic process by which that function is compromised. An individual's response to sickness is in large part determined by his or her cultural background, social standing, educational and economic status, the opinions of the family about the sickness, and the individual's anticipation of functional compromise. In the SH, you will want to know about these features.

8. **Review of systems (ROS).** You will find that doing the review of systems, which is an exercise in completeness, will become easier if you have asked all the necessary questions in the HPI and included the individual's positive and negative replies in the HPI. Then you are left with the important but not immediately applicable data about current other system function and malfunction. If your patient has a chief complaint involving the gastrointestinal system, the review of the GI system should logically be included in the history of present illness. Similarly, if the patient has diabetes, much of the ROS will be included in the HPI as pertinent positives and negatives, since diabetes may involve almost any system. Then, when you come to write this section, under each systemic subsection you will simply say "See HPI."

a. **General.** Fever, chills, weight change, anemia.

b. **Head.** Headaches, dizziness.

c. **Eyes.** Acuity, diplopia, blurring, pain, discharge.

d. **Ears.** Acuity, past infections, tinnitus, pain, discharge.

e. **Nose.** Epistaxis, discharge, odd odors.

f. **Throat and mouth.** Dental repair, sore tongue, frequent sore throats.

g. **Chest.** Cough, pain, shortness of breath, wheeze, hemoptysis, production of sputum (amount, appearance). Last chest x-ray. Last skin test for TB. Breast masses, pain, discharge.

h. **Cardiovascular.** Chest pain, palpitations, shortness of breath, orthopnea, history of heart murmur, of heart attack, of rheumatic fever as a child, claudication, Raynaud's phenomenon.

i. **Gastrointestinal.** Appetite, nausea, vomiting, diarrhea, constipation, change in character of stool (caliber, consistency, color), jaundice, dark urine, abdominal pain, hematemesis, melena, hematochezia, heartburn. Any laxative or antacid use?

j. **Genitourinary**. Hesitancy, dribbling, difficulty starting stream, dysuria, frequency, urgency, gross hematuria, nocturia, incontinence. Any history of venereal disease? Sores on genitals? Any history of urinary tract infections?

k. **Menstrual**. Menarche, menopause. Interval between periods, duration of periods, regularity. Amount of flow. Any pain? Date of last period. Number of pregnancies, abortions, term deliveries. (A shorthand you may use is G = gravida, P = para, A = abortus. Thus, a woman pregnant four times with three live children and one miscarriage would be designated "G4P3A1.")

l. **Neuromuscular**. Syncope, vertigo, weakness or paralysis, numbness or tingling, seizures, psychiatric difficulties, "moodiness," arthritis, edema, cyanosis.

m. **Skin**. Rashes, hives, eczema, bruising.

THE PHYSICAL EXAMINATION

The trouble with doctors is not that they don't know enough, but that they don't see enough.

SIR DOMINIC J. CORRIGAN
(1802–1880)

A physical examination that follows a logical sequence maximizes both your efficiency and the patient's comfort. A minimum number of position changes, especially in the sick individual, is obviously desirable. Note with each step where you position yourself with respect to the patient. Incidentally, a considerable amount of the historical review of systems can be done during the physical examination, as you touch upon each major area of the body.

SEQUENCE OF EXAMINATION

Step I
Note **general appearance** (Chap. 4) as you take the history and when initiating the physical examination, usually with the patient sitting. **Vital signs** (Chap. 5) may be taken at this time, and a survey of the **skin** (Chap. 6) may be started.

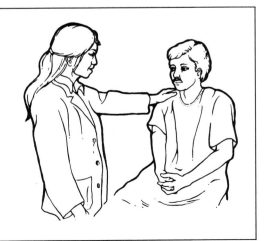

Step II
Examine the **head and neck** (Chaps. 8–10), including **cervical nodes** (Chap. 7). **Thorax** (Chaps. 11, 12), **breast** (Chap. 13), **supraclavicular** and **axillary nodes** (Chap. 7), and initial **cardiovascular examination**, including **upper extremity pulses** and **neck vein** observation (Chap. 12), are done next.

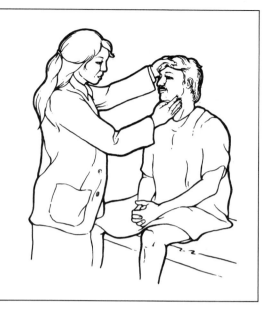

Step III
Move to the rear and station yourself on the **left**. Examine the **posterior lung fields** (Chap. 11) and **back** (Chap. 17). A posterior palpation of the **thyroid gland** (Chap. 10) is often done. Observe the **skin** of the back (Chap. 6).

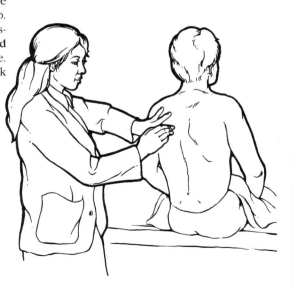

Step IV
With the patient supine, station yourself on the **right**, and continue **cardiac examination** (Chap. 12), including reexamination of the **neck veins**. Palpate the **breasts** (Chap. 13). Examine the **abdomen** (Chap. 14), including **kidneys** (Chaps. 14, 15) and **aorta** (Chaps. 12, 14). Palpate the **inguinal nodes** (Chap. 7) and **femoral pulses** (Chap. 12). Observe the **external genitalia** (Chaps. 15, 16). **Peripheral pulses in the lower extremities** (Chap. 12) and parts of the **musculoskeletal examination** (Chap. 17) are done in this position.

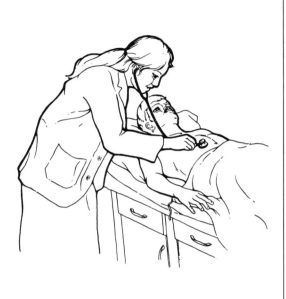

Step V
With the patient again sitting, examine the remainder of the **musculoskeletal system** (Chap. 17). As part of the **neurologic examination**, the cranial nerve, motor, reflex, cerebellar, and sensory examinations are done now (Chap. 18).

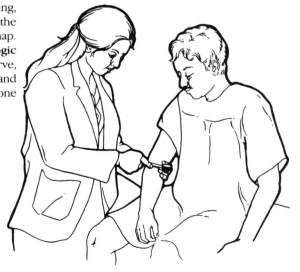

Step VI

The patient stands for the rest of the neurologic examination (station and gait, Romberg's sign) (Chap. 18). In men, examine the **external genitalia**, including **hernia** (Chap. 15).

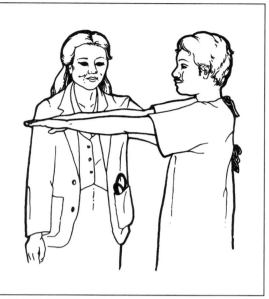

Step VII

In women, the **pelvic examination** (Chap. 16) is done last, with the **rectal** (Chap. 14) conducted as part of this examination. In men, the **rectal** (Chaps. 14, 15) completes the physical.

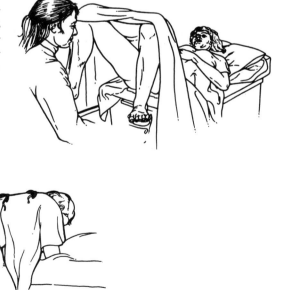

Though of less diagnostic help than a well-taken history, a pertinent physical is obviously very important. You will find the physical examination more interesting if you direct it to the elucidation of those points touched upon in the history. For example, if you suspect that your patient has infective endocarditis, you should look for physical hints of this disease when you do the examination. Then, instead of writing "eyes normal," you will say "no conjunctival petechiae, no Roth's spots." You will specify either that there are no murmurs or that one is present. You will look at the fingers and specify whether or not there is clubbing, splinter hemorrhages, Osler's nodes, or Janeway lesions. You will specify whether or not there is splenomegaly. Knowing that all these physical features correlate with your diagnostic suspicion makes the physical more than a routine and will help you to bolster your diagnostic acumen.

For patients who have potentially rapidly changing disease, it is important to put down the time at which your physical examination was performed.

OUTLINE OF THE PHYSICAL EXAMINATION

1. **General appearance.** Well or poorly developed or nourished. Color (black, white, jaundiced, pale). In distress (acutely or chronically)?
2. **Vital signs.** Blood pressure (which arm or both, orthostatic change). Pulse (regular or irregular, orthostatic change). Respirations (labored or unlabored, wheeze). Temperature (axillary, rectal, or oral). Weight. Height.
3. **Skin, hair, and nails.** Pigmentation, scars, lesions, bruises, turgor. Describe or draw rashes.
4. **Nodes.** Any cervical, supraclavicular, axillary, epitrochlear, inguinal lymphadenopathy? If so, size of nodes (in cm), consistency (firm, rubbery, tender), mobile or fixed.
5. **Head.** Scalp, skull (configuration), scars, tenderness, bruits.
6. **Eyes**
   a. **External eye.** Conjunctivae, sclerae, lids, cornea, pupils (including reflexes), visual fields, extraocular motions.
   b. **Fundus.** Disc, blood vessels, pigmentation.
7. **Ears.** Shape of pinnae, external canal, tympanic membrane, acuity, air conduction versus bone conduction (Rinne's test), lateralization (Weber's test).
8. **Nose.** Septum, mucosa, polyps.
9. **Mouth and throat.** Lips, teeth, tongue (size, papillation), buccal mucosa, palate, tonsils, oropharynx.
10. **Neck.** Suppleness. Trachea, larynx, thyroid, blood vessels (jugular veins, carotid arteries).
11. **Chest and lungs**
    a. **Inspection.** Contour, symmetry, expansion.
    b. **Palpation.** Expansion, rib tenderness, tactile fremitus.
    c. **Percussion.** Diaphragmatic excursion, dullness.
    d. **Auscultation.** Rales, rhonchi, rubs, wheezes, egophony, pectoriloquy.
12. **Heart**
    a. **Inspection.** Point maximal impulse, chest contour.
    b. **Palpation.** Point maximal impulse, thrills, lifts, thrusts.
    c. **Auscultation.** Heart sounds, gallops, murmurs, rubs.

13. **Breasts.** Symmetry, retraction, lesions, nipples (inverted, everted), masses, tenderness, discharge.
14. **Abdomen**
    a. **Inspection.** Scars (draw these), contour, masses, vein pattern.
    b. **Auscultation.** Bowel sounds, rubs, bruits.
    c. **Percussion.** Organomegaly, hepatic dullness.
    d. **Palpation.** Tenderness, masses, rigidity, liver, spleen, kidneys.
    e. **Hernia.** Femoral, inguinal, ventral.
15. **Genitalia**
    a. **Male.** Penile lesions, scrotum, testes. Circumcised?
    b. **Female.** Labia, Bartholin's and Skene's glands, vagina, cervix. Bimanual of internal genitalia.
16. **Rectum.** Perianal lesions, sphincter tone, tenderness, masses, prostate, stool color, occult blood.
17. **Extremities.** Pulses (symmetry, bruits, perfusion). Joints (mobility, deformity). Cyanosis, edema. Varicosities. Muscle mass.
18. **Back.** Contour spine, tenderness. Sacral edema.
19. **Neurologic**
    a. **Mental status.** Alertness, memory, judgment, mood.
    b. **Cranial nerves** (I–XII).
    c. **Cerebellum.** Gait, finger–nose, heel–shin, tremors.
    d. **Motor.** Muscle mass, strength deep tendon reflexes. Pathologic or primitive reflexes.
    e. **Sensory.** Touch, pain, vibration. Heat and cold as indicated.

ROUTINE LABORATORY STUDIES

The sequential recording of laboratory data (the least important of the information you have gathered to date because laboratory data only serve to confirm or deny what you have found on history and physical) is best done in orderly fashion.

1. **Hemogram** (hematocrit, hemoglobin, white count, differential and peripheral blood smear).
2. **Urine analysis.**
3. **Serologies** (electrolytes and other indicated studies).
4. **X-rays.** Describe these, rather than just noting that they are "WNL" (within normal limits). Be specific in your descriptions.
5. **ECG.** This also should be recorded in a logical manner. In order, one notes the rate, the rhythm, intervals (PR, QRS, QT), axis, P wave configuration, QRS configuration, T wave configuration, abnormal configurations, interpretations.

   Only by reading the ECG in the preceding way (which gives much more information than "abnormal ECG" or "within normal limits") can a reader compare a cardiogram taken at a later time with the one that was present during your workup.

Include in the laboratory findings only those data that pertain to your patient. There is no intrinsic virtue to any lab study. If laboratory data disagree with clinical judgment, you would probably be correct in ignoring the laboratory data.

IMPRESSIONS

*It is an old maxim of mine that when you have excluded the impossible,
whatever remains, however improbable, must be the truth.*

> Sherlock Holmes, as quoted by
> Sir Arthur Conan Doyle
> (1859–1930)

The next step is to take the information that you have gleaned from the history, the physical examination, and laboratory studies and resynthesize it into a cogent explanation of your patient's status, along with your best advice as to how to further understand it, and what to do about it.

List your impressions (or the patient's problems) in the order of their importance to the patient and to you. Under each impression write a description of the rationale behind the diagnosis and what you plan to do about it. This description may take many forms, including the problem-oriented approach or one of the more traditional forms (e.g., differential diagnosis). The problem-oriented medical record (POMR) attempts to provide an ongoing system by which data, problems, plans, and follow-up are ordered in a logical sequence that, according to its promoters, lends itself to analysis more readily than does the classic history and physical. Which form you use may not really matter so long as the description is clear and complete. A single-paragraph summary is often included at the end.

Examples of both the traditional and POMR approaches to the history and physical are presented in Chapter 24. (A complete review of the POMR may be found in Weed, L. L., *Medical Records, Medical Education, and Patient Care.* Cleveland: Case Western Reserve University Press, 1981.)

PROGRESS NOTES

As you follow your patient each day, new information will have to be recorded. This information may consist of new history (remembered by patient, family, or brought to light by the arrival of a medical record), new events occurring in the hospital, changes in physical examination (the pertinent features of which must be repeated *at least* once a day, and often more frequently), and consultative or laboratory data. To this new information you should append any changes in diagnosis or therapy that you have instituted and the reasons why. Progress notes must be brief, relevant, and always dated and timed (things may change rapidly in hospital). They must, of course, be legibly signed. An example of progress notes follows.

9/18/82 5 p.m. Hospital day #3

Feels better on penicillin therapy, instituted yesterday at 10 p.m. Myalgias and headache are less and appetite improved. Temperature has fallen from a high of 102°F orally at 3 a.m. today.

P.E. T (PO) 99°F, pulse 78 and regular, BP 130/85. R 12 and unlabored. She has no splinting (an improvement over yesterday evening). Her chest is clear to percussion.

Auscultation shows scattered inspiratory rales at the left base, unchanged from 9/17/82.

Lab from this morning shows wbc = 7800 with a normal differential.

Chest x-ray this noon shows no change in her fluffy left lower lobe infiltrate.

Sputum cultures of 9/15/82 are growing *D. pneumoniae*.

Impression: Pneumococcal (left lower lobe) pneumonia improving on penicillin therapy.

Plan: Continue procaine penicillin G (6 million units IM bid).

John Smith
(MS III)

(John Smith)

ORAL PRESENTATIONS

Physicians teach each other medicine mainly by the "case method." Simply put, doctors orally describe the history, physical examination, and laboratory findings on their patients so that listening doctors can learn (and teach) about the patient's problem. The oral presentation may be brief or lengthy, depending on the circumstance in which it is given. The least formal presentations occur when students or physicians chat with their colleagues over dinner about the interesting patient of the day: "I saw a 34-year-old woman with angina today. She'd had rheumatic fever as a kid. She's got a fantastic aortic insufficiency murmur. . . ." The most formal presentations are those given to the Senior Physician in formal rounds, when the student details chief complaint; history of present illness; past, social, and family history; and review of systems. The physical examination is described in its entirety, including pertinent negatives, and salient laboratory studies are detailed. The purpose of this exercise is to make as much information available to the Senior Physician as possible, so that he or she can knowledgeably discuss the case. Such a detailed presentation may take up to 10 minutes, but should never be much longer than that.

In either of these extremes, or in the multitude of variations between them, the oral presentation should be clear, logical, entertaining, and pertinent. Giving such a presentation takes considerable practice.

CHAPTER 3

THE PATIENT'S HISTORY

Maxim: The treatment begins with the history.

The search for what sickness threatens the patient almost always begins by taking a history—listening to the patient's story of the illness. The interesting thing about a history is that it not only allows posing the question, but it begins to provide the answer. The general form of the diagnostic question asks what threatens this patient's functioning at this time, so the answer will be incomplete if it stops at the *what*—the disease.

Understanding what the history of an illness actually is, makes it clear why it is so useful—why no other diagnostic technology can take its place.

When patients are asked what is the matter, they usually answer with a story. For example:

Yesterday, when I got up I noticed this pain in my side, which I thought was my back because I've had a lotta trouble with my back. But later on it moved over into my stomach and I felt sick, so I thought it must be my gall bladder or something. When it got so bad, I thought I better come to the emergency room—I haven't got my own doctor—but I put it off 'cause I don't like going to doctors. I took two aspirin—which I never do because I don't like to take medicine—but it didn't help. So it began to hurt real bad and in my groin and all and I got frightened so I came.

Last week my wife and I were on vacation and I got the runs, which I've had plenty of times before. Anyway, when we came back they didn't get better, and I started to have a fever so I thought I better come in.

As these brief examples illustrate, medical stories, like all stories, have a cast of characters, take place somewhere, and evolve over time. You can see in both of the examples that the patients recounted the occurrence of physical symptoms over a period of time, while at the same time describing their reaction to them. If we employed 20 instead of two examples, the same basic characteristics would be present. This is because a medical story differs from others in that it always has at least two characters—the patient and the patient's body. The symptoms—pain in the first instance and diarrhea in the second—are the story of what is happening to the patient's body over time as reported by the patient.

To see why getting the most out of taking a history requires keeping this qualifier in mind, we must look briefly at how symptoms arise. Dyspnea is a good example. Dyspnea occurs, in the simplest case, when the metabolic demand for oxygen exceeds the ability of the lungs to meet the increased need at that moment. A moment's reflection will serve to demonstrate that that condition happens commonly to everyone. Walking briskly up the stairs you find yourself breathing more heavily, especially if you are carrying packages. A lifetime of experience with the capacities of your body allows you to factor in the number of stairs, the briskness of your pace, and even the weight of the package to arrive at an estimate of the correctness of your breathing. Although, strictly speaking, your shortness of breath qualifies for the symptom, "dyspnea-on-effort," you do not consider yourself to have a symptom of illness. Instead, the heavy breathing is interpreted as being due to the stairs.

Persons with early congestive heart failure also become short of breath while climbing stairs, but their rate and depth of respiration will be (slightly in the beginning, more so later on) greater than is usual for them with the same stair-climbing effort. This change in their dyspnea is directly related to the pathophysiology of congestive heart failure. The report of the symptom, shortness of breath, is *not* directly related to the pathophysiology of heart failure, however, because of the person's need to interpret the body sensation. The chances are that in the beginning the person will not bring to conscious awareness the fact of heavier breathing because it is so slight. As it worsens and the person is forced to acknowledge it, it becomes an event to be explained, to be given meaning. All events, everything that comes to awareness, large and small, must be given meaning. Meaning has at least two components, the first is significance and the second importance. Heavy breathing on the stairs might signify (to the person as he or she experiences it) steeper stairs, heavier burdens, lesser physical conditioning, tiredness, or malfunctioning of the body. Each of these assignments of significance is more or less consequential to the person, that is, has one or another kinds and degrees of emotion attached to it. According to the emotional charge assigned to the interpretation of the heavy breathing, the next moment's self-observation of breathing will be influenced because the occurrence and interpretation of symptoms is a process taking place over time. It is characteristic of the interacting process of perception and interpretation (assignment of meaning) that other facts will be mustered to bolster the dominant interpretation while perceptions at odds with the interpretation will be suppressed.

Because to become a symptom, body sensations must reach awareness and be interpreted as due to illness, they are usually not direct, one-to-one expressions of pathophysiology. It is these facts that sometimes lead physicians to give up on histories because they believe them to be unreliable indicators of disease. It is these same characteristics, however, that make the history of an illness the invaluable diagnostic aid that it is.

Once you understand that a symptom is not the disease talking, but the patient talking about the illness (about what the disease is doing to the patient), you can see that properly taking a history offers you at least five kinds of information. First, it provides evidence about what pathophysiologic process or disease is present (diminished pulmonary oxygenation in the example given). Second, it provides the context in which the illness occurred and factors related to its onset and course (congestive heart failure, probably due to ischemic cardiomyopathy, in a cigarette-smoking steel-mill worker with a large family, for example). Third, it gives insight into the meaning of existing symptoms to the patient and thus predicts the meaning the patient will attach to future events (every man in this patient's family died of heart disease and he expects to do the same, to continue the example). Fourth, it tells you about the various types of impact the disease process is having on the patient (he is forced to stop working and go on disability, with a major reduction in income, and his older son is beginning to act like the head of the household).

Finally, taking the history offers the opportunity of finding out what kind of a person the patient is (this man is stubborn and opinionated and knows better than others what is best for him). Too frequently in the past, physicians extracted from the history the information that pointed to the disease process and actively rejected the remainder as an obstruction to diagnosis. Yet these further facts are essential for making a complete diagnosis, including finding out the extent of the threat to the patient, planning treatment, determining the causal chain that led to the illness, and predicting its future.

Our brief description of the origin of a symptom should make it clear that the spontaneous stories of their illnesses related by patients themselves will not provide all the information that can be obtained. In fact such reflexive histories may, in themselves, be relatively valueless! Taking a history is an active process. It is an interaction between doctor and patient in which the doctor's attitude facilitates the flow of information and his or her questions probe for details and specifics. Histories remain only potentially valuable unless they are interactively elicited by the history taker.

One frequently hears from physicians early in their training that the patient misled them or provided information that was incorrect or incomplete. You must ask yourself why patients would purposely do such things. In the vast majority of doctor patient interactions the patients' intention is not to mislead but to help their doctors help them. Despite that fact, patients' spontaneous histories may be extremely misleading. This is exemplified in the statement:

This is the time of year when I get my allergies, and it happened as usual except last week I developed bronchitis and I hoped you could give me some antibiotics for it.

In this fragment of a history, the patient tells us no symptoms, but only her diagnoses. We presume that she had symptoms and that her diagnoses are based on them. The physician who bases his or her actions on the patient's self-diagnosis may indeed be misled, but the patient should not be held responsible. The skill in taking a history lies in using questions to obtain information about the disordered body sensations that led to the patient's interpretations and self-diagnoses. This is possible because despite the fact that patients' conclusions, misperceptions, reactions to the symptoms, illness, and medical care introduce distortions in reportage, *the memory of the body sensations remains available for recall by the patient and reinterpretation by the doctor.*

Obtaining diagnostically useful information is made easier because the factors that lead to the patients' distortion are relatively few in number and are identifiable.

HABITUAL EXPERIENCE

Recall that a body sensation becomes a symptom because it rises into awareness, is perceived as alien, and because it is assigned a meaning in the person's category of illness. Sometimes patients who are actively coughing while you take the history will say no when asked whether they have a cough! If you ask them about the cough you just heard, they may say that it is not a cough, it is a cigarette cough. "Cigarette cough" has become part of them, like age wrinkles. Patients with long-standing disease may become acclimated even to severe symptoms such as dyspnea. Unless their breathing has recently changed, they may misinterpret your questions about it. In such instances, if the information is important to you, you must search for the details of the impairment in their function (e.g., exercise capacity). *It is your knowledge of pathophysiology that should guide your questions.* Taking a good history depends for accuracy on your knowledge of how organ dysfunctions are reflected in the dysfunction of whole persons in their everyday environment. An attentive physician does not require much experience in taking histories before he or she begins to know what degree of diminished oxygenation will make a patient stop after walking two blocks or one flight of stairs. We wish to stress that if you have obtained a history of diminished exercise tolerance that has stood the test of repeated questions and yet all your test results are normal, *do not make the error of concluding that the patient was not telling the truth.* Something is wrong or the patient would not have diminishing exercise tolerance. Either your questions were misunderstood, you misunderstood the answers, the test results are incorrect (or mislabeled), or the patient has another difficulty that you have not yet uncovered. Most experienced clinicians have discovered the hard way that tests are more often incorrect than are patient's answers untrue.

"HOMEOSTASIS" AND "DENIAL"

We put quotation marks around both words to indicate that the mechanism that induces patients not to report dire symptoms, or even to forget them, is unclear. It is true, however, that patients appear to suppress information whose import, if they faced it squarely, would make them aware that they were seriously ill. When this occurs, doctors are frequently incredulous that a patient could be so dumb. We suggest that you be more generous with such behavior against the time when you become ill and do it yourself. Patients seem genuinely unaware of the significance of the symptoms that they are playing down or forgetting, even though when the information is brought to their awareness, they know its meaning. We employed the word *homeostasis* because one of the reasons for this behavior appears to us to be the attempt not to bring matters to awareness that will cause major changes in the person's life, disturbing its equilibrium. The importance of the phenomenon to you is that digging out the information is more difficult, and the patient seems to be actively resisting you when that is not their conscious intent.

Physicians should be careful to guard against the same human trait affecting their diagnostic performance. On occasion, a patient says something, which, if true, suggests a diagnosis or a disease severity at odds with what the doctor wants to believe. It is much too common, in these circumstances, for the disturbing information to be dismissed rather than followed up. Similarly, oncologists often see patients with tumor masses that are so large that a child would have detected them, yet the patient had been previously examined and the mass overlooked. It is generally believed that doctors do not respond to the dire symptom or register the ominous mass because, without conscious intent, they too shy away from having to confront the terrible meaning of the findings or the need to discuss them with the patient.

THE ASSIGNMENT OF VALUE

It is of the highest importance in the art of detection to recognize out of a number of facts, which are incidental and which are vital.

Sherlock Holmes, as quoted by
SIR ARTHUR CONAN DOYLE
(1859–1930)

The adjectives, verbs, nouns, adverbs, and pronouns that patients use in describing their symptoms tell the careful listener not only what the symptoms are, but how the patients feel about them. Even the nonword portions of utterances—pause, pitch, speech rate, and intensity—contribute to our knowledge of the speaker's beliefs and values. It follows that it is virtually impossible for a patient to report a symptom as an "objective fact" in the manner of the computer. The adjectives that are used in describing pain, nausea, shortness of breath, or any other symptoms not only tell us the patient's attitude towards the symptom, they place it on a scale of relative values for that patient. Because we are concerned with the severity of symptoms, we must disengage this information from the patient's scale of values and give it a rating on our "medical scale." How is this to be accomplished? The language the patient uses to describe other events allows us to learn what palette of emotional colorings is usual for the person. If a patient states that the pain in the chest is "not so bad" but also uses toned-down language for everything else, we should suspect that by our medical standards the pain may be worse than reported. On the other hand, if a pain is described as excruciating, but everything else is "horrible," "terrible," "simply awful," "magnificent," or "sensational," we may be justified in pausing before surgery.

When knowing the severity of a symptom is crucial to the diagnosis, then the clue provided by language usage must be supported by other information. This is true of all diagnostic information; the more important a fact is, the more evidence must be sought that bears on it. This can be accomplished, on occasion, by asking the patient to discuss previous illness and pains. The language employed for the current symptom can be compared to previous usage. The assignment of value can be both idiosyncratic and shared. Certain kinds of pain—pressure on a nerve root for example—will be described by most patients employing the same kinds of adjectives, e.g., boring, searing, burning, like a toothache, deep, "I can't get away from it," gnawing, exhausting, or nagging. Such commonality allows descriptive language to enter the diagnostic process, much like an objective referent.

Sometimes patients will use language that suggests very severe distress even though the symptom ultimately turns out to be mild and such strong language is unusual for them. This occurs because language use is conditioned not only by the body sensations themselves, but by the meaning ascribed to them. Thus if a patient suspects life-threatening disease, he or she may describe the symptoms as the patient believes they would feel if the disease is present. When this occurs, and the physician is able to demonstrate it, then the disparity is a clue to the patients' fears—in themselves important information because they must ultimately be addressed for cooperation to be obtained and reassurance to be successful. This can be uncovered by questions such as, "Would this symptom bother you if you didn't think it meant heart disease?"

THE EXPERIENCE OF OTHERS

Patients' reports of symptoms are influenced by their association with the experiences of significant others, primarily family members. What the patient knows of illness and health through the experience of the patient's family, friends, or other laypersons is far more influential in the assignment of meaning to alien body sensations than any other sources of information, including physicians. Thus patients will ascribe their symptoms to food or the environment, link symptoms simply because they occur on the same side of the body, lump together sebaceous cysts, breast "cysts," and ovarian cysts as evidence that they are "cyst formers," when none of these categories has any standing among physicians. These beliefs may significantly influence how symptoms are reported, but they cannot be brushed aside without risking errors in history taking. The symptoms must be teased away from the connections the patient has made. When doctors make fun of their patients' conceptions of disease because they are not scientific or accurate they are, in essence, belittling the persons.

THE SPACE-TIME DIMENSION OF EXPERIENCE

People vary enormously in their ability to report details about time and place. In part this seems to be idiosyncratic; some remember when and where everything happened like a television newscaster, whereas for others everything before yesterday is the hazy past. Because illness stories take place over time and in places, this variability introduces a distortion in history taking that must be overcome. Thus questioning must establish when things happened and in what order with some precision if the march of the disease is to be correctly interpreted. The best way to do this is to tie questions to known anniversaries (holidays, birthdays, and summer vacations are good time-posts) or known places or activities (the job site, home, while watching a ball game).

ILLNESS IS A TEMPORAL OBJECT

There is another feature of illness that introduces distortion. Illnesses are what the philosopher Husserl called temporal objects, things that are complete and self-contained in time as other objects are complete and self-contained in space (e.g., a vase or a stone). In this respect, a melody is an object in time. Even though the sounds that make up the melody go zipping into the past, the listener combines the sounds and makes of them a complete temporal object, the melody. The story of an illness is similar; it is a cohesive object created out of a combination of parts occurring through time; in other words, the illness, like the melody, is an object with a temporal dimension. People do not like it when you break apart their illness, something they have formed into a temporal object, by asserting that it is really two different objects, and consequently they are resistant to the reconstitution of the story of their illness into a different temporal object. Thus, when your questions attempt to obtain information that is *not* part of the illness object as they have formed it, you meet resistance. The difficulty does not arise because *the patient* is resisting you, but because it is in the nature of thought processes to form temporal objects out of stories, and in the nature of perception to maintain objects of perception intact.

These and the other distortions of the patients' stories of illness discussed earlier might seem enough cause for despair about ever getting at the real disease underlying the symptoms by talking to the patient. Earlier (p. 36) we discussed the various kinds of information that are only available from the history; your need for these, if you are a clinician, requires that you learn how, artfully, to overcome the distortions that are inevitable in the history-taking process.

There is another reason that has to do with the meaning of the words *real disease*. What is the real disease in a patient with, for example, acute myocardial infarction? Is it the disorder of lipid metabolism that results in the atherosclerotically narrowed segment of a coronary artery, or is it the afflicted artery itself? Atherosclerosis, a widespread ailment, is the focus of dietary and pharmacologic maneuvers for prevention of the disease. Coronary artery disease, which occurs frequently in patients who never develop myocardial infarction, is the point of attack for angioplastic and surgical attempts at revascularization. Is it the fresh thrombus that seems to precipitate the event and is currently open to attack by thrombolytics, or is it the loss of viable muscle that contributes to the reduction in ventricular function? We could go on delineating every feature of an acute myocardial infarction to demonstrate that myocardial infarction is the name for a thing that is not a "thing" at all: it is a moment in a pathophysiologic process. In the lives of some patients, it is their final moment, whereas in others it never even troubles their awareness. For doctors, what is considered the real disease differs depending on their own perspective; it is one thing for autopsy pathologists, another for clinical pathologists, yet another for electrophysiologists, and different still for cardiac surgeons.

The point of view that clinicians must take about myocardial infarction is distinct from that of all other physicians, although it must share their knowledge of pathology, laboratory findings, electrophysiology, and therapeutic possibilities. For clinicians, the real disease is the pathophysiologic process as it unfolds in *this individual patient*. When we add the fact that what is of interest is what is happening in an individual patient, then we have implicitly added the factors associated with the individual patient from environmental to psychodynamics that modify the pathologic process. And these factors, as we hope we have made abundantly clear, can be discovered from no other source as well as from a history of an individual patient.

THINKING INTO THE FUTURE

The clinician is also unique in that he or she is always viewing any event that befalls a patient in light of the future. Not merely what has happened, but what will happen. With some illnesses, that is easier to demonstrate than others, for example, when a patient throws a pulmonary embolus. Even in the presence of severe pain, dyspnea, hemoptysis, and other dramatic occurrences, the clinician's overriding concern must be the next embolus. If, as we talk about it, the patient is still alive, then survival is most probable. What about the next embolus, however? If that occurs, survival is by no means a certainty! Whenever we are worried about our patients, our fears are not for now, they are for what we fear may be coming.

The layperson's everyday idea of the future is what is to happen in years to come (as in futurology), but the next moment is also the future, as is a minute, hour, day, week, month, year, decade, and old age from now. It is in all these different dimensions of the future that clinicians must think. Most clinical research involves intermediate futures, from days to the usual maximum of about 5 years (durations determined more by the realities of grant funds than any other factor). It is reasonable to ask which future concerns us. Obviously, it is the patient's future rather than just the future of the heart (to stay with myocardial infarction) that is our focus. It is one of the wonderful things about our work, however, that clinicians must never lose sight of what is happening to the heart as well as what is happening to the patient. We are always involved in predictions about both.

When clinicians think about the future, they are always translating predictions from the general to the particular, from the statistical to the individual. To understand this, contemplate two different ways in which predictive statements are frequently made for patients. For example, suppose the average life expectancy after a diagnosis of a certain disease is 3 to 5 years. Those numbers sound pretty similar, considering that the life expectancy from birth of a woman in this country is over 80 years, unless you are living it, in which case there is a big difference between 3 and 5 years—and the difference may be even larger depending on the quality of the years. If there is some sick person living those years, then there is some clinician sharing the difference between 3 and 5 with that patient.

Another way in which prognoses are given is in the form of a death rates per year. For example, for patients with (say) stable angina, a death rate of one percent per year may be quoted. For the clinical researcher, the number is derived from a variably sized cohort that has been followed for a few years with the deaths in the group smoothed out over time as a result of some statistical projection technique. The implication is that the speed of the progress of the disease is uneven, slower in some and faster in others. Clinicians must translate the statistical outcome to the pace and rhythm of the disease as they experience it in *this* individual patient as opposed to another. They must learn about these variable disease velocities from their individual patients. They must consider how the pace of disease in this individual patient varies in relation to the statistical mode of patients in general. If they think only about the individual patient, then the discoveries of medical science about the natural history of disease are closed to them. If they think only about the generalizations of medical science, then the care of the individual patient suffers through either overtreatment or undertreatment. Both exclusive approaches have real risks, especially in this era of potent therapeutics, pharmacologic and invasive.

As you probably recognize, we have been discussing an aspect of clinical judgment. *There is no highly developed clinical judgment in the absence of a highly developed sense of timing.* Every distortion about time that afflicts patients as they tell their stories influences the clinician's ability to evaluate the pace and rhythm of the patient's illness and, thus, the future of the patient. Further, clinicians, being human, are as subject to the same time distortion as are their patients. For example, patients tend to behave as though the imminence of a complication of disease is dependent upon its seriousness rather than on the pace of the disease. When you explain that one reason for treating hypertension is that many years of untreated hypertension may lead to stroke, some patients will feel threatened with immediately impending stroke with every transient rise in pressure. For physicians, the strongly felt need to treat immediately on the discovery of a serious disease is often the result of the same type of time distortion. The matter is important because choosing *when to treat* is as important as deciding *how to treat;* consequently, it is essential that the urgency of treatment be generated by the pace and timing of the disease process and the patient, rather than by the fears of the physician. The best protection against error here, as elsewhere, is an awareness of how the decision for treatment is generated and a disciplined resolve to remain rooted in clock and calendar time, rather than subjective time, when decisions are made involving timing.

THE ASSIGNMENT OF CAUSE

Just as no event can be experienced without a search for meaning, so too, no event can be experienced without a search for cause. Events are not merely caused, they cause other things to happen—they have consequences. Our beliefs about objects, events, relationships and people, including the event that is a symptom, include ideas about where the event comes from and what will follow. When someone develops a pain that is attributed to carrying something heavy, more goes with that assignment of cause than merely an explanation of the source. Beliefs about cause have prognostic implications as well. This kind of pain comes from "muscles." The quotes around the word are to distinguish the patient's use of the word from the medical term, *muscle.* "Muscle" pains are usually short-lived, go away without treatment, and portend nothing serious. Ideas of cause may be used to explain away the symptoms as in the layperson's word, "virus"—a generally short-lived illness with variable symptoms and variable duration that is not life-threatening. The physicians' word virus refers to a specific group of disease agents, e.g., coxsackie, simian B virus, varicella-zoster, adenovirus, or human immunodeficiency virus (HIV), some of which *are* dangerous while others cause trivial illness. Doctors also recognize the meanings and make use of the word "virus" as it is employed by patients.

Causes may have antecedent causes as in, "Because I've been under so much strain at my job, I got run down, which is why I developed this virus." The chain of events may include psychological determinants or even moral factors, such as when patients believe that their illnesses are a punishment for their sins.

When symptoms are assigned a nonthreatening cause, such as "virus," they can be dismissed from the mind. When the cause assigned is something dire—cancer, for example—then the matter *cannot* be dismissed from the mind, and the patient's thoughts will go around and around, finding other evidence that supports the awful belief. Whether the cause that is seized upon is trivial or serious, once the patient has fixed on the idea, evidence to the contrary will be suppressed.

It should be clear now why the history *as given,* without interaction and interpretation by the clinician, is almost always valueless and in fact can mislead. It could not be otherwise even if a physician were the patient. *The patient does not have the option nor the interest to relate things objectively when his or her illness is concerned.* To process the sense data of experience, the patient *must* assign meaning. When reporting the details of causality and timing, and when choosing words to describe events, the patient can only reflect the meaning of these events in his or her own spatiotemporal, causal, and value terms.

Patients generally give their histories in one of three ways; as a causal chain, as a series of diagnoses, or as a group of symptoms.

Of course my throat got bad because I had to be out in the cold.

Because my arthritis has flared up, I have a pinched nerve in my arm. Either that or it's my old bursitis back again.

I wrote these down so I shouldn't forget any of them. I noticed some brown spots on my face I want you to look at. I've been very tired lately. I think my digestion isn't as good as it used to be because I have so much gas lately—my husband says he's going to divorce me unless you do something about the gas. My hands are kind of funny looking, shiny-like. And I wonder whether you think its time to do something about my hemorrhoids.

In none of these common presentations is there enough symptoms on which to base much more than a diagnostic guess. The first diagnosis may be the sore throat of an upper respiratory infection, or *Candida* pharyngitis in someone with HIV infection. The second may be what the patient believes it is or carcinoma of the lung with Pancoast's syndrome. The third may be a healthy patient with some ordinary complaints or someone with scleroderma. However, *each of these patients has the answers to the questions which, if asked, will lead to the correct diagnosis.* The patient's history achieves its central role in medical care, not in the form as given, but as the result of the interaction of doctor and patient. The art of history taking is the art of asking questions and listening to and interpreting the answers.

APPROACH TO THE PATIENT
Maxim: [We repeat] *the treatment begins with the history.*

COOPERATION
Taking a history should be approached as a cooperative venture between a physician and a patient, both of whom have a mutual goal in mind—helping the patient. The atmosphere is almost invariably benevolent. When it is not, it can usually be made benevolent with effort. Ill persons are usually concerned for their health or even frightened. They try to do and say the things that will most help the doctor. That it sometimes does not come out that way should not obscure their attempts to be helpful. For example, in the ambulatory setting, all the way to the doctor's office patients commonly rehearse what they are going to say in order not to forget anything that seems important—obscuring, in the process, other facts such as those whose import is unknown to them. Similarly, in order to have been admitted to the hospital, the patient must have already told someone the history, and, because a previous history taker has unavoidably communicated the importance of some particulars over others, the patient may emphasize certain answers and forget oth-

ers. Patients may be afraid you will think that they are wasting your time or that they are really not sick so they may want to impress you with their symptoms. Conversely, they may get the idea that you think that they are sicker than they initially believed and as a consequence they may deemphasize some crucial aspect of their story.

All these "helpful" behaviors (and others described earlier) and perhaps the doubting attitude of one of their teachers lead too many physicians and students away from a cooperative attitude and into believing that you cannot trust what patients tell you—that generally patients intentionally mislead, misinform, or lie. But, why would patients want to do that? They have come to you to get better. It is a cultural maxim that you are not supposed to lie to your doctor because he or she is trying to help you, a maxim that most people follow *if they perceive that the doctor is not judging them, but rather is trying to help them.* If you are demonstrating that your intention is to help rather than to judge, your maxim should be: *patients speak the truth until proven otherwise.* If you want patients to trust you, you must trust them. If you are sceptical, remember three things. First, this cooperative approach to history taking in which the patient is trusted comes from generations of practicing physicians who have taken care of patients just as tough or down and out as any you may be seeing. Second, you are training yourself to take care of the sick, not to do battle with a world of deceit and connivance. Finally, the alternative (not trusting patients) condemns you to a sea of uncertainty. There is enough uncertainty in medicine in the best of circumstance, with the patient as your ally, without making it worse.

SITTING DOWN

Sit down in a chair by the bedside or (in ambulatory settings) opposite the patient. Try not to stand over the patient or emphasize your size or the fact that you are upright (against their smallness or the fact that they are in bed). Look the patient directly in the eyes when you ask questions or wait for answers. Eye contact tells people that you care and can be trusted. If, because of your own personal habits, or preferences, you have difficulty making eye contact, learn how.

Ask your questions in the most direct and simple language that you can find while still sounding friendly. This is not an ordinary social conversation, where circumlocutory and indirect usage is conventional; it is a doctor taking a history. Early in your training it is perfectly acceptable to refer to notes or the history-taking form used in your hospital. Similarly, it is better to take notes about the answers then to forget them. But most of your time should not be spent in writing or using your note pad to avoid looking at the patient. Sometimes physicians are intentionally rude, as if bad manners with patients denoted their indifference to death and gore. Nonsense. Bad manners just puts patients off, wastes time, and diminishes the physician's effectiveness. Even John Wayne said, "Howdy, mam." Remember the maxim that introduced this chapter. Do not throw away your therapeutic advantage just for the sake of looking good!

Make sure the patient's position in the bed or chair is comfortable and that looking at you does not require looking into the light. As the history progresses stay alert to the patient's comfort. Usually what helps the patient helps you. You are there, however, to get a good history, something that serves the best interests of the patient. This is your primary objective, to which other issues, including the patient's comfort, must temporarily be secondary.

ASKING QUESTIONS ABOUT THE BODY

A doctor who cannot take a good history and a patient who cannot give one are in danger of giving and receiving bad treatment.

PAUL DUDLEY WHITE
(1886–1973)

Ask questions to find out the story of the progressive dysfunction of the patient's body or its parts. *We cannot state this rule too strongly; do not ask questions to fill out your mental questionnaire about a particular disease.* For example, if the first symptoms suggest peptic ulcer disease, *do not* only ask questions that satisfy the remainder of the criteria for ulcer disease. The reason for our emphasis results from an understanding of how doctors' minds function when they elicit symptoms. Within moments of hearing the patient's first symptoms, some idea about what is wrong leaps into the doctor's consciousness. This is exactly the equivalent of the patient assigning meaning to alien body sensations that have reached awareness. In both instances, the assigned meaning may be correct. But what if it is not? For the doctor, this means making a mistake and possibly endangering the patient.

This means that the diagnostic idea of which you suddenly become aware should be greeted as just what it is, an idea, hypothesis. All your scientific education has taught you (correctly) that *only the null hypothesis can be proven.* Do not let your training desert you at this crucial point. When this hypothesis occurs to you ("this patient's got an ulcer") start to accumulate the evidence that will disprove it. Here is a typical example.

Physician: How can I help you?

Patient: I get this pain in my stomach that feels like an ulcer. (Please promise *never* to ask a patient, "What brought you to the hospital." It is a silly question unless you work for a transportation company. In the hospital you might start with, "Please tell me the story of your illness." For long or difficult illnesses, a successful opening question is, "When were you last entirely well?")

Physician: When you eat, what happens to the pain?

Patient: It feels much better.

Physician: Does it matter what you eat?

Patient: No, almost anything I put in my stomach makes me feel better.

Physician: How long does it take the food to make you feel better?

Patient: Almost immediately.

Physician: Do you wake up in the middle of the night with pain?

Patient: Yes.

Physician: If you take an antacid, say Tums or Alka-Seltzer, what does that do?

Patient: Sometimes it helps me. (If you had been filling out a mental questionnaire, this answer might have been okay, but since you have been alert to answers that disprove the hypothesis of peptic ulcer, the lack of positiveness is suspicious. So you ask . . .)

Physician: What does that mean?

Patient: Well, sometimes when I take Maalox, after a while I feel better, but sometimes it doesn't help much. (Now your suspicions are fully raised. Food relieves pain in ulcer disease because it functions as an antacid. If antacids themselves do not relieve the pain in a particular patient, perhaps there is alternative explanation for why food helps, but not antacids. Perhaps the pathophysiologic process is something other than hyperacidity. Maybe you had better go back and check some details. *Remember, you are not suspicious of the patient, you are suspicious of your hypothesis.* You are not "checking up" on the veracity of the patient, but on whether you have sufficient detail to know what the food actually does when it relieves this patient's pain.)

Physician: When you say that the pain wakes you up, tell me what you mean.

Patient: Well, I wake up and I feel the same pain or ache, or whatever, in my stomach.

Physician: What is the feeling like?

Patient: Like a big emptiness, like I'm hungry, like an ache, or a hunger pang. (Is the discomfort the effect of unbuffered excess acid or is it the effect of a stomach that is not full enough to satisfy this patient? You had better keep asking until you find the question that will settle the issue. The difference is the difference between a GI series and endoscopy or someone [maybe yourself] dealing with an eating disorder. That is a big difference.)

Physician: What do you do when you get that feeling?

Patient: I eat anything I can get my hands on. It could be salad, or even once I ate uncooked spaghetti and it did the trick. (This does not sound like ulcer disease. Keep on asking questions until you are satisfied that you *know* what is happening to her. Knowing means that you have found an hypothesis that will stand up to repeated attempts to disprove it. In this case, we would suggest that you go back and find out not only when the discomfort started, but when she had to eat just to make herself feel better. Of course, at this point you have shifted hypotheses, so you now have something new to disprove. Take your time. Remember, if she has an eating disorder she may have embarrassment about aspects of it, such as inducing vomiting, so your questions will have to be gentle and friendly while they persist in their attempt at finding out what threatens her now.)

In your mind's eye you are trying to "see" inside the body to find out what is going on. Your knowledge of pathophysiology is your guide. As time goes on, you will be increasingly better at correlating everyday activities with organ function. Each question provides some further detail about body function in *this* patient. Although the answer to one question may lead to another, you are not simply building a linear chain of inference. The answer to every question implies something that can *only be true* under certain circumstances but not others. Your job is to come to a rounded picture of the patient and body circumstance in the light of which the answer makes sense. Every question should help round out that picture. In the beginning you will find that you waste questions—asking those that do not contribute to your picture—or have trouble finding the correct question. As you become more experienced, your questions will be more parsimonious and less ambiguous, producing more useful information. Watching a skilled questionner in action is a treat. As the artist's brush paints a picture, so does the practiced clinician's questions. The questions and their answers add a detail here, erase a doubt there, making first one diagnosis and then another seem improbable in the universe of *this* patient. When questioning is done best, the diagnosis that emerges may seem self-evident. The diagnosis may be the name of a disease; a pathophysiologic process (unstable angina); the chain of events that led to the patient's symptom (the patient develops pain in the neck or shoulders after using a computer with a poorly placed monitor); a behavior of the patient that is producing the symptom (as in the woman with abdominal pain above); a threatening meaning that a patient has assigned to an otherwise innocuous event or process, or a clear-cut indication of the next action that the doctor should take.

Any question is a good question if it gets the information you need! You will frequently hear that direct questions are bad because they lead the patient. There are no bad questions, only inexpert questioners. If you ask a direct question you must be alert to the possibility that the patient will try to please (or displease) you with the answer. Alertness means being attentive to every word, pause, pitch, intonation, or nuance of timing in the patient's speech. If every previous answer has been definite, but in response to your direct question, "So you had diarrhea with the pain?", the answer is, "Diarrhea, yeh, maybe a little," you must (if the answer is important to the picture you are building) re-question. "What do you mean by diarrhea, frequent watery bowel movements, or what?" "No, maybe they were a little loose that day; I really don't remember."

There is a type of question that is extremely useful in taking a history that is not syntactically correct. It is the open-ended question of the type, "And your fever . . .?" "And your pain. . .?" Use such questions when you are stumped. The central symptom seems to be dyspnea on effort, yet you have had trouble pinning its degree to the effort expended in any particular activity. Perhaps the patient does not want to face the degree of disability implied in his answers; perhaps he is not as disabled as he appeared at first. Repeated questions have failed to get a consistent picture. You know that dyspnea, when it is related to inadequate oxygenation, is consistently related to effort (unless great anxiety is present). Switch tactics. Ask for a detailed account of yesterday's events. Sooner or later he will tell about some physical activity that, if he is inadequately oxygenating, should have produced shortness of breath. Then ask, "And your breathing. . .?", rather than, "Were you short of breath when you did that?"

Physicians are wary of open-ended questions because they are afraid that the patient will never stop talking. That is usually not the difficulty. But if it happens, it can be ended by saying, "I'm interested in that, and I will be coming back to talk more about it with you, but right now I need to know about your bowel movements."

THE PAIN LITANY

Questions about pain, so central to the story of many illnesses, demonstrate a fact that must not be forgotten. Although nobody but the patient knows what the patient has experienced, the patient may not have the language to express the way the pain feels. In the instance of pain, and frequently for other symptoms, we must supply a vocabulary that permits the patient to explain what body sensations he or she has experienced. Pain has certain characteristics that often allow its source to be known with great accuracy.

CHARACTER

Is the pain burning, sharp, dull, achey, tooth-achey, knifelike, like needles sticking in, throbbing, pressing, squeezing, boring, gnawing? Is it really a pain or is it a discomfort? Do not insist upon the word pain (which patients may deny), but shift to the word discomfort instead. "Is your discomfort more like a needle-stick or like someone sitting on your chest?"

CONSTANCY

Does the pain or discomfort come and go? Is it never varying night and day? Does it come in waves? Do other activities distract the patient from the discomfort? This aspect of pain is so important that you should not leave the questions until you really know.

SEVERITY

Is it annoying, agonizing, unpleasant, terrible, discomfitting, unendurable? How does the patient's language for the pain compare to language about other things? How does the pain rate on an analog scale? Hold your hands about a foot apart and say, "My left hand stands for the least pain and my right hand stands for the worst pain you ever had, *show me* (not, tell me) with your finger where this pain stands in relation to my right and left hand." You can do the same thing with a piece of paper. It is a good technique for comparing pain severity from one day to the next.

DURATION

Did (or does) the pain last for moments, minutes, hours, days or weeks? Note how a little change in this parameter can alter the hypothesis about source. "Where is your pain?" "Right over the center of my chest. It feels like someone is sitting on my chest." "How long has it been there?" "For days, maybe even a couple of weeks." Or, conversely, "When do you get the pain in your chest?" "Whenever I walk fast or if I get upset." "How long does it last?" "A couple of seconds, maybe." "And if you keep walking?" "Still, a couple of seconds at the most, but it scares me because my father died when he was younger than me."

ONSET

Exactly (details count) when and how did the pain or discomfort start? Avoid accepting generalities such as, "At work." When, what was the patient doing, what else happened—be *very* specific.

RECURRENCES

Is this the first episode? If not, get the details of the previous episodes. Nothing relieves a doctor's mind like discovering that the dangerous-sounding symptoms reported by the patient have been occurring for years without apparent harm to the patient.

ASSOCIATED SYMPTOMS

Is there nausea, vomiting, diarrhea, sweats, fever, and so on? These are important because, for example, pain in the abdomen with *no* associated gastrointestinal symptoms and no relief from belching, flatus, vomiting, or bowel movements makes one wonder whether the pain arises from an intraabdominal process.

WHAT MAKES IT WORSE? WHAT MAKES IT BETTER?

Is it aggravated by food, position, deep-breathing, work, having sex, lifting pack-ages, walking fast, or other activity? Does lying down or pulling the knees up on the abdomen relieve the pain or discomfort? Does belching, the passage of flatus, urinating, vomiting, or moving the bowels change the discomfort? Is it worse when first awakening or does it worsen as the day goes on? Does the pain ease while running or exercising only to return as the patient cools down. These questions can frequently be asked in such a manner that the patient can try out the maneuver on the spot. This makes it possible to "do a physical" over the telephone. "Sit up straight. Push your arm on the side of the pain straight out in front of you as hard as you can. Does that aggravate your chest pain?" That maneuver mobilizes the scapula and puts the intraspinatus on stretch. If the pain in the chest is muscular in origin, it will be worsened. If it is intrathoracic in origin, there will be no effect on the pain. It is useful to develop a whole set of maneuvers that can be turned into questions.

WHAT DID YOU DO FOR THE PAIN?

Was the pain relieved by aspirin, Alka-Seltzer, Tylenol, a heating pad, other anal-gesics or medications? Does the speed and degree of relief seem appropriate to the modality? It may not be the aspirin itself if relief followed 30 seconds after taking the pills.   .

WHAT HAVE OTHER DOCTORS SAID?

If the pain (or any other symptom) is of long duration, other doctors may have been consulted. They have probably done diagnostic studies or tried treatments. If you are lucky they have done all the work. When it seems that every other doctor was wrong, but that you have the answer, *be careful.* When nothing worked before, there is always a good reason. In these circumstances, if you always assume that every previous physician was smart, you probably will not end up looking dumb.

It is not generally necessary to go through every point in the pain litany before you recognize the origin of the pain sufficiently to offer yourself an hypothesis to try knocking down. Nonetheless, the pain litany should be committed to memory. There is something that must be said about pain that holds for many other symp-toms as well. *Only the patient knows whether pain is present. Only the patient knows the severity of the pain. There are not and there cannot be any objective measures of pain!* This cannot be stated too strongly. Although the presence of other symptoms, behaviors, or measures may help in the evaluation of pain, ulti-mately you must believe or disbelieve the patient! Learning to believe patients about their pain will save you from many embarrassing errors and, more impor-tantly, save you from permitting or causing unnecessary pain. Whenever doubt exists, ask yourself about the alternatives. "What follows if I believe the patient?" "What follows if I do not believe the patient?"

ESTABLISHING A TIME LINE

Illness is a process, not an event; therefore, it inevitably unfolds over time. As in-dicated earlier, because illness is frequently considered by the sick as a temporal object whose temporal dimensions are fixed, establishing the time line of the process may be difficult and require persistent questioning. Be patient. Use holidays and shared public experiences as dating signposts to translate the patient's experience of time into clock and calendar time. Here, especially, do not leave the line of questioning until *you are sure* you know the sequence of events. Seemingly small matters such as whether the nausea or the pain came first, whether the pain started while the patient was still on vacation and before returning to work, and how many years back the whole illness started (not just, "along time ago") will pay off in diagnostic accuracy. Remember that the case you are constructing out of the circumstances of patient and body (that will make sense of events) *always* has a temporal dimension.

THE PERSONAL HISTORY, SOCIAL HISTORY, AND PAST HISTORY

The diagnostician who has uncovered what is wrong with the patient's body to produce the symptoms of the illness has solved only the first of the four problems presented by any sick person. Three more remain to be investigated. The first of the remaining three concern things internal to the patient—who the patient is, and how that person and his or her behaviors interact with the pathophysiology to produce this specific illness. Second, there must be an attempt to discover what external factors—familial, social, occupational, or environmental—have played a part in making the patient sick. Third, there is the definitional problem: the clinician must discover how the patient defines the problem and what has to be corrected before the patient will consider the problem solved. When all this has been accomplished, you will understand what is the matter, why it threatens the patient, and why it happened when it did. Because you have defined the problem both in your own (medical science) terms as well as in the patient's, you are in a position to plan treatment for the disease that is suited to the individual and, almost as important, comprehensible by the patient.

The language that patients use, that is, word choice and paralanguage (pause, pitch, speech rate, and emphasis), as well as their beliefs and values as revealed in the history have provided the opportunity for you to know much about each of them as persons. However, in these sections of the history (personal history, social history, and past history) you will discover much more about them that is essential to understanding their relationships to their illnesses. Here, however, you are not merely trying to understand *this* person, but rather the personal, social, and other outside forces that may have acted on the individual and his or her diseases. Sometimes disease occurs because of occupational exposures of 20 years earlier (for example, mesothelioma), which the person has long forgotten. Other times, ethnicity and associated dietary habits may be responsible (fish tapeworm from eating raw fish). The present epidemic of the acquired immunodeficiency syndrome (AIDS) has reminded physicians once again that the epidemiology of disease may be intimately related to sexual behaviors or illegal drug use. All these facts and many more can be discovered in a well-taken personal and social history.

The basic principle of questioning in these areas, however, is very different. In taking the history of the present illness, the principle that underlies questioning is that any question is a good question if it elicits the information (with appropriate checks to ensure accuracy). In contrast, in the personal and social history the principle is to *employ fixed and unchanging questions* at the start of each category. The reason for this change in the method of questioning can be explained best using the example of finding out how much alcohol the patient consumes. It is well known that denial is a constant feature in those who abuse alcohol (or other drugs). Simply asking how much a patient drinks may get little reliable information. Since we cannot know for sure how much the patient drinks compared to others, we substitute the next best thing, knowing how the patient answers the question about alcohol use compared to others. To know this, you must employ *the same question* asked *in the same manner* at the *same point* in the history. The necessity for exact duplication is known from survey research, where it has been shown that varying the order or wording of questions influences the answers. Thus here, as in every feature of the personal and social history, you will be developing and memorizing the order and wording of your questions. Variation in patient answers should depend on the patient, not the manner in which the questions were asked or their wording. The principle is the same as in the physical examination where it is your knowledge of the normal body that allows you to know when something is abnormal.

You might ask the question, "How much do you drink alcohol?" It is a seemingly silly little question considering how important a drinking history can be. However, after you have asked it hundreds of times you will be alert to answers that make you want to ask more questions. Then you may pursue the issue using questions that get at both quantity and chronicity of drinking. You may even end with a question like, "Do you drink a quart of whiskey (or a case of beer, or a gallon of wine) a day?" Allow the patient to deny such excess ("Maybe a fifth a day, but never a quart"). Starting with that question, however, will offend many (and make you sound like an adversary unnecessarily) and perhaps not produce more information. Thus, the innocuous opening question is used.

You should start out employing the questions suggested by us or your institution. As your knowledge grows and your self-mastery increases, you may change the wording to better fit your particular needs and style. We suggest that whenever you change questions, you experiment with a new wording for awhile until you settle on the new form of the question and then *do not change it again without good reason.* When the standard question points to a source of information worth pursuing, once again, use any question that will get the information you want.

You are trying to find out who this patient is. The background knowledge that helps you interpret the patient's answers is your knowledge of the world. Patients' histories are not only helpful in finding out about them and their illnesses, but in educating yourself. When a patient does a kind of work with which you are unfamiliar, allow the patient to tell you about it. In this manner you will show the patient that you care about him or her, find out about its relevance to their illness, and enlarge your knowledge of the world. Patients will teach you about marriage and divorce, child-raising, being orphaned, having an alcoholic parent, intravenous drug abuse, ethnic behaviors, pouring steel, gambling, what it is like to have multiple sclerosis or any other disease, and an endless amount about what it means to be human. All you have to do is ask, and then *listen* to the answer. *Everything* that clinicians know is relevant to the care of the sick.

THE QUICK AND DIRTY HISTORY

There is *never* a time when a physician does not need to know something about a sick person. No matter how terrible the emergency, no matter how self-evident the problem, if the patient can speak (or otherwise respond) some history must be obtained. The following few questions can be asked after you have found out how the accident happened or the illness started:

1. Do you take any medicine regularly, even vitamins?
2. Do you have any allergies?
3. Are there any foods or drugs that make you sick, make you break out, give you pain in your abdomen, or which you avoid for any reason?
4. Have you ever been operated on?
5. Have you ever been in a hospital for any physical or mental problem?
6. Do you have any other illnesses at this time?
7. Have you ever been seriously ill?
8. When is the last time you saw a doctor for anything?

Again and again, serious errors are committed because the patient was not asked whether the present illness had occurred previously or was not asked even the few questions listed here. Not taking a history is as grievous a fault as not examining a patient.

SECTION II

GENERAL EXAMINATIONS

4. GENERAL APPEARANCE

5. VITAL SIGNS
   Faith T. Fitzgerald
   John C. Floyd, Jr.
   Richard D. Judge
   John G. Weg

6. SKIN
   Peter J. Lynch

7. HEMATOPOIETIC SYSTEM
   Alan D. Campbell
   Max S. Wicha

The physician should have
.... *mercy on the sick and*
pledge himself to relieve
suffering among all
classes.... All are to be
treated equally. He should
look upon the misery of
the patient as if it were his
own.
CHINESE CANON OF MEDICINE
200 BC–200 AD

1. Observe your patient, including skin.
2. Examine the hands.
3. Take the temperature.
4. Count pulse and respirations.
5. Take the blood pressure.
6. If the lymph nodes are enlarged, examine them all at this time. If not, do them regionally.

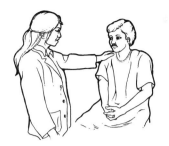

CHAPTER 4

GENERAL APPEARANCE

In all experimental knowledge there are three phases: an observation made, a comparison established, and a judgment rendered.

CLAUDE BERNARD
(1813–1878)

From the moment you meet your patient, and throughout the interview, you should be constantly observing him or her in an orderly and scientific way. The ability to observe accurately is a great asset in most fields of endeavor; it is indispensable in the practice of medicine. The physical examination is simply a series of observations.

Yet as Goethe said, "We see only what we know." The first step is to perceive. The second is to relate the sensory stimuli to relevant knowledge or past experience. Both abilities are indispensable, and both are irrevocably interdependent. From reading, from lectures and clinical experience, we accumulate the body of knowledge that gives significance to what we perceive. This background is concerned with more than the simple interpretation of findings; it is part of the act of observing. Let us consider an example.

An inexperienced student at the foot of the bed of a patient with clubbed digits is asked to describe anything he sees that might be significant. Rarely, he may point out the peculiar rounded appearance of the nails without being able to explain its significance. Far more often, however, the finding will go unnoticed. It does not register because it has no meaning for him. The lesson here is a simple one. In your eagerness to begin clinical work, do not lose sight of the importance of your preclinical scholarship. Without basic knowledge derived from careful study, you cannot expect to be an artful observer. You see only insofar as you understand. Medical observation is complex; it must therefore be deliberate and systematic. It requires concentration. An ill-timed distraction may cause an oversight; the oversight, a missed diagnosis. It is always helpful to focus your attention on one thing at a time. Looking at the hand is not enough. You must scrutinize in turn the nails, the skin texture, the color, the hair distribution, and so forth. Use of a disciplined system helps in this respect by limiting your field of observation. It makes you less susceptible to errors of omission.

The mental phase of observation may be both conscious and subconscious. What attracts us more than anything else is change. Like the continuous sound that is "heard" only when it suddenly stops, the physical abnormality captures our attention almost automatically. At this point we begin to think. We look more carefully. We may reposition the patient, have him breathe more deeply, or perform some other maneuver aimed at accentuating the finding or facilitating its analysis. We also begin to think ahead, for one finding may be a signpost that tells us to look carefully for other specific possibilities. One or two spider angiomas (indicating liver disease) noticed during history taking tells the experienced observer to watch particularly for an enlarged liver, palmar erythema, clubbing, splenomegaly, testicular atrophy, dilated abdominal veins, external hemorrhoids, hyperactive reflexes, or a flapping tremor. Of course, the first signpost on the way to diagnosis is the patient's history itself.

PREPARING THE PATIENT

The physical examination should be made as easy as possible for the patient, who usually expects it to be a relatively distasteful experience. If the physician is considerate and gentle, the patient should feel, when it is all over, that most of his or her fears on that score were unfounded. The ideal examining room is private, warm enough to avoid chilling, and free from distracting noise and sources of interruption. Adequate (preferably fluorescent or natural) light is essential. The examining table may be placed with its head against the wall, but both sides (particularly the right) and the foot should be accessible to the examiner.

The first crisis concerns the problem of undressing. In the outpatient department the patient disrobes while the physician is out of the room. It is always stressed that the patient must disrobe completely; it is folly to try to examine the heart through a nightgown or the abdomen through a slip. But it is equally true that respect for the patient's modesty is an important factor that greatly affects the subsequent physician-patient relationship. Tell the patient to leave on his or her underpants. They can be moved aside later, when necessary. This simple concession will not interfere with 90 percent of the examination, and it will greatly reduce anxiety. In addition, a sheet should always be available to drape the patient from the waist down. A towel or special gown may be used to cover the female chest (Fig. 4–1). This combination allows complete examination without prolonged, embarrassing exposure.

Begin and end the examination by washing your hands. When possible, do this in the patient's presence. Your movements should be deliberate and methodical but always gentle. Your attitude should be basically objective but not serious. An occasional smile or distracting comment is a great help to relieving tension. Try to avoid surprise. Preface each maneuver with a simple direction or explanation. When the time comes to inspect the breasts, prepare the patient with a simple statement such "Now we must remove this towel for a moment." The same is true for examining the abdomen. This gives a sense of purpose to your actions that practically eliminates embarrassment. The pelvic examination, of course, takes special preparation, and a female attendant should always be present if the examining physician is a man.

At times it will be necessary to cause the patient some discomfort. In these instances it is particularly important to explain the necessity of going ahead. For example: "I'm sorry if this hurts but it's important." The examiner should not hold back because of pain, but on the other hand he must balance the importance of the observation against the degree of discomfort and proceed as deftly as possible.

HISTORY

Changes in general appearance, especially gradual changes, may go unnoticed by the patient. It is often valuable to obtain a photograph of the patient from 1 or 2

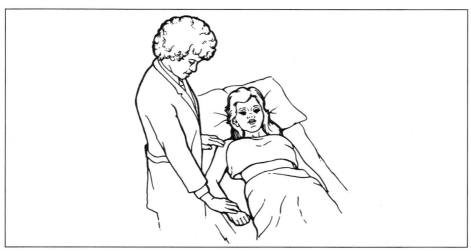

FIGURE 4–1
Woman draped for examination.

years before, to compare with current appearance. Most individuals, in our pound-conscious era, can tell you if they have gained or lost weight over recent months. If they cannot, old records (hospital charts, identification cards, some driving licenses) can be consulted for past weight.

Unaccustomed clumsiness or acquired "accident-proneness" may be the only historical clue to neurologic disease. Decrease in accustomed activity may signal progressive weakness.

Close friends, relatives, and neighbors may be more aware of changes in general appearance and activity than the patient. You should not hesitate to ask for their opinions and to incorporate these judiciously into your history.

PHYSICAL EXAMINATION

1. Observe your patient.
2. Examine the hands.

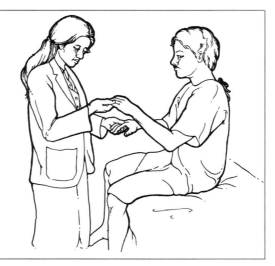

It has been observed, that the height of a man from the crown of the head to the sole of the foot, is equal to the distance between the tips of the middle fingers of the two hands when extended in a straight line.

PLINY THE ELDER
(23–79)

Even before the formal physical you will begin making observations that may alert you to disease. Throughout the history and physical, these cumulative observations form the basis for logical diagnostic deductions.

As the patient moves into the examining room, you might note the **gait**. Is it painful (antalgic)? Is there evident favoring of one side of the body, as in stroke? Is it rigid, bradykinetic, as in Parkinson's disease? Is the movement slow, the posture slumped, as in depression? Is the patient unsteady, as in weakness, middle-ear disease, or cerebellar dysfunction?

A wealth of information can be gained by **shaking hands** with the patient. Warm, moist hands may suggest hyperthyroidism (Fig. 4–2). Are they the painful, swollen hands of the arthritic? The cold, moist hands of the anxious patient? The calloused hands of the manual laborer or the softer fingers of the scholar? Is the ring loose, as with weight loss, or tight, as with edema?

When the patient speaks, does the tone of his **voice** suggest the hoarseness of laryngeal cancer; the weakened, thickened, and lowered voice of hypothyroidism; the "vocal ataxia" or "scanning speech" of multiple sclerosis or cerebellar disease? Is slurred speech the result of central nervous system injury or oropharyngeal pathology? Do an elderly person's dentures click, suggesting weight loss or dehydration, or are the ill-fitting dentures themselves a cause of weight loss? Are words "hard to find," as in the aphasia following some cerebral vascular occlusive events? Is the speech monotonal or emotionless as in certain psychiatric disorders?

The **face** has always been the mirror of the mind. It shows pain, fear, anxiety, and sadness. It is in the face that we first notice whether our patients are pale, ruddy, cyanotic, or icteric. Thickened features suggest hormonal imbalance—e.g., of the thyroid or growth hormone. Fullness may be a consequence of edema, obesity, or a result of excess corticosteroids. A malar flush may signal *lupus* or *mitral stenosis*. Shiny skin and tight features first alert us to possible *scleroderma*. Cranial nerve dysfunction may be manifested by ptosis, strabismus, or facial asymmetry.

Habitus refers to your patient's general shape—his or her body build. *Cachexia* is an extreme thinness and debility caused by some serious disease, such as cancer or chronic infection. Signs of recent weight loss, such as loose clothes, newly punched belt holes, and redundant skin folds and striae (stretch marks), clue the clinician to a loss of flesh or fat that may or may not have been noticed by the patient.

Simple *obesity* is a deposition of body fat in excess of some arbitrary standard and is partly culturally defined. Pathologic obesity is deposition of body fat to the point of physiologic compromise of the individual, who may have respiratory, cardiac, or orthopedic difficulty. In these conditions excess fat is apportioned generally around the body—face, trunk, buttocks, and extremities. Deposition of fat

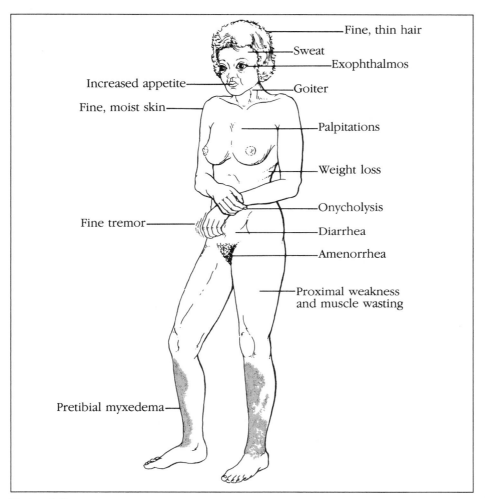

FIGURE 4–2
Hyperthyroidism. A diagnosis you can make by observation.

around the trunk, with thin extremities in which muscle wasting is evident, may suggest hypercorticosteroidism.

Develop the habit of closely observing the patient's **hands**; they are highly informative. It is said that when a physician was called to the harem to treat one of the sultan's wives, he was allowed to examine only the hand of the patient extended between the folds of a curtain. This procedure was not entirely without diagnostic value. One need only watch a concert pianist to recognize the close relationship between brain and hand. Speech is intimately associated with the hand, and gestures may convey more meaning than words. The types of rings (and other jewelry) have a special message. Nicotine stains also convey a certain impression, as does the general hygiene.

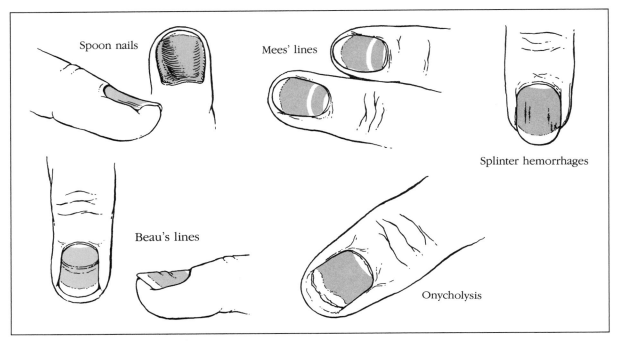

Figure 4–3
Some nail signs of systemic disease.

Observe the nails closely (Fig. 4–3). *Beau's lines* are transverse furrows that begin at the lunula and progress distally as the nail grows. They result from a temporary arrest of growth of the nail matrix occasioned by trauma or systemic stress. If all the nails are involved, a period of general catabolism, such as infection, childbirth, and toxicity, may be postulated (local nail trauma seldom involves more than one or two digits). Knowing that the nail grows about 0.1 mm/day, one can, by measuring how far Beau's lines are from the cuticle, approximately date the stress. For example, if the line is 4 mm out, some serious event occurred about 40 days before.

Spoon nails (koilonychia) may occur in a form of iron deficiency anemia, as well as in a variety of other disorders (coronary disease, syphilis) and with the use of strong soaps.

Subungual splinter hemorrhages may provide a clue to bacterial endocarditis or *Trichinella spiralis* infestation in the febrile patient.

The nails may reflect metabolic disturbances. *Terry's nails* are the white nails with normal pink tips described in patients with cirrhosis. *Mees' lines* are paired, white, parallel transverse bands seen in individuals with hypoalbuminemia. *Lindsay's (half and half) nails,* in which the proximal portion of the nail is white and the distal 20–50 percent is red, are associated with renal failure. None of these is specific, but all give useful hints. *Onycholysis* or destruction of the nails, may be

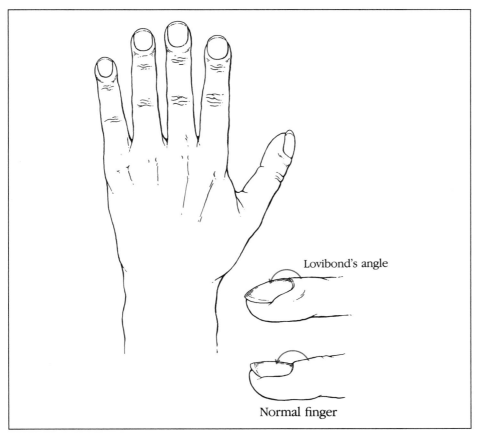

Lovibond's angle

Normal finger

FIGURE 4—4
Clubbing.

seen with hyperthyroidism, fungal nail infection, or in association with psoriasis. In the latter condition, a less severe change may be seen, namely, pitting of the nails.

Clubbing of the nails may occur in association with cardiovascular disease (congenital, cyanotic), subacute bacterial endocarditis, pulmonary arteriovenous fistula, and pulmonary disease (bronchiectasis, abscess, empyema). Clubbing is not associated, generally, with simple emphysema or nonsupperative chronic lung disease. One sees a bulbous enlargement of the distal portion of the digits (Fig. 4–4). The angle made by the proximal nail fold and the nail plate (Lovibond's angle) exceeds 180°. The cause of clubbing is still uncertain, although it is probably related to increased blood flow through multiple arteriovenous shunts in the distal phalanges (Table 4–1).

Extreme redness (erythema) of the palm is common in cirrhosis of the liver and in women who have borne children. Pallor of the palm, especially the creases,

TABLE 4–1. Some Causes of Clubbing

I. Symmetric clubbing
  A. Cardoivascular disease
    1. Congenital, cyanotic
    2. Subacute bacterial endocarditis
    3. Pulmonary arteriovenous fistula
  B. Pulmonary disease
    1. Severe, chronic inflammatory
      a. Bronchiectasis
      b. Abscess
      c. Empyema
    2. Asbestosis
    3. Neoplasm
      a. Carcinoma, primary
      b. Pleural mesothelioma
    4. Interstitial fibrosis
    5. Cystic fibrosis
  C. Extrathoracic disease
    1. Gastrointestinal
      a. Sprue
      b. Ulcerative colitis
      c. Regional enteritis
      d. Dysentery
    2. Hepatic
      a. Biliary cirrhosis
      b. Liver abscess
      c. Amyloidosis
    3. Toxic
      a. Arsenic
      b. Phosphorus
      c. Alcohol
      d. Silica or beryllium
    4. Familial
    5. Miscellaneous
      a. Chronic pyelonephritis
      b. Syringomyelia
      c. Chronic granulocytic leukemia
II. Asymmetric clubbing
  A. Unidigital
    1. Median nerve injury
  B. Unilateral
    1. Aneurysm of innominate artery
    2. Recurrent subluxation of shoulder
  C. Unequal
    1. Anomalous aortic arch
    2. Reverse patent ductus

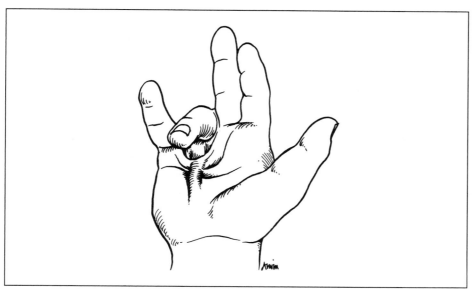

FIGURE 4-5
Dupuytren's contracture.

suggests anemia. *Dupuytren's contracture,* a fibrosis and contraction of the palmar fascia, is seen with liver disease, trauma, epilepsy, and simple aging (Fig. 4–5).

Arthritic changes in the hands will be discussed more fully under the joint examination.

Examine, by quick but thorough observation, the **entire body** of your patient before you begin a regional examination. Overall *hair distribution,* for example, not only differs according to age and sex (Fig. 4–6) but may signal disease (Table 4–2).

"Educated" observation may lead to a suspicion of diagnosis even before the patient speaks, as evidenced particularly in the endocrine disorders illustrated in Figures 4–7 through 4–10.

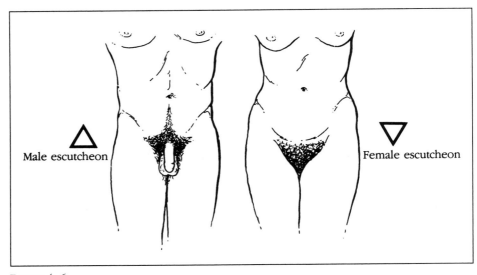

FIGURE 4–6
Normal sexual hair distribution in adult men and women. Changes may signal hormonal abnormalities.

TABLE 4–2. Some Causes of Hirsutism

Racial and familial
Puberty, pregnancy, menopause
Drugs
    Phenytoin
    Diazoxide
    Corticosteroids
    Progestagens
    Androgens
    Minoxidil
Endocrine abnormalities
    Adrenal hyperplasia
    Adrenal adenoma or carcinoma
    Stein-Leventhal syndrome
    Ovarian tumors
    Pituitary tumors
Congenital sex anomalites

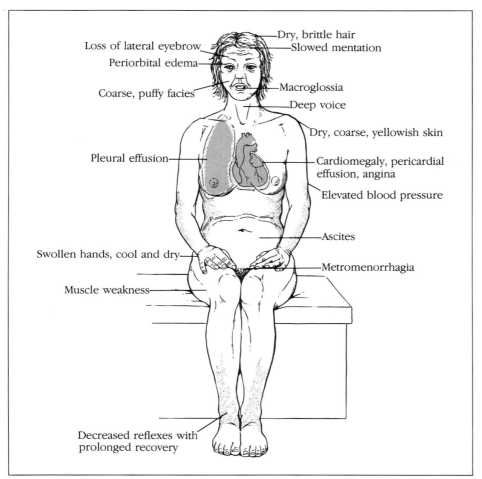

Loss of lateral eyebrow
Periorbital edema
Coarse, puffy facies
Dry, brittle hair
Slowed mentation
Macroglossia
Deep voice
Dry, coarse, yellowish skin
Pleural effusion
Cardiomegaly, pericardial effusion, angina
Elevated blood pressure
Ascites
Swollen hands, cool and dry
Metromenorrhagia
Muscle weakness
Decreased reflexes with prolonged recovery

Figure 4–7
Myxedema. A diagnosis you can make by observation.

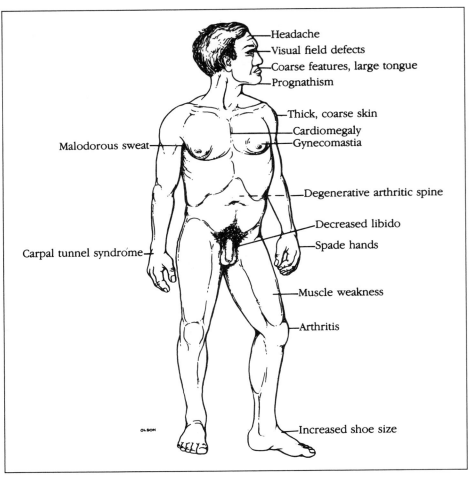

FIGURE 4–8
Acromegaly. A diagnosis you can make by observation.

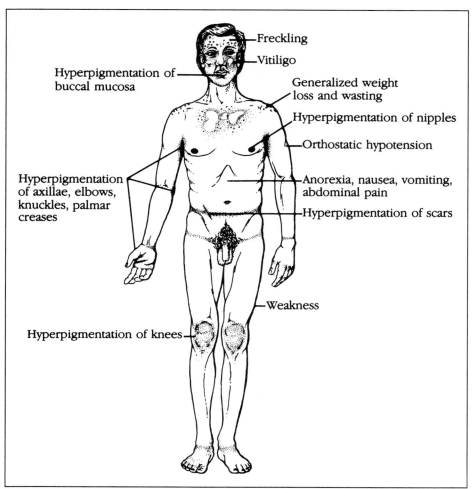

FIGURE 4–9
Adrenocortical insufficiency (Addison's disease). A diagnosis you can make by observation.
Hyperpigmentation does *not* occur with pituitary adrenal insufficiency.

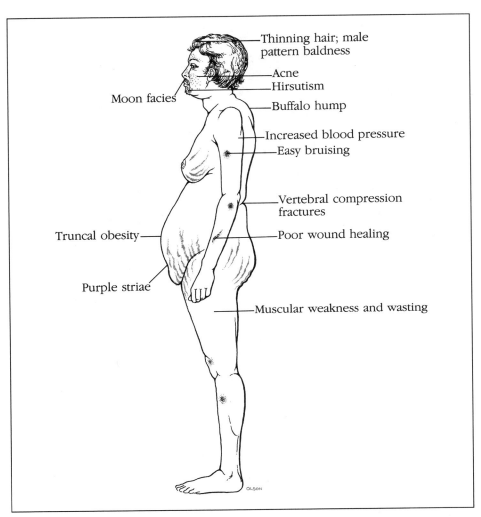

FIGURE 4–10
Adrenocortial excess (Cushing's syndrome). A diagnosis you can make by observation.

CHAPTER 5

VITAL SIGNS

It is better that a fever succeed to a convulsion, than a convulsion to a fever.
HIPPOCRATES
(460?–377? B.C.)

Because a heartbeat, breathing, and body warmth are the clinical signs of life (the absence of which signaled death in the era before the advent of modern laboratory aids such as the electroencephalogram), the so-called vital signs (pulse, respiratory rate, temperature, and blood pressure) continue to be the most frequently examined of all physical findings.

HISTORY

Abnormalities in vital signs touch on all disease states. Certain symptoms (e.g., sweats with fever) may form a patient's isolated initial complaint. Conversely, a significant abnormality in vital signs (e.g., high blood pressure) may be asymptomatic.

Because of the pervasive nature of variations in the vital signs in health and disease, history regarding subjective awareness of changes in pulse, respirations, and temperature is correlated with each patient's total picture, no matter what the chief complaint might be.

PHYSICAL EXAMINATION

1. Insert oral thermometer.
2. Count radial pulse.
3. Count respirations.
4. Take blood pressure, both arms.
5. Remove and read thermometer.

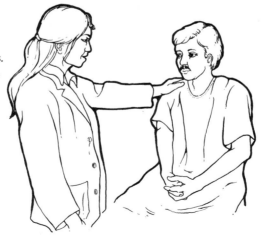

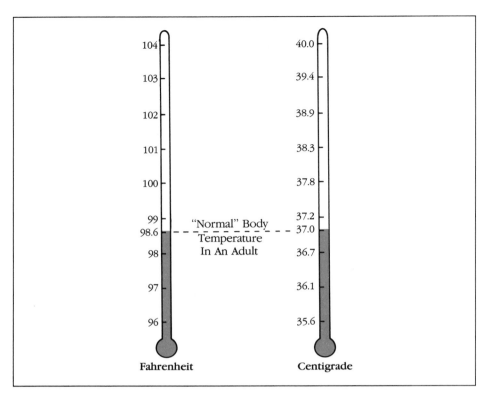

FIGURE 5–1
A comparison of the temperature scales commonly used in United States hospitals.

TEMPERATURE

The temperature is generally taken by placing the bulb of a well-shaken thermometer under the patient's tongue for 3 minutes. Newer instruments may allow the oral temperature to be recorded by thermistor in less than 60 seconds. The temperature may be taken orally or rectally, and in the United States the Fahrenheit scale is usually used (Fig. 5–1). When fever is present the mercury column climbs quite rapidly (15 to 30 seconds) to within a few tenths of the final reading. Falsely low levels may result from incomplete closure of the mouth, breathing through the mouth, leaving the thermometer in place for too short a time, or the recent ingestion of cold substances. Falsely elevated levels may result from inadequate shaking down of the thermometer, previous ingestion of warm substances, smoking, recent strenuous activity, or even a very warm bath.

In most persons there is a diurnal (occurring every day) variation in body temperature of 0.5° to 2°F. The lowest ebb is reached during sleep, at which time the temperature may fall as low as 96.5° to 97°F. As the patient begins to awaken, the temperature slowly rises.

There is a well-known temperature pattern in the menstruating woman that reflects the effects of ovulation. The morning temperature falls slightly just prior to menstruation and continues at this level until the midpoint between the two periods. There may be a further drop 24 to 36 hours prior to ovulation, and coincident with ovulation the morning temperature rises and remains at a somewhat higher level until just before the next menses.

You will note that the upper limit of normal on the standard thermometer is 98.6°F. It must be remembered that this is an arbitrary value that applies primarily to patients at bed rest. Many normal people show higher levels when active, and on a hot summer day in the outpatient clinic, readings of 99.4°F are not at all uncommon in perfectly normal individuals. Even higher values can be recorded in children following hard play.

Rectal temperatures are usually 0.5° to 1°F higher than oral temperatures, but they tend to be less subject to alteration by the oral factors mentioned above and are generally more constant and reproducible. It is an error to believe that rectal temperatures are more accurate than oral temperatures in the sense that rectal temperatures are more reflective of "core" temperature than are oral readings. It is probably the case that the thermoregulatory centers in the hypothalamus are directed in their control of body temperature by temperatures that more closely approximate those in the anatomically neighboring mouth than those in the more distant rectal core. Axillary temperatures are so inaccurate that they will not be discussed further.

Fever is an elevation of body temperature due to disease. It is one of the oldest and still most useful signs in clinical medicine. Pyrogens, both exogenous (e.g., endotoxin from bacterial cell walls) and endogenous (interleukin 1) act to "reset" the hypothalamic thermoregulatory centers at a higher "set point." The generation of heat to achieve this newly directed set point may be by the mechanism of violent muscular exertion—the shaking chill or "rigor." Attempts to dissipate extra body heat in febrile states are seen by the clinician as sweating (diaphoresis) and cutaneous vasodilation, the fever "flush." Increased body temperature of whatever origin increases heart rate and metabolic rate in general.

Fever patterns (e.g., intermittent, remittent, relapsing) are seldom diagnostically useful.

Hypothermia, or an oral temperature of less than 94°F, may be missed because most clinical thermometers do not go below 94°F. If you suspect a lower temperature, you must check it again with a special long thermometer or thermistor. Abnormally low temperatures may occur with severe brain injury, hypoglycemia, thiamine deficiency, starvation, exposure, sepsis, burns, hypothyroidism, hypoadrenalism, a variety of drug intoxications, and extremes of age. All these conditions have a common pathophysiology. They interfere either with central thermoregulation in the hypothalamus or with peripheral generation and retention of body heat.

PULSE

The radial pulse is best taken at the base of the patient's thumb (Fig. 5–2). If the examiner uses two or three fingers along the course of the artery, he or she may determine the pulse contour as well as the rate (see Chap. 12, Cardiovascular System).

Initially, and *always* if the pulse is irregular, the examiner should count the pulse for a full 60 seconds. If the pulse rate is between 60 and 100, and the rhythm is absolutely regular, many physicians will "shortcut" and count the pulse for 30 seconds, then multiply by two.

If the radial pulse is poor or irregular, the pulse may be taken by listening to or palpating the apex of the heart (the *apical pulse*). The normal resting pulse rate ranges from 60 to 100. It may be in the 50s in a conditioned athlete, or 100 or over in an excited patient. Rates less than 60 are often referred to as *bradycardia* (literally, "slow heart"), and rates over 100 as *tachycardia* ("fast heart").

The lability of the pulse rate is well known to all. Usually the rhythm is relatively regular. Occasional premature beats are so common that they are not necessarily considered abnormal. They are perceived as transient skips or breaks in rhythm. Sinus arrhythmia can be identified in most patients under the age of 40. It refers to a transient increase in pulse rate with inspiration, followed by a slowing with expiration. This phenomenon can be rather marked in some normal patients.

The pulse rate and rhythm should be recorded, and if abnormal contour is discovered, that too must be noted.

RESPIRATIONS

When man grows old . . . there is much gas within his thorax, resulting in panting and troubled breathing.

> HUANG TI (the Yellow Emperor)
> (2697–2597 B.C.)

Many physicians find it of value to count the respirations while appearing to take the pulse, since the natural tendency of the patient is to breathe awkwardly under observation. Normal respiratory rate is between 8 and 14 per minute in adults and is somewhat more rapid in children.

Note abnormalities of respiratory rate and rhythm (Fig. 5–3). Extremely slow respiration usually indicates central nervous system respiratory depression due to disease or drugs. Periodic or *Cheyne-Stokes respiration* occurs with serious cardiopulmonary or cerebral disorders. It is characterized by a periodic, regular, sequentially increasing depth of respiration followed by periods of apnea and is due to a loss of the normal fine-tuning of the respiratory centers to levels of arterial carbon dioxide. The PCO_2 rises during the apneic phases, stimulating vigorous breathing. As the patient breathes, however, he blows off so much carbon dioxide that apnea is induced until PCO_2 rises again. In contrast, *Biot's respiration* is irregularly irregular, almost spasmodic, with longer periods of apnea than of breathing; it is almost always associated with hypoventilation. It is generally associated with central nervous system disease. Deep slow breathing *(Kussmaul's respiration)* characterizes acidosis, a state in which the physiologic response to increased metabolic acid in the blood is a compensatory "blowing off" of carbon dioxide. Extreme tachypnea is present during many acute illnesses. It may be due to chronic or acute pulmonary or cardiac disease or systemic disorders, such as shock, severe pain, and aci-

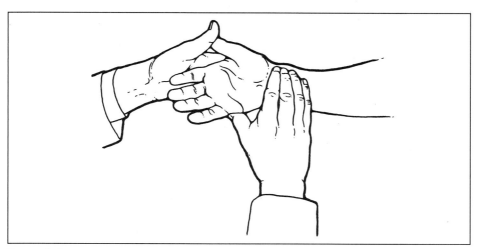

FIGURE 5–2
Palpating the radial pulse.

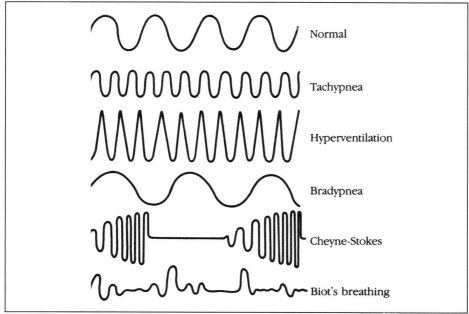

FIGURE 5–3
Patterns of respiration.

dosis; although it may represent undue excitement or nervousness, especially when accompanied with sighing, an organic cause should be excluded.

The patient's preferred position is important. Can he lie flat comfortably? Patients with congestive heart failure prefer the sitting position, as do patients with pulmonary disease during acute attacks of infection or bronchospasm. Patients with pericarditis often sit and lean forward. Although cardiac patients often awaken dyspneic several hours after reclining (due to redistribution of excess blood volume into the lungs [paroxysmal nocturnal dyspnea]), people with large amounts of sputum frequently awaken shortly after reclining to clear retained secretions. Preference for lying on one side or the other may point to the localization of pathologic processes; secretions or foreign bodies may be aspirated into a specific area because of position.

BLOOD PRESSURE

At the moment the heart contracts, and when the breast is struck, when in short the organ is in its state of systole, the arteries are dilated, yield a pulse, and are in a state of diastole.

WILLIAM HARVEY
(1578–1657)

The normal adult blood pressure varies over a wide range. The normal systolic range varies from 95 to 140 mm Hg, generally increasing with age. The normal diastolic range is from 60 to 90 mm Hg. Pulse pressure is the difference between the systolic and diastolic pressures. Mean pressure can be approximated by dividing the pulse pressure by three and adding this value to the diastolic pressure. Routine measurements should be made with the patient sitting and recumbent. If you find an abnormality, compare the determination in both arms with the patient supine, sitting, and standing. Any reliable sphygmomanometer may be employed, but the bladder, or inflatable bag encased in the cuff, should be long enough to encircle the limb. In obese or very muscular patients, a leg cuff can be used.

Fit the cuff evenly around the upper arm, with the lower edge 1 inch above the elbow and the air bladder over the brachial artery. The palpation method is first employed to determine the systolic pressure (Fig. 5–4A). Rapidly inflate the cuff until the radial pulse disappears, and then deflate it slowly. The level at which the radial pulse first reappears is the systolic pressure. A gross estimate of the diastolic pressure is sometimes possible by palpation, for with further deflation of the cuff, the radial pulse assumes a bounding quality and then abruptly becomes normal. This point of change, when evident, roughly approximates the diastolic pressure. The auscultatory method is then employed to estimate both the systolic and diastolic pressures (Fig. 5–4B).

Place the stethoscope lightly over the brachial artery and inflate to 20 or 30 mm above the palpable systolic pressure. The highest level at which sounds are heard (phase 1 of Korotkoff) is the systolic pressure. With further lowering by decrements of 2 or 3 mm, the sounds are replaced by a bruit (phase 2) and then by loud, sharp sounds (phase 3). Finally the sounds suddenly become damped (phase 4), and a few millimeters below this they disappear. The point of complete disappearance

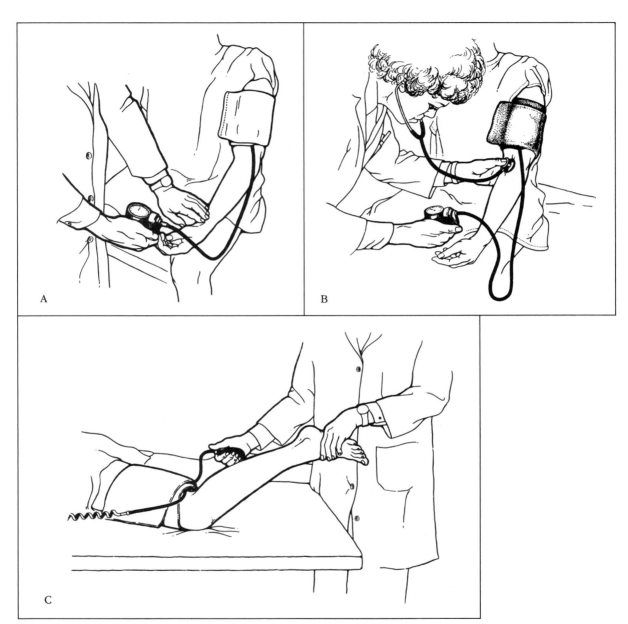

FIGURE 5–4
Blood pressure measurement. A. *By palpation*. Pump up the cuff to the point where the radial pulse is no longer felt. With decreasing cuff pressure, mark where the radial pulse reappears. This is the palpable systolic pressure. B. *By auscultation*. Auscultate the systolic and diastolic pressure over the brachial artery. C. *By palpation of blood pressure in the leg*. Palpate the dorsalis pedis pulse. Use a leg (oversized) cuff.

TABLE 5–1. Causes of Marked Asymmetry (>10 Torr Difference) in Blood
Pressure of the Arms

Errors in measurement
Thoracic outlet syndromes (e.g., cervical rib)
Embolic occlusion of an artery
Dissection of the aorta
External arterial occulsion (e.g., tumor, hematoma)
Atheromatous occlusion
Coarctation of the aorta
Marked difference in arm size (e.g., secondary to unilateral edema or withered arm)
Takayasu's arteritis
After Blalock-Taussig surgical procedure

of sound is considered the best index of diastolic pressure. Under hemodynamic conditions in which sound does not cease, the point of muffling should be taken as the diastolic pressure, with the point of total disappearance recorded as well (e.g., 140/60–0).

The pressure should be determined in both arms, at least on the initial evaluation. One may have a normal variation of up to 10 mm Hg (10 torr) between the two arms (Table 5–1). When it is advisable to measure the blood pressure in the leg, such as when a congenital narrowing (coarctation) of the aorta or dissecting aortic aneurysm is suspected, the palpation method should be employed with the patient prone (Fig. 5–4C). Apply the cuff to the calf or thigh and estimate the systolic level by palpating the posterior tibial or dorsalis pedis artery. The systolic level in the leg is normally equal to or higher than that in the arm (it is never critical to measure the diastolic pressure in the leg). Applying the standard cuff to the thigh and listening for sounds over the popliteal artery in the average adult is not only mechanically difficult but also may result in falsely elevated readings.

The patient's assuming an erect position may not necessarily affect the arm pressure taken at heart level. It is, however, not uncommon for the systolic pressure to fall by 10 to 15 mm Hg on standing, and about half of the time the diastolic pressure will rise slightly (by 5 mm Hg).

Orthostatic blood pressure changes should be sought in any patient in whom there is suspicion of (1) *volume loss* (bleeding, dehydration), (2) *nervous system dysfunction* (e.g., Parkinson's disease or diabetes, which may affect the autonomic nerves), and (3) *drug therapy* (e.g., antihypertensive drugs have their therapeutic effect by inducing orthostatic changes). Such orthostatic drops in blood pressure should obviously be sought in patients who complain of dizziness on assuming an erect posture.

Concomitant pulse rate must be measured with orthostatic blood pressure. Obviously, one who maintains a blood pressure of 120/80 only by increasing the pulse rate 25 beats per minute on rising may be volume deficient, even though the blood pressure does not drop noticeably.

Anxiety may raise the blood pressure, and multiple careful measurements over time should be taken before applying the diagnosis of hypertension to an individual with modest elevations.

Low blood pressure (hypotension) may of course be present in shock states or may accompany cachexia, prolonged bed rest, dehydration, and adrenal insufficiency among other causes. In an asymptomatic patient with no other complaints, systolic blood pressures as low as 80 to 90 torr may be perfectly normal. Shock cannot be said to be present unless there is evident decreased regional blood flow (e.g., syncope, oliguria, and pallor). Decreased regional blood flow is associated with dizziness, visual blurring, sweating, and, at times, syncope.

Irregular rhythms, especially atrial fibrillation, may lead to wide variations in the measured blood pressure. The flow (stroke output) and peripheral resistance in these arrhythmias may be different from beat to beat. Several blood pressure determinations in this circumstance are useful to get an *average* reading.

The *auscultatory gap* is a silent period between the systolic and diastolic pressures that may be appreciated in some patients with hypertension. Using the palpation method prior to auscultation to determine systolic pressure, and carefully listening throughout the descent of the mercury column, will prevent underestimation of the systolic or overestimation of the diastolic pressure.

Widened pulse pressure is common to all conditions producing an *increased stroke volume*. Simple bradycardia widens the pulse pressure by raising the systolic pressure (e.g., 150/70) as do fever, anemia, and hypermetabolic states. These disorders all have in common an increased stroke volume. Incompetence of the aortic valve widens the pulse pressure due to lowering of the diastolic pressure (e.g., 150/30). With aging, the elasticity of the great arteries diminishes, producing an increase in the systolic pressure at times referred to as "systolic hypertension" (e.g., 165/80).

The following common errors in the determination of blood pressure should be recognized and avoided:

1. Discrepancies between the relative cuff size and limb size may result in false reading. For example, an obese arm yields falsely elevated pressures when measured with a normal cuff. In obese patients you may check the systolic level with the cuff on the forearm, palpating the radial artery. Similarly, a standard cuff on an emaciated arm or the small arm of a child may give falsely low values.
2. Applying the cuff too loosely will give falsely elevated values.
3. The anxious patient may have an elevated level. If it is high, always leave the cuff in place and recheck the blood pressure several times. Never rely on a single determination.
4. It is possible to fail to recognize an auscultatory gap. Sounds may disappear between the systolic and diastolic pressures and then reappear. If the cuff pressure is raised only to the range of the gap, the systolic reading will be falsely low. This error is eliminated by first determining the systolic level by palpation.
5. Feeble Korotkoff's sounds may make your determination unreliable. In this event, deflate the cuff and have the patient elevate his arm, reinflating the cuff in this position. Then lower the arm and repeat. The sounds may be louder now because of diminished venous pressure. If they are not, you may have to settle for a palpable systolic pressure only.

CHAPTER 6

SKIN

The skin possesses the closest relations with the general economy, as shown by the observation that there are comparatively few so-called general diseases in which it . . . is not at some period involved in a slight or a marked degree.

LOUIS A. DUHRING
(1845–1913)

What portion of the physical examination could be easier than the examination of the skin? The skin is directly visible both in color and in three dimensions; it is directly palpable; and it is so thin that even the deepest cutaneous pathology is only a few millimeters away from the examiner. But this easy accessibility also creates some problems, in that it provides a great quantity of information, much of which is unimportant or unrelated to the patient's presenting problem. This abundance is complicated by the fact that we are so accustomed to viewing the skin that we really do not "see" it at all. Most of us, in performing the physical examination, consequently ignore all the information provided by the skin rather than make the effort to sort the important from the unimportant. This chapter is designed to assist the examiner in the sorting process.

ANATOMY

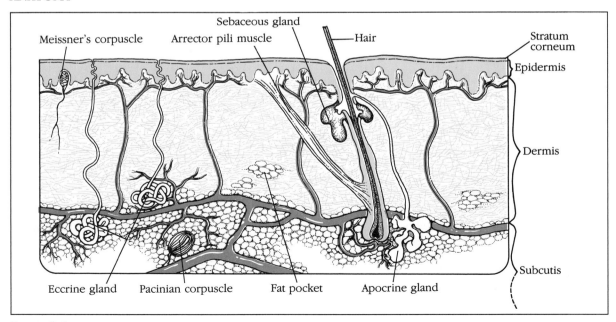

FIGURE 6–1
Cross-section of the skin and appendages.

TABLE 6–1. Pruritus

I. Pruritus with visible skin disease
  A. Excoriations may be present
    1. Eczematous skin disease (atopic/neurodermatitis, contact dermatitis, stasis dermatitis, anogenital pruritus, seborrheic dermatitis, dyshidrotic eczema)
    2. Scabies
    3. Dermatitis herpetiformis
    4. Psoriasis (scalp and intertriginous areas)
    5. Superficial fungal disease (feet and intertriginous areas)
    6. Pinworm infestation (perianal)
    7. Psychogenic causes (prurigo nodularis, neurotic excoriation)
  B. Itching with little or no excoriation
    1. Urticaria
    2. Erythema multiforme
    3. Lichen planus
    4. Drug reactions*
    5. Pityriasis rosea
    6. Urticaria pigmentosa (mastocytosis)
    7. Pruritic papules of pregnancy
II. Pruritis without visible skin disease
  A. Associated with internal conditions
    1. Uremia
    2. Liver disease (especially biliary cirrhosis and obstructive jaundice)
    3. Lymphoma (especially Hodgkin's disease)
    4. Polycythemia vera
    5. Pregnancy
    6. Miscellaneous (pruritus is often stated as being associated with diabetes mellitus, thyroid disease, parathyroid disease, iron deficiency, and internal carcinomas, but most reports are anecdotal)
  B. Not associated with internal disease
    1. Pediculosis pubis
    2. Pinworm infestation
    3. Xerosis (asteatosis)
    4. Psychogenic causes

---

*Drug reactions generally result in urticaria or erythema multiforms.

HISTORY

Two important **symptoms** signal cutaneous pathology: **pruritus** and **pain**. These two symptoms are related insofar as the respective sensations are both carried by the peripheral nervous system via its cutaneous branches.

Pain occurs under several sets of circumstances. Most commonly it appears when the skin around the nerves is no longer intact, exposing the sensitive nerve endings to the dry hostile environment outside the body. Pain may also occur as a direct effect of biochemical mediators in some kinds of cutaneous inflammatory reactions. Finally, pain may be the result of simple nonpenetrating external trauma. Usually these situations are clinically apparent; thus pain is more often a therapeutic problem than a diagnostic one.

Little is known regarding the pathophysiology of **pruritus,** but for the purpose of this chapter it suffices for us to know that itching is carried by the small nerve fibers of the skin. The first step in assessing patients with pruritus is to determine whether the itching is associated with visible disease of the skin or whether it is occurring in skin that is apparently normal (Table 6–1). The itching of specific skin diseases varies both in intensity (quantity) and in the degree to which it provokes a response of scratching (quality). Thus eczematous disease, especially in those who are genetically atopic, is usually associated with the presence of excoriation, whereas most other pruritic processes lack prominent scratch marks. Pruritus, occurring in patients without visible primary lesions, may reflect the presence of various systemic diseases, dry skin (xerosis), or functional disability.

Pruritus causes several problems for the patient. First, the itching often disturbs sleep patterns and during daytime hours may almost literally "drive a patient crazy." In fact, the sensation of itching may be so disturbing that a patient may compulsively scratch until the resultant pain of excoriation supplants the awareness of pruritus. Second, scratching may intensify the itching leading to even more vigorous scratching, thus creating a vicious circle which continually worsens the process which initiated it. This habitlike scratching (the itch-scratch cycle) is one of the most vexing therapeutic problems in dermatologic disease.

Of course, the dermatologic history should not exist in isolation from the rest of one's history taking. In many patients, the observable cutaneous disease may reflect the presence of serious underlying systemic disease. Thus, information regarding time of onset, periods of exacerbation and remission, presence or absence of lesions in family members, and response, or lack thereof, to various therapies may provide clues to the presence and nature of internal illness. An example of this relationship of skin to the rest of the body, specifically to internal malignancy, is presented in Table 6–2, but other processes such as the purpura of coagulation disorders, cutaneous infections as a sign of depressed immune response, and the multifarious skin lesions of diabetes are certainly of equal importance. In many ways, then, it is very true that "the skin is the mirror of the body."

PHYSICAL EXAMINATION

1. Inspection
   a. General
   b. Specific
2. Characterize each abnormality by size, shape, quality, distribution of lesions.
3. Look specifically for skin findings associated with diagnoses suggested by history.

Examination of the skin is carried out through inspection and palpation. Inspection requires both adequate lighting and adequate exposure of the patient's skin. Bright, diffuse, overhead fluorescent light is the best way to achieve adequate lighting. Daylight and incandescent light can be used, but light from these sources is usually insufficiently bright and is too directional.

Proper exposure of the patient's skin for a general clinical examination requires the removal of clothing at least down to the underwear, over which may be worn a hospital examining gown of the type that opens at the rear. I cannot emphasize too strongly that inadequate exposure is almost always the fault of the examiner rather than that of the patient.

TABLE 6–2. Some Cutaneous Manifestations of Internal Malignancy

I. Cutaneous malignancy with frequent internal spread
    A. Melanoma
    B. Squamous cell carcinomas arising from old scars, x-ray–damaged skin, and mucosal surfaces
    C. Mycosis fungoides
    D. Kaposi's hemorrhagic sarcoma
II. Internal malignancy with extension or metastases to skin
    A. Breast carcinoma
    B. Leukemia and lymphoma cutis
    C. Miscellaneous manifestations (occasional metastases to the skin are seen with gastrointestinal, genitourinary, and pulmonary malignancies)
III. Pigmentary changes
    A. Hypermelanosis (especially with melanoma and polypeptide-secreting tumors)
    B. Acanthosis nigricans (especially with gastrointestinal carcinoma)
    C. Sign of Leser-Trélat (rapid appearance of multiple seborrheic keratoses)
    D. Peutz-Jeghers syndrome
    E. Jaundice (primary tumors of biliary tract and pancreas, liver metastases from other tumors)
    F. Purpura (mostly leukemias)
IV. Flushing and facial erythema
    A. Carcinoid
    B. Mastocytomas
    C. Pheochromocytomas
    D. Cushing's disease
V. Specific skin lesions sometimes signaling internal malignancy
    A. Dermatomyositis in adults
    B. Bullous disease in adults (pemphigus and pemphigoid)
    C. Bowen's disease on non–sun-exposed areas
    D. Arsenic keratosis of palms and soles
    E. Paget's disease of nipple or groin
    F. Basal cell nevus syndrome
    G. Urticaria and erythema multiforme of the chronic types
    H. Acquired ichthosis (lymphomas)
    I. Exfoliative erythrodermatitis

First, with the patient sitting on the edge of the examining table, examine the exposed areas, including the scalp, hair, face, mouth, neck, arms, hands, and fingernails (Fig. 6–2). Place a second folded sheet such that it covers the waist. Ask the patient to pull the hospital gown out from under the covering sheet so that the gown is bunched over the breasts or shoulders, allowing examination of the abdomen, lower chest, anterior surface of the lower legs, feet, and toenails (Fig. 6–3). Then ask the patient to stand facing away from you and examine the back, buttocks, and posterior legs (Fig. 6–4). Unfortunately, nonconsecutive viewing of the skin in a piecemeal fashion during the physical examination often leads to incomplete and inadequate information regarding the skin.

Most of us have acquired, on a nonmedical basis, significant knowledge regarding the appearance of normal skin, but this knowledge is probably insufficiently organized to be useful. This section will attempt to put that knowledge into appropriate perspective.

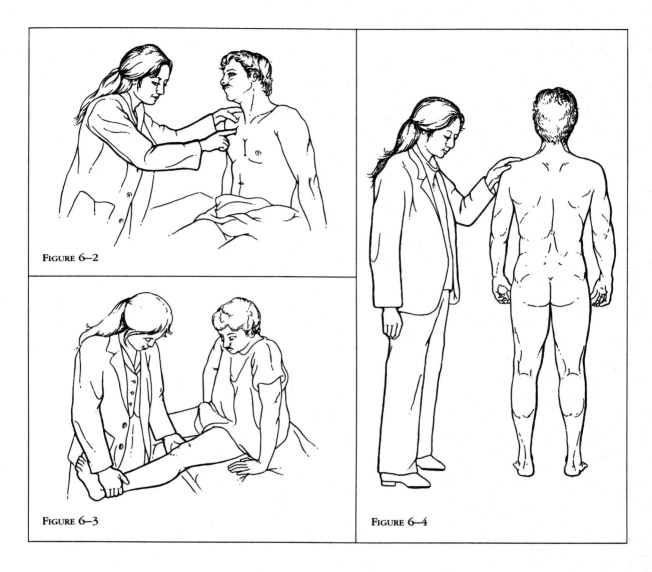

FIGURE 6–2

FIGURE 6–3

FIGURE 6–4

TABLE 6–3. Generalized Cutaneous Color Changes

  I. Brown
     A. Addison's disease
     B. Hemachromatosis (may be gray-brown)
     C. Porphyria cutanea tarda
     D. Scleroderma
     E. Neurofibromatosis (café au lait spots)
     (See also Table 6-2)
 II. Yellow
     A. Jaundice
     B. Anemia (especially pernicious anemia)
     C. Carotenemia (sclerae are not yellow)
     D. Quinacrine (Atabrine) usage
III. Gray or blue-gray
     A. Gold deposition (secondary to intramuscular gold therapy)
     B. Silver deposition (argyria)
     C. Phenothiazine usage (long-term, high-dose therapy)
     D. Minocycline
     E. Amiodarone
 IV. Hypopigmentaion
     A. Albinism
     B. Vitiligo
     C. Pallor of anemia
  V. Purpura
     A. Intravascular defects (e.g., thrombocytopenia, hemophilia)
     B. Vascular wall destruction (various types of vasculitis)
     C. Extravascular defects (steroid purpura, senile purpura, etc.)
 VI. Red and blue hues (these color changes generally depend on vascular flow and are
     too variable to identify specific diseases)

COLOR

The range of color that can be considered normal is great and depends on many variables, such as race, nationality, and degree of sun exposure. Physiologically, skin color is derived from three major sources: (1) erythematous hues that come from oxygenated hemoglobin contained in the cutaneous vasculature, (2) brown hues that come from melanin pigment produced by the melanocytes of the epidermis, and (3) yellow hues that come from the natural color of nonvascularized collagen and from bile and carotene pigments. Cutaneous color changes, whether pathologic or physiologic, are related to changes in the balance of these three hues.

The range of normal skin color is wide, and the simple presence of one color or another is not necessarily significant; but the fact that the presenting color represents a change from what existed before is important. Changes in color may be generalized or localized. Small localized areas of color change are called *macules;* larger areas are called *patches.* The major kinds of color change include the following (Table 6–3):

BROWN

Generalized darkening of melanin pigmentation is an important clue to some types of pituitary, adrenal (Fig. 6–5), liver, and other diseases (Fig. 6–6). Localized in-

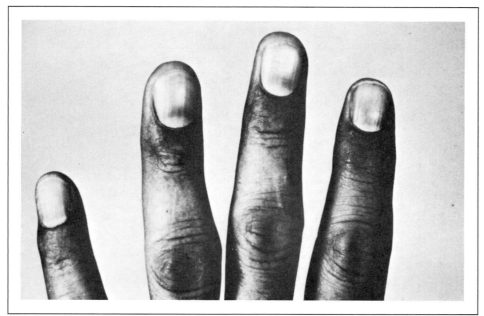

FIGURE 6–5
Hyperpigmentation of the fingers and nails in adrenal insufficiency (Addison's disease). Note accentuation of pigmentation at the knuckle folds.

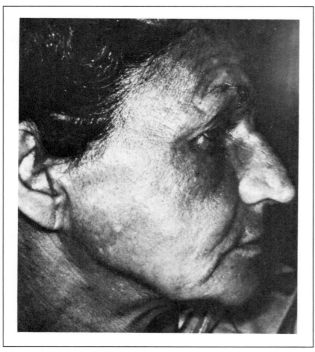

FIGURE 6–6
Hyperpigmentation in porphyria cutanea tarda.

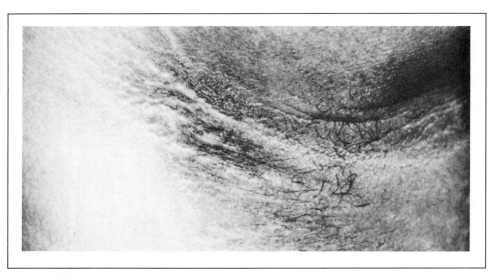

FIGURE 6–7
Acanthosis nigricans of the axilla.

crease in melanin pigmentation may be seen in the brown macules or patches of café-au-lait spots, freckles, lentigines, nevi, and areas of postinflammatory hyperpigmentation. Acanthosis nigricans, a velvety black pigmentation in axillae and groin, is associated with obesity, endocrine disorders, and certain tumors (Fig. 6–7).

WHITE
Absence of melanin gives the skin a white color. Generalized hypopigmentation may be seen in albinism, and localized areas of hypopigmentation may be seen in the macules or patches of vitiligo (Fig. 6–8), scars, postinflammatory hypopigmentation, and a variety of other cutaneous diseases.

YELLOW
Generalized yellowness of the skin due to an increase in cutaneous bile pigment may be seen in liver failure, in which case it is known as jaundice or icterus. More rarely, diffuse yellowness occurs in hypothyroidism and vegetarians as a result of increased carotene pigmentation. Finally, a pale yellow color may be seen in anemia, in which the contribution of the red oxygenated blood decreases, allowing accentuation of the normal yellow color of collagen. This latter phenomenon is particularly prominent in pernicious anemia and in anemia of chronic renal disease.

ERYTHEMA
Increased cutaneous blood flow, most commonly as a component of inflammation, leads to increasing redness of the skin. Thus, generalized erythema may occur with drug eruptions, viral exanthems, and urticaria. Localized inflammation and redness occur nonspecifically in a vast array of cutaneous diseases. Noninflammatory red-

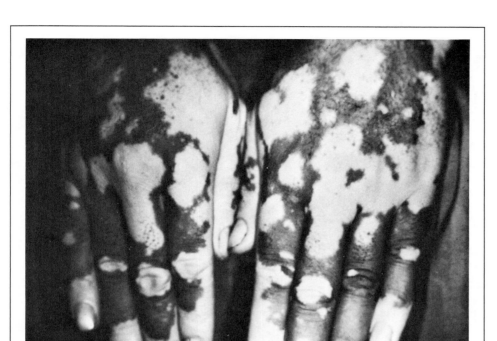

FIGURE 6–8
Vitiligo of the hands.

ness occasionally occurs due to an increased number of intravascular red blood cells (polycythemia). Flushing sometimes occurs with carcinoid tumors, pheochromocytoma and systemic mastocytosis.

OTHER COLORS
Rarely, some medications that are injected or ingested contribute their own color to the skin. Examples include the blue-gray color due to phenothiazines, minocycline, and amiodarone and the yellow color due to quinacrine. Cyanosis, the bluish color of unsaturated hemoglobin, may occur with decreased oxygen, decreased blood flow (Fig. 6–9); and certain drugs (nitrates).

TEXTURE
The characteristic "feel" of skin depends on a number of physiologic processes. These include softness, as provided by the layer of fat cells that abuts the lower portion of the dermis; moisture, as provided by water diffusion through the skin and by sweating onto the surface of the skin; lubrication, as provided by the sebaceous glands; warmth, as provided by the circulation of internally warmed blood; and the presence or absence of roughness, depending on the amount of scale (keratin) produced by the epidermal cells. Balance among these factors depends on the patient's age, sex, and, of course, on the region of the skin being examined.

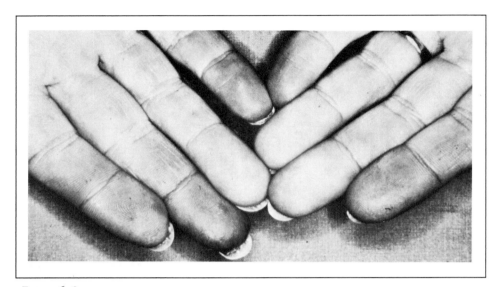

FIGURE 6–9
Cyanosis of the fingers in Raynaud's phenomenon.

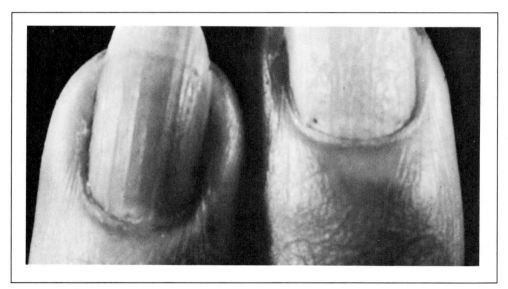

FIGURE 6–10
Pitting of the fingernails in psoriasis.

TABLE 6—4. Nail Changes

   I. Nail pitting
      A. Psoriasis
      B. Alopecia areata
  II. Nail dystrophy
      A. Trauma
      B. Psoriasis
      C. Fungal infections
      D. Arteriosclerotic changes (toenails only)
 III. Curvature without clubbing
      A. Raynaud's phenomenon
      B. Scleroderma
  IV. Clubbing
      A. Chronic pulmonary disease
      B. Pulmonary malignancy
      C. Cardiovascular disease with cyanosis
   V. Onycholysis (Separation of nail plate from the nail bed)
      A. Candidiasis (moniliasis)
      B. Tetracycline (photo-onycholysis)
      C. Hyperthyroidism
      D. Trauma
  VI. White banding (Terry's nails, Mee's lines)
      A. Hypoalbuminemia
      B. Cirrhosis
      C. Renal failure
      D. Chronic arsenic exposure
 VII. Spoon nails (koilonychia)
      A. Iron deficiency anemia
      B. Familia, without associated disease
VIII. Transverse grooving (Beau's lines)
      A. Severe infection
      B. Myocardial infarction
      C. Trauma
  IX. Splinter hemorrhages (present in 20% of healthy individuals)
      A. Subacute bacterial endocarditis
      B. Trichinosis
      C. Collagen vascular disease
      D. Trauma

CHANGE IN TEXTURE

After puberty the scalp and face of most patients will feel oily (a condition known as seborrhea), but there are no pathologic states specifically associated with an increase in sebaceous secretion. On the other hand, decreased lubrication (dryness, chapping, or xerosis) is common after the age of 60 and occasionally occurs in younger people as a result of too-frequent bathing. Rarely, xerosis reflects a deficiency of thyroid or sex hormones. Dryness to the point of ichthyosis may occur in some patients with lymphoma.

As a result of thermal stimuli (such as fever or an overly warm examining room), patients may develop a palpable moistness of the skin associated with generalized sweating. Emotional stimuli, on the other hand, cause sweating on the forehead, palms, soles, axillae, and groin. Rarely, moist skin may be a reflection of the increased metabolic rate that occurs in hyperthyroidism.

Increased warmth of the skin occurs when an increase in cutaneous blood flow delivers body heat to the surface of the skin, where it is then lost by convection, conduction, and radiation. This may occur with fever or following exercise. Localized areas of increased warmth may accompany the increased blood flow seen with cutaneous inflammation. Coolness of the skin reflects decreased blood flow, such as is seen in the lower legs of patients with peripheral arteriovascular disease.

Finally, the skin may lose its elasticity, or feel tough, when it is distended by edematous fluid, when the cutaneous fat is replaced by collagen (as in scleroderma), or when normal collagen is replaced by scar tissue.

MUCOUS MEMBRANES

Mucous membranes are characteristically pink in color and moist to palpation. Mottled brown or black melanin pigmentation may be present on the oral mucous membranes of black patients. Increased oral pigmentation may occur in adrenocortical insufficiency disease.

HAIR

Normal hair distribution is well appreciated by most examiners and need not be considered here. However, it should be remembered that facial, axillary, and pubic hair depend on the presence of sex and other hormones and thus is related to both the sex and the age of the patient. Scalp hair should be specifically examined for length, texture, fragility, sheen, and the ease with which hairs can be manually removed from their follicles. Scalp hair normally grows about 0.3 mm per day or, in more practical terms, about 0.5 inch per month. Some causes of hair loss can be seen in Figures 6–11 through 6–12 and in Table 6–5.

SPECIFIC CUTANEOUS LESIONS

Thus far we have talked primarily about functional changes that occur in the normal components of the skin. In this section we will discuss structural changes, that is, the development of lesions that, strictly speaking, always represent cutaneous pathology. In some instances the pathology has little significance (e.g., nevi and senile angiomas), but the experienced examiner should consider the presence of any of these structural changes as potentially important until he or she has become familiar with those that can safely be ignored. The patient, because of the ready visibility of skin lesions, may be concerned about cutaneous changes out of proportion to their actual importance. These concerns should, of course, be addressed. The most common structural changes are shown in Figure 6–14 and are discussed below.

NONPALPABLE LESIONS

These circumscribed flat changes in skin color are called macules (if less than about 1 cm in diameter) and *patches* (if larger). Freckles, for example, are macules, and large areas of hypopigmentation may be referred to as vitiliginous patches.

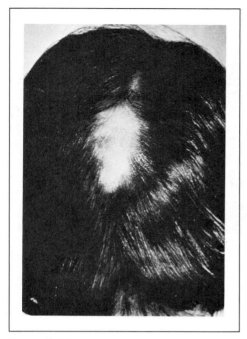

Figure 6–11
Alopecia areata. The area of hair loss is sharply marginated, and the exposed scalp appears normal.

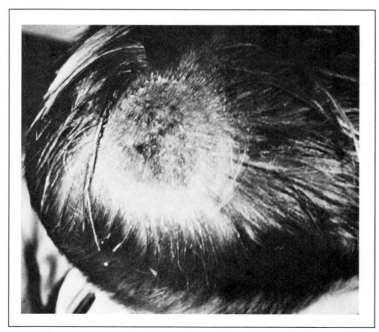

Figure 6–12
Tinea capitis. A fungal infection of the scalp.

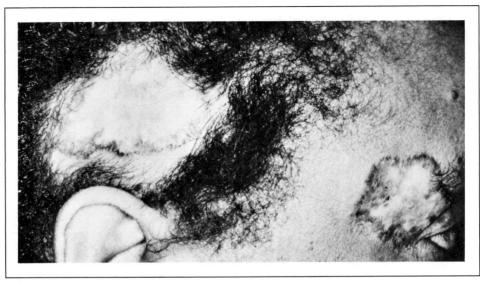

Figure 6–13
Discoid lupus erythematosus. Typical scarring plaques are found on the scalp.

Table 6–5. Some Causes of Hair Loss

I. Generalized alopecia
   A. No underlying scalp disease
      1. Telogen effluvium (especially postpartum and after severe illness)
      2. Alopecia totalis
      3. Some cases of male and female pattern alopecia
      4. Thyroid disease
      5. Drug induced (mostly birth control pills and cancer chemotherapeutic agents)
      6. Congenital hair defects
   B. With underlying scalp disease
      1. Seborrheic dermatitis (hair loss is mild)
      2. Contact dermatitis (permanents, bleaches, and dyes)
II. Localized or patterned alopecia
   A. No scalp disease
      1. Alopecia areata
      2. Male and female pattern alopecia
      3. Trichotillomania
      4. Secondary syphilis
      5. Traction alopecia
   B. With scalp disease
      1. Tinea capitis
      2. Lupus erythematosus (discoid type)
      3. Psoriasis (hair loss is mild)

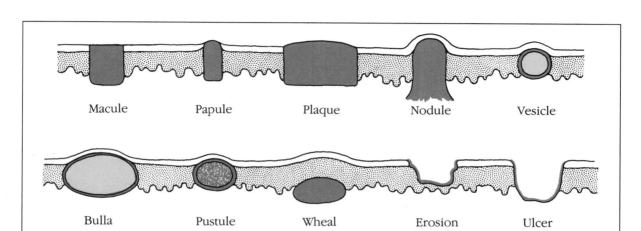

FIGURE 6–14
Most common structural changes in the skin.

PALPABLE LESIONS

These are localized lesions that have substance or mass, are always palpable, and are usually elevated above the surface of the skin. Small palpable lesions are called *papules,* and large papules are called *nodules.* A confluence or centrifugal enlargement of papules or nodules, resulting in a large flat-topped lesion, is called a *plaque.* The palpable substance of papules, nodules, and plaques occurs as a result of one or both of the following processes: (1) proliferation of the various cells normally found in the skin (e.g., nevus cells, fibroblasts) inflammatory cells, metastatic tumor cells, and leukemic cells; or (2) the accumulation of fluid within the skin. Fluid accumulating within the skin may be present in a diffuse fashion (e.g., a hive or wheal) or in a loculated fashion (as in a blister). Small blisters are known as *vesicles,* and large blisters are known as *bullae.* Vesicles or bullae that contain many polymorphonuclear leukocytes appear cloudy or white and are called *pustules.*

Extravasation of red cells into the skin (purpura) may present with red or reddish purple punctate lesions 1 to 5 mm in size *(petechiae)* or larger confluent bruises *(ecchymoses).*

EROSIONS AND ULCERS

Superficial loss of skin is called an erosion, whereas deep loss is termed an ulcer. In both situations the barrier function of the skin is lost, and serum, together with inflammatory cells, exudes to the surface as "weeping" or "oozing." When this exudate dries, it forms crusts. It is important to distinguish between the light gray flakes of scale and the yellow-brown friable granules of crusts, inasmuch as the former represents epithelial proliferation and the latter represents epithelial loss.

Erosions and ulcers arise in three major ways: (1) as a result of external trauma, most commonly scratching; (2) from the unroofing of vesicular or bullous lesions; or (3) from the necrotic effect of vascular ischemia. Ability to determine which of

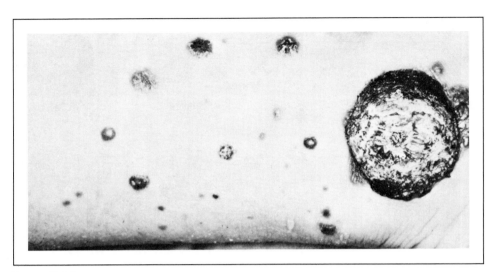

FIGURE 6–15
Malignant melanoma with satellite cutaneous metastases.

these three mechanisms is responsible for an ulcer greatly simplifies the preparation of a differential diagnosis.

Some characteristic lesions of the skin are illustrated in Figures 6–15 through 6–20. In addition to describing the lesions by color, type, size, and distribution, the student (and those who read the workup) will find value in drawing the lesions, as illustrated in Figure 6–21.

Once examiners have learned to recognize the kind of pathologic conditions described above and can use appropriate terms in their written or verbal descriptions, they are ready to formulate differential diagnoses. To assist the student in this task, many dermatology textbooks are arranged or organized according to the different patterns of cutaneous pathology; the student then may go directly from his own descriptions of the lesions to the appropriate textbook chapter.

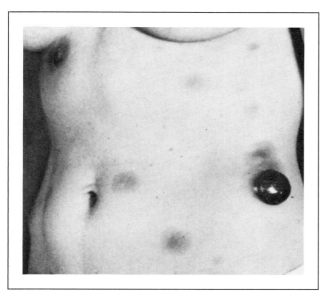

FIGURE 6—16
Lymphoma cutis. Each of the large nodules represents a cutaneous aggregation of atypical lymphocytes.

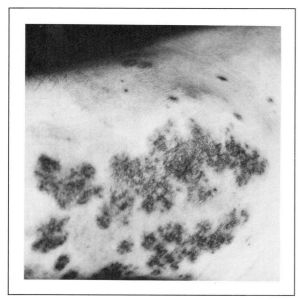

FIGURE 6—17
Purpura of the foot in vasculitis.

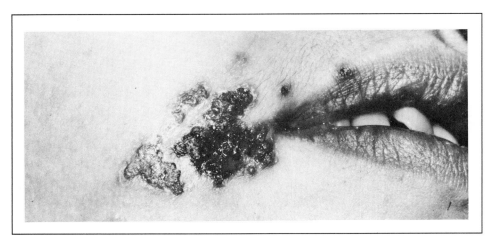

FIGURE 6–18
Impetigo. A crusted weeping, infectious lesion common in children.

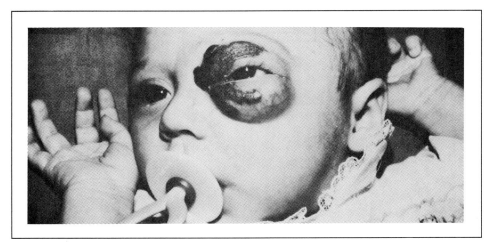

FIGURE 6–19
Hemangioma of the eye.

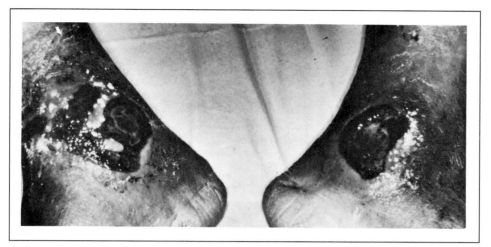

FIGURE 6–20
Bilateral stasis ulcers with surrounding dermatitis.

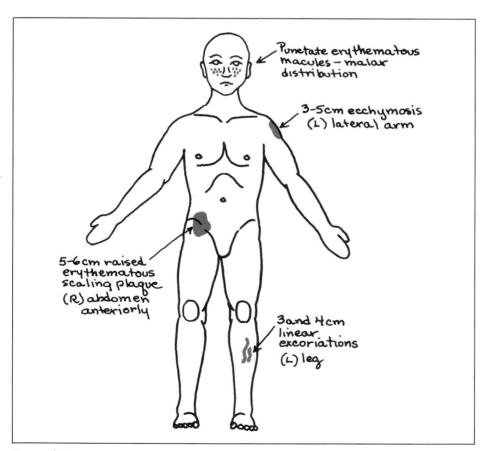

Punetate erythematous macules – malar distribution

3-5cm ecchymosis (L) lateral arm

5-6cm raised erythematous scaling plaque (R) abdomen anteriorly

3 and 4cm linear excoriations (L) leg

FIGURE 6–21

CHAPTER 7

HEMATOPOIETIC SYSTEM

She was very anaemic. Her thin lips were pale, and her skin was delicate, of a faint green colour, without a touch of red even in the cheeks.

W. SOMERSET MAUGHAM
(1874–1965)

The major components of the lymphohematopoietic system—lymph nodes, bone marrow, and the circulating blood—can be considered together because the cellular components of these tissues all arise from a common pluripotential stem cell. Our understanding of the basic cell and molecular biology of many hematologic disorders has changed dramatically in recent years. Despite these rapid changes in our knowledge of pathophysiology, the clinical manifestations of hematologic disease have remained constant. Detecting these clinical signs requires a broad familiarity with the disorders of the lymphohematopoietic system and the painstaking application of a few simple skills. The clinical information thus gained can then direct the physician to more specialized laboratory tests or to a specific diagnosis.

ANATOMY

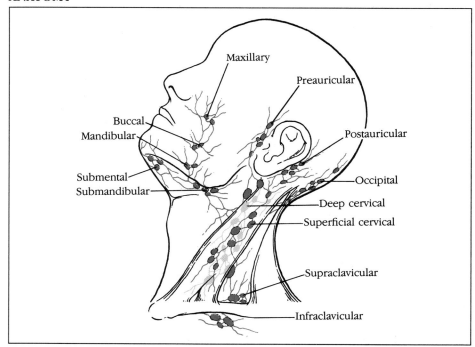

FIGURE 7–1
Cervicofacial and supraclavicular lymph nodes.

101

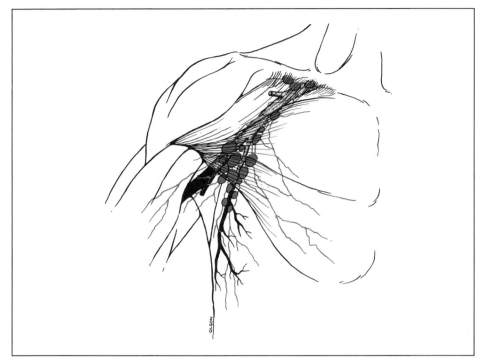

FIGURE 7–2
Axillary lymph nodes.

HISTORY

Symptoms arising from lymphohematopoietic disease may originate from a decrease in the formed elements of blood (anemia, thrombocytopenia, leukocytopenia), an increase in these cells (erythrocytosis, thrombocytosis, leukocytosis), or an enlargement of the lymph nodes (lymphadenopathy). Oxygen delivery to tissues is directly related to the hemoglobin concentration of the circulating blood. Decreased hemoglobin concentration such as that found in anemia of any cause therefore results in symptoms of deficient tissue oxygenation: easy fatiguability, muscular weakness, lassitude, and shortness of breath. The severity of these symptoms strongly depends on the rapidity with which the anemia develops: acute blood loss generally causes more severe symptoms, for example, than does pernicious anemia of equivalent degree. Thrombocytopenia does not cause symptoms in itself, unless bleeding supervenes. In such cases patients may complain of easy bruising or bleeding, epistaxis, excessive gum bleeding after brushing the teeth, or petechiae, especially over the lower extremities and around areas of constriction from tight-fitting clothes. Leukocytopenia also does not cause symptoms in itself but granulocytopenia predisposes the patient to infection, primarily from bacteria. This will cause symptoms depending on the site of infection. Common sites in granulocytopenic patients are the lung, skin, and oropharyngeal and perirectal areas.

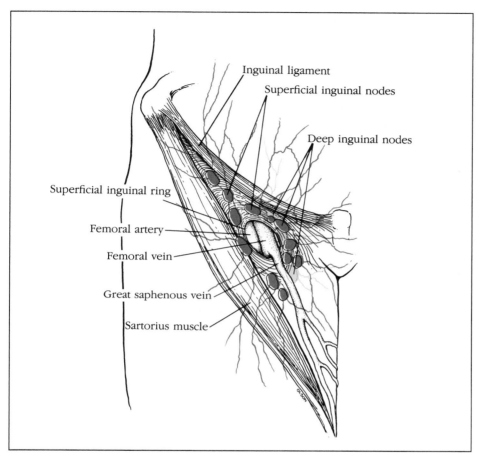

Figure 7–3
Inguinal and femoral lymph nodes.

Excessive red cell concentration in the peripheral blood (erythrocytosis) results in symptoms related to increased blood viscosity such as dyspnea, headache, mental clouding, and fatigue. In addition, pruritus may be prominent. Thrombocytosis does not cause symptoms unless platelet counts are high enough to result in pathologic thrombosis, in which case symptoms will be related to the site involved. Leukocytosis does not cause symptoms in and of itself unless it is related to a leukemic process. In such cases, if the peripheral white cells are mainly immature, microcirculatory "sludging" may occur, giving rise to symptoms such as dyspnea, mental status abnormalities, and visual changes.

Lymphomas and leukemias generally cause symptoms related to abnormal numbers of red cells, platelets, and white cells. In addition, enlargement of lymph nodes

nodes may cause pain, depending on the rapidity with which it develops, and obstruction to lymph flow may cause swelling distal to the obstruction, producing a complaint of foot swelling, for example. Lymphadenopathy in certain critical locations may cause characteristic constellations of symptoms. Mediastinal and hilar adenopathy may cause compression of a major bronchus or trachea, with resulting dyspnea, cough, or cyanosis. Obstruction to lymphatic and venous drainage of the head due to adenopathy within the superior mediastinum may cause swelling of the face, a sensation of head fullness, visual blurring, and mental status changes (superior vena cava syndrome). Retroperitoneal adenopathy may cause lower extremity swelling secondary to poor lymphatic drainage (lymphedema).

Constitutional symptoms associated with neoplastic disorders of the lymphatic tissue include fever, night sweats, and weight loss. These symptoms may be related to release from lymphoid cells of tumor necrosis factor, a hormone recently shown to function as an endogenous pyrogen that inhibits normal fatty acid metabolism, promoting weight loss. Some hematologic disorders, such as multiple myeloma, cause major abnormalities in serum protein concentration, resulting in symptoms of hyperviscosity and other symptoms related to deficient antibody-mediated immunity (susceptibility to infections, especially bacterial). Others, such as acquired immunodeficiency syndrome (AIDS) cause major disturbances in cell-mediated immunity and susceptibility to fungal, viral, and psoriatic infections because of deficient function of the T4 helper T cell, which is central to normal immunoregulation.

Disorders of coagulation, such as the hemophilias, mainly cause symptoms of excessive bleeding, often delayed in onset, after minimal or no trauma. Such bleeding is often deep (such as in joints or in the thoracic or abdominal cavity) and results from deficiency or deficient function of one or more coagulation proteins in plasma. Coagulation disorders can also result from a deficiency or the deficient function of platelets, in which case the bleeding manifestations are more commonly superficial, such as in mucous membranes and skin.

LYMPH NODES

Lymph nodes are distributed throughout the body but for most purposes can be divided into five major groups: cervicofacial-supraclavicular, axillary, epitrochlear, inguinal, and femoral (see Fig. 7–1 to 7–3). Other lymph node groups that occasionally become pathologically enlarged are the suboccipital, postauricular, suprasternal, and popliteal. Evaluation of the numerous lymph nodes of the mediastinum, abdomen, pelvis, and lower extremities must be done by computed tomography (CT) or lymphangiography.

Lymph nodes are examined by palpation. In general the tips of the first four fingers are used, and five major qualities of the nodes are noted: location, size in centimeters (using a ruler), degree of tenderness, fixation to underlying tissue, and texture (hard, soft, etc.).

Normal lymph nodes are not palpable. However mild enlargement (< 1 cm) of the inguinal nodes is quite common, and probably results from repeated superfi-

PHYSICAL EXAMINATION

1. Palpate head and neck nodes.
2. Palpate epitrochlear and axillary nodes.
3. Palpate inguinal nodes.
   a. When looking specifically for lymphadenopathy, these examinations for regional nodes are done one directly after another. Otherwise, lymph node examination is often done as part of the regional examination of the head and neck, breast, abdomen, and extremities.
   b. Examination of the spleen is usually done as part of the abdominal examination (see Chap. 14).

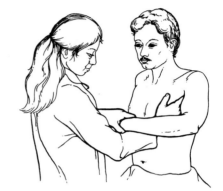

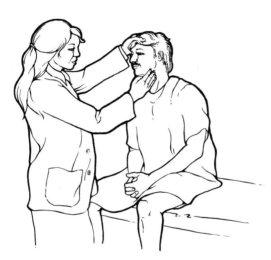

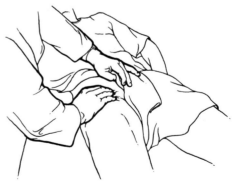

TABLE 7–1. Clinical Lymphadenopathy

Lymph Node	Region Drained	Causes of Enlargement
Submental	Lips, mouth, tongue	Oral infections, tumor
Submandibular	Face	Facial, oral infections, tumor
Preauricular	Ears, temporal scalp	Infection
Postauricular	Scalp	Scalp infections, injury
Occipital	Scalp	Viral, local infections
Superficial cervical	Ears, parotid	Infection, tumor
Deep cervical	Tongue, larynx, thyroid, trachea, esophagus	Infection, tumor
Supraclavicular	Neck, axillae, GI tract (left)	Infection, tumor
Inguinal	Lower extremities, pelvis	Infection, tumor
Axillary	Chest, upper extremities	Infection, tumor

cial infections of the feet and legs. These nodes are soft, nontender, and movable, with normal overlying skin. Femoral node enlargement, in contrast, is more likely to be of clinical significance. Similar small, soft, movable nodes are also found in children in the cervicofacial and axillary areas as a result of exposure to upper respiratory pathogens and superficial infections of the upper extremities.

Lymphadenopathy may be either localized or generalized. The former is generally associated with a local infectious process in the anatomic area drained by the nodes in question, or neoplasm (Table 7–1). Texture, size, tenderness, and fixation can all weigh in favor of one or the other of these possibilities; hard nodes favor neoplasms, as do greatly enlarged (> 3 cm), nontender, and fixed nodes. Small, soft, tender, red, and movable nodes are more often a result of inflammation or some other type of antigenic challenge. Location is also of importance; isolated occipital, postauricular, or epitrochlear lymphadenopathy is unusual in primary lymphoma and more commonly results from localized inflammation. Posterior or anterior cervical, supraclavicular, mediastinal, or intraabdominal adenopathy is more commonly associated with neoplasia.

CERVICOFACIAL AND SUPRACLAVICULAR

The patient should be seated comfortably with the examiner standing in front. The postauricular and preauricular nodes are palpated first, followed by the submental, which lie in the midline between the digastric muscles, and the submaxillary, which lie beneath the angle of the mandible close to the submaxillary gland (with which they can be confused). Often these node groups can be better appreciated bimanually by placing a gloved finger in the floor of the mouth. Next the jugular chain nodes are examined. For this it is usually preferable for the examiner to stand behind or to the side of the patient, with the patient's neck slightly flexed to relax the sternocleidomastoid (Fig. 7–4). The nodes are palpated by placing the thumb and index finger posterior and anterior to the superior aspect of the sternocleidomastoid muscle and proceeding gradually downward using a circular motion of the fingers. The carotid body lies near the bifurcation of the common carotid artery deep to the jugular chain of lymph nodes. Care must be taken in

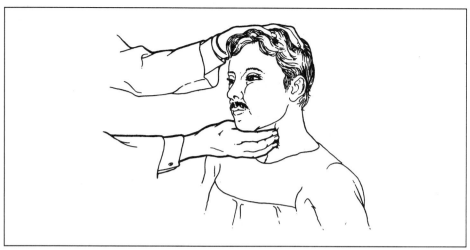

FIGURE 7–4
Palpation of anterior cervical nodes.

palpating this structure, which may be confused with a lymph node. Simultaneous bilateral palpation of the carotid body should be avoided, because reflex bradycardia and hypotension, with resultant syncope, may result. Following examination of the jugular chain nodes, the supraclavicular fossae are examined, and finally the suprasternal notch, which may contain a palpable pretracheal node. The Valsalva maneuver can often make nodes in these areas more easily palpable.

AXILLARY AND EPITROCHLEAR
The patient should be seated comfortably with the examiner in front. The patient must be relaxed. The patient's left arm should be supported by the examiner's left hand, while the examiner probes high into the axilla with the right hand. The reverse process is done on the patient's right side (Fig. 7–5).

Next the epitrochlear nodes are palpated. This is done by holding the patient's elbow slightly flexed with one hand while gently palpating slightly proximal to the lateral and medial epicondyles (Fig. 7–6).

INGUINAL AND FEMORAL
Lymph nodes in this region are found in relation to the external iliac and femoral veins in the inguinal areas, above and below the inguinal ligament. They are palpated using the tips of the fingers in a rotary motion. The inguinal area often contains palpable lymph nodes because of the frequency of superficial infections of the toes and feet in the general population and, in such cases, the mildly enlarged nodes (< 1 cm) are of little significance.

Generalized lymphadenopathy is usually due to a generalized inflammatory process or neoplasm. Systemic viral (infectious mononucleosis or rubella), fungal (histoplasmosis, coccidioidomycosis), parasitic (malaria, schistosomiasis), or protozoal

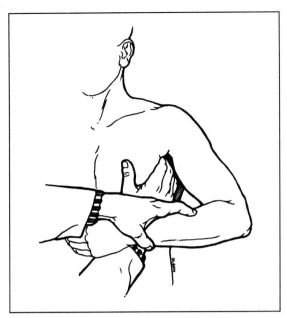

Figure 7–5
Palpation of axillary nodes.

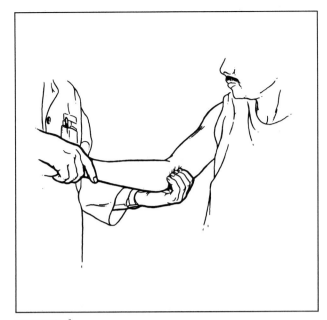

Figure 7–6
Palpation of epitrochlear nodes.

(toxoplasmosis, amebiasis) infections may cause systemic adenopathy as part of the normal immune activation in response to infection (Table 7–2). Again, such nodes are usually soft, small, movable. Generalized lymphadenopathy may also be a manifestation of lymphoma or leukemia. In such cases the nodes are larger, nontender, often not easily movable, and matted together. Chronic leukemia tends to produce more striking lymphadenopathy than the acute leukemias, and lymphocytic types produce more than myelocytic types.

SPLEEN

Splenomegaly may signal disease of the hematopoietic system. Since the spleen is usually considered a part of the examination of the abdomen, the technique of that examination and the significance of abnormalities are treated in Chapter 14.

SKIN

Hematologic disorders can cause a variety of cutaneous abnormalities. Pallor is often seen in anemia, though it is an unreliable measure of severity when the anemia is mild. Pale nail beds and conjunctivae are also seen in anemias. Rubor, the opposite of pallor, is seen in polycythemia vera. This is particularly apparent in the face and may be accompanied by suffusion of the conjunctivae (bloodshot eyes). Petechiae are punctate cutaneous or mucosal hemorrhages (< 0.5 mm diameter), which result most often from thrombocytopenia or dysfunctional platelets. They characteristically are nonblanching and tend to occur in dependent areas or

TABLE 7–2. Some Causes of Generalized Lymphadenopathy

Lymphatic leukemia
Lymphoreticular malignancy
Secondary syphilis
Measles
Juvenile rheumatoid arthritis
Infectious mononucleosis
Plague
Tuberculosis
Sarcoidosis
Toxoplasmosis
Scabies
Acquired immunodeficiency syndrome (AIDS)
Amyloidosis
Serum sickness

areas associated with tight-fitting clothes. Ecchymoses are larger cutaneous hemorrhages (> 0.5 mm) that are violaceous, flat, and irregular (synonymous with the common "bruise").

MUCOSA

Atrophy of the lingual mucosa and papillae may occur in iron-, folate-, or B_{12}-deficiency anemias, making the tongue appear smooth rather than normally papillated. In pernicious anemia, the tongue classically appears smooth and beefy red (Fig. 7–7). Angular stomatitis, or fissuring at the corners of the mouth, may be seen in the deficiency anemias. Gingival swelling and violaceous discoloration is often seen in monocytic leukemia (Fig. 7–8).

BONE

Localized bone tenderness to palpation, particularly in the sternum, is seen in the hematopoietic disorders characterized by uncontrolled proliferation of blood cell progenitors in the marrow. Such tenderness is commonly believed to result from increased intramedullary pressure due to cellular proliferation.

OPTIC FUNDI

Examination of the fundi is often useful, especially in hyperviscosity syndromes and disorders of hemostasis. In the former, a distinctive "sausage-link" appearance of the retinal veins, consisting of alternate bulges and constrictions, may be seen, as well as retinal vein tortuosity. In disorders of hemostasis, retinal hemorrhages may be seen, most commonly associated with thrombocytopenia.

SPECIAL TECHNIQUES

The examination of a well-stained *peripheral blood smear* is an integral part of the evaluation of the hematopoietic system. It is the safest, least expensive, and most

TABLE 7–3. Some Causes of Anemia

I. Decreased production
  A. Marrow suppression
    1. Toxins
    2. Chronic infections
    3. Uremia
    4. Hepatic disease
  B. Marrow destruction
    1. Fibrosis
    2. Toxins
    3. Infiltration (neoplasm, infection)
  C. Deficiency states
    1. Folic acid
    2. Vitamin B_{12}
    3. Vitamin B_6
    4. Iron
    5. Copper
    6. Zinc
    7. Phosphorus
  D. Defective hemoglobin synthesis
    1. Thalassemia
    2. Sickle cell
    3. Other hemoglobinopathies
II. Hemolysis
  A. Red cell defects
    1. Hemoglobin (e.g., sickle cell anemia, vitamin B_{12} deficiency)
    2. Membrane (e.g., spherocytosis)
    3. Energy systems (e.g., glucose 6-phosphate dehydrogenase deficiency, phosphorus deficiency)
  B. Red cell toxins
    1. Bacterial hemolysins (e.g., clostridial toxin)
    2. Antigen-antibody complexes (e.g., drug hemolysis)
    3. Erythrophagocytosis (certain tumors)
  C. Red cell parasitism
    1. Malaria
    2. *Borrelia*
    3. Babesiosis
III. Increased loss
  A. Gastrointestinal bleeding
  B. Uterine blood loss
  C. Pregnancy
  D. Hematuria
  E. Epistaxis
  F. Hemoptysis
  G. Trauma

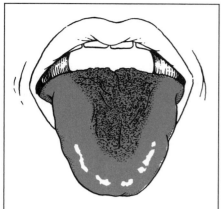
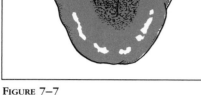

FIGURE 7–7
Tongue in pernicious anemia.

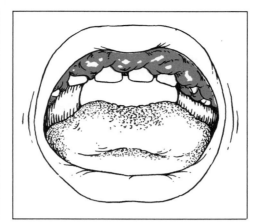

FIGURE 7–8
Gums in leukemia.

easily obtained biopsy available to the clinician. Many disorders of leukopoiesis, erythropoiesis, and thrombopoiesis can be diagnosed directly from the smear, and in many other cases the smear may point to other more conclusive laboratory studies.

BONE MARROW ASPIRATION
This is also a relatively easily obtained specimen, which is of great value in the diagnosis of many hematopoietic disorders, especially leukemias, thrombocytopenic states, certain anemias, and myeloproliferative and myelodysplastic disorders.

LYMPH NODE BIOPSY
This is an absolute requirement in the definitive diagnosis of most neoplastic disorders of the lymphoid system. Standard hematoxylin and eosin staining gives crucial information regarding the overall architecture of the node, as well as some information regarding the type of lymphoid cell involved in the neoplastic process. Special immunologic techniques such as immunoperoxidase staining can often give important information regarding monoclonality of the cells, which can help distinguish benign from malignant processes and B cell origin from T cell origin.

X-RAY FILMS
Routine posterior-anterior and lateral views of the chest can provide important information regarding mediastinal adenopathy. Plain abdominal films are much less helpful in evaluating abdominal adenopathy. Lymphangiography, in which radiopaque dye is injected into the lymphatic vessels of the feet and used to opacify the lymph nodes of the iliac and retroperitoneal areas, is far superior. Node size and contour, and even abnormal architecture within the node, can then be assessed. CT scans are also invaluable in assessing intrathoracic and intraabdominal

adenopathy. With this technique, upper abdominal nodes can be better visualized than they can with lymphangiography.

FLOW CYTOMETRY

In this technique, cells can be separated quickly according to DNA content or cell-surface antigenic characteristics. It is often used to identify the cell lineage (granulocytic versus lymphocytic, B cell versus T cell lymphocytic) or degree of maturation of neoplastic lymphohematopoietic cells.

SECTION III

HEAD AND NECK

8. EYE
   Terry J. Bergstrom
9. HEAD
   Gilbert S. Small
   William W. Montgomery
10. NECK
    Faith T. Fitzgerald
    John C. Floyd, Jr.

If nature had only one fixed standard for the proportions of the various parts, then the faces of all men would resemble each other to such a degree that it would be impossible to distinguish one from another; but she has varied the five parts of the face in such a way that although she has made an almost universal standard as to their size, she has not observed it in the various conditions to such a degree as to prevent one from being clearly distinguished from another.

LEONARDO DA VINCI

(1452–1519)

1. Examine regional lymph nodes and skin.
2. Inspect the head.
3. Examine the eye.
   a. Visual acuity
   b. External eye
   c. Pupils
   d. Extraocular movements
   e. Visual fields
   f. Fundi

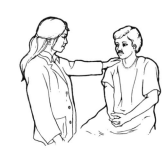

4. Examine the ear.
   a. External ear
   b. Auditory acuity
   c. Middle ear
   d. Sinuses
5. Examine the nose.
6. Examine the mouth and throat.
7. Observe the neck and check range of motion.

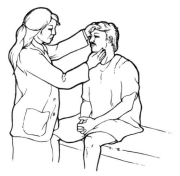

8. Palpate (cervical nodes)
   a. Trachea
   b. Thyroid
   c. Carotids
9. Auscultate the neck.
   a. Thyroid
   b. Carotids

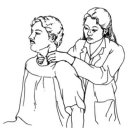

CHAPTER 8

EYE

O loss of sight, of thee I most complain!
JOHN MILTON
(1608–1674)

The eye is a transparent, superficial organ readily accessible to direct examination. The evaluation of the visual system not only reveals ocular abnormalities but also provides clues to a variety of local and systemic disorders. The eyes may reflect central nervous system, metabolic, vascular, and infectious diseases.

Because the importance of vision to the patient should always be considered, this portion of the physical examination must be accomplished with great care and tact.

ANATOMY

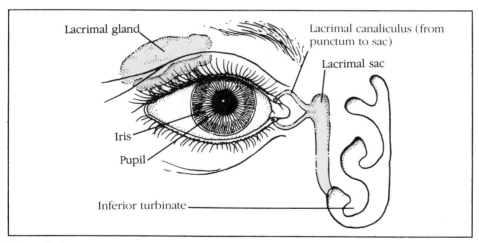

FIGURE 8–1
External eye and lacrimal apparatus.

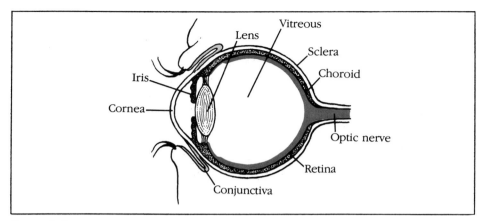

FIGURE 8–2
Cross-section of the eye.

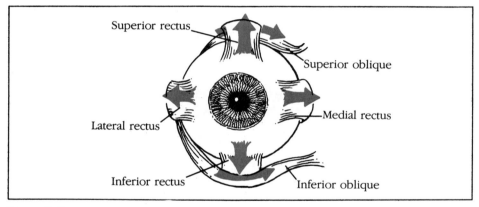

FIGURE 8–3
Extraocular muscles (right eye).

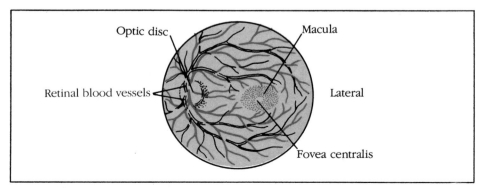

FIGURE 8–4
Ocular fundus (left eye).

HISTORY

The historical review of systems concerning symptoms of the eyes may be done as you do the physical examination. In addition to the symptoms listed below, be sure to record when the patient last had his eyeglasses changed (some people buy their eyeglasses off the counter in a discount store) and when he or she last had a glaucoma check.

PAIN

The complaint of pain in or about the eyes must be evaluated as to location, duration, type, and mode of onset. It may be related to a specific incident, as in the case of an injury to the eye. Pain in the eyes and forehead may be the result of uncorrected refractive error or ocular muscle imbalance, in which case it will often follow use of the eyes. Almost all patients with headache will ask whether the eyes are involved, but eye diseases are among the least common causes of headaches; on the contrary, a typical unilateral migraine headache, which will often include ocular pain on that side, is unrelated to eye pathology.

Very severe localized pain in one eye usually suggests surface ocular disease, such as a foreign body or corneal abrasion. A dull throbbing pain is more typical of iritis or of acute glaucoma and may be worse when the patient is lying down. Deep pain in the orbit may not be associated with local signs but may indicate neighboring disease, such as sinus disease or intracranial sensory nerve involvement. Irritation of the meninges or increased intracranial pressure may produce orbital pain.

VISUAL LOSS

This may range from blurring of vision to complete blindness in one or both eyes. The earliest signs of double vision may be recognized by the patient only as a visual blur related to the overlapping images. A reduction in visual acuity can reflect systemic disease, such as early diabetes, where a shift to myopia may occur. The early symptoms of senile cataract may include visual blurring, especially for distance, and the ability to read without glasses ("second sight" due to myopia).

Sudden loss of vision usually signals retinal or optic nerve disease and may be related either to inflammation or to vascular embarrassment. Transient visual loss (amaurosis fugax) may signal occlusion (by atherosclerosis or emboli) or spasm of the great vessels of the neck or vessels in the eye itself. Central visual loss must be distinguished from that of the peripheral vision; the patient is usually much more aware of loss of central reading acuity than of a peripheral narrowing of the visual field.

Reduced vision is a significant finding and suggests either local or general disease, especially when the loss has been sudden or when relatively recent glasses no longer aid. A reason must be sought for any instance of reduced vision. Causes can range from local ocular pathology (e.g., cataracts, retinal detachment, and vitreous or retinal hemorrhage) through optic nerve involvement as a part of neurologic disease. Sudden changes may suggest circulatory insufficiencies of various types, such as cerebral hemorrhage, major carotid occlusions, and the like. Poor vision in one eye may be noted in many patients who had a strabismus in childhood, with resulting suppression of central vision (amblyopia). Visual field defects of intracranial disease may be associated with complaints of visual loss, but the central acuity often may be normal and visual field examination then becomes necessary.

Any case of reduced vision, either unilateral or bilateral, demands an explanation.

DOUBLE VISION

Visual confusion is characteristic of the patient with double vision (diplopia). He will often close or cover one eye for relief. In certain cases of incomplete paralysis of an eye muscle, he may assume an unusual head position in order to maintain single vision; for example, head turning to the left, with the eyes directed to the right, in the case of a partial paralysis of the left lateral rectus muscle. Diplopia usually signifies either muscular or neurologic disease. A lack of parallelism of the eyes may not be associated with double vision when it is the result of a "lazy" or amblyopic eye dating from a muscle imbalance in childhood. Monocular diplopia usually indicates either corneal or lens changes.

PHOTOPHOBIA

Sensitivity to light varies considerably among normal individuals, but where it is significant there is usually disease of the cornea or of the anterior segment of the globe. In acute cases, a corneal foreign body, corneal ulcer, or iritis may be suspected, although old corneal scarring and vascularization may also produce a hypersensitivity to light.

HALOS

Distortions around point sources of light described as halos or rainbow-like fringes are visual symptoms of corneal edema, often caused by an abrupt rise in intraocular pressure, as in acute glaucoma. Other, less serious causes of light distortion, such as spokes around lights, may be caused by tearing problems or cataracts.

BURNING, ITCHING

Many relatively minor ocular abnormalities manifest themselves by burning, itching, or uncomfortable eyes. Irritations from tear insufficiency or mild conjunctivitis are common causes. Itching sensations of the eye should arouse suspicions of an allergic cause, particularly seasonal allergies or reactions to eye make-up or eye drops.

"FLOATERS"

Patients, particularly older ones, may notice small specks or lines of various shapes that pass across the visual field, lagging slightly behind ocular movements. They are more commonly observed when looking at a clear blue sky, a blank page of a book, or a blank well-illuminated wall. They are usually images of small vitreous opacities and disappear when the eyes are closed. The sudden appearance of a large floater or multiple floaters may indicate a serious problem such as a retinal hole or detachment, vitreous detachment, or vitreous hemorrhage.

DISCHARGE

Material emerging from the eye as either watery or more viscid discharge usually suggests either conjunctival disease or difficulty in the lacrimal drainage system. In acute infections it may be more purulent and may collect on the lid borders. Where the lacrimal drainage system is occluded, tearing may be continuous, and mucus may collect in the tear sac so that pressure over this structure causes regurgitation of material into the eye. In allergic conjunctival disease the consistency of the discharge is stringy and tenacious. Increased tearing may also be a part of the light-sensitivity response of a diseased eye.

REDNESS

Vascular congestion, or redness of the eyes, must be evaluated in terms of other findings and may represent infective or allergic conjunctivitis, inflammation of the iris, or acute glaucoma. The latter must be kept in mind as a diagnostic possibility in all cases of redness of the eye if precipitous blindness is to be prevented. In certain florid individuals, redness of the eye may not be significant unless other findings support the diagnosis of disease (Table 8–1).

TABLE 8-1. Differential Diagnosis of "Red-Eye"

	Conjunctiva	Iris	Pupil	Cornea	Anterior Chamber	Intraocular Pressure	Appearance
Acute glaucoma	Both ciliary and conjunctival vessels injected. Entire eye is red	Injected	Dilated, fixed, oval	Steamy, hazy	Very shallow	Very high	
Iritis	Redness most marked around cornea. Color does not blanch on pressure	Injected	Small, fixed	Normal	Turgid	Normal	
Conjunctivitis	Conjunctival vessels injected, greatest toward fornices. Blanch on pressure. Mobile over sclera	Normal	Normal	Normal	Normal	Normal	
Subconjunctival hemorrhage	Bright red sclera with white rim around limbus	Normal	Normal	Normal	Normal	Normal	

"EYE STRAIN"

This commonly used term is not sound from a medical standpoint and should not be used to denote the symptom of fatigue. "Strain" connotes damage, but eye use in itself never produces irreversible change. If there is discomfort with use of the eyes (asthenopia), a search should be made for ocular problems, such as refractive error or ocular muscular imbalance.

PHYSICAL EXAMINATION

1. Check visual acuity with and without glasses.
2. Inspect.
   a. Lids
   b. Lacrimal system
   c. Conjunctivae
   d. Sclerae
   e. Corneas
3. Test extraocular movements.
4. Test pupillary responses.
5. Check visual fields by confrontation.
6. Perform funduscopy.
7. Check intraocular pressure.

VISUAL ACUITY

Accurate estimation of the patient's visual acuity is the most important measure of ocular function. In cases involving head trauma or injury of the face or eyes, the vision must be measured and recorded, not only to help determine the extent of the damage to the visual system, but also in case of future compensatory or legal action.

The patient should be comfortably seated 20 feet from an eye chart, such as a Snellen's chart (in which the letters subtend an angle of 5' of arc) (Fig. 8–5). The eyes are covered one at a time, and the patient is asked to read the letters starting from the top and proceeding down the chart, from the larger to the smaller letters. The last row in which the patient is able to read the majority of the letters should be recorded. The lower figure in the designation of visual acuity (20/**20**) represents the distance at which the normal eye would see the letter, the upper figure (**20**/20) refers to the distance (in feet) that the patient is seated from the chart. For

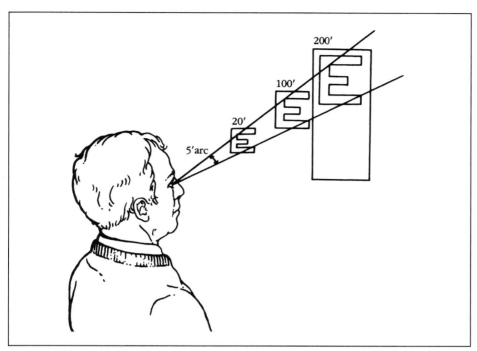

FIGURE 8–5
Measuring visual acuity.

example, the notation of 20/40 vision indicates the standard chart distance (20 feet) from the patient and the fact that the subject cannot read past the line that a normal individual would be able to read from 40 feet away. The numbers are in no sense a fraction.

Ask the patient to cover one eye and read down the chart, preferably with distance glasses on. If the patient reaches the 20/30 row and misses two letters, the record notation is: 20/30-2. The cover is shifted to the other eye, and if the patient reads through the 20/40 row and reads only two letters in the next row, the record notation is: 20/40 + 2. The result is written "O.D. (right eye) 20/30 − 2: O.S. (left eye) 20/40 + 2." If glasses are worn, note "with correction"; if not, "without correction."

If none of the letters on the chart are seen at 20 feet, gradually move the patient closer until the large letter at the top of the chart can be seen. If this is 5 feet from the chart, write "5/200" (because the upper figure designates the distance of the patient from the letter). The designation "5/200'" means the patient can see at 5 feet what a normal individual can see at 200 feet. If no letters can be read, hold up your fingers and ask the patient to count them; record the distance at which this occurs (e.g., "counts fingers at 2 feet"). If the patient cannot see (or count) your fingers, check for the ability to see moving objects or the direction from which your flashlight beam is shining on his eye; record "moving objects" or "light projection." "Light perception" may be recorded if the patient is unable to recognize direction but knows that the light is on. Do not record the eye as blind unless no light is perceived.

In some cases it may be desirable to record the near vision. Special graded reading cards are available for this, but in a general examination ordinary newsprint will suffice for your records.

For general purposes a vision of 20/30 or better in each eye can be accepted as normal. Be sure that the patient is wearing glasses if a refractive error is present. In normal individuals there usually is no more than a one-line difference between the vision of the two eyes. It is normal for persons over 40 years of age to begin to have near-vision difficulty because of presbyopia and to require glasses for reading.

EXTERNAL EXAMINATION

Before and while you are checking the visual acuity, you should be observing the patient's face and eyes along with general physical characteristics. Clues to systemic disease may be evident in the facial and ocular expression, the general appearance of the face and eyelids, the prominence of the eyes, and the alert or dull expression that they may convey.

The overall appearance of the eyes and face may reveal a staring expression,

TABLE 8–2. Some Eye Signs of Thyroid Disease

Eponym	Description	Appearance
Stellwag's sign (or stare)	Retraction of the upper lid due to spasm of levator palpebrae (in hyperthyroidism)	
Graves' exophthalmos	Protrusion of the eye(s) from the orbit (in Graves' disease)	
von Graefe's sign	Lagging of the lids upon looking downward, with visible sclera above the iris	

with retraction of the upper lids and prominence of the eyeballs in hyperthyroidism (Table 8–2). Unilateral prominence of an eye (proptosis) (Table 8–3) may indicate a space-occupying lesion of some type in the orbit, and bilateral prominence may be associated with thyroid abnormalities (which may also give unilateral proptosis), chronic lung disease, and genetic factors (American blacks may have more prominent eyes than whites do). Drooping upper lids (ptosis) may indicate extreme debility or neuromuscular disease. Partial ptosis can be part of Horner's syndrome, with involvement of the cervical sympathetics (Table 8–4). More marked ptosis of an upper lid associated with decreased pupillary light reaction may be the earliest indication of oculomotor paralysis (Fig. 8–6).

Always remember the order in which observation of external findings should be made: eyelids, lacrimal apparatus, conjunctiva, sclera, cornea, anterior chamber, iris. If each of these is thought of in turn, findings will not be overlooked.

Table 8–3. Some Causes of Unilateral Exophthalmos (Proptosis)

Graves' disease (may be asymmetric)
Orbital hemorrhage
Orbital cellulitis
Orbital tumor
Orbital vein thrombosis
Sphenoid wing meningioma
Carotid-cavernous fistula
Orbital von Recklinghausen's disease

Table 8–4. Some Causes of Ptosis

Congenital
Paralysis of cranial nerve III
Cervical sympathetic paralysis (Horner's syndrome)
Myasthenia gravis
Inflammation of lid
Progressive external ophthalmoplegia

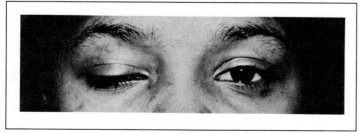

Figure 8–6
Ptosis (oculomotor paralysis).

EYELIDS

Note the appearance of the **eyelids** (Table 8–5). There may be edema, changes in the skin, and differences in height of the palpebral lid fissures; a staring expression may be evident or the upper lids may be pulled upward in a retracted position. Eversion of the lid (ectropion) may result from scar tissue or from senile laxity and is associated with overflow of tears (epiphora). Inversion (turning inward) of the lid border (entropion) causes irritation by abrasion of the lashes against the cornea and may be due to lid spasm or to contraction of scar tissue. Many structural variations may fall within the normal range. A slight difference in the palpebral fissures is usually not significant unless associated with unequal pupils. Differences in the depth of the upper lid fold may occur. Normal racial differences can be expected.

The appearance of the eyelids themselves may reveal systemic edema in advance of more noticeable changes elsewhere (Table 8–6). The skin may be involved in either local or generalized dermatologic conditions.

LACRIMAL DRAINAGE SYSTEM

Inspect the **lacrimal drainage system**. Observe the position and patency of the punctum at the inner end of each lid. The puncta should be turned backward slightly to contact the pool of tears in the inner canthus. Tears should also not spill over onto the cheek (epiphora). Gently palpate each lacrimal sac and note whether any material regurgitates back into the eye. Conjunctival inflammation that is greater in the inferior fornix may be associated with lacrimal obstruction or tear sac infection. A mass in the lacrimal gland may be a solid tumor or lymphoma.

CONJUNCTIVAE

The **conjunctiva** covers the entire anterior eyeball (other than the cornea) and is reflected back onto the posterior lid surfaces (see Fig. 8–2). Its appearance (edema, pallor, vascular injection) should be noted. The palpebral conjunctivae and the fornices must be seen, because foreign bodies may lodge here. To examine the conjunctiva of the lower lid, place your index finger firmly over the midpoint of the lid just above the bone of the lower orbital rim and pull downward. This everts the lower fornix; changing the position of your fingers will expose different areas.

In order to see the superior fornix and the conjunctiva of the upper lid, the eyelid must be everted (Fig. 8–7). Ask the patient to look downward, grasp the upper lashes gently with the thumb and forefinger of one hand, using a cotton swab to form a fulcrum just at the upper border of the tarsal plate (lid fold). By pushing down at this point and pulling inward on the lashes, you will evert the upper lid, exposing the posterior surface. As long as the patient keeps looking downward, the lid will remain in this position. After inspection, ask the patient to look upward, and the lid will flip over to its normal position.

There is considerable normal variation in the degree of vascularity of the conjunctivae. In general, the more florid the patient's complexion, the more likely that the eyes will appear to be "red" and congested. A small amount of discharge present in the inner canthus merely reflects the "wastebasket" function of the tear drainage mechanism and is to be expected, more so in patients with oily skin and greater meibomian secretions.

TABLE 8–5. Some Lesions of the Lids

Name	Description	Appearance
Ectropion	Eversion of the lid margin	
Entropion	Rolling inward of the lid margin	
Hordeolum (stye)	Inflammation of an eyelash follicle	
Chalazion	Chronic granuloma of a meibomian gland	
Xanthelasma	Raised yellow cholesterol plaque at inner canthal area	
Dacryocystitis	Painful swelling of tear sac	
Blepharitis	Inflammation of the lid margin	
Epicanthal fold	Fold of skin across inner canthus	

TABLE 8–6. Some Causes of Edema of the Lids

Local lesions of the lid or eye
Acute sinusitis
Acute allergic reactions
    Angioneurotic edema
    Urticaria
Dermatitis of the face
Cellulitis of the face
Measles
Mononucleosis
Hypoproteinemia
    Nephrotic syndrome
    Malabsorption
    Starvation
Congestive heart failure
Trichinosis
Thyrotoxicosis
Myxedema
Cavernous sinus thrombosis

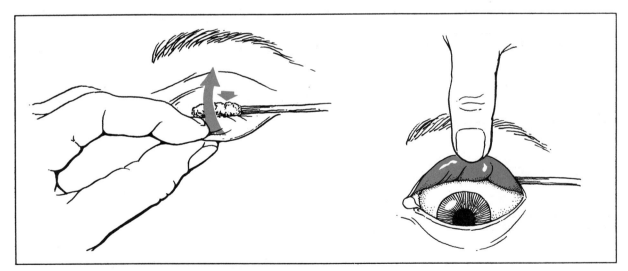

FIGURE 8–7
Technique of eversion of the eyelid.

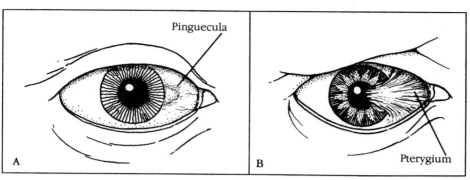

FIGURE 8–8
Lesions of the conjunctiva. A. Pinguecula. B. Pterygium.

Almost all disease affecting the conjunctivae produces both injection (dilation) of the vessels and discharge. In conjunctivitis of infectious origin, the injection usually increases in the fornices, and secretions are present. More severe involvement produces small hemorrhages beneath the conjunctivae. Spontaneous limited hemorrhages may also occur beneath the conjunctivae in otherwise healthy patients and usually have no significance unless signs of a bleeding tendency are present elsewhere.

Boggy conjunctivae may occur in patients with systemic fluid retention or as a manifestation of endocrine exophthalmos, local inflammation, or vascular stasis.

A localized degenerative process of the conjunctiva (pinguecula) may invade the superficial cornea, where it is called a *pterygium* (Fig. 8–8).

SCLERAE

The sclera gives the eye its white appearance. Yellowness of the **sclerae** may precede clinical jaundice of the skin in the hyperbilirubinemic patient. A "muddy" color of the sclerae is common in dark-skinned people and should be distinguished from jaundice.

CORNEA

Observe the **cornea**. It should be shiny and bright when illuminated by your flashlight. Any break in this clear continuity, such as scarring, vascularization, or ulceration, will dull the reflection. The size (horizontal diameter 11 to 13 mm) and curvature should be noted. In elderly patients, a partial or complete white ring about the periphery of the cornea (arcus senilis) is not unusual.

Pain in the eye is usually severe in acute disease of the cornea. Photophobia, manifested by the patient's evident discomfort in light, also occurs in most corneal diseases. In abrasions and ulcers of the cornea there is often increased redness of the globe around the corneal limbus. Loss of the bright surface reflection occurs in surface lesions, and at times a surface area of involvement will cast a shadow on the underlying iris if the flashlight is directed at the proper angle. Enlargement of the cornea is the most common finding in infantile glaucoma and is usually associated with a cloudy appearance of the cornea and photophobia. Edema of the cornea may be a part of local disease or of acute glaucoma.

Any vascularization or visible white scarring of the cornea is indicative of disease. A white arcus occurring around the limbus in younger individuals may indicate an abnormality of lipid metabolism. A brown ring of pigment occurs around the corneal limbus in hepatolenticular degeneration (Wilson's disease) and is known as a Kayser-Fleischer ring (Table 8–7).

ANTERIOR CHAMBER

Observe the depth of the **anterior chamber.** There should be adequate clearance between the cornea and iris, with no irregularities in depth. The depth varies somewhat among normal persons, but if the iris appears to bulge forward and the space is very shallow, you should immediately think of the possibility of acute glaucoma. Anything other than clear aqueous humor occupying the anterior chamber is abnormal.

Blood may be present after injury (hyphema) (Fig. 8–9), or pus may level out in the lower chamber in association with corneal infection (hypopyon). The chamber may be lost in perforating wounds with aqueous leakage.

IRIS

Findings involving the **iris** and pupil often are associated. An irregular pupil may be due to adhesions of the iris to the lens (synechiae) as the result of prior iritis. Congenital abnormalities, such as multiple or displaced pupils, must be differentiated from tears of the iris base (iridodialysis) due to prior trauma. Localized elevation of the iris is immediately suspect for possible tumor, especially if the iris is darkly pigmented.

Iritis is a nonspecific inflammation of the iris. The patient notes throbbing pain and visual blurring. There is circumcorneal injection with a small pupil. The eye is usually quite soft to palpation and is tender.

Abnormalities of the position of the pupils and irregularities in shape or difference in size between the two (anisocoria) should be recorded (Table 8–8). The size of the pupils varies in normal individuals. Large pupils are generally found in myopic (near-sighted) eyes and in younger patients. Smaller pupils are more common in patients with hyperopia (far-sightedness) and in older individuals. A small difference in pupil size between the two eyes is usually not significant unless accompanied by abnormal reflexes or change in consciousness.

Remember that when you are looking at the pupillary opening in the iris, you are also inspecting the **lens** of the eye, which is normally transparent. Any visible clouding of the lens as seen through the pupil is indicative of cataract formation. A cataract may also be seen as a dark shadow against the light reflex of the fundus in the beginning of the ophthalmoscopic examination. If the lens has been removed by cataract surgery, or is dislocated, the normal support of the iris will not be present and the iris will "flutter" with ocular movements (iridodonesis).

TABLE 8–7. Some Lesions of the Cornea

Name	Description	Appearance
Arcus senilis	Concentric gray depositions of lipid around the cornea. May or may not suggest hyperlipidemia	
Band keratopathy	Horizontal band of subepithelial calcification, most marked at the periphery of the cornea (at 3 and 9 o'clock) and fading toward the center. Occurs in hypercalcemic states and in degeneration of the globe	
Keratoconus	Congenital condition but often not manifest until after puberty	
Keratitis	Inflammation of the cornea May be infective, toxic, or allergic	
Keratoconjunctivitis sicca	Defect in lacrimation leading to drying of conjunctiva and cornea Associated with certain forms of arthritis	
Corneal ulcer	Acute or chronic lesion, due to trauma or infection	
Kayser-Fleischer ring	Pericorneal deposition of copper salts seen in Wilson's disease, biliary cirrhosis, and chronic copper toxicity	

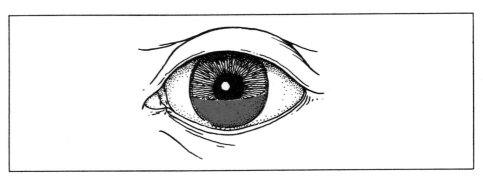

FIGURE 8–9
Hyphema.

EXTRAOCULAR MOVEMENTS

Seat yourself facing the patient and hold your flashlight in the midline between yourself and the patient, with the patient looking directly at the light. Observe the position of the reflection of the light on each of the corneas with respect to the location of the pupils (corneal light reflex). Then cover one eye (with the patient still looking at the light). Remove the cover quickly and notice whether the eye moves to regain fixation on the light (cover-uncover test). This test may demonstrate a drift of the eye behind the cover, which can indicate muscle imbalance. Perform the cover-uncover test on the other eye. Then shift the cover from one eye to the other and back again, always observing the movement that the uncovered eye makes to regain fixation (alternate cover test). If weakness or paralysis of one of the horizontal rectus muscles is present, a horizontal shift will occur. If one of the elevator or depressor muscles is involved, a vertical movement will be noted.

The maintenance of parallel eyes (and therefore of corneal light reflexes that are equally centered) occurs in most patients because of the fusion reflex, which makes binocular vision possible. If deviation of the eye occurs behind the cover, and then recovers when both eyes are uncovered, you are dealing with *phoria,* a latent tendency to deviation that is held in check by fusion (Fig. 8–10 A, B). If, on the other hand, the deviation of the eye behind the cover continues when both eyes are uncovered, the muscle imbalance is called a *tropia* (Fig. 8–10 C, D).

It is normal to find a small amount of horizontal shift of the visual axes with the alternate cover test, provided the eyes regain a parallel position as soon as the cover is removed. It is more common to find a small outward deviation (exophoria) than a minor inward deviation (esophoria). In both instances parallelism is regained. Usually any vertical shift behind the cover is abnormal.

In evaluating possible weaknesses of individual extraocular muscles and consequently their innervation (in most cases), it is helpful to use a system of "diagnostic positions of gaze" to unravel the complexities of movement of 12 muscles (six on each eye) acting in concert (Fig. 8–11).

In each of the diagnostic positions, two muscles are evaluated. The muscle pairs indicated are known as "yoked muscles," because they are yoked together by in-

TABLE 8–8. Some Pupillary Abnormalities

Condition	Causes	Appearance
Anisocoria	Cranial nerve III paralysis Sympathetic paralysis Ocular disease (ciliary spasm)	UNEQUAL PUPILS
Horner's syndrome (small pupil is the pathologic one)	Unilateral (generally) sympathetic paralysis, usually due to trauma or tumor along the sympathetic train in neck or brain	Ptosis Miosis Anhidrosis Pseudoenophthalmos
Dilated, fixed pupil (large pupil is the pathologic one)	CNS disease, cranial nerve III palsy, Adie's pupil	No direct or consensual reaction
Argyll Robertson pupil (small pupil is the pathologic one)	Syphilis, diabetes, CNS disease due to involvement of the Edinger-Westphal nucleus	Small, irregular pupil Reacts to accommodation but not to light
Miotic pupils	Drugs (pilocarpine or other parasympathetic stimulants), sympathetic blockade, narcotics	PINPOINT PUPILS
Mydriatic pupils	Drugs (atropine, catecholamines) Brain death	FIXED AND DILATED
Irregular pupils Postsurgical	Iridectomy for cataract	
Postinflammatory	Syphilis, occular inflammation (synechiae)	

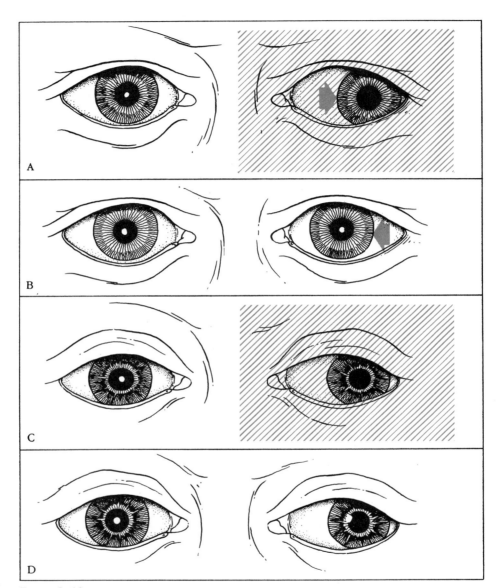

FIGURE 8–10
Alternate cover test. A and B. Exophoria. C and D. Exotropia.

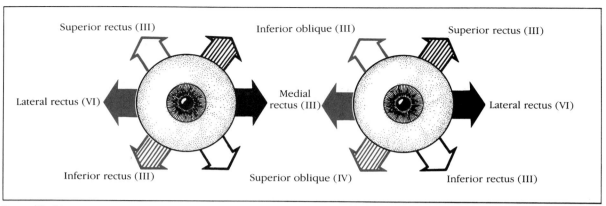

FIGURE 8–11
Extraocular movements and their controlling nerves. Cranial nerves in parentheses.

TABLE 8–9. Yoked Muscles

Right Eye	Left Eye	Turn Eyes
Medial rectus	Lateral rectus	Left
Lateral rectus	Medial rectus	Right
Superior rectus	Inferior oblique	Up and right
Inferior rectus	Superior oblique	Down and right
Superior oblique	Inferior rectus	Down and left
Inferior oblique	Superior rectus	Up and left

nervation to act in unison (see Table 8–9 and the pairs of "yoked" muscles with similarly colored arrows in Fig. 8–11). Remember, the eye that is turned out is in position to evaluate the superior and inferior recti, and the eye that is turned in is in position to evaluate the obliques.

Ask the patient to follow your light with his eyes, and observe him in each of these diagnostic positions: (1) up to the right, (2) directly to the right, (3) down to the right, (4) down to the left, (5) directly to the left, (6) up to the left. Notice the position of the corneal light reflexes in each eye and make sure they are parallel. If the eyes cease to be parallel in a certain position, the lagging muscle can be designated directly. In addition, ask the patient whether he sees two lights in any of the positions (diplopia, or double vision). This will give you a clue regarding the muscle pair that should be analyzed further.

Any lack of parallelism in these six diagnostic positions of gaze is beyond the range of normal. Any tropia (constant deviation from parallel) is abnormal. A transient jerking movement of the eyes in the *extremes* of horizontal gaze (nystagmus) ordinarily falls within normal limits, though marked nystagmus is abnormal and suggests drug toxicity, thiamine deficiency, or congenital, vestibular, or neurologic disease.

Paralysis of the specific nerve supply to any of the extraocular muscles produces characteristic findings (Fig. 8–12A). In abducens (cranial nerve VI) paralysis, the involved eye will be turned in toward the nose because of unopposed action of the normal medial rectus, and the esotropia will be greater when looking in the direction of the normal action of the paralyzed lateral rectus muscle. The patient with an oculomotor (cranial nerve III) paralysis will have his eyes turned down and out, with ptosis of the upper lid. Diplopia will not occur because of the closure of the lid (Fig. 8–12 B, C). The patient with trochlear (cranial nerve IV) palsy will complain of difficulty with vision in the lower field, as in reading (Fig. 8–12D). If he has been able to maintain single binocular vision, his head will be tilted toward the shoulder opposite the side of paralysis.

Isolated involvement of ocular muscles may occur with certain neuromuscular diseases, may follow orbital or facial fracture, or may be part of the findings of the endocrine exophthalmos of thyroid disease.

PUPILLARY TESTING

The presence of **pupillary reflexes** denotes integrity of cranial nerves II (optic) and III (oculomotor). Cranial nerve II must be intact to perceive and transmit the presence of light to the brain stem. Cranial nerve III must be intact to effect pupillary constriction (Fig. 8–13). An easy mnemonic device for this is "In two, out three." Note that in cortical blindness (damage to the occipital visual cortex of the brain) the pupillary reflexes will be intact, but the patient will still be blind.

Shine your light quickly into one eye and observe the response of both eyes. The illuminated eye shows constriction of the pupil (direct light reaction), and the pupil of the other eye also constricts an equal amount (consensual light reaction). Then shine the light into the other eye and observe the same reactions. Ask the patient to look at a distant target (over 10 feet away) and then at your finger or an object (such as a pen) held a few inches in front of the patient's nose. When focusing for this near object, both pupils will constrict (the "near reaction" or pupillary reaction in accommodation) (Fig. 8–13B).

Avoid confusing the light and near reaction by shining your light into the eye from the side rather than from directly in front of the patient (Fig. 8–13C). (Some patients, if the light is in front, will look directly at the light, and their accommodative pupillary response may be mistaken for an intact direct light reaction).

The rapidity of response of the pupillary reflexes varies considerably in normal patients. Usually the presence of the response is sufficient, as long as it is equal in the two eyes. Older patients who have difficulty with accommodation often show a normal slowing of the near reaction.

Loss of the pupillary light reaction is always important (Table 8–10). When it is unilateral due to blindness, neither a direct reflex nor a consensual reflex will occur when the blind eye is tested. When the loss is bilateral in a nonblind patient, neurologic disease is usually present. An example is the Argyll Robertson pupil of central nervous system syphilis, in which the light reflexes are gone but the near reflex in accommodation is present. As the old clinical saw has it: "An Argyll Robertson pupil is like a prostitute—it's accommodating but doesn't react."

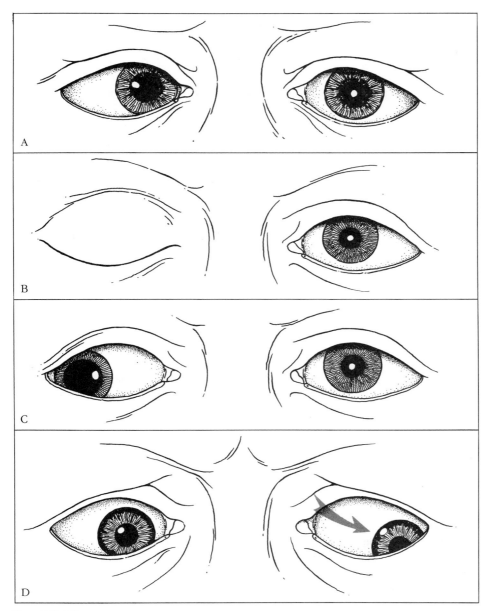

FIGURE 8–12

Extraocular motor palsies. A. Right cranial nerve VI palsy: patient looks straight ahead; affected right eye turns nasally. B and C. Right cranial nerve III palsy: Lid closed and open. Eye is ptotic. If lid is lifted, affected eye turns out and down, with dilated pupil. D. Right cranial nerve IV palsy: patient cannot look downward nasally.

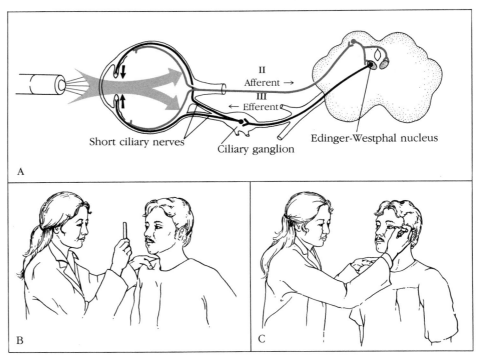

FIGURE 8–13
Pupillary reflex pathway. A. Physiologic pathways: The afferent (II) and the efferent (III) loops of the pupillary reflex pathway. B. Checking accommodation. C. Checking the light reflex.

Pupils that resemble the Argyll Robertson pupil may also occur in diabetes mellitus, midbrain lesions, myotonic dystrophy, and familial amyloidosis. In midbrain involvement, the pupils are enlarged, in contrast to the Argyll Robertson pupil.

A unilaterally fixed, dilated pupil may be the result of local trauma to the eye, but more often it is a serious sign in a patient with a recent head injury because it indicates the beginning involvement of the oculomotor nerve. A miotic pupil associated with partial drooping of the upper lid may indicate disease of the cervical sympathetic system on that side and is part of Horner's syndrome (see Table 8–8).

VISUAL FIELDS BY CONFRONTATION

The peripheral (side) vision may be grossly determined by a confrontation visual field technique. Position yourself about 2 feet in front of the patient so that your face is level with the patient's face. To test the right eye, have the patient look at your left eye and cover the patient's left eye with your right hand or an occluder such as an opaque reading card. Close your right eye so that your own visual field is roughly superimposed on that of the patient. Bring your wriggling index finger slowly from the side until the patient perceives it. Then check each of the four

TABLE 8–10. Some Abnormal Pupillary Reflexes

Name	Finding	Suggested Condition
Amaurotic pupil	Light in affected eye gives no direct and no consensual reflex Light in normal eye gives both direct and consensual reflex	Blind eye, without light perception
Marcus Gunn pupil (afferent pupillary defect)	Light in affected eye gives minimal direct, normal consensual reflex Light in normal eye gives brisk direct and consensual reflex If, after the normal eye is checked, the light is quickly returned to the abnormal eye, the pupil of the abnormal eye appears to dilate (since the direct response is less constrictive than the abnormal eye's consensual response)	Optic nerve disease but not blindness
Hutchinson's pupil	Dilated, fixed, unresponsive to light	Neurologic disease (e.g., herniation, aneurysm impinging on cranial nerve III)
Adie's pupil	May be unilateral or bilateral Pupil shows minimal reaction to light, slow reaction to near vision Occurs in women 20–30 years old and is associated with decreased knee and ankle reflexes	Ciliary ganglion dysfunction

quadrants of the patient's peripheral vision, comparing his visual field to your own (Fig. 8–14). When examining children, asking the patient to tell you how many fingers are seen in each quadrant may be helpful.

Because significant neurologic field defects often show a difference on either side of the vertical midline, the use of two red objects to test fields (such as the tops of two eye-drop bottles) may show subtle differences in color saturation across the midline, even though the visual confrontation test is normal.

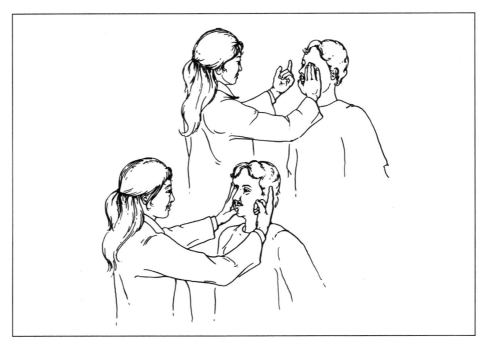

FIGURE 8–14
Visual fields by confrontation.

TABLE 8–11. Abnormalities of Visual Fields

Condition	Causes	Appearance	
		Left	Right
1. Blind eye	Lesions of the optic nerve	○	●
2. Homonymous hemianopsia	Lesion contralateral optic tract, optic radiation, or occipital cortex	◗	◗
3. Homonymous quadrantanopsia	Partial lesion contralateral optic tract, optic radiation, or occipital cortex	◵	◵
4. Bitemporal hemianopsia	Lesion of the optic chiasm	◖	◗

Note: Conditions are caused by lesions shown in Figure 15 with corresponding numbers (1 through 4).

To evaluate a more central field defect, ask the patient to look at your nose and tell you whether a part of your face is missing.

Next, to evaluate the patient's left visual field, have the patient look into your right eye and cover the patient's right eye with your left hand. With your left eye closed, repeat the above procedure in all four quadrants.

Abnormalities of the visual field are shown in Table 8–11 with corresponding lesions in the optic pathway shown in Figure 8–15. If any visual field defect is suspected as a result of the confrontation technique, a formal field examination by an ophthalmologist using specifically designed instruments should be requested. Because visual field defects occur early in cases of uncontrolled chronic glaucoma, serial examinations are necessary to assess the response of the disease to treatment.

FUNDUSCOPIC EXAMINATION

Evaluation of the ocular fundus will often aid in the general physical evaluation of the patient. Constant practice with the ophthalmoscope is necessary and most rewarding.

Seat the patient comfortably and dim the room lights. Ask the patient to look straight ahead. Hold the instrument with your right hand and stand on the patient's right side. Examine the right eye with your right eye; the reverse holds for the left eye. A +8 lens (black numbers of the dial) is placed in the instrument aperture, and the pupil is observed from a distance of 6 to 8 inches. This illuminates the retina, and any opacity or obstruction to the emerging light will be seen as a dark spot or shadow against an orange-red background. Gradually move closer to the patient, hold the upper lid open gently with the thumb of your free hand, resting your hand on the patient's forehead. The lens wheel of the ophthalmoscope is turned (toward zero on the dial) until the lighter color of the optic disc is seen just nasal to the center of the retina. Then refocus your instrument until details of the optic nerve head are seen clearly (Figs. 8-16–8-18).

Although dimming the lights is sufficient preparation for ophthalmoscopic examination in most patients, a mydriatic drop is often useful. In the vast majority of patients a mydriatic drop may be used safely, but you must be aware of the possibility of inducing a rise in intraocular pressure (glaucoma) in a predisposed eye. This is more often the case in patients over 40 years of age. Always question the patient regarding any previous diagnosis of glaucoma, observe the optic nerve head for abnormality, and, if there is any question, measure the intraocular pressure. The presence of a cornea that is small in diameter with a shallow anterior chamber increases the possibility of causing an acute rise in intraocular pressure. After checking for these points, instill 1 drop of a mild mydriatic (among others, 0.5% Mydriacyl or 2.5% Neo-Synephrine) into each eye. If this is done early in the physical examination, you may return to the funduscopic examination later after the drops have had adequate time to cause sufficient dilation of the pupils. *Note:* If there is acute neurologic disease, especially a recent brain hemorrhage or head trauma, the observation of serial changes in the pupils is crucial in planning treatment. In order to avoid masking important changes, *do not* dilate the pupils. Also do not dilate the pupils if the patient has had intraocular lens implantations.

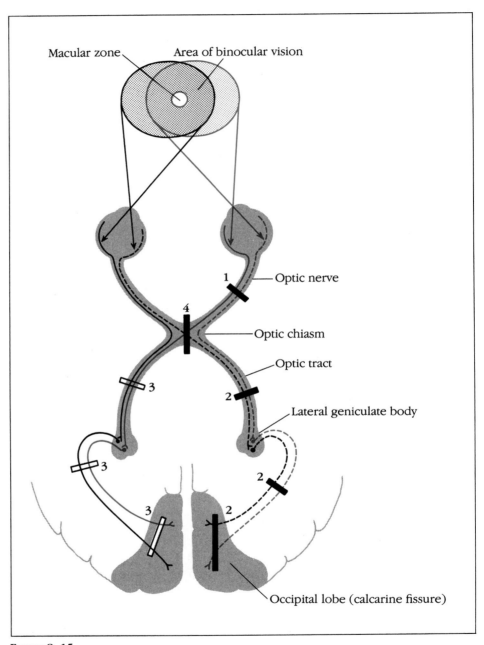

FIGURE 8–15
Optic pathways from retinas to occipital lobes. Numbered lesions cause visual field defects shown in Table 8–11 (complete lesions are indicated by solid bars and partial lesions by open bars).

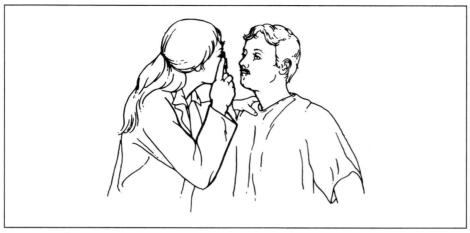

FIGURE 8–16
Ophthalmoscopy.

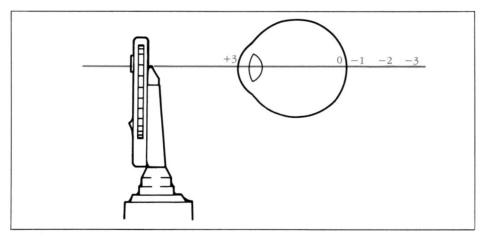

FIGURE 8–17
Sites of focus (with normal eyeball).

You must follow a definite order of examination of the retina, always reserving the central or macular area until last. This avoids "dazzling" the patient early in the examination and will ensure better cooperation for prolonged viewing.

A blurred image of the fundus that will not clear with proper focus of the ophthalmoscope is usually due to clouding in the media of the eye (i.e., the cornea, lens, or vitreous). Vitreous haziness is present in intraocular inflammation. *Cataract* in the lens or *corneal scarring* may also blur visualization of the fundus. In an occasional patient with a high refractive error, the fundus may be difficult to see, and in this case you should attempt funduscopy through the patient's correcting lenses.

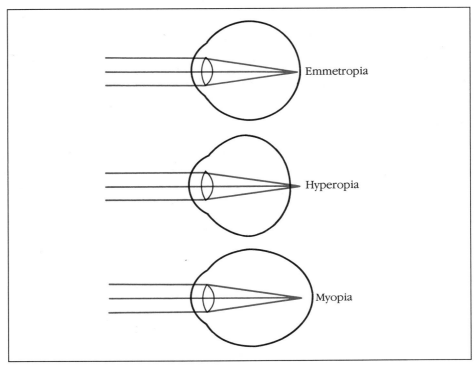

FIGURE 8–18
Common defects in the optical system of the eye. Emmetropia denotes a normal-sized eye. A shortened eyeball gives rise to hyperopia (farsightedness). An abnormally long eyeball may characterize myopia (nearsightedness). Adjustments should be made in the lens selection on the ophthalmoscope for these anatomic differences.

The blood vessels of the retina (Fig. 8–19) emerge from and enter the disc in four main pairs. Examine the superior nasal vessels first, following them out as far as possible without having the patient turn his eye. This is followed in order by the inferior nasal, inferior temporal, and superior temporal pairs. The retina adjoining each of these pairs is inspected at the same time. Then ask the patient to look up, up and in, directly in toward the nose, down and in, straight down, down and out, directly outward, and then up and out. This covers eight successive overlapping zones of the peripheral retina, and each zone joins the margins of the more central retinal areas seen along with inspection of the vessels. The central retina and macular area are visualized last; ask the patient to look directly at the light if necessary. The foveal pit in the macula is seen as a small bright dot produced by light reflection from the indentation.

The position of the vessels on the nerve head may vary. The retinal vessels are usually gently sinuous in their courses, with approximate right angles at division points. They usually cross each other without noticeable indentations. The veins

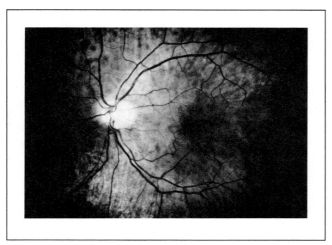

FIGURE 8–19
Normal ocular fundus.

TABLE 8–12. Keith-Wagener-Barker Classification of Hypertensive Retinopathy*

Group	Description
I	Moderate arteriolar narrowing, often with focal spasm and accentuated arteriolar light reflex
II	Arteriolar narrowing, arteriovenous nicking Hard exudates and small hemorrhages
III	Marked arteriolar narrowing Retina appears wet, edematous Soft exudates and hemorrhages
IV	Signs in group III *and* papilledema

*It is always preferable for the examiner to *describe* fully the changes seen in the fundus rather than to classify them arbitrarily.

are somewhat darker than the arterioles and are about one-third wider. Both can be traced almost to the visible periphery in the eye with a widely dilated pupil.

Evaluation of the retinal vessels is helpful in assessing the patient with arteriosclerosis or hypertensive disease (Table 8–12 details one of the systems for classifying hypertensive retinopathy). The normal retinal arteriole is seen only as a blood column (Fig. 8–20A). When thickening of the wall occurs, a shinier reflection is noted (Fig. 8–20B). It may be copper-colored in less advanced sclerosis but will appear like a silver wire in advanced disease. This change is due to visibility of the vessel wall, and at times the wall itself may be seen along the edge of the blood column. In addition, where an involved artery crosses a retinal vein, it may indent the vein and even cause evidence of back pressure in the vein distal to the crossing (AV nicking) (Fig. 8–20 C, D). The disappearance of the vein on both sides of the

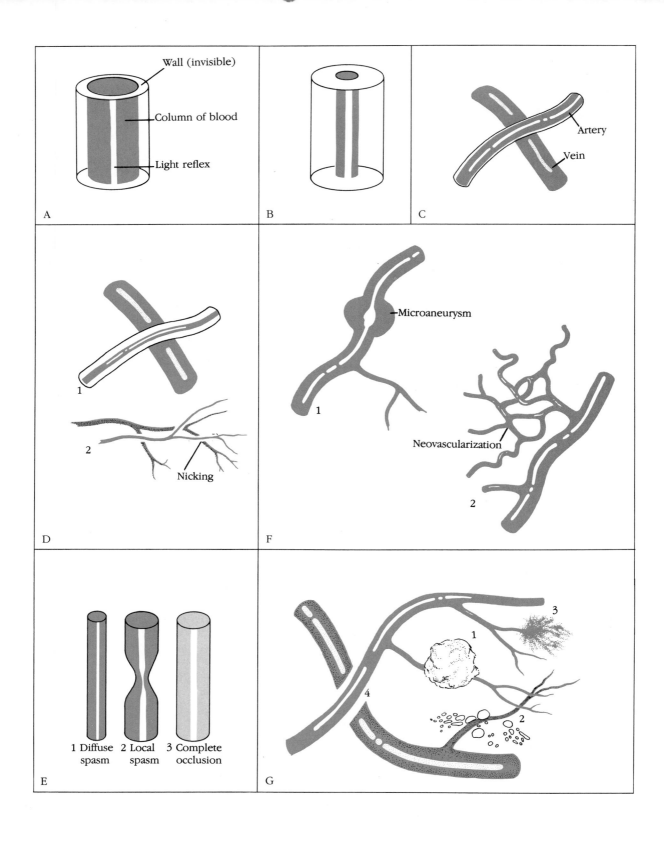

A

Wall (invisible)

Column of blood

Light reflex

B

C

Artery

Vein

D

1

2

Nicking

F

Microaneurysm

1

Neovascularization

2

E

1 Diffuse spasm   2 Local spasm   3 Complete occlusion

G

blood column representing the arteriole is a measure of thickening of the arteriolar wall.

With hypertension there is localized or generalized narrowing of the arteriolar blood column (Fig. 8–20E). This is identified by a change in the ratio of arteriolar to venule size. In tracing out the smaller branches toward the periphery, the arterioles will disappear earlier than the veins. In the more severe degrees of hypertension, leakage of the vascular walls will lead to hemorrhages and deposits in the retina, and papilledema may ensue (Fig. 8–21).

Hemorrhages and exudates in the retina are always important signs of disease (Figs. 8-21–8-24). The shape of the hemorrhages indicates the depth of the retina at which it occurs. Superficial hemorrhages are flame-shaped or splinterlike in contour and lie in the nerve fiber layer of the retina (Fig. 8–21). They usually occur when venous back pressure is present, such as in occlusion of the central retinal vein or one of its branches, or in association with papilledema. In contrast, closure of the central retinal artery or a branch results in ischemic edema of the area involved; where the artery is completely closed, the retina is pale and edematous, with the thinner macular area shining through as a cherry-red spot. Hemorrhages that are located in the deeper retinal layers are rounder or blotchier in contour and are often associated with exudates (Fig. 8–22). These latter deposits represent residues of edema and of blood substances that are incompletely absorbed due to poor retinal circulation. Sharply defined yellow or white deposits should be distinguished from more fuzzy cotton-wool patches, which are small ischemic infarcts in the nerve fiber layer (see Fig. 8–20G).

The association of hemorrhages and exudates occurs in advanced hypertension, severe renal disease, certain of the collagen diseases, diabetes, the blood dyscrasias, retinal venous occlusion, and acquired immunodeficiency syndrome (AIDS). The early hemorrhages of diabetic retinopathy may be punctate or clusterlike, because they are really venous microaneurysms (see Figs. 8–22 and 8–20F). They are usually present only in the macular area and surrounding posterior pole of the eye.

FIGURE 8–20
Blood vessels of the fundus. A. Normal artery. B. Arteriolosclerosis. Note that light reflex *appears* broader (relative to the visible column of blood) in the sclerotic arteriole. Since arteriolar wall is not seen, early arteriosclerosis is perceived as a narrowing column of blood and widened light reflex. C. Normal arteriovenous crossing. Note that arteriole is from two-thirds to three-fourths the size of the vein. D. Arteriovenous nicking. As the arteriolar wall thickens (1), it cuts off vision of the underlying vein. The obstruction (2) makes it appear as though there were a gap between the arteriolar column of blood and the underlying vein. E. Vasospastic disease. In hypertension, spasm may be complete and diffuse along the arteriole (1) or may be local or segmental (2). If atheroma has totally occluded the vessel, it appears whitish, the "silver wire" phenomenon (3). F. In diabetes, weakening of the arteriolar wall may give microaneurysms (1). New-vessel formation (neovascularization) (2) may, in this disease, be mistaken for hemorrhage unless careful observation is made. G. Soft exudates (1) are fuzzy, gray patches thought to represent infarcts in areas of arteriolar insufficiency. Hard exudates (2) are dense, gray localized infiltrates probably caused by venous stasis. Hemorrhages (3) may occur as well as arteriovenous nicking (4).

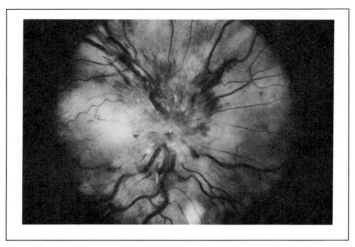

FIGURE 8–21
Hypertensive retinopathy with papilledema and superficial hemorrhages.

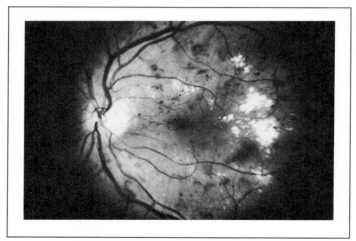

FIGURE 8–22
Diabetic retinopathy with hard exudates and deep hemorrhages.

Later retinal changes in diabetes mellitus may include soft and hard exudates, hemorrhages, and hypertensive changes (Fig. 8–20G) as well as the ominous findings of neovascularization (Figs. 8–20F and 8–23). A significant difference between the two eyes in hemorrhages and exudates may indicate carotid occlusive disease.

When blood extravasates in front of the retina (preretinal hemorrhage), it will obscure the underlying details and may show a gravitational fluid level (Fig. 8–24). Such bleeding is associated with sudden intracranial hemorrhage.

When round blotchy hemorrhages occur that are noted to have white centers

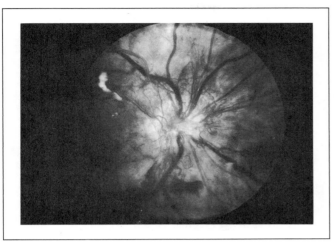

FIGURE 8–23
Neovascularization.

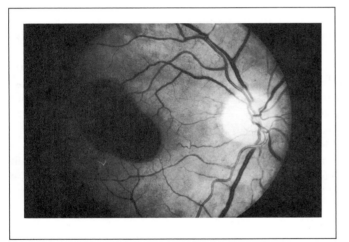

FIGURE 8–24
Preretinal hemorrhage.

(Roth's spots), one must think of blood dyscrasias or of the embolic lesions of subacute bacterial endocarditis (Fig. 8–25).

Note that the background color of the fundus may be dark in brunettes, very light in blonds; and in the latter the deeper choroidal vessels may shine through. The healthy retina is transparent and produces no visible findings except for highlights, which often follow the expected pattern of the retinal nerve fibers.

Considerable variation in the size and shape of the *nerve head* (optic disc) may occur. If the disc is small the nasal border may be blurred. If the eye is myopic

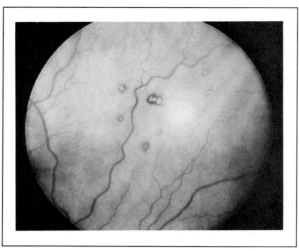

FIGURE 8–25
Roth's spots.

there may be an arc of pallor along the temporal side. The physiologic depression may vary from highly prominent to nonexistent. Pigment may be noted along the disc border.

Note the size, shape, color, margins, and physiologic depression of the optic nerve. Any elevation can be measured by focusing on the highest part of the disc. Then throw the light beam about two disc diameters nasally to the nerve head and refocus on the retina. Note the number of clicks as the lens wheel is turned to refocus; then read the difference directly from the dial.

Major abnormalities of the optic nerve are optic atrophy, cupping of the disc in glaucoma, and papilledema. In optic atrophy the color of the disc is paler than normal and may be chalky white in advanced cases (Fig. 8–26A). There may be associated superficial scar tissue or loss of substance, and usually there is resultant decrease in vision.

The cupping of the disc that occurs in glaucoma (Fig. 8–26B) consists of an exaggeration of the physiologic depression (Fig. 8–26C) on the temporal side that extends to the temporal border. The cup may be deep and is bluish white; the emerging retinal vessels may disappear behind the shelf at the edge of the cup, then emerge over the edge to reach the retina. Cupping of the disc is expressed as a ratio of the cup diameter to the horizontal disc diameter (C/D ratio). While no exact C/D value differentiates physiologic from abnormal, a ratio greater than 0.3 or an asymmetry between the two eyes should be viewed with suspicion.

Swelling of the nerve head (papilledema) (Fig. 8–26D) may be unilateral in localized optic nerve disease or bilateral in the "choked" disc of increased intracranial pressure. The amount of elevation should be measured with the ophthalmoscope for estimation of future change. Early papilledema is difficult to determine, but filling in of the physiologic depression, blurring of the margins of the disc, fullness of the retinal veins, and loss of spontaneous venous pulsation on the disc

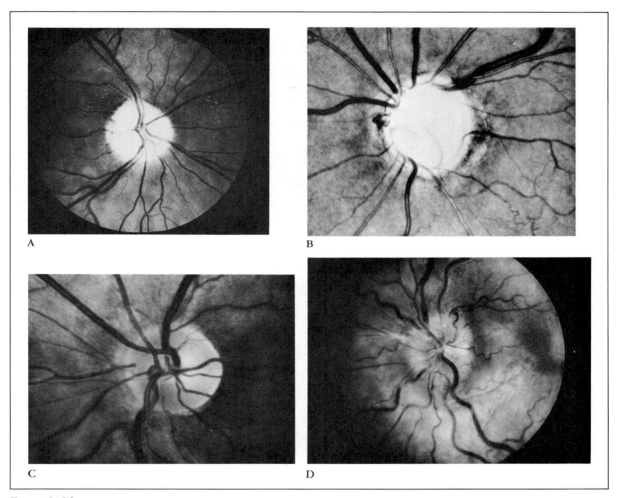

FIGURE 8–26
Optic disc. A. Optic atrophy. B. Advanced glaucomatous cupping. C. Physiologic cupping. D.
Papilledema.

are early signs. Where the process is more advanced, superficial hemorrhages and
exudates around the disc make diagnosis more certain.

Any area of retinal elevation is significant. A solid mass indicates tumor growth,
usually arising in the choroid. If it has a dark color it is likely to be melanoma (Fig.
8–27), and if lighter, one must think of metastatic malignancy. When the elevation
is transparent and wrinkled, retinal detachment must be considered.

Areas of localized chorioretinal scarring are recognized by irregular pigment
deposition around a paler center (Fig. 8–28). If they are clear-cut and sharp in
outline, no current inflammatory activity is suspected; but if they have fuzzy borders, hemorrhages along the margin, or associated clouding in the vitreous, an

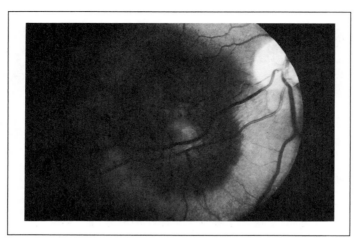

Figure 8–27
Choroidal melanoma.

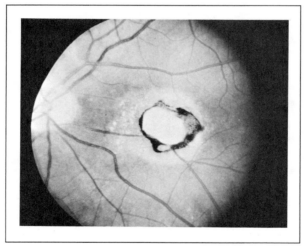

Figure 8–28
Chorioretinitis (congenital toxoplasmosis).

active process may be suspected. Irregular mottling of pigment and scar tissue change in the macular areas may be seen in older patients who are suffering from senile macular degeneration (Fig. 8–29), and associated decrease in central vision will be found.

INTRAOCULAR PRESSURE

Intraocular pressure measurement should be considered in every complete physical examination, and many clinicians refer patients who are over 40 years of age to ophthalmologists for this essential yearly test. A simple screening instrument,

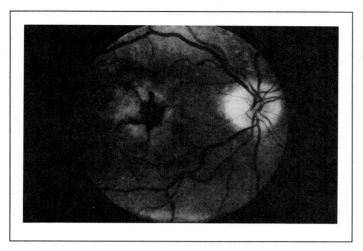

FIGURE 8–29
Macular degeneration.

the Schiotz tonometer, can be used to measure intraocular pressure. It measures the indentation of the cornea caused by a weighted plunger fitted into a curved footplate. The movement of the plunger is transmitted to a leverscale. The scale reading is translated into millimeters of mercury. The procedure for measuring intraocular pressure using the Schiotz tonometer is as follows. Make the patient comfortable in a reclining position and instill 1 drop of a local anesthetic, such as 0.5% tetracaine, into each eye. When the eyes are anesthetized, direct the patient to look straight above him, fixing either on his extended finger or on a target on the ceiling. Hold the instrument lightly in one hand, and separate the lids gently with the fingers of the other hand. Rest the footplate on the cornea and take the reading from the scale. A small rhythmic deviation in the pointer is observed (transmitted pulse pressure) to ensure a proper reading. Repeat the procedure for the other eye. Care must be taken not to exert pressure on the lids, and the instrument must be kept meticulously clean. The normal range of intraocular pressures is between 8 and 21 mm Hg. Any elevation of intraocular pressure is abnormal and requires a formal evaluation for glaucoma by an ophthalmologist. Glaucoma can occur at any age but is more common in older patients. It is the greatest single cause of blindness in patients over 40 years of age even though it can be controlled by proper treatment if discovered early. Acute glaucoma is uncommon but is associated with pain in the eye, a cloudy, edematous cornea, a moderately dilated pupil, and systemic symptoms, such as severe headache, nausea and vomiting, and prostration. Abdominal symptoms have led to misdiagnosis of an acute abdomen in rare instances. The more common chronic glaucoma may cause only variable visual blur, minor headache, and peripheral vision loss or may be entirely silent. Clues here are the findings of moderately elevated intraocular pressure and early cupping in the optic nerve head. More precise tonometry and detailed evaluation of the visual fields must be done.

CHAPTER 9

HEAD

Nature has given man one tongue, but two ears, that we may hear twice as much as we speak.

EPICTETUS
(62–120)

Headache, alterations of hearing, nasal and sinus disorders, and oropharyngeal diseases are among the most common of patient complaints in practice. The seriousness of head and neck disorders that are detectable by careful history and physical examination ranges from the trivial (though discomforting) viral upper respiratory tract infection to the malignant tumor. Complaints of headache, tinnitus, nasal discharge, change in voice, sores in the mouth, and masses about the head and neck, though commonplace, are never treated lightly by the good physician.

The variety of structures in the head, though obviously integrally interconnected, will be presented separately in order to clarify the anatomy, history, and physical examination of each.

EARS

ANATOMY
The auricle usually forms a 30-degree angle with the side of the head. Its lateral surface is irregularly concave (Fig. 9–1). The concha of the auricle receives its sensory innervation, as does the external auditory canal, from the auricular branch of the trigeminal nerve and the vagus (Arnold's nerve). In contrast to that of lower animals, the auricle of higher animals does not serve to direct and amplify sound. Its usefulness seems to be limited to "leading around little boys and hanging earrings."

The outer one-third of the canal contains hair follicles, sebaceous glands, and cerumen glands. At the junction of the middle and inner thirds of the canal is located a bony narrowing called the isthmus (Fig. 9–2).

The tympanic membrane is usually found on a slanted plane (Fig. 9–3). The anteroinferior quadrant is the farthest away from the examiner. This accounts for the triangle of light that is reflected anteroinferiorly from the umbo.

HISTORY
The historical review of systems concerning the ear may be done as you examine your patient. Remember that "**earache**," a common malady, may reflect pathology in the jaw (temporomandibular joint disease) as well as a problem with the ear. Wax (cerumen) in the ears is not a pathologic condition unless hearing is compromised by its buildup. Many patients poke sharp objects into their ears, such as hairpins and wooden sticks, to clean out the wax, risking injury to the drum. Chil-

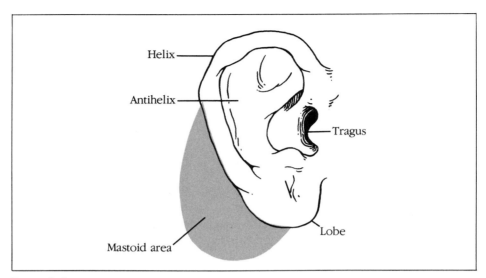

FIGURE 9–1
External ear (auricle).

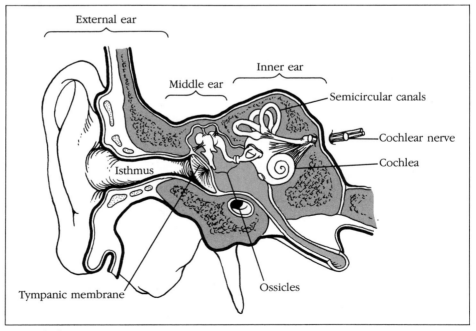

FIGURE 9–2
Cross-section of the ear.

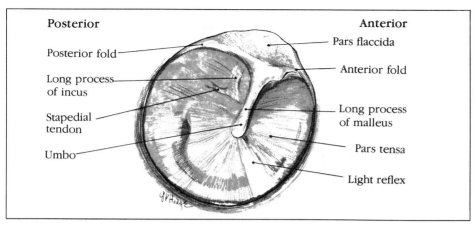

FIGURE 9–3
Right tympanic membrane showing important landmarks.

dren put things in their ears because they are children, and a complaint of decreased hearing in one ear in a child may follow the impaction of anything from bugs to peanuts in the ear canal. Ask specifically about a history of frequent childhood ear infections, ringing in the ears (tinnitus, which suggests disease or drug toxicity to cranial nerve VIII), and **discharge** from the ears. Any discharge should be classified as serous, mucoid, purulent, putrid, or sanguineous. A putrid, foul discharge may indicate mastoid disease with bone destruction. A sanguineous discharge can occur with acute otitis, but neoplasm or injury also are possible.

Vertigo is the specific sensation of the room spinning, rather than the less discrete "light-headedness" or dizziness. Vertigo often occurs with disease of the labyrinth and may be associated with nausea and vomiting.

Hearing loss is a frightening symptom for anyone. There are three basic types of hearing losses (Table 9–1):

1. *Conductive hearing loss* applies to any disturbance in the conduction of sound impulse as it passes through the ear canal, tympanic membrane, middle ear, and ossicular chain to the footplate of the stapes, which is situated in the oval window. As a general rule, a person with conductive hearing loss speaks softly, hears well on the telephone, and hears best in a noisy environment.
2. *Sensorineural hearing loss* applies to a disturbance anywhere from the cochlea, through the auditory nerve, and on to the hearing center in the cerebral cortex. A person with a sensorineural hearing loss usually speaks loudly, hears better in a quiet environment, and hears poorly in a crowd and on the telephone. He often states that he hears but does not understand (i.e., hears sounds but they are garbled), which is indicative of poor discrimination.
3. *Mixed hearing loss* is a combination of conductive and sensorineural loss.

TABLE 9–1. Common Causes of Hearing Loss

Conductive
    Blockage of the external canal by foreign body, wax, tumor, inflammation with swelling
    Middle ear disease (otitis media), acute or chronic
    Rupture of the tympanic membrane
    Otosclerosis (fixation of the ossicles due to bony overgrowth)

Sensorineural
    Toxins (e.g., aspirin, quinine, aminoglycosides, diuretics)
    Viral disease of the inner ear
    Syphilis
    Cerebellopontine tumor
    Congenital defect
    Ménière's disease
    Trauma to cranial nerve VIII
    Very loud noises, chronic or acute
    Aging
    Late otosclerosis

PHYSICAL EXAMINATION

1. Observe the external ear.
2. Otoscopic examination of the ear canal and tympanic membrane.
3. Check hearing; Weber's test.
4. Rinne's test.

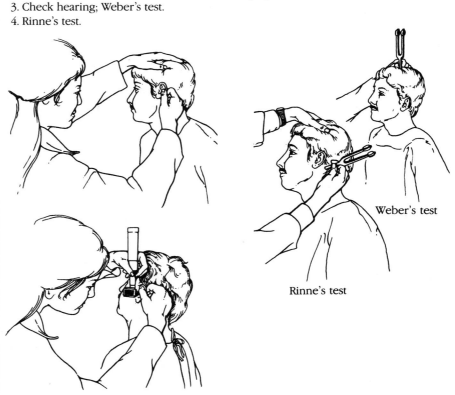

Weber's test

Rinne's test

Abnormalities in the **external ear** may reflect systemic disease, as in alterations of configuration or acuity associated with renal disease and mental retardation. Gouty tophi may occur on the pinna. Pigment or calcium deposition in the ears may give clues to other metabolic disorders.

Examine the lateral and medial surfaces of the auricle, and palpate the mastoid process. The auricle is commonly affected by frostbite, eczema, and sebaceous cysts. Tenderness in the external auditory canal usually indicates furunculosis or external otitis. The external canals may become obstructed by cerumen or foreign bodies, or by certain tumors, particularly exostoses, cysts, and malignant neoplasms. Exostoses (benign bony projections usually associated with prolonged swimming in cold water) are commonly found in the canal; however, these are rarely significant.

The ear canal and tympanic membrane are best examined with a head mirror and ear speculum. However, the battery otoscope is used by most non-otorhinolaryngologists and is adequate. It may be somewhat cumbersome when instrumentation is necessary. The pneumatic otoscope tests the mobility of the tympanic membrane and provides magnification. To obtain proper visualization of the canal and tympanic membrane, *the auricle must be pulled upward and backward.* In infants and small children, the auricle is pulled straight back. The reason for this is that the outer one-third of the canal is directed upward and backward, while the inner two-thirds is directed downward and forward.

The **tympanic membrane** mirrors past and present middle ear disease. With bulging, the landmarks become obscure, and there is usually some thickening and erythema, indicating acute otitis media (Fig. 9–4A). With retraction the landmarks are accentuated. This usually indicates obstruction of the eustachian tube or old scarring from past otitis. An amber-colored membrane indicates serous otitis me-

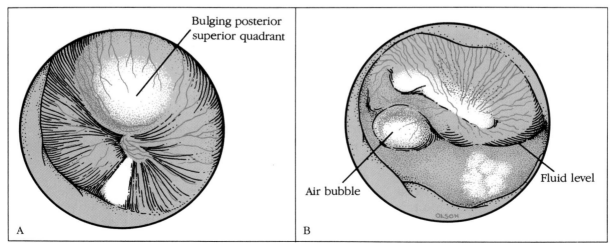

FIGURE 9–4
A. Acute otitis media. B. Serous otitis media. Both are shown in the left drum.

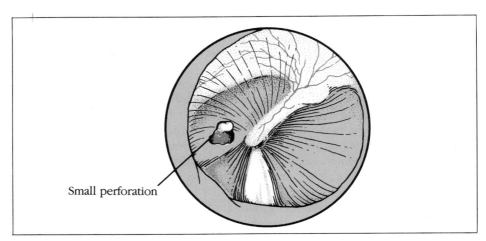

Small perforation

FIGURE 9–5
Perforated drum (*right*).

TABLE 9–2. Tuning Fork Tests

Hearing	Weber's	Rinne's
Normal	Midline	AC > BC bilaterally
Conductive loss	Lateralizes to affected ear	BC > AC affected ear AC > BC normal ear
Sensorineural loss	Lateralizes to normal ear	AC > BC both ears

AC = air conduction; BC = bone conduction.

dia, and air bubbles or a fluid level can at times be seen (Fig. 9–4B). Perforations vary in size and usually point to old inflammatory disease (Fig. 9–5). They may be central (usually benign), anterior, or marginal. Pearly white cholesteatomas may occur in chronic otitis media.

WHISPERED AND SPOKEN VOICE TEST

The test is performed in a quiet room, with the examiner facing the ear to be tested. The other ear is blocked with the examiner's hand. A rough hearing test is then performed 1 foot from the patient's ear. If the patient cannot hear a whispered voice at 1 foot, he has at least a 30-decibel loss. This loss is 60 decibels if he cannot hear a spoken voice at 1 foot.

WEBER'S TEST

This test is accomplished by placing the vibrating tuning fork on the vertex, forehead, or front teeth. With a conductive loss the sound lateralizes to the diseased ear. The reason is that the conductive loss is masking some of the environmental noise, and thus the cochlea is more efficient on the diseased side. The lateralization of the sound or vibrations to the better-hearing ear signifies sensorineural hearing loss in the poorer-hearing ear.

RINNE'S TEST

This test is a comparison of the duration of air conduction with that of bone conduction. The tuning fork is struck against a rubber object with maximum force so that the results will be consistent. It is first held against the mastoid bone. The fork is then held approximately 1 inch from the ear canal opening. Have the patient compare the loudness of the sound with the tuning fork 1 inch from the ear canal (air conduction) to the sound with the tuning fork pressed on the mastoid (bone conduction). Air conduction should normally be louder than bone conduction (AC > BC). Air conduction that is equal to or less than bone conduction indicates a conductive hearing loss.

Another good test is to strike the tuning fork lightly and compare the patient's air and bone conduction with your own. There are many other methods to test the hearing, such as electric audiometry, speech audiometry, and evoked response audiometry.

NOSE

Know that I glory in this nose of mine,
For a great nose indicates a great man—
Genial, courteous, intellectual,
Virile, courageous.

> *Cyrano de Bergerac*
> EDMOND ROSTAND
> (1868–1918)

ANATOMY

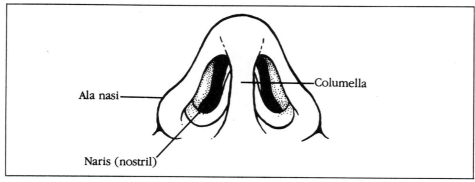

FIGURE 9–6
Frontal view of the nose.

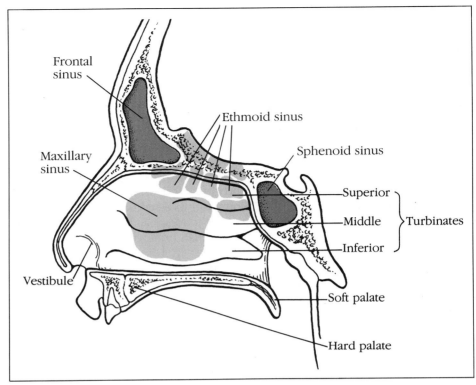

FIGURE 9–7
Lateral view of the nasal cavity.

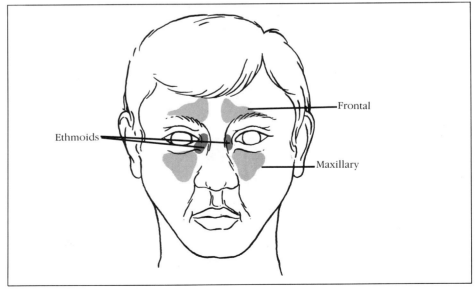

FIGURE 9–8
Paranasal sinuses.

HISTORY

Rhinitis, as in the common cold, is a frequent complaint. Inflammatory disease of the nose is usually on an infectious, allergic, or vasomotor basis. Nasal allergy results in sneezing, watery rhinorrhea, stuffiness, and epiphora. With infections, watery rhinorrhea suggests a viral cause, whereas a thick purulent discharge points to probable superimposed bacterial infection.

Sinusitis rarely, if ever, causes generalized headache. More frequently there is pain and tenderness over the involved sinus. There are numerous orbital complications of sinus disease that are a first sign or symptom (for example, proptosis, pain, diplopia, epiphora, swelling of lid(s), and tumor mass). A purulent nasal discharge is frequently present. Fever and prostration may occur.

Nasal obstruction may be unilateral or bilateral. Unilateral obstruction suggests deviated septum, foreign bodies, or neoplasm. Bilateral obstruction is usually the result of rhinitis. In children, adenoid hypertrophy is a common cause of bilateral obstruction. A deviated septum which is S-shaped may actually obstruct both airways. Nasal polyps are another common cause of bilateral obstruction.

Perforation of the nasal septum may be on a traumatic or infectious basis. Anterior perforation occurs with tuberculosis, while posterior perforation is more common with syphilis. Other causes of septal perforation are lupus erythematosus and the use of catecholamine nasal sprays and cocaine. When **epistaxis** occurs it may arise posteriorly from a branch of the sphenopalatine artery or superiorly from an ethmoid vessel. By far the most common site of epistaxis, however, is the anterior septum (Kiesselbach's plexus), which is easily accessible to the examiner.

PHYSICAL EXAMINATION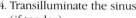

1. Inspect the external nose.
2. With a nasal speculum examine:
    a. Vestibule
    b. Septum
    c. Nasal mucosa
    d. Turbinates
3. Palpate for sinus tenderness.
4. Transilluminate the sinuses (if tender).

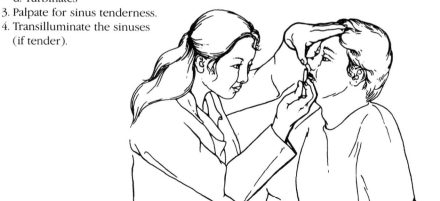

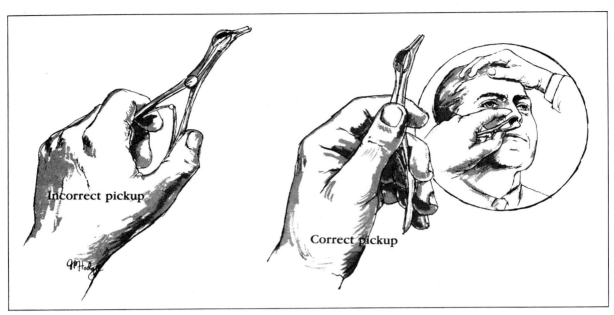

FIGURE 9–9
Use of the nasal speculum.

Begin by examining the **external nose**. The examiner may stand or sit beside and face the patient. Observe and palpate for any loss of structure or support. A nasal speculum is necessary for adequate **intranasal examination** (Fig. 9–9). Be sure not to overdilate the external nasal orifice or to touch the nasal septum with the tip of the speculum, for this will be quite painful. Observe the nasal vestibule; determine the adequacy of the airways. Observe carefully for a deviation of the nasal septum. Check the color of the nasal mucosa and determine whether the turbinates are normal, hypertrophic, edematous, erythematous, or atrophic. If you spray the nose with 0.25% Neo-Synephrine or 1% ephedrine solution and reexamine after a few minutes, the posterior aspect of the nasal cavities and the superior nasopharynx can be visualized in most cases.

Examine the **sinuses** by *palpation* of the roof of the orbit, the ascending processes of the maxillae, and the canine fossae. Tenderness may be elicited, or masses may be palpated.

TRANSILLUMINATION OF THE SINUSES

Transillumination of the sinuses is used as a diagnostic tool for frontal and maxillary sinus disease (Fig. 9–10). The light is placed under the intraoral hard palate for the maxillary sinus and under the supraorbital rim for the frontal sinus. The test is not of true diagnostic value, for the frontal sinus is often underdeveloped. A

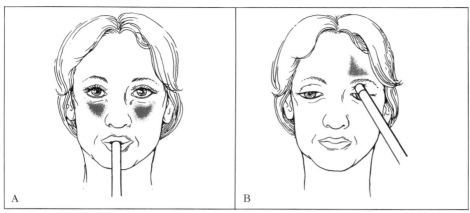

FIGURE 9–10
Transillumination of the sinuses. A. Maxillary. B. Frontal.

sinus filled with clear fluid may transilluminate fairly well, but thickness of soft tissue and bone will interfere with transillumination. This test is used mostly to follow the patient's progress once a clinical and x-ray diagnosis has been made. Transillumination must be carried out in a dark room.

The **internal nose** is the conditioner for inspired and expired air. There are two openings posteriorly, known as choanae, which lead into the nasopharynx and are sometimes referred to as the *posterior nares*. Usually the sinus orifices cannot be visualized during routine rhinoscopy, for they are located in the meati and obscured from vision by the turbinates.

A mucous blanket of viscid secretion covers the entire lining of the nasal cavities. This functions to collect debris and bacteria from the inspired air. The mucous secretion is continuously carried to the nasopharynx by ciliary action. When it reaches the pharynx, it is either swallowed or expectorated.

As the air enters the nasal cavities it is warmed by heat from blood in the cavernous spaces in the turbinates. You will notice that one side of the nose remains more patent than the other at any given time. Blood entering and leaving the cavernous spaces is controlled by the autonomic nervous system. Air is also moistened as it enters the nasal cavities. The parasympathetic supply (vidian nerve) affects turbinate swelling and mucous secretion.

The *olfactory organ* is a small yellowish area on the roof of the nasal cavity and is very difficult to visualize by ordinary rhinoscopy. There are two theories of olfactory function: (1) the undulation theory—that energy waves, similar to light, impinge on the olfactory nerve endings; and (2) the chemical theory—that odorous substances initiate a chemical reaction in the olfactory epithelium.

ORAL CAVITY

Diseases enter by the mouth.

JAPANESE PROVERB

ANATOMY

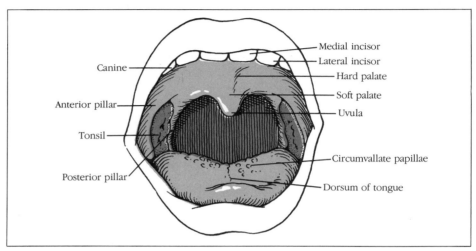

FIGURE 9–11
Anatomy of the mouth.

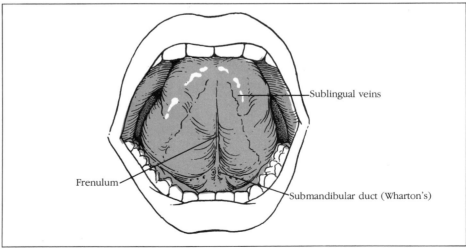

FIGURE 9–12
Sublingual view of the mouth.

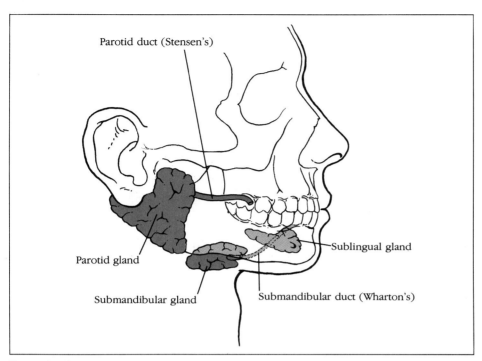

FIGURE 9–13
Salivary system.

HISTORY

The oral cavity is the most accessible body orifice and may reveal significant local diseases as well as signs of systemic diseases. Few areas of the body are exposed to the degree of continuous insult to which the oral tissues are subjected. Constant, mechanical, thermal, chemical, and microbiologic stress makes the tissues of the oral region a significant index of tissue tolerance and systemic defense. Systemic diseases, such as hematologic disorders, diabetes, and exanthematous disease, that reduce tissue tolerance often have oral manifestations. Lesions reactive to local injury also are common in the mouth.

MOUTH AND JAWS

The patient's history is as important to the examination of the mouth as to that of any other part of the body. However, minor discomfort in the oral region is apt to be a common and transient experience. The fact that significant oral pathology may present only slight discomfort should stimulate the examiner to inspect this region with critical interest. Although the mouth and jaw region is commonly examined and treated by the dentist on a periodic basis, it is important for the physician to recognize normality, common abnormalities, and the oral manifestations of systemic diseases. Many conditions will prompt the referral of the patient to a dental specialist for appropriate treatment.

COMMON SYMPTOMS IN THE MOUTH

DRY MOUTH (XEROSTOMIA). This condition is seen with atrophy of salivary glands in senility, disease states, radiation, and as a side effect of many drugs that decrease salivary function.

EXCESS SALIVA (PTYALISM). This is a response of salivation to any mucosal irritation, heavy-metal toxicity, or pilocarpine-like drug action.

COMMON SYMPTOMS AFFECTING THE LIPS

ULCERS. These chiefly occur secondary to vesicular lesions of viral origin and to trauma.

NUMBNESS. In the lower lip, sensory deficit is due to anesthesia or damage to the inferior alveolar nerve in the mandible resulting from trauma, inflammation, or neoplasm.

DROOLING. This is a result of motor loss due to facial nerve paralysis, either peripheral or central.

SWELLING. A rather pronounced response to any inflammatory process, it is sometimes subtle, as in angioneurotic edema and other allergic phenomena.

COMMON SYMPTOMS OF THE TONGUE

COATED TONGUE. Thickening of mucosal keratin, with filiform papillae hypertrophy, is found in response to irritation and immobility and in association with poor oral hygiene.

BURNING TONGUE. Causes of glossodynia are not well defined and include anemias, diabetes, hormonal imbalance, vitamin deficiencies, psychogenic factors, myofascial referred pain, and possible changes in the immune system.

ABNORMAL MOTILITY. Neuromuscular disorders such as stroke and myasthenia gravis induce tongue muscle changes and may cause speech disturbance from faulty tongue action. A fixed, firm tongue may result from infiltration by scar tissue or malignant neoplasm, usually squamous cell carcinoma. Excess frenulum attachment may limit tongue motion (ankyloglossia).

COMMON SYMPTOMS AND SIGNS AFFECTING GUMS AND TEETH

GINGIVAL BLEEDING. This results from local inflammation and infection or hemorrhagic disorders.

GINGIVAL RECESSION. Gingivae recess to a low position on the roots of the teeth with increased age, as a result of trauma from incorrect brushing, and from chronic periodontitis.

GINGIVAL SWELLING. A common sign of odontogenic infection, which also may produce sinus tracts draining dentoalveolar abscesses. *Note:* Enlargement of the gingivae may be seen in a generalized form in conditions of chronic inflammation, pregnancy, endocrine disturbance, phenytoin medication (Dilantin), blood dyscrasias, and as a familial tendency to gingival fibromatosis.

NASOPHARYNX

The nasopharynx may be the site of inflammatory, neoplastic, or congenital disease. Polyps and cysts are not uncommon. When there is obstruction, there may be a change in the quality of the voice because normal voice resonance is produced by the nasopharynx. The student should remember that inflammatory and neoplastic disease of the nasopharynx almost always produce obstruction of the eustachian tube orifice, which will result in hearing loss and otalgia. The resultant negative middle ear pressure causes transudation of serum into the middle ear space.

OROPHARYNX

"Sore throat" is among the most common of patient complaints and may suggest viral or bacterial infection, toxic irritation (as from smoking or thermal injury), trauma, or tumor.

Dysphagia, or difficulty in swallowing, may rarely result from neuromuscular dysfunction of the oropharynx as part of more systemic neurologic disease (e.g., diphtheria, polio, multiple sclerosis, botulism). More commonly, dysphagia is esophageal in origin.

The sensation of a *mass* in the throat can never be ignored, and tumor must be assiduously sought. Globus hystericus, or the feeling of a lump in the throat as a neurotic manifestation, is always a diagnosis of exclusion. Malignant and benign tumors may arise from the buccal mucosa, the tonsils, and the nasopharynx itself.

LARYNGOPHARYNX

The most common indication for careful laryngeal examination is *hoarseness* of more than 2 weeks' duration (Table 9–3). Hoarseness may occur as a result of acute inflammation (laryngitis). Hoarseness may also result from chronic laryngitis due to repeated infections, voice abuse, smoking, tuberculosis, or poor nasal respiration. Hoarseness may occasionally result from congenital abnormalities or benign tumors. It is an extremely important symptom of carcinoma of the larynx. Stridor, dysphagia, severe pain, halitosis, hemoptysis, and cervical adenopathy are advanced symptoms. Hoarseness may be the only early symptom.

Paralysis of the vocal cords causes hoarseness when incomplete. Cord paralysis indicates interruption of the recurrent laryngeal nerve on the same side. This can result from a large number of traumatic, operative, inflammatory, neoplastic, or vascular abnormalities. It is occasionally a symptom of central nervous system disease as well.

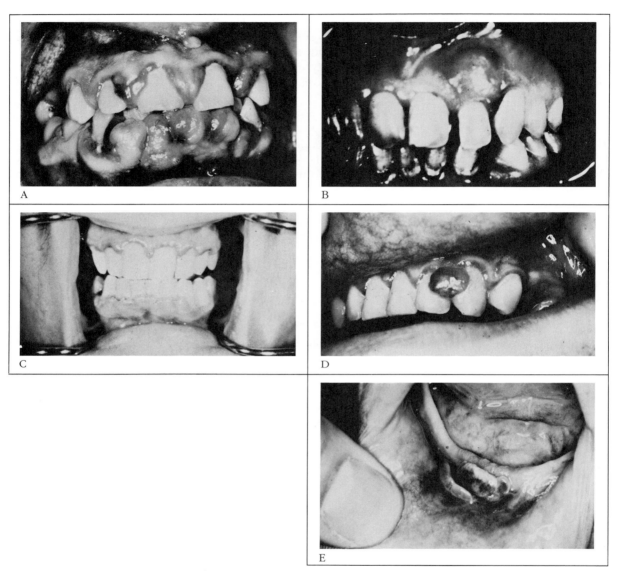

Figure 9–14
Lesions of the gums. A. Normal gingiva. B. Periodontal disease with abscess. C. Vincent's stomatitis. D. Gingival fibroma. E. Fissure from denture irritation.

TABLE 9–3. Some Causes of Hoarseness

Traumatic
    Foreign body
    External injury to larynx
    Voice abuse (singer's nodes)
    Irritant gases (tobacco and other smoke)
    Aspiration (acid, alcohol)

Infectious
    Virus
    Diphtheria
    Syphilis
    Leprosy

Idiopathic
    Sarcoidosis
    Lupus erythematosus
    Cricoarytenoid ankylosis in rheumatoid arthritis

Neurologic
    Recurrent laryngeal nerve injury
    Bulbar palsy
    Myasthenia gravis

Other
    Weakness
    Myxedema
    Acromegaly

PHYSICAL EXAMINATION

1. Inspect the lips, gums, and teeth.
2. Inspect the buccal mucous membrane, including Wharton's and Stensen's ducts.
3. Inspect the hard palate, soft palate, and uvula with and without phonation.
4. Inspect the protruded tongue, both ventral and dorsal surface.
5. Palpate the intraoral structures, including salivary glands.
6. Gently percuss the teeth.
7. Palpate the temporomandibular joint and inspect the range of mandibular motion.
8. Do mirror examination of the nasopharynx (when suggested by symptoms).
9. Do mirror examination of the laryngopharynx (when suggested by symptoms).
10. A quick cranial nerve examination may be done at this time.

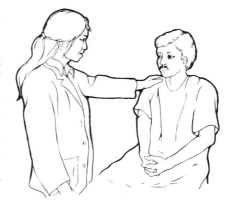

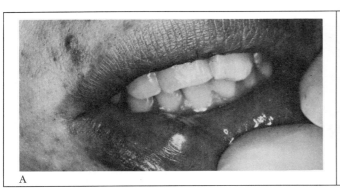
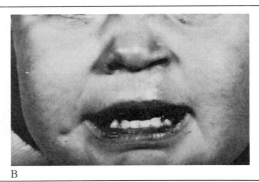

FIGURE 9–15
Lesions of the lips. A. Mucocele of the lip. B. Repaired cleft lip.

MOUTH AND JAWS

The examination of the mouth and jaws is carried out by inspection, palpation, percussion, and transillumination.

Seat the patient comfortably and, if possible, stabilize the head with back support.

Observe the symmetry in form and function of the **lips** in pursing action. The function of the lips in speech, oral intake, control of secretion, and contributing to facial expression is governed by the orbicularis oris muscles. Sensory nerve supply is abundant, and there is a rich blood and lymphatic supply. Accessory salivary glands under the inner aspect of the lips provide lubrication. Because the lips closely cover the hard tooth structure, they are easily injured.

The vermilion surface of the lips in the young shows slight vertical linear markings and a smooth pliable surface. Atrophic changes of the vermilion with age erase the striated pattern and lose the sharp definition at the mucocutaneous junction. Surface keratosis, induration, and ulceration in older individuals should suggest the changes of solar cheilitis, dyskeratosis, or squamous cell carcinoma. Herpetic vesicles, or ulcers of the lip, are common. Fissures with inflammation at the angle of the mouth from loss of dental structures may be seen in the aged, and also may be a feature of nutritional deficiency. Superficial accessory salivary glands of the lip occasionally develop retention cysts (mucocele) (Fig. 9–15A) following injury. Congenital anomalies include folds of the double lip and parasagittal scars in the upper lip from congenital cleft lip repair (Fig. 9–15B). The rich blood and lymphatic supply contributes to rapid edema collection with inflammation of the lips.

Ask the patient to remove any dental appliances. With the patient's mouth only slightly open, retract the lips and cheeks with the tongue blade, and with direct light inspect the inner lip and cheek surfaces and all recesses of the **gingivobuccal fornices** and **gums** (Fig. 9–16).

Attachment of the upper and lower lips in the midline to underlying bone is demonstrated in the normal frenula extending toward the attached gingiva. Posteriorly, similar frenula represent muscle attachments to the alveolar process of the

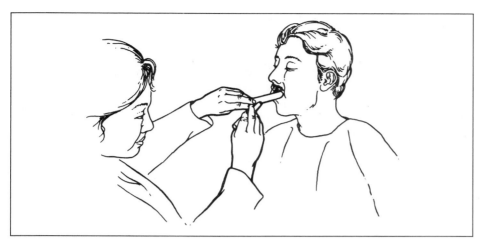

FIGURE 9–16
Examination of the mouth.

jaws. Buccal mucous membrane inspection may reveal a horizontal white line extending from the commissure of the mouth to the retromolar pad, indicating the contact made by the occluding surfaces of the teeth. This may be a zone of hyperkeratotic reaction and shaggy superficial slough when cheek-biting habits are present. A generalized prominence of the posterior buccal mucosa with fairly large buccal fat-pad structures may be seen. There often are small yellow macules or papules indicative of normal sebaceous gland deposition (Fordyce's spots). Recent trauma of the buccal mucosa may produce small spots of submucosal hemorrhage, and similar lesions are produced readily in patients with blood dyscrasias with bleeding tendency.

The **parotid duct orifice** (Stensen's duct) is found in the posterior mucosal surface of the cheek opposite the maxillary second molar. The posterolateral recess behind the tuberosity of the maxillary alveolar process requires mirror inspection for complete vision.

Next, ask the patient to open his mouth wide and tilt his head back so that the **hard and soft palates** can be seen. Depress the dorsum of the tongue with a blade and request "ah" phonation to observe midline uvula elevation and coordinated pharynx constriction. The **tonsils**, aggregated lymphoidal tissue between the anterior and posterior fauces, may be atrophic in adults or surgically absent. Painless enlargement is also common. Lesions of the tonsils include acute tonsillitis, chronic tonsillitis, peritonsillar abscess, tuberculosis of the tonsil(s), and lymphoma.

Morphologic and functional aspects of the hard and soft palates are quite different. The hard palatal vault is composed of underlying body processes of the maxilla covered by dense fibrous tissue and mucosa. In the anterior one-third of the hard palate, specialized ridges of normal palatal rugae are noted, with a midline anterior palatine papilla just behind the central incisor teeth. Cysts in this area are associated with the nasopalatine canal.

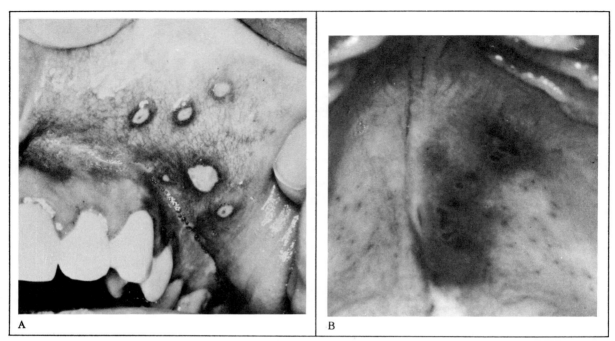

FIGURE 9–17
A. Aphthous stomatitis on movable tissues. B. Herpetic ulcers on immovable tissues.

The most common variation in hard palate structure is seen as a midline hard swelling or exostosis (torus palatinus) (Fig. 9–18). It occurs in 20 percent of the adult population. Such bony growths are benign and are significant only when the surface mucosa becomes ulcerated, or when dental prosthetic requirements necessitate their removal. The soft palate is muscular and has abundant submucosal accessory salivary glands. The normal central position of the soft palate is demonstrated by elevation and reflex.

Soft palate function is coordinated with the pharynx in a constrictor mechanism functioning as the velopharyngeal valve. These actions are essential for normal swallowing and speech.

The palatal vault beneath a maxillary artificial denture may indicate changes of nodular papillomatosis from irritation. Congenital clefts involve both the hard and soft palates and may extend through the alveolar ridge between the canine and lateral incisor teeth. Degrees of original congenital deformity or scar tissue from surgical repair may be noted in these regions of potential cleft. A bifid uvula (Fig. 9–19) may be featured as part of a submucosal cleft palate, which usually includes hypernasal speech.

The chronic irritation of nicotine stomatitis may produce inflammation of the accessory salivary glands with red dilated orifices, in contrast to general white mucosal hyperkeratosis. Palpation of the posterior palatal vault may reveal submucosal

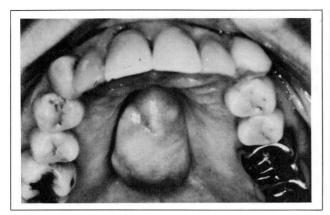

FIGURE 9–18
Torus palatinus.

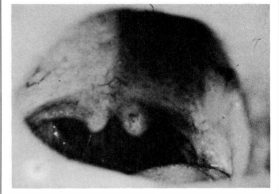

FIGURE 9–19
Bifid uvula.

nodular swelling as the only sign of neoplasm in this region.

Inspect the **oral mucous membranes**. The oral mucosa has a rich vascular supply and a resilient, flexible epithelial surface. Except for the vermilion tissue of the lips, the oral mucosal surfaces are kept moist by numerous submucosal accessory salivary glands adding to the major salivary gland secretions.

Normal mucosal surfaces are pale coral pink. Bright red surfaces generally indicate the erythema of inflammation, while pallor indicates localized ischemia or generalized anemia. Cyanotic color changes may indicate local congestion or many systemic states that produce hypoxemia. The oral mucous membranes are normally pigmented and variations in generalized and local melanin may occur on the basis of race. Local deposits of brown pigment in the mucosa also are seen in some metabolic disturbances, such as hypoadrenalism (Addison's disease). Linear pigmentation of the terminal capillary beds of the gingival margin may indicate heavy-metal absorption, which may correlate with toxic symptoms. Localized bluish pigmentation in the gingival areas that is not related to underlying vascular abnormality may be due to the accidental implantation of metal dental filling materials (amalgam tattoo).

The most frequent surface changes of the oral mucous membranes are ulcers and white patches. Increase in the layer of mucosal keratin produces white, thickened patches. Candidal infection will also produce white plaques. Ulceration is indicative of trauma or secondary lesions following initial vesicles of viral or other primary disease lesions. AIDS-related complex (ARC) markers in the oral regions include hairy leukoplakia (Fig. 9–20B), Kaposi's sarcoma, and candidiasis. Herpetic ulcers generally occur on the attached tissues of the palate or gingiva, whereas canker sores occur on movable mucosal tissues (see Fig. 9–17, A, B).

Swelling of the oral mucosa and submucosa may be found on the basis of inflammation, reactive hyperplasia, cysts, congenital deformities, and neoplasm, in that order of frequency. Many submucosal swellings are detected only by careful palpation.

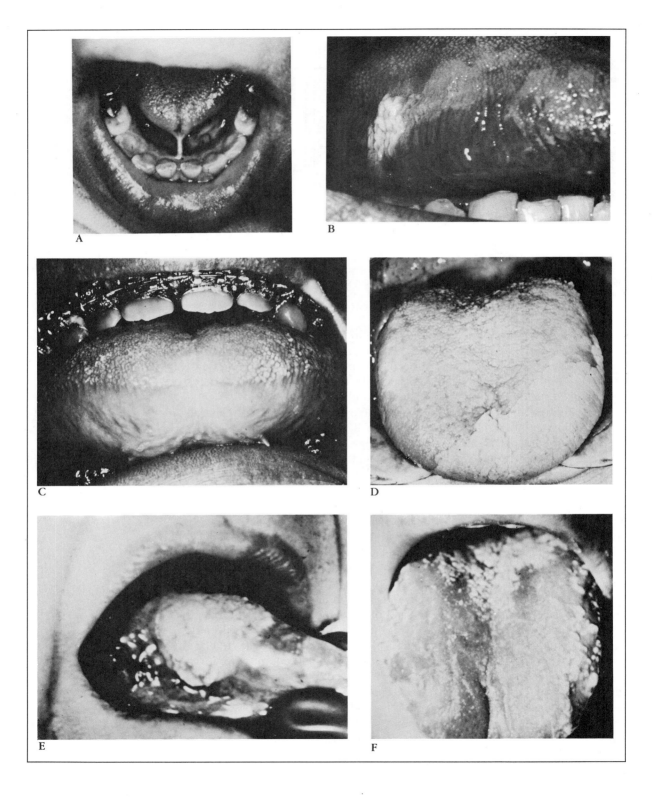

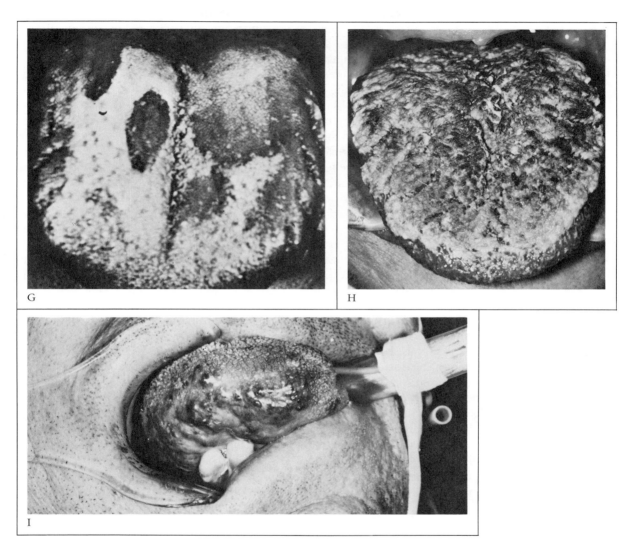

FIGURE 9–20
Some lesions of the tongue. A. Lingual frenulum (ankyloglossia). B. Hairy leukoplakia (AIDS). C. Macroglossia. D. Leukoplakia. E. Cancer of the tongue. F. Candidiasis. G. Geographic tongue. H. Black hairy tongue. I. Hemangioma of the tongue.

The examiner should look for bleeding from any surface. Such a finding dictates great care in locating the source of bleeding and the tissue characteristics of the bleeding source (inflammatory or neoplastic).

Have the patient resume the original head examination position and protrude the **tongue**. Note here the symmetry and muscle coordination of midline protrusion as well as the dorsal surface characteristics of the tongue (Fig. 9–20). Complete the inspection of the oral cavity by retracting the patient's tongue laterally to view its posterior surface and the floor of the mouth. The importance of this maneuver lies in the frequency of malignancy in this area. Ask the patient to touch the hard palate with the tip of the tongue in the open-mouth position. Observe the ventral surface of the tongue and structures in the anterior floor of the mouth. Tongue mobility and function are essential to speech, mastication, taste, and swallowing.

The specialized mucosa of the dorsum of the tongue presents papillae of filiform, fungiform, and circumvallate types; at the posterolateral borders of the tongue, ridges of foliate papillae are noted. Many variations of the pattern of papillae are seen. Atrophy leaves a red, smooth surfaced appearance suggesting nutritional deficiency or pernicious anemia. Hypertrophy and hyperkeratosis of the filiform papillae may present a furred, hairy surface. Such a thick coat, which may be pigmented, is a condition associated with poor oral hygiene. A midline elevated area in the posterior dorsum of the tongue represents the congenital benign lesion of median rhomboid glossitis. A striking pattern of arcuate variations in papillary distribution is seen in transient forms in the benign condition known as geographic tongue. The dorsum of the tongue is deeply furrowed in a congenital morphologic variation in some 5 percent of the population (fissued tongue). Macroglossia may be indicative of hypothyroidism as well as a number of inflammatory, cystic, congenital, and neoplastic variations (Table 9–4). Lesions that produce asymmetric tongue enlargement are hemangioma, lymphangioma, and neurofibroma.

Ventrally the **lingual frenulum** is noted at the midline attached to the gingiva at the symphysis of the mandible. The sublingual caruncles at the orifices of the submandibular ducts are noted and the flow of secretion is observed. The floor of the mouth may be the site of retention cysts of the sublingual glands, producing soft translucent swellings (called a ranula). Occasionally a localized stone in the course of the submandibular duct (Wharton's) may be palpated and will produce obstructive symptoms. Exostosis of the mandible is seen as a hard mass projecting toward the floor of the mouth from the region of bone supporting the premolar teeth (torus mandibularis) (Fig. 9–21). Similar hard swelling may be noted in the midline of the mandible at the position of the genial tubercles, which are especially prominent when teeth are gone and the alveolar process has atrophied.

Begin palpation by asking the patient to stick out his tongue, which is then grasped between layers of gauze. With this control, use the index finder of the opposite hand, covered with a finger cot, to palpate the soft, smooth tongue surfaces gently but firmly. Release the tongue and continue palpation of the floor of the mouth. Palpate these sublingual structures, with the opposite hand supporting the submental and submandibular tissues. Bimanually palpate between oral mucosa and facial skin in the cheek and lip regions. Conclude palpation with the hard

TABLE 9–4. Macroglossia

Acute
  Injury with hemorrhage or edema
  Hemorrhage without injury (bleeding disorders)
  Toxic insect sting to tongue (e.g., bee sting)
  Angioneurotic edema
  Infections (streptococcal—Ludwig's angina)
  Pemphigus
Chronic
  Generalized enlargement
    Hypothyroidism (cretinism)
    Down syndrome
    Acromegaly
  Local enlargement
    Irritation (e.g., by tooth)
    Tumor
    Gumma
    Tuberculosis
    Actinomycosis
    Calculus in sublingual salivary gland
    Angioma
    Lipoma
    Amyloidosis

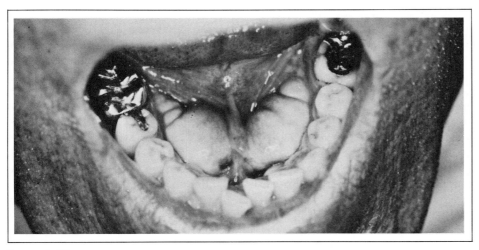

FIGURE 9–21
Torus mandibularis.

TABLE 9–5. Some Causes of Parotid Enlargement

Acute
  Infection
    Virus (especially mumps)
    Bacteria
  Recurrent mucus plugging Stensen's duct
  Calculi in Stensen's duct
  Trauma
Chronic
  Lead or mercury poisoning
  Iodides
  Thiouracil
  Lymphoma
  Lymphoblastoma
  Solid tumors of parotid
  Chronic alcoholism
  Diabetes mellitus
  Sarcoidosis
  Actinomycosis
  Chronic insufflation (trumpeter's parotitis)

and soft palate areas. Note the flow and secretion from the orifices of the submandibular and parotid ducts.

The **submandibular gland** can be palpated directly under the ramus of the mandible about halfway between the chin and the angle of the jaw. It has a firm, irregular consistency. This gland can be more accurately palpated bimanually. Place the index finger of one hand on the floor of the mouth, between the lateral aspect of the tongue and the teeth. With the other hand, palpate the gland externally. An overlying lymph node can also often be palpated. The submandibular glands descend and become more prominent with advancing age; this is frequently misinterpreted as enlargement of the glands. The **parotid gland** is located anterior to and below the auricle. It normally extends from the sternomastoid muscle anteriorly to the masseter muscle (Table 9–5 presents some causes of parotid enlargement). Unless they are abnormal, the numerous sublingual glands cannot be palpated with any degree of accuracy. When infiltrated with neoplastic tissue, the sublingual gland becomes well defined and indurated.

Examine the **gingivae**. The gingival tissues covering the alveolar process normally have a pale coral-pink color and slightly stippled surface. (See Fig. 9–14A). Normal gingivae attach to the teeth, and gingival projections fill the interdental spaces as papillae. Gingivitis is a common inflammatory reaction that may result from local factors of irritation and infection. The most common irritant to this region is the deposition of dental calculus around the necks of teeth. This hard deposit is particularly abundant in the anterior mandibular teeth and the maxillary molar teeth near the orifices of the major salivary gland ducts. The epithelial attachment of the gingivae to the necks of the teeth is lost in the lesions of periodontal disease, with the production of pocket lesions adjacent to the teeth and loss of supporting soft tissue and bone (chronic periodontitis). The presence of pocket

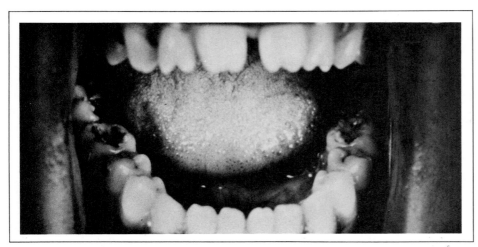

FIGURE 9–22
Hutchinson's incisors.

lesions and the level of gingival attachment are determined with a fine probe. A combination of painful gums with bleeding from the free gingival margins, pseudomembrane, and loss of interdental papillae are seen in ulcerative gingival stomatitis (Vincent's infection). Although the acute symptoms of this process may be attenuated by antiinfective medication, comprehensive dental treatment is required to eliminate the disease process. The most common localized gum inflammation is around the impacted mandibular third molar (pericoronitis). Local care and prompt removal of the third molar are required and may prevent the extension of infection into the fascial spaces of the neck.

Examine the **teeth** for their form, function, and support in the jaws. Light percussion with a mirror handle may be helpful in localizing painful dental conditions. The normal white enamel surface of the crowns of teeth becomes dark with surface stains and also with devitalization of the pulp of teeth through trauma or disease. The crowns of teeth may be irregular in form because of congenital hypoplasia, may become reduced in length by attrition, and may be broken down by destructive phases of dental caries. Classic hypoplasia of the incisors in congenital syphilis creates the notched and barrel-shaped Hutchinson's incisor (Fig. 9–22).

Normally the teeth are firmly anchored in the alveolar process by the periodontal membrane. Hypermobility of permanent teeth (adult) may be due to injury but is most frequently seen in advanced periodontal disease. Localized hypermobility of teeth should alert the examiner to consider alveolar bone destruction by neoplastic disease (primary or metastatic).

Observe the excursions of the mandible and occlusion of the teeth that determine the functional potentials of the masticating system. Palpate the condyles of the temporomandibular joint by placing your fourth ("little") fingers in the external auditory canals during jaw excursions. Palpate over the condylar head of the

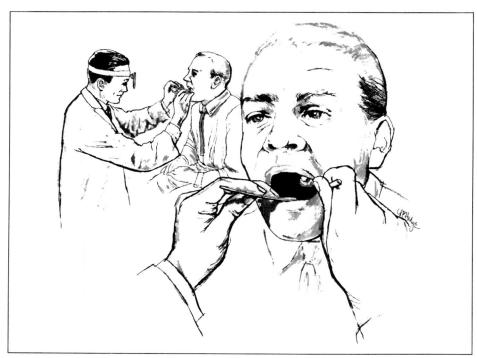

FIGURE 9–23
Technique of examination of the nasopharynx.

joints during opening and closing. Also palpate the condylar neck. Note and isolate painful responses in these three areas. Movement should be symmetric and painless. Auscultate both joints for crepitus, which may indicate abnormal coordination of meniscal movements. Lateral excursions of the joints should be similarly painless. Determine if there is a history of locking in either open or closing movements. The normal excursion of the jaws will admit the width of three contracting fingers of the patient's hand (3.5 to 4.5 cm).

The excursions of the mandible should be smooth and gliding in type. Restriction of the mandible may be caused by disturbances in the temporomandibular joint, extra-articular restriction by scar tissue, trismus from spasm of the elevating muscles of mastication from any inflammatory cause, and the specific contractions of hysteria or tetanus. Findings of crepitus or pain may be indicative of disturbances in the temporomandibular joint.

NASOPHARYNX

Although it is not part of a routine physical examination, the student should familiarize himself with the technique of looking into the nasopharynx (Fig. 9–23). A size 0 through 3 mirror is used. The mirror is warmed by a flame, by being im-

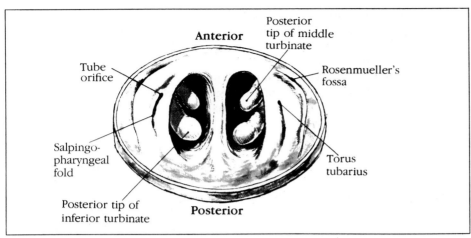

FIGURE 9–24
Mirror view of the nasopharynx.

mersed in hot water, or by being held over an electric light bulb. If no heat is available, place a thick soapy solution on the mirror and wipe it off without rinsing. Both of these techniques prevent fogging of the mirror by the patient's breath. The patient sits directly in front of the examiner. The examiner's and the patient's heads should be at the same level. Ask the patient to sit erect and well back in the chair with his head projected slightly forward.

Depress the tongue into the floor of the mouth with the left hand, making sure not to extend the tip of the tongue blade posterior to the middle third of the tongue. Light is reflected into the pharynx with a head mirror. Grasp the mirror with the right hand as one would hold a pencil and slip it behind and to one side of the uvula. Encourage the patient to breathe naturally and not to hold his breath; asking the patient to breathe through his nose or to hum often relaxes a tense palate and opens the nasopharynx for examination. Be careful not to touch the base of the tongue. When necessary, 2% tetracaine (not to exceed 80 mg) or 4% cocaine (not to exceed 20 mg) solution may be sprayed into the pharynx to control the gag reflex. Figure 9–24 shows the important landmarks.

The nasopharynx extends from the choanae to the inferior border of the soft palate. Looking anteriorly from the nasopharynx into the nose, the posterior border of the nasal septum dividing the two choanae can be seen. In each choana, the posterior tips of the middle and inferior turbinates can be visualized.

Adenoid tissue is present on the posterior wall (usually absent by age 16 years). This mass of lymphoid tissue is also known as the pharyngeal tonsil. The adenoid is connected with the palatine and lingual tonsils by a band of lymphoid tissue extending down the lateral pharyngeal wall. This entire lymphoid complex is known as Waldeyer's ring.

The mucous blanket passes from the nose into the oropharynx by way of the nasopharynx. Under normal conditions, the nasal mucosa produces approximately a quart of seromucous fluid a day. When this amount is decreased as a result of nasal or environmental factors, the mucous blanket becomes greatly thickened. It is then referred to as postnasal drip, and the patient is quite conscious of this concentrated form of secretion. Smoking and air pollutants tend to thicken the mucus and intensify the symptoms of postnasal drip, which at times is seen as white or yellow strands or webs in the nasopharynx.

LARYNGOPHARYNX

Inspection of the laryngopharynx is not considered part of the routine physical examination. It should be done if the patient complains of prolonged hoarseness or change of voice. To examine the laryngopharynx, a size 4 through 6 mirror is used (Fig. 9–25). The mirror is prepared as described in **Nasopharynx**, above. Instruct the patient to sit erect, with his head projected slightly forward. Grasp the tongue with a piece of folded gauze. It is important that the thumb be on top of the tongue and the second finger be underneath the tip of the tongue. The index finger elevates the upper lip. Insert the mirror after testing the temperature on the back of the left hand. Place it in the oropharynx so that it elevates the uvula. Touching the lateral walls, tonsils, or back of the tongue will cause gagging. If the patient has a hypersensitive gag reflex, discontinue the examination and spray the pharynx with 2% tetracaine or 4% cocaine solution. Cetacaine spray is also useful and has a more rapid onset of anesthesia. Wait 4 or 5 minutes before resuming the indirect laryngoscopy.

First ask the patient to breathe quietly and not to hold his breath. Especially reassure the patient that you will not obstruct his airway. Then ask him to say "a-a-a-a-a" and "e-e-e-e-e." This will bring the larynx up and back to facilitate visualization. Observe the landmarks, listed below (see also Fig. 9–26).

1. Base of tongue—lingual tonsils
2. Epiglottis
3. Arytenoids
4. Aryepiglottic folds
5. True and false vocal cords
6. Trachea
7. Hypopharynx
8. Pyriform sinuses
9. Mouth of the esophagus

The intrinsic muscles of the larynx act on its cartilaginous framework to tense, relax, abduct, and adduct the vocal cords. This action can be observed during indirect laryngoscopy. The sphincteric action of the laryngopharynx can also be noted during swallowing. The trachea is guarded by three layers of sphincters: the epiglottis and aryepiglottic folds, the false cords, and the true cords.

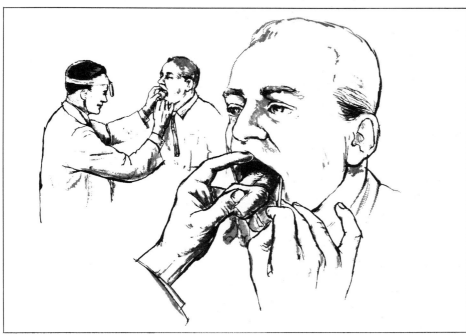

FIGURE 9–25
Technique of examination of the laryngopharynx.

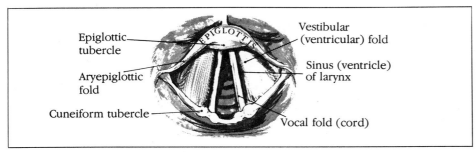

FIGURE 9–26
Mirror view of the laryngopharynx.

TABLE 9–6. Quick Cranial Nerve Examination

Cranial Nerve	Observation
I	Smell. Is there sense of smell? (seldom useful)
II	Vision.
III, IV, VI	Extraocular movements and pupillary responses.
V	Muscles of mastication. Ask the patient to clench his teeth, and feel the masseter contract.
VII	Facial muscles. Ask the patient to smile, and watch his face for symmetry.
VIII	Hearing.
IX	Muscles of soft palate and palatal symmetry. Watch motion when the patient says "Ah-h-h."
X	Muscles of pharynx and larynx. Is the patient hoarse? Is his swallowing normal?
XI	Trapezius muscles. Ask the patient to shrug his shoulders.
XII	Muscles of tongue. Ask the patient to stick out his tongue.

CRANIAL NERVES

Before leaving the examination of the head, you may wish to complete the cranial nerve examination that has been partially done already as a normal component of examination of the eyes, ears, nose, and throat. Any historical suggestion of cranial nerve dysfunction would, of course, dictate a far more thorough cranial nerve examination than that outlined in Table 9–6.

CHAPTER 10

NECK

*The enlargement of the thyroid, of which I am now speaking, seems to be
essentially different from goiter in not attaining a size at all equal to that
observed in the latter disease. Indeed, this enlargement deserves, rather, the name
hypertrophy.*

ROBERT JAMES GRAVES
(1795–1853)

Pain in the neck, a common joke, is not funny to those who have it. It may indicate
disorders of musculoskeletal function but also may accompany infection of the
meninges or intracranial bleeding—grave medical emergencies. Symptoms in the
neck may suggest pathology of the structures therein (thyroid, trachea, esophagus,
muscles), may signal disease in head or chest (nodes, referred pain, meningitis),
or may be a feature of systemic illness (tetanus, myopathies).

ANATOMY

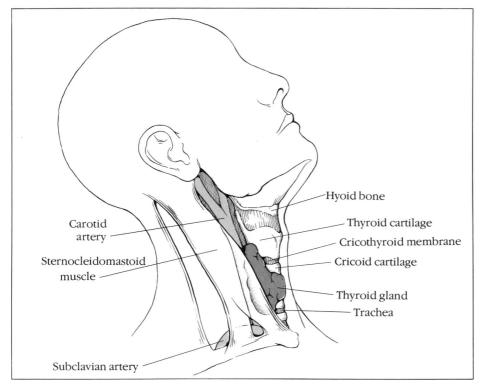

FIGURE 10–1
Structures of the neck identifiable by palpation.

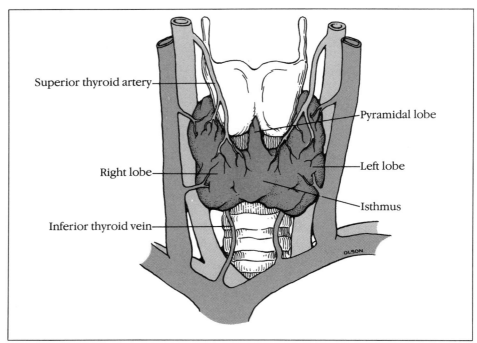

Figure 10–2
Anatomy of the thyroid gland.

HISTORY

NECK

Cervical muscle spasm is a frequent cause of so-called tension headache, characterized by predominantly occipital pain. The rapid onset of a **stiff neck**, especially if accompanied by fever and headache,* is a symptom that calls for immediate evaluation for *meningitis* (other causes of stiff neck are given in Table 10–1). Neck pain may occur as one of the referred pain patterns of *acute myocardial infarction.*

Masses in the neck may be lymph nodes (as with Hodgkin's disease, cancers of the mouth and throat, and thyroid cancer), infections producing enlarged nodes and/or abscess (pharyngitis, tuberculosis [scrofula], actinomycosis), or cysts. Inflammatory or neoplastic disease of the salivary glands may present as a painless or painful neck mass.

THYROID

The thyroid gland may enlarge as a result of iodine deficiency or as a result of the action of goitrogens, with or without other clinical evidence of thyroidal dysfunction. Neoplastic and inflammatory disease may also produce enlargement of the thyroid.

---

*Abrupt stiff neck with excruciating basilar headache ("the worst headache ever," according to the patient) warns of subarachnoid hemorrhage.

TABLE 10–1. Some Causes of Cervical Muscle Spasm (Stiff Neck)

Exposure to cold, as with a draft

Strain (physical or emotional)

Abnormal positioning of the head for protracted periods (attending altered vision, poor sleeping posture, prolonged reading, etc.)

Enlarged lymph nodes, abscesses, tumors of the neck

Inflammation of muscles of the neck

Cervical spine arthritis or radiculitis (traumatic, inflammatory, infectious, neoplastic)

Muscle disease (parkinsonism, phenothiazines, myotonia)

Tetanus

Acute thyroiditis

Congenital wryneck (torticollis)

TABLE 10–2. Thyrotoxicosis: Thyroid Physiology and Pathophysiology

I. Physiology

TRH = thyrotropin-releasing hormone
TSH = thyroid-stimulating hormone
T_3 = triiodothyronine
T_4 = tetraiodothyronine

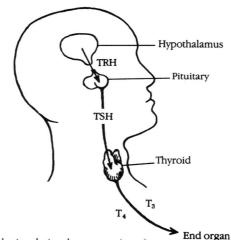

II. Pathophysiology of thyrotoxicosis
  A. Diffuse enlargement of the thyroid
    1. Graves' disease
    2. Due to activity similar to that of thyroid-stimulating hormone (rare)
      a. Choriocarcinoma
      b. Hydatidiform mole
      c. Hepatoma
      d. Pituitary adenoma secreting thyroid-stimulating hormone
  B. Nodular, enlarged thyroid
    1. Graves' disease (unusual)
    2. Toxic multinodular goiter (Plummer's disease)
    3. Toxic uni-nodular goiter (functional thyroid adenoma; thyroid gland itself may not be enlarged)
  C. Tender, enlarged thyroid
    1. Subacute thyroiditis
    2. Hashimoto's thyroiditis (occasionally tender)
    3. Irradiation thyroiditis
    4. Iodine thyroiditis (Jod-Basedow) (occasionally tender)
  D. Nonpalpable thyroid
    1. Factitious hyperthyroidism—ingestion of excess thyroid hormone
    2. Struma ovarii
    3. Metastatic thyroid carcinoma
    4. Graves' disease (gland may be nonpalpable)

Thyrotoxicosis, the metabolic expression of overproduction of thyroid hormone(s), usually is accompanied by clinical thyroidal enlargement (Table 10–2) and weight loss/with disappearance of subcutaneous fat. Other symptoms may include intolerance heat, easy sweating, increased emotional lability, wakefulness, tremulousness, palpitations, easy fatigability, diarrhea, and double vision (see Chap. 4).

Hypothyroidism, the metabolic expression of underproduction of thyroid hormone, often is accompanied by clinical thyroid enlargement. Myxedema, the result of severe and often prolonged hypothyroidism, presents characteristic symptoms. The patient may feel "puffy" and complain of continual coldness. He may note a dry skin, hoarsening and deepening of the voice, thinning and increased brittleness of the hair, fatigue, slowing of thought and movement and chronic constipation (see Fig. 4–7).

It should be appreciated that these are descriptions of symptomatic, classic, or fully developed states of thyroid dysfunction in the adult. Hypothyroidism in the child may result in dwarfism, in which case body skeletal proportions tend toward the infantile.

PHYSICAL EXAMINATION

1. Inspect for symmetry, pulses, masses.
2. Check range of motion, passive and active.
3. Palpate nodes, trachea, carotids, thyroid.
4. Auscultate thyroid, carotids, supraclavicular arteries.

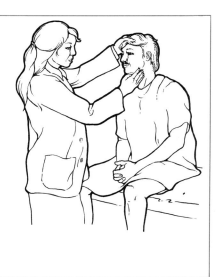
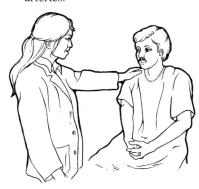

The glands in the neck had assumed the form of large, smooth, ovoid masses connected together merely by loose cellular membrane and minute vessels; when cut into they exhibited a firm cartilaginous structure, of a light colour and very feeble vascularity, but with no appearance of softening or suppuration.

THOMAS HODGKIN
(1798–1866)

NECK

With the patient sitting and his neck illuminated obliquely, if possible with day light, inspect the neck for symmetry, pulsations, masses, and range of motion. Have the

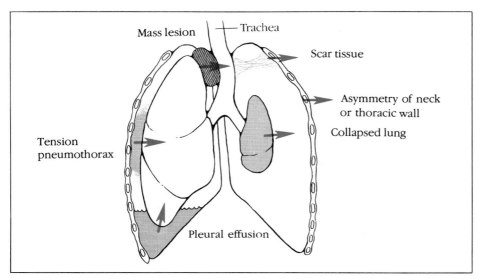

FIGURE 10–3
Causes of tracheal deviation.

patient touch his chin to his breastbone. If he must open his mouth to do this, some degree of stiffness or pain in the neck is suggested. Touching the ear to the shoulder tests lateral flexion. Hyperextension of the neck tests mobility and, in addition, throws the thyroid gland and trachea into more prominent view. Hyperextension should not be attempted in an individual with severe rheumatoid arthritis, however, as this may cause serious harm because of involvement of axial cervical joints by synovitis. Both normal and abnormal structures are further evaluated by gentle palpation.

The **trachea** is midline, and any deviation to either side must be noted (Fig. 10–3). Such deviation may be caused by a pulling of the trachea to right or left, as by scar tissue, tumor, or ipsilateral collapse of lung; the trachea may be pushed to the contralateral side by a mass lesion in the neck or increased pressure in the chest (e.g., tension pneumothorax). The "tracheal tug" of aortic aneurysm is the pulsation of the aorta transmitted through the trachea, felt when the examiner palpates the cricoid cartilage and extends the patient's neck.

Palpation of the **lymph nodes** in the neck is systematically done (see Chap. 7) as part of the neck exam or, as you prefer, as a segment of general nodal examination.

Palpation of the **carotid pulses** should be done with gentle care (Fig. 10–4). Carotid pressure receptor reflexes may slow the heart if massage is too vigorous. Moreover, especially in the elderly, vigorous massage may occlude blood flow to the brain or break off an atheromatous plaque, sending the fragment as an embolus to the cerebral cortex and precipitating a stroke. Always ask the patient whether he is left- or right-handed and begin by palpating the carotid on the side of handedness because the cerebral hemisphere on that side is nondominant. In this way, if

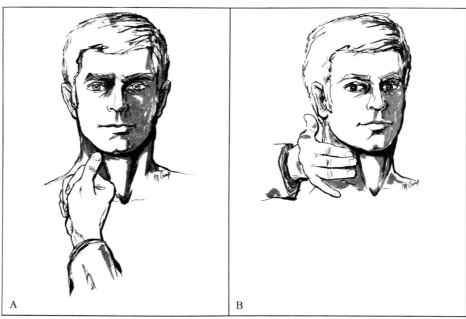

FIGURE 10–4

Technique of carotid palpation. A. Some examiners prefer to stand in front of the patient and use the thumb on the carotid artery for analysis of the arterial pulse contour. This also allows one to examine the neck veins easily without changing position while using the carotid pulse for timing purposes. B. Others prefer to use three fingers from behind or at the side of the patient.

embolism or occlusion results (fortunately, extremely rare), the nondominant hemisphere will be affected.

An aneurysm of the carotid artery may produce a striking pulsatile enlargement on one side of the neck. Any high-output state (aortic insufficiency, thyrotoxicosis, fever) may also result in dramatic pulsations of both carotids.

To auscultate the carotid in the neck, ask the patient to hold his breath (to eliminate airway sounds), and listen with the diaphragm of the stethoscope over each carotid. The supraclavicular fossae should be auscultated for bruits in the same way. Don't forget to tell your patient to begin breathing again after you've finished!

Venous pulsations in the neck, a valuable clue to cardiac function, are discussed in Chapter 12. They are observed both during examination of the neck (with the patient sitting) and again as part of the cardiac examination (with the patient supine).

Torticollis or wryneck causes deviation of the head to one side. This often very painful condition may be a consequence of drugs, congenital disease, muscle strain, or infection.

THYROID

The **thyroid gland** is examined by inspection, palpation and auscultation. This is best accomplished with examiner and patient seated facing one another. When the thyroid is located substernally it frequently is enlarged, in which case it may be detected by percussion of the chest at the manubrium (restrosternal dullness). Movement of the thyroid, produced by the act of swallowing, aids in its inspection and palpation. Sips of water allow repetitive swallowing. Face the patient and observe the base of the neck as he swallows. Repeat the observation with the patient slightly extending his neck. The normal thyroid gland usually is not visible. An enlargement may be evident as a subtle fullness that glides upward transiently on swallowing. Such movement is more easily appreciated when the neck is slightly extended and illuminated by obliquely directed natural light. Turn off the artificial light and raise the window shades.

The thyroid gland is frequently not palpable in normal patients. However, in the average asthenic individual it is felt as a vague layer of tissue that glides briefly beneath the fingers, rising slightly with swallowing. The isthmus can usually be felt as a soft transverse band below the cricoid cartilage.

The examiner may palpate the thyroid gland from a position in front of or behind the patient (Fig. 10–5). In either case relaxation of the muscles of the patient's neck and shoulder greatly eases the examination; relaxation results from a gentle shake of the patients shoulder(s) and a word of encouragement. Flexion of the patient's neck toward the lobe being examined results in relaxation of the corresponding sternocleidomastoid muscle, and this facilitates palpation. When the examiner is behind the patient, he lightly places the tips of the first two or three fingers of both hands on either side of the patient's trachea, slightly below the level of the thyroid cartilage. First, explore for the thyroid isthmus by palpating over the anterior surface of the trachea from the cricoid cartilage downward to the thoracic inlet; an enlarged isthmus is most often accompanied by enlargement of the lateral lobes. Both lobes are then surveyed simultaneously as the patient swallows. A light, rotary motion of the examiner's fingers will help to delineate nodules and irregularities. Next, palpate each side separately. Flex the neck to the side being examined. The first two fingers of the left hand are used to palpate the right lobe, while the right hand is placed behind the sternocleidomastoid muscle to evert the gland as much as possible. The left lobe is similarly examined with the neck flexed slightly to that side. With each maneuver the patient is asked to swallow. Palpation should be gentle because vigorous pressure may cause soreness, choking, or cough, and tension of the neck muscles, making further examination difficult.

Seated in front of the patient, examine the right lobe. Use the right thumb to displace the larynx and the gland to the side being examined. With the left first and second fingers placed behind the sternocleidomastoid muscle, attempt to palpate the underlying thyroid tissue between these fingers and the thumb of that hand. The left side is examined by exchanging the relative positions of the examiner's hands.

A variation of this technique that is useful for smaller goiters is to rest the hand on the base of the neck and palpate the thyroid with the thumb. The right hand is

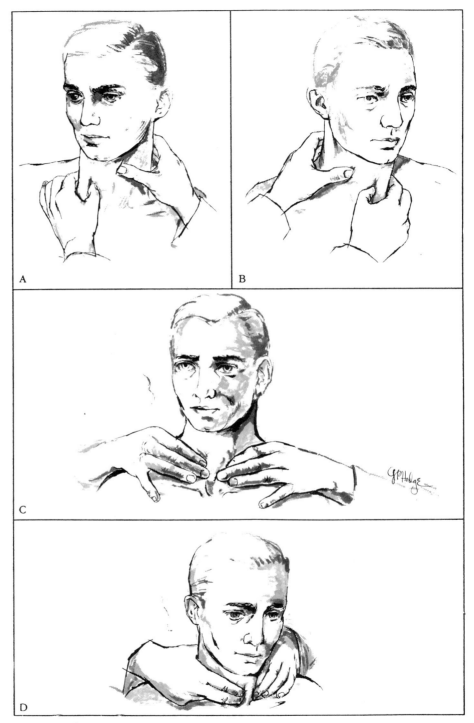

FIGURE 10–5
Examination of the thyroid gland. A. Anterior (lateral deviation to the right). B. Anterior (lateral deviation to left). C. Posterior. D. Lateral deviation posterior.

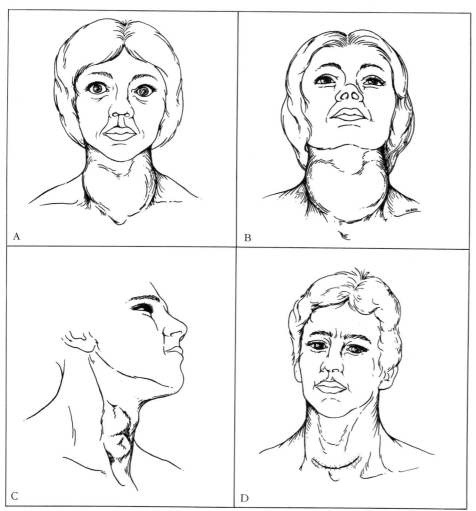

FIGURE 10–6
Thyroid abnormalities. A. Diffuse toxic goiter (Graves' disease). B. Diffuse nontoxic goiter. C. Nodular goiter. D. Thyroidectomy scar.

used to examine the left lobe; the left hand, the right lobe. Experienced examiners may use only the thumb of one hand. Patients appreciate this gentle approach.

Enlargement of the gland into the thoracic inlet may prevent palpation of the lower poles. An enlarged gland that has descended into the thoracic inlet may occasionally be made to rise into the neck and become visible when the patient performs the Valsalva maneuver. Percussible retrosternal dullness can also help in delineating such enlargement.

Auscultate the thyroid with the stethoscope. Because of the increased thyroidal blood flow that occurs with thyrotoxicosis due to hyperthyroidism, a hum or systolic bruit—sometimes accompanied by a thrill—may be detectable over the gland. If there is a goiter or thrill, or historical suspicion of hyperthyroidism, examine the skin, which is classically warm and moist with a fine velvety texture. The eyes may protrude. The eye findings in thyrotoxicosis (Table 8–2) result from:

1. Retraction of the lids, which produces widening of the palpebral fissures, exposure of more sclera, especially evident inferiorly, a staring expression, and lid lag.
2. Swelling of the extraocular muscles and other orbital contents, which produces forward displacement of the globe.
3. Swelling of the conjunctivae (chemosis), due in part to orbital swelling and in part to the effects of trauma to the exposed globe.
4. Weakness of the extraocular muscles, with limitation of upward gaze. Later, convergence and lateral movement may be impaired.

There may be a fine tremor of the hands, onycholysis (more commonly of the fourth and fifth fingers), and exaggeration of the deep tendon reflexes in the **hyperthyroid** patient. The pulse rate is almost invariably elevated, and the pulse has a bounding quality. The pulse pressure is widened due to an elevation of the systolic pressure, the result of increased cardiac stroke volume. Cardiac arrhythmias are common. The heart sounds are loud and hyperactive (particularly the first sound), and a functional systolic murmur may be present. In Graves' disease, warmth and elevation of skin over the shins may occur (pretibial myxedema).

The most common cause of **hypothyroidism** in the United States is Hashimoto's thyroiditis. The gland characteristically is moderately enlarged, the isthmus and the lateral lobes, and is firm and bumpy to feel. Its upper and lower extents can easily be delineated by palpation. It is the feel of the gland that is so characteristic of this condition. If hypothyroidism is very long-standing or caused by iodine-131 treatment, the gland may not be palpable. The hypothyroid patient (see Chap. 4) presents a puffy face, particularly noticeable in the eyelids. The lips and tongue may be thickened. The speech is slow and the voice deep. The skin is thick and dry and frequently has a yellowish cast, with rough scaly texture and appearance. There may be thinning of the hair, which is coarse and brittle. The body temperature is usually subnormal. The pulse rate is slow. Blood pressure is usually normal but may be increased. Heart sounds are soft and muffled. The deep tendon reflexes are characteristically hypoactive, with a slow recovery phase.

Some, all, or none of these findings may be present in any given individual with thyroid disease, depending on the severity of the disorder and whether the rate of release from the gland of thyroid hormone(s) is abnormal.

SECTION IV

CHEST

11. RESPIRATORY SYSTEM
   John G. Weg
12. CARDIOVASCULAR SYSTEM
   Bruce J. Genovese
   Ron J. Vanden Belt
   Richard D. Judge
13. BREAST
   George D. Zuidema

The physician observing a disease in different circumstances, reasoning about the influence of these circumstances, and deducing consequences which are controlled by other observations—this physician reasons experimentally, even though he makes no experiments.

CLAUDE BERNARD
(1813–1878)

Patient Sitting
1. Examine the regional lymph nodes and skin.
2. Inspect the thorax and accessory muscles of respiration.
3. Inspect and palpate the breasts.
4. Palpate the bony thorax, anterior and posterior.
5. Percuss the spine and costovertebral angle.
   Check for sacral and flank edema.
6. Check expansion and diaphragmatic excursion.
7. Percuss the chest. Check vocal fremitus.
8. Auscultate the lungs.
9. Inspect, palpate, and auscultate the precordium.

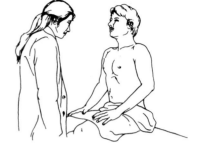

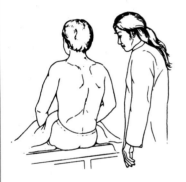 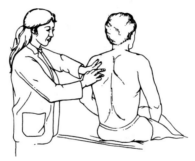 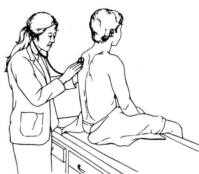

Patient Supine
10. Inspect the precordium.
11. Palpate the precordium and concurrently inspect the neck
    vein.
12. Auscultate the heart.
13. Palpate the breasts.

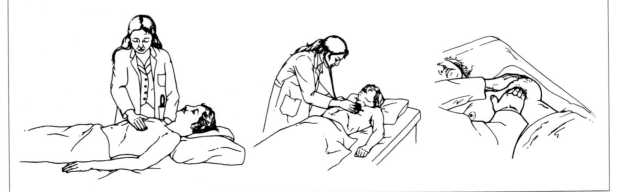

CHAPTER 11

RESPIRATORY SYSTEM

The crepitus rattle is the pathognomonic sign of the first stage of peripulmonary [lobar] pneumonia. It is perceptible from the very invasion of the inflammation; at this time it conveys the notion of very small, equal-sized bubbles, and seems hardly to possess the character of humidity.

RENÉ THÉOPHILE HYACINTHE LAËNNEC
(1781–1826)

Examination of the respiratory system consists primarily of examination of the chest.

To master physical diagnosis of the chest, it is only necessary to have good eyes, good ears, one stethoscope . . . a good roentgenographic unit, a ration of intelligence, a measure of determination and a mess of patients.*

Traditionally the four components of the examination are inspection, palpation, percussion, and auscultation. To these must be added the study of the chest roentgenogram, spirometry, and arterial blood gases. The student must sharpen perception to learn the normal and appreciate the abnormal findings. You must first learn what to look for; later, you must avoid the pitfall of prejudiced perception because of prior experience. Look for nothing specifically, yet see what is actually there. Develop a thorough, systematic routine that is the same for each patient you see. Think of the pathologic changes, rather than specific diseases, that may account for the abnormalities elicited. Diagnosis awaits the correlation of clinical, roentgenographic, and laboratory findings.

ANATOMY

Knowledge of the underlying anatomy of the lungs is essential to a properly conducted examination, because each bronchopulmonary segment must be checked (Table 11–1). The sketches and roentgenograms with bronchopulmonary anatomy superimposed in Figures 11–3 through 11–6 may be helpful. The angle of Louis is a prominence in the sternum at the second chondrosternal junction; it is a helpful landmark for counting ribs and then identifying segments from which abnormal findings arise. Other helpful topographic aids are a series of imaginary lines, names of which are self-explanatory, projected onto the chest wall (Figs. 11–1, 11–2).

Robert A. Green, M.D., Professor of Internal Medicine, Pulmonary Division, The University of Michigan Medical School, Ann Arbor, was sole author of this chapter in the first two editions, (1963 and 1968) and co-author of the last two, (1974 and 1982). His extraordinary knowledge and skill in clinical, roentgenographic, and pathologic correlations, along with his truly unique ability to implant them in medical students, house officers, fellows, and colleagues are evident on almost every page of this edition. Hopefully, these pages will in some small way replicate the joy of learning he has given to so many.
*J. J. Waring. Physical examination, helps and hindrances. *Ann. Intern. Med.* 28:15, 1948.

TABLE 11−1. Summary of the Lobes of the Lung[a]

Right Lung	Left Lung
Upper lobe	Upper lobe (superior division)
1. Apical segment (B-1)	1−2. Apical-posterior segment[c] (B-1 and B-3)
2. Posterior segment (B-3)	3. Anterior segment (B-2)
2′. Axillary subsegment[b]	Lingula (inferior division)
3. Anterior segment (B-2)	4. Superior lingular segment (B-4)
3′. Axillary subsegment[b]	5. Inferior lingular segment (B-5)
Middle lobe	Lower lobe
4. Lateral segment (B-4)	6. Superior segment (B-6)
5. Medial segment (B-5)	7−8. Anteromedial basal segment[d] (B-7 and B-8)
Lower lobe	9. Lateral basal segment (B-9)
6. Superior segment (B-6)	10. Posterior basal segment (B-10)
7. Medial basal segment[c] (B-7)	
8. Anterior basal segment (B-8)	
9. Lateral basal segment (B-9)	
10. Posterior basal segment (B-10)	

[a]The Jackson and Huber nomenclature is used. The Boyden numerical system is indicated in parentheses.
[b]These axillary subsegments are listed as such because of the frequency with which they are diseased together, without the remainder of their respective segments.
[c]The medial basal segment does not present on the surface of the lung under the chest wall.
[d]The apical-posterior and anteromedial basal segments on the left are considered segments with subsegment subdivisions because they are supplied by a single segmental bronchus. In some classifications the posterior segment is referred to as (3) and the anterior segment as (2).

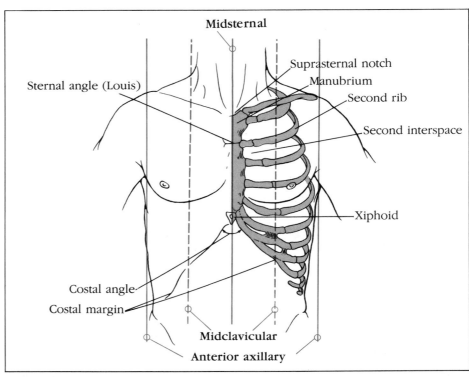

FIGURE 11−1
Landmarks on the chest wall (anterior).

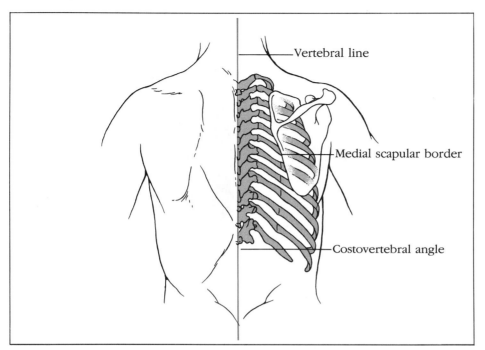

FIGURE 11–2
Landmarks on the chest wall (posterior).

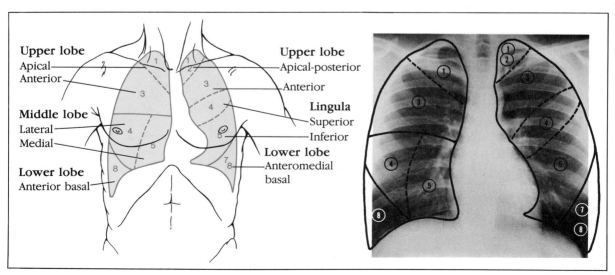

FIGURE 11–3
Segmental pulmonary anatomy (anterior).

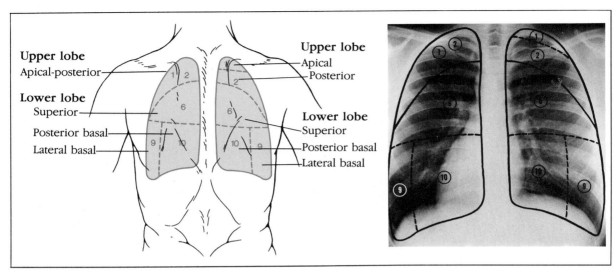

FIGURE 11–4
Segmental pulmonary anatomy (posterior).

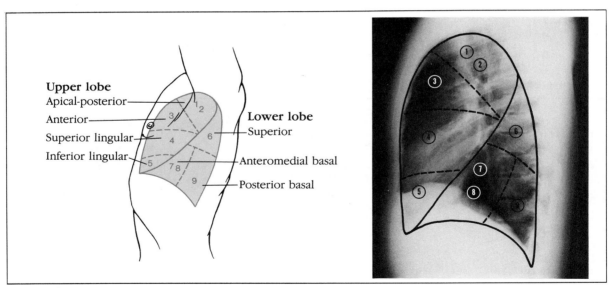

FIGURE 11–5
Segmental pulmonary anatomy (left lateral).

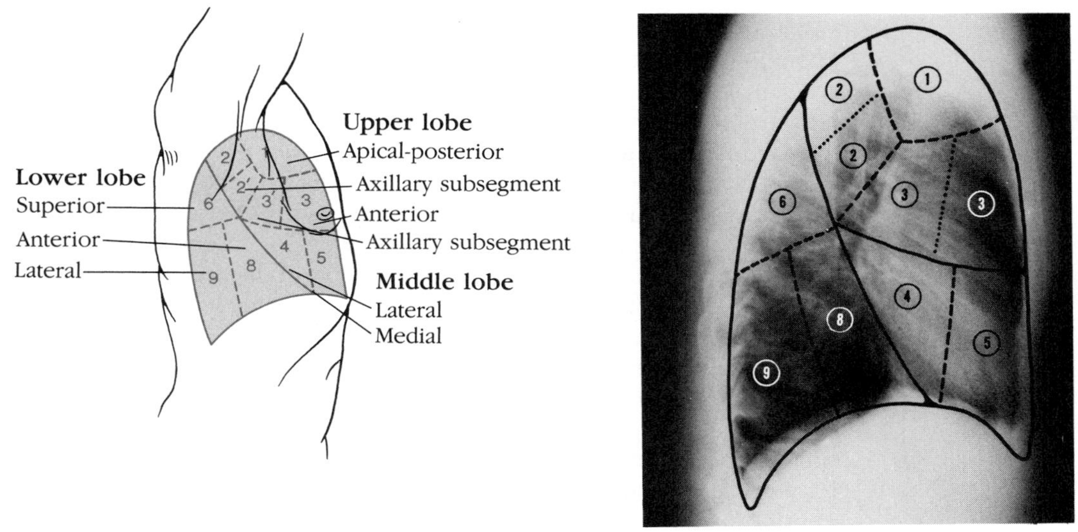

FIGURE 11–6
Segmental pulmonary anatomy (right lateral).

Record your findings by their relation to these lines, ribs, and interspaces. For example, crackles may be heard 3 cm to the right of the midsternal line at the level of the fourth anterior intercostal space. Record the finding as such; later you will interpret the crackles as arising from the medial segment of the right middle lobe.

The bronchopulmonary segments are outlined on the roentgenograms as they project on the surface of the lung and thus on the chest wall where their physical findings would present separately. The lines do *not* necessarily represent the roentgenographic projection of each entire segment. All projections on the external chest are drawn to correspond to the position in which the associated roentgenogram is taken. The continuous lines represent interlobar fissures; the interrupted lines represent segmental planes. The bronchopulmonary segmental nomenclature is dependent on the anatomy and nomenclature of the supplying bronchi.

HISTORY

Love and a cough cannot be hidden.

LATIN PROVERB

Cough is the most common symptom of pulmonary disorders. A normal person coughs rarely, and hardly ever more than twice in a bout. Cough may occur as a response to an inhaled irritant or aspirated material. It is preceded by a deep inspiration; the glottis then closes as the expiratory muscles contract. With the abrupt opening of the glottis, air is expelled at high flow rates along with secretions or other material in the airways. Stimulation of irritant vagal-afferent receptors, that are particularly prominent in the large airways, initiates the cough reflex through the medulla to vagal efferent nerves, the phrenic nerve, and other spinal motor nerves. Cough may also be initiated by abnormalities in the upper respiratory tract. It occurs with focal anatomic pulmonary lesions anywhere in the respiratory system and is also frequently due to diffuse airway or parenchymal abnormality. Coughs should be characterized as productive or nonproductive of sputum, paroxysmal, brassy, loud and high-pitched, or whooplike in character.

Sputum production often accompanies cough when irritation or inflammation of any portion of the pulmonary system leads to transudation or exudation of fluids. Expectoration of sputum (phlegm) is abnormal. The tracheobronchial tree's normal secretions of 60 to 90 cc/day are swallowed. The nature and quantity of sputum should be recorded. Note the volume, color, odor, turbidity, and consistency. Some sputum is colorless, clear, and watery. Mucoid sputum is gray-white, translucent, and slimy. Globs of thicker white mucus or pus may be intermixed (mucopurulent sputum). Purulent sputum is thick and opaque; it may be green, yellow, or brown, and mixed varieties are common. Sputum may be so viscous that it sticks to the inverted specimen container.

For adequate gross sputum examination, the patient must save his secretions, because estimates of both the quantity and the quality are commonly very poor. Expectoration should be directly into clear plastic or glass-capped containers. The patient's course should be followed by daily measurements of volume or weight as well as the changes in the sputum character. A Gram stain of sputum should be part of the initial evaluation.

Sputum may vary in amount from a few teaspoons daily, raised predominantly in the morning, to a pint or more. Patients often are unaware of even copious sputum production if it has increased gradually. They should be asked about it in several ways: inquire about smoker's cough, clearing the throat in the morning, raising phlegm while brushing the teeth, and so forth. Morning expectoration usually implies accumulation of secretions during the night and is common to many chronic bronchopulmonary suppurative disorders. Sputum may be mucoid, as occurs commonly in bronchitis, or may be largely purulent with superimposed infection. A large volume of purulent sputum expectorated into a glass jar ordinarily settles into four distinct layers. At the bottom is amorphous debris; a translucent layer of thin pus, mucus, and saliva is next; above this, pus globules float freely and hang suspended from the surface, which is covered with a layer of froth. Sputum of this type usually results from pulmonary destruction and suppuration and is common in lung abscess and bronchiectasis.

Note the presence of black anthracotic particles, concretions. In answer to direct questioning the patient may describe the expectoration of sand or small stones—broncholiths, casts of bronchioles (little wormlike solid pieces), and foreign material.

Sniff the opened sputum jar. Most sputum is neither foul nor offensive to the patient or to the examiner. However, with certain necrotizing infections (especially with anaerobic organisms) an extremely fetid odor is present, often at a considerable distance from the patient or his sputum jar.

Note specifically whether blood is present. Copious bleeding results in bright-red, frothy sputum; blood may present as small streaks on the surface or as tiny globules of darker blood intermixed with the sputum. The brighter the blood, the fresher the bleeding. Note whether the specimen is pure blood or blood mixed with pus or mucus.

Hemoptysis is frequently due to a single anatomic lesion, proximal or distal, that inflames or destroys the lung or bronchus involved (Table 11–2 outlines some causes of hemoptysis). It can occur with diffuse increase in pulmonary capillary pressure, as in cardiac disease. Blood loss into the lung can be great despite minimal external evidence of bleeding. Blood streaking of sputum commonly accompanies diffuse or localized inflammatory disorders and can be associated with paroxysmal coughing. Acute respiratory tract infections are the most common cause. Careful questioning and examination are required to separate hemoptysis from hematemesis (Table 11–3).

Chest pain (Table 11–4) due to pulmonary disease most often results from involvement of nerve endings in the parietal pleura, as the pulmonary parenchyma itself is insensitive. Pain can arise from major bronchial and peribronchial disease, in which case it tends to be constant, deep, and aching. Pleural pain, which varies with respiration, is sharp and intermittent. Characteristically, pleuritic pain is described as abruptly "cutting off my breath" on inspiration. Chest pain due to pulmonary hypertension may simulate angina pectoris. Pain may also arise from the chest wall; it is usually associated with localized tenderness.

Dyspnea is the patient's perception of shortness of breath or difficulty in breathing in an inappropriate setting. Shortness of breath after running a mile ("breathlessness") is appropriate and thus not dyspnea, whereas shortness of breath in a young person after walking up a flight of stairs is dyspnea. Although all symptoms require quantitation, this is essential in describing dyspnea. Each occurrence of dyspnea should be recorded in relation to everyday activity, with precise details of respiratory rate and length of activity, time to recovery, and progression over time. Because dyspnea is subjective, special care is necessary in understanding the patient's description; he may complain only of fatigue or of a tightness or heaviness in the chest. The respiratory rate is almost always increased with dyspnea of an organic nature, while a normal rate associated with sighing usually indicates an anxiety state. Although the mechanisms of dyspnea are not fully defined, it appears that reflexes originating in the lung and chest wall (that reflect the perception of inappropriate or excessive work such as with a stiffened lung, a low compliance, obstructed airways, or an increased resistance) and central mechanisms (mandating regular respiratory cycles) play the most critical roles. Increasing carbon dioxide tensions or decreasing pH also causes increased ventilation and dyspnea. Despite common belief, however, hypoxemia (a low oxygen tension) does *not* cause dyspnea. When inspired oxygen tensions are reduced, such as in simulating high

TABLE 11–2. Some Causes of Hemoptysis

Infections
  Acute bronchitis
  Pneumonia
  Bronchiectasis
  Lung abscess
  Tuberculosis
  Fungal infections (histoplasmosis,
    coccidioidomycosis, aspergillosis)
  Parasites (paragonimiasis,
    sechistosomiasis, ascariasis,
    amebiasis, ecchinococcosis,
    strongyloidiasis, etc.)

Neoplastic
  Bronchogenic carcinoma
  Bronchial adenoma
  Metastatic neoplasms

Traumatic
  Lung contusion
  Bronchial rupture
  Postintubation

Vascular
  Pulmonary infarction
  Pulmonary vasculitis
  Arteriovenous fistula
  Anomalous vessels

Cardiovascular
  Pulmonary edema
  Mitral stenosis
  Aortic aneurysm

Parenchymal
  Diffuse interstitial fibrosis
  Systemic diseases and vasculitis Wegener's granulomatosis, rheumatoid arthritis, systemic lupus erythematosus,
    Goodpasture's syndrome, etc.
  Sarcoidosis and hemosiderosis
  Other diffuse lung diseases

Other
  Cystic fibrosis
  Endometrial implants
  Broncholiths
  Coagulopathies (with generalized bleeding)
  Nonrespiratory tract (esophagus, stomach)
  Spurious

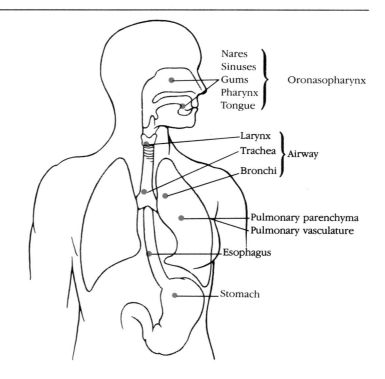

TABLE 11–3. Distinctive Characteristics of Hemoptysis and Hematemesis[a]

Hemoptysis	Hematemesis
1. Blood coughed up	1. Blood vomited up
2. Blood may be frothy	2. Blood not frothy
3. Blood mixed with sputum	3. Blood mixed with food
4. Blood is bright red	4. Blood is dark ("coffee grounds")
5. Stools may be tarry black (melena) if enough blood is swallowed	5. Stools often tarry black
6. History of chest disease	6. History of gastrointestinal disease
7. Patient says blood from lungs[b]	7. Patient says blood from stomach
8. Hemosiderin-laden macrophages in sputum	8. No hemosiderin-laden macrophages in sputum

[a]If the amount of blood is very large, patient will often swallow some blood which may be vomited; likewise some blood may be aspirated with massive hematemisis and subsequently coughed up.
[b]Patients are sometimes remarkably perceptive in this regard and may even tell you the area of the lung the blood is coming from.

TABLE 11–4. Some Sources of Chest Pain

Extrathoracic
  Migraine
  Cervical arthritis
  Subdiaphragmatic disease (e.g., appendicitis, hepatitis, splenic infarct, pancreatitis, ulcer, gallstones)
Chest wall
  Rib fracture, neoplasm
  Intercostal muscle spasm, inflammation (Bornholm disease)
  Herpes zoster
  Costochondritis
  Thoracic vertebral pain
  Thoracic nerve disease (radiculitis)
Pleura
  Pleurisy (infectious, neoplastic, vasculitic, irritative)
Lung parenchyma
  Pneumonia }
  Neoplasia } (pain uncommon with pure parenchymal lesions)
Lung vasculature
  Pulmonary infarction
  Pulmonary hypertension
Mediastinal structures
  Lymph nodes (pain with lymphoma, cancer)
  Esophagitis
  Aortic dissection
  Tracheobronchitis
  Pericarditis
  Myocardial pain (angina, infarct)

altitude, one is aware of no unpleasant sensation. Rather, one just very pleasantly lapses into unconsciousness. It was graphically described by Tissandier during a high altitude balloon flight in 1875:

... at 24,600 feet the condition of torpor that overcomes one is extraordinary. Body and mind become feebler.... There is no suffering. On the contrary one feels an inward joy ... one rises and is glad to be rising.... All at once I shut my eyes and fell down powerless and lost all further memory.*

The balloon ascended to 23,820 feet and then descended on its own. Tissandier recovered but two companions died. Hypoxemia can be a silent killer.

Other symptoms of particular importance in chest disease are **hoarseness**, which may indicate damage to a laryngeal nerve by tumor or inflammation or which may be secondary to vocal cord trauma with severe coughing; **fever**, which is indicative of inflammatory or neoplastic disease; chills or a **rigor** (a shaking chill); **weight loss**; and **edema**.

Snoring is common, and brief periods of apnea (no air flow for 10 seconds or more) during sleep are normal. This common snoring has a very low frequency, 40 to 60 Hz. In contrast, individuals with the sleep apnea syndrome may have extremely loud snoring—loud enough to be heard in other rooms, with a frequency of 1000 to 3000 Hz. Obstructive sleep apnea is characterized by episodes of apnea followed by progressively louder snorting (snoring) until normal breathing is resumed. A spouse will often give this history when asked. In contrast, central apnea is not associated with these intermittent snorting events. The combination of central and sleep apnea is common. Patients with sleep apnea may complain of frequent awakenings (even requesting help for insomnia), mental fuzziness and headaches on awakening in the morning, daytime hypersomnolence, decrease in mental functioning, personality changes, and impotence. In adults under 55 years, more than five apneic episodes/per hour is considered abnormal. In older individuals, especially men, 30 to 60 percent of normal individuals, without sleep or respiratory complaints, may meet this criterion.

A past history of pneumonia in childhood, recurrent pneumonia, or whooping cough may indicate a predisposition to respiratory tract infection, chronic obstructive pulmonary disease, bronchiectasis, or congenital anomalies. A history of recurrent respiratory tract infections may indicate an underlying genetic disorder, e.g., cystic fibrosis immunoglobin abnormality, etc. The use of oily nose drops, poor oral hygiene, a recent dental extraction, alcoholism, or unconsciousness may predispose to aspiration pneumonia or lung abscess, or both. A history of close exposure to infectious tuberculosis, occupational exposure to certain mineral or organic dusts, travel to areas with endemic fungal infections, or inhalant allergy (e.g., hay fever) provides potentially important diagnostic information.

*Quoted in H. G. Armstrong, Principles and Practice of Aviation Medicine. Baltimore: Williams and Wilkins, 1939. Pp. 2–3.

PHYSICAL EXAMINATION

1. Inspect for respiratory rate, rhythm, symmetry of chest and expansion.
2. Palpation for expansion (degree and symmetry), vocal fremitus, rib tenderness or deformity. Supraclavicular nodes and trachea may be done here.
3. Percuss systematically for note, borders, diaphragms.
4. Auscultate systematically for breath sounds, egophony.

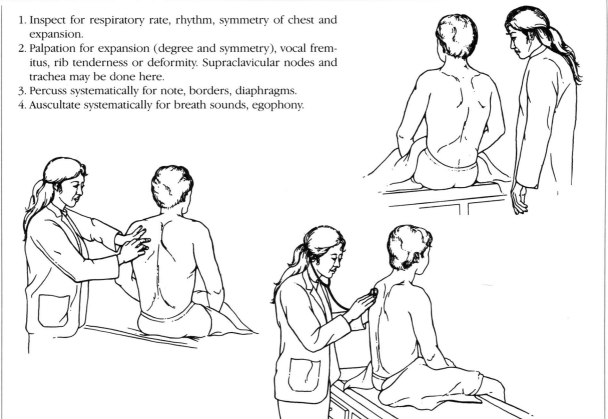

Peripneumonia and pleuritic affections, are to be thus observed: If the fever be acute, and if there be pains on either side, or in both, and if expiration be attended with pain, and the sputum expectorated be of a blond or livid color ... the physician should proceed thus.

HIPPOCRATES
(460?–377? B.C.)

GENERAL EXAMINATION

A routine physical examination allows excellent evaluation of the ventilatory function of the respiratory tract; it permits an estimate of the volume of exchanging gas and of the rate and distribution of air flows. The other functions of the lung—that is, diffusion, perfusion, and the relation of ventilation to perfusion—cannot be well evaluated; however, the clinical findings in disease states in which these are involved are often characteristic.

Have the patient sit upright. If the patient is too ill to sit upright by himself, have an aide support him in the sitting position, because examination with the patient on his back or side may introduce numerous undesirable variables.

The patient is stripped to the waist; a drape is used for female patients. Inspect the patient from the front, from behind, from the side, and while standing behind the patient and looking down over his shoulders at the anterior chest.

INSPECTION

Inspection has its major value in observation of abnormalities in respiration and symmetry, both of ventilation and structure, of the two sides of the thorax.

First and most important is the respiratory rate. Is it increased or decreased? Is it irregular? What is the length of inspiration? Of expiration?

The respiratory rate in the normal resting patient varies between 12 and 16 breaths per minute, although rates as high as 25 have been considered normal. Respiration is regular and quiet; the inspiratory phase lasts half again as long as the expiratory (see Chap. 5). Respirations should be counted for 30 seconds.

Is the patient in pain? Is he in respiratory distress, or is respiration noisy? Observe the chest during quiet respiration. Note the status of the skin and breasts, the muscular development, the state of nutrition, localized areas of bulging or retraction, the presence of thoracic deformities, especially if unilateral, the position of the apex impulse, scars or sinus tract openings, evidence of vascular pulsation or dilation. What are the size and shape of the chest? Pay special attention to chest contour, as it may influence other physical findings and interpretation of the chest roentgenograms. Note the angle of the costal margins at the xiphoid, the angle that the ribs make posteriorly with the vertebrae, and the slope of the ribs. Note whether the interspaces retract or bulge generally or in limited areas during ventilation. Does one area lag or flare more than another? Is respiration predominantly costal or abdominal?

After inspecting the chest in quiet breathing, ask the patient to take in a maximum breath and force it out with his mouth wide open until his lungs are completely empty (i.e., a forced vital capacity [FVC] maneuver). This should be preceded by a demonstration, and the patient should perform the maneuver two or three times to ensure maximum effort and complete emptying. The examiner should measure and record, in seconds, the time to complete this maneuver (i.e., the forced expiratory time [FET]), by listening near the mouth or with the stethoscope placed over the cervical trachea. A normal person can empty his lungs in 3 seconds or less. A prolonged FET (4 seconds or greater) provides a most sensitive and semiquantitative clinical measure of diffuse airways obstruction (Fig. 11–7).

The hallmark of normal inspection is symmetry—both of structure and of movement. Due to the frequency of scoliosis in the normal population, however, symmetry is rarely perfect (Fig. 11–8). The thorax is broader from side to side than from front to back, and its shape varies with the build of the individual; it is short and broad in the stocky person, and long, flat, and narrow in the asthenic person. Minor variations from the normal structure of the thorax include a funnel-shaped depression of the lower portion of the sternum (pectus excavatum) and the reverse condition in which the sternum projects beyond the frontal plane of the abdomen (pectus carinatum, or pigeon breast). Slight thoracic kyphosis (increased spinal

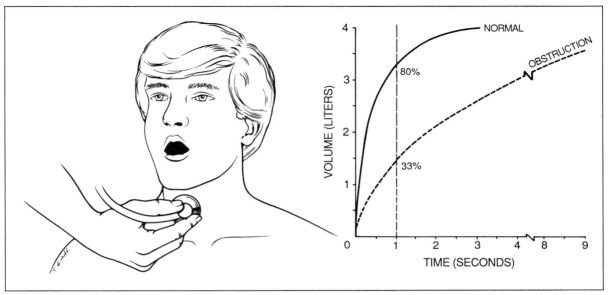

FIGURE 11–7
Forced expiratory time (FET). A. Patient forcibly exhaling from full inspiration with mouth wide open; the examiner times expiration by placing the stethoscope over the trachea. A normal FET is approximately 3 seconds. An FET of 4 seconds or more is a very sensitive measure of airway obstruction. B. Spirometric recording of forced vital capacity maneuver; volume is measured in liters on the ordinate and time in seconds on the abscissa. A normal person can exhale approximately 80% of his vital capacity in 1 second; the forced expiratory volume at 1 second divided by the forced vital capacity is recorded as $FEV_1\%$.

convexity as viewed from the side) resulting from poor posture is not uncommon and is often associated with scoliosis (lateral spinal deviation as viewed from the rear).

Normally the interspaces between the ribs do not particularly retract or bulge during inspiration. The subcostal angle is less than 90 degrees and widens with inspiration. The ribs themselves make an angle of approximately 45 degrees with the vertebral column.

Both men and women usually breathe predominantly with their thoracic cage, which expands on inspiration when they are erect. When the person is supine, respiration is largely abdominal with the abdomen moving out and intraabdominal pressure increasing (identified by palpating the abdomen). Inward movement of the abdomen with a decrease of intraabdominal pressure is paradoxical. If not voluntary, it indicates severe respiratory muscle (in particular, diaphragmatic) fatigue; it may also be seen with diaphragmatic paralysis. The entire rib cage moves laterally and upward with inspiration, gently rising with each breath. Ventilation is symmetric in onset and depth.

Inspection for respiratory disease requires inspection of more than the thorax. Clubbing, cyanosis, use of accessory respiratory muscles, respiratory distress, and

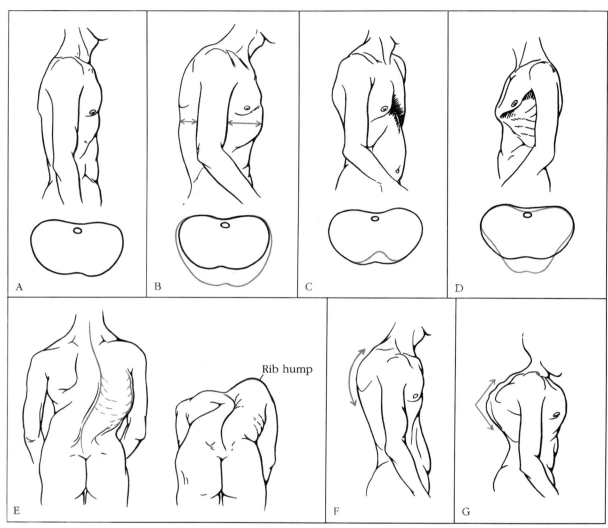

FIGURE 11–8
Chest wall contours. A. Normal. B. Barrel chest (emphysema). C. Pectus excavatum (funnel chest). D. Pectus carinatum (pigeon breast). E. Scoliosis. F. Kyphosis. G. Gibbus (extreme kyphosis).

marked sweating are important extrathoracic signs of intrathoracic disease. Poor veins with scarring may indicate drug addiction; peripheral thrombophlebitis may correlate with chest pain and dyspnea in pulmonary embolic disease; a rash following an intercostal nerve root distribution suggests herpes infection; a prominent bulging of the dorsal spine in a kyphotic individual, or a gibbous deformity, suggests tuberculosis; the presence of Horner's syndrome (see Chap. 8), with pain in the shoulder radiating into the arm with muscle atrophy, suggests malignancy in the lung apex; a prominent venous pattern of the chest wall may indicate vena caval obstruction; and so on.

Clubbing of the fingers is especially important (see Chap. 4). If the syndrome of pulmonary osteoarthropathy accompanies the clubbing, the periosteum over the ends of the long bones of the forearm and leg may be palpably tender. This is almost always a manifestation of carcinoma of the lung. Clubbing is commonly associated with diffuse interstitial fibrosis of the lung (idiopathic) and is almost always seen in patients with cystic fibrosis. It is not a manifestation of asthma, chronic bronchitis, or emphysema. Dilated veins may indicate compression of the venous flow within the mediastinum, and subcutaneous swellings may represent metastatic tumor nodules, abscesses, or the pointing of an empyema. Sinus tract openings or scars similarly suggest underlying infection.

Asymmetry due to localized prominence of the chest wall will occur occasionally with large tumors or large pleural effusions; in chronic conditions in which considerable scarring of the lung and pleura has occurred, localized contraction is not uncommon. Scoliosis must be eliminated as the cause of such asymmetry. A barrel-shaped appearance of the chest is common in older patients and those with emphysema. The ribs are more horizontal, and the subcostal angle is greater than 90 degrees without variation during respiration; thus, this is neither a specific nor a sensitive finding. Localized areas of diminished ventilation may reflect either local disease or the effects of severe pain with splinting on thoracic motion. Local inspiratory retraction of the intercostal spaces indicates local bronchial obstruction; generalized retractions are common in symptomatic chronic obstructive pulmonary disease, asthma, chronic bronchitis, and emphysema.

PALPATION

Palpation is the best method for evaluation of the degree and symmetry of expansion with respiration, as well as for appreciation of the transmitted vibrations of the spoken voice. It is complementary to inspection in evaluation of respiratory excursion. Use both hands simultaneously, and palpate symmetric areas of the thorax (Fig. 11–9). The examiner's hands must be warm. Standing behind the patient, place the hands on the lower chest with the thumbs adjacent near the spine. Tell the patient to inhale deeply, and compare the symmetry of onset and depth of inspiration. Place the hands similarly over the lower lateral chest. Then, standing behind the patient, place them over the shoulders onto the anterior chest below the clavicles. This procedure also can be performed over the low anterior chest but is of less value there.

Costal expansion of 4 to 6 cm is considered normal. Limited costal expansion indicates diffuse obstruction or fibrosis, muscle weakness, or ankylosing spinal disease.

Palpate the chest wall and note any masses. Note the general turgor of the skin, its temperature, moistness, or the presence of edema. Note the character of the musculature. Palpate each rib, noting whether tenderness is elicited. A costal cartilage may be exquisitely tender when inflamed (Tietze's syndrome). Far from requiring severe trauma, rib fractures may occur from so ordinary a stress as heavy coughing. Firm anteroposterior compression of the chest (sternum to vertebrae)

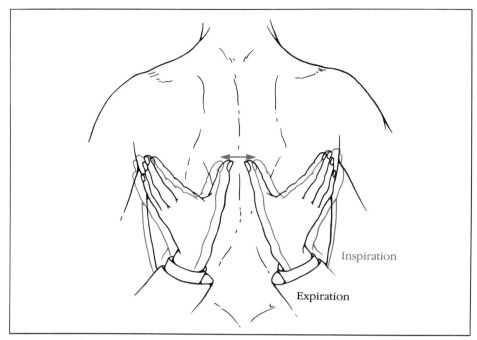

FIGURE 11–9
Palpation for expansion.

will often cause severe pain at the site of rib fracture. Note both the position of the trachea in the episternal notch relative to the midline and the distance of the trachea from the posterior surface of the sternum. This is ascertained most accurately by standing behind the patient and letting each index finger slide off the head of the clavicle deep into the sternal notch on either side of the intrathoracic trachea (Fig. 11–10).

The trachea is in the midline, admitting almost an index finger on either side at the episternal notch when palpated from behind the patient; the space between it and the sternum does not allow more than one finger at the episternal notch. The lower palpable trachea may deviate slightly to the right in older patients.

Supraclavicular lymph nodes can be sought at the same time you palpate the trachea. Nodes in this area, such as those that occur with sarcoid and neoplasia, may be brought up to the examining finger by having the patient perform the Valsalva maneuver.

With the palmar aspect of the fingers or the ulnar aspect of the hand, appreciate tactile fremitus by asking the patient to phonate (Fig. 11–11). It is standard practice to have the patient repeat "one, two, three" or "ninety-nine" to elicit fremitus; "blue moon" is also a helpful phrase. As with other chest examinations evaluate vocal fremitus over all lung segments, and note its comparative increase or decrease or its absence. It will be elicited again during auscultation; you should check your tactile findings with the auscultatory findings at this point.

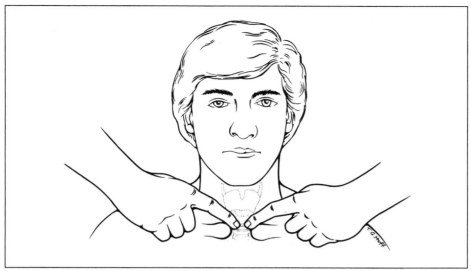

Figure 11–10
Palpating the intrathoracic trachea. When the fingers slide down and posterior to the clavicular heads, the normal trachea can be felt in the midline.

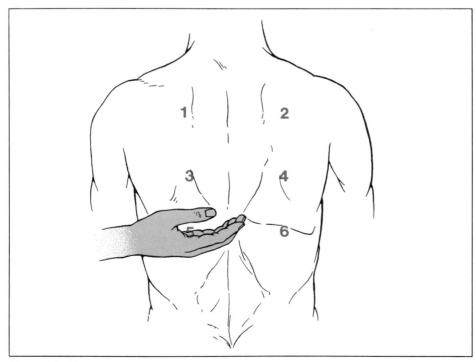

Figure 11–11
Evaluation of tactile fremitus.

Sound vibrations are best transmitted to the examiner's hand in patients with thin chest walls and deep voices. Fremitus is most prominent over areas where the bronchi are relatively close to the chest wall. It increases as the intensity of the voice increases and as its pitch drops. It is normally symmetrical except for a slightly greater intensity over the right upper lobe than over the left.

Notice if coarse vibrations associated with noisy respiration are palpable. This finding, termed *rhonchal fremitus,* implies the presence of exudate in the trachea or larger bronchial tubes, which will also produce rhonchi on auscultation. Auscultation and palpation are both necessary to differentiate rhonchal fremitus from a pleural friction rub. The pleural rub is more grating in quality and is commonly associated with pain. Palpable rhonchi are predominantly inspiratory whereas rubs involve both phases of the respiratory cycle. Rhonchi may clear with cough; rubs are unaffected. Rubs are usually more localized, are heard or felt unilaterally, sound close to the ear, and are accentuated by pressure of the hand or stethoscope, features that are all absent with rhonchi.

The evaluation of tactile or vocal fremitus is at times unreliable. Take special care to compare symmetric areas of the chest, as symmetric decreases or increases in fremitus are rarely significant. Localized diminution of fremitus occurs when the transmission of the voice sound from the trachea through the vibrating lung to the examining hand or finger is interfered with by any cause. It is therefore absent in patients with an obstructed bronchus, when air or fluid in the pleural space is interposed, or when the chest wall is considerably thickened or edematous. Generalized diminution in fremitus occurs with diffuse bronchial obstruction. Localized areas of increased fremitus occur with consolidation—denser lung with a patent bronchus—and occasionally when the lung is compressed above a pleural effusion. Increased fremitus over consolidated lungs is appreciated only if the increased density of the lung extends to the pleural surface.

Remember that the intensity of fremitus and the breath sounds are influenced in the same direction by the same physical factors. They should therefore correlate at all times (e.g., diminished fremitus with diminished breath sounds, increased fremitus with loud or bronchial breathing). Minor differences in correlation may occur in the absence of pathological changes. The auscultatory findings are generally more reliable.

Before leaving palpation of the chest, notice if subcutaneous emphysema is present. If it is present, the fingers palpate a peculiar crackling sensation of bubbles of air underneath the skin, indicating a leak somewhere from the lung or other air-containing viscera. It is usually felt earliest in the supraclavicular area but may spread into the neck and face, over the trunk, and into the scrotum; sometimes it can be heard more easily with the stethoscope than felt. This finding may occur spontaneously or with trauma; it is usually associated with mediastinal emphysema, pneumothorax, or both.

PERCUSSION

The signs of hydrops of the chest on one side of the thorax, besides the general signs which I have just presented, the affected side (if it is not entirely filled with fluid) is weakened and is perceived to be less moveable on inspiration.

Moreover on percussion, there is no resonance in any part.
But if it is half filled with fluid, a greater resonance is obtained in that part
which is not filled with fluid.

LEOPOLD AUENBRUGGER
(1722–1809)

Percussion has its greatest value in determining the relative amount of air and
solid material in the underlying lung and in delimiting the boundaries of organs
or portions of the lung that differ in structural density. Direct percussion involves
tapping the chest with the middle or ring finger. It is especially valuable in percussing over the clavicle. Mediate percussion is more popular and is best learned
by direct demonstration by an instructor. Figure 11–12 shows the basic method for
mediate, or indirect, percussion.

Place the distal two phalanges of the middle finger of the left hand (the finger is
then pleximeter) firmly against the chest wall in the intercostal spaces parallel to
the ribs. Strike the distal interphalangeal joint with a quick, sharp stroke with the
tip of the middle finger (which becomes the plexor) of the right hand, one or two
rapid staccato blows in succession. Hold the forearm stationary and make the striking motion with the wrist. Note both the sound elicited and the sense of resistance
and vibration underneath the finger. Percuss from side to side, comparing symmetrical areas of the chest. Percuss gently though firmly, making a special effort to
apply equal force at all points. It will be necessary to percuss more firmly in individuals with thick chest walls, more lightly in the thin. Skillful percussion requires
much practice, until the technique becomes automatic and the examiner can concentrate completely on the sounds and sensations he elicits.

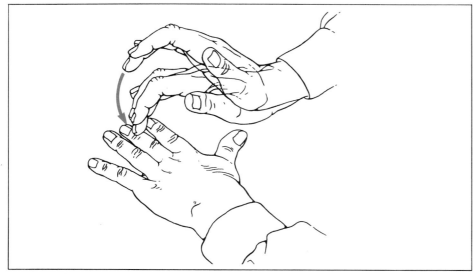

FIGURE 11–12
Mediate percussion of the chest.

Percuss the lower margins of the lungs and the width of the heart and upper mediastinum. The extent and equality of diaphragmatic excursion are well evaluated in most patients by percussion. Tell the patient to inhale deeply and hold his breath. Note the line of change in the percussion note between the resonant lung and the abdominal viscera posteriorly. Then ask the patient to exhale completely and hold his breath. The lower level of pulmonary resonance has now moved upward (Fig. 11–13). The distance between these two points represents the extent of diaphragmatic excursion. The lower lung margin may vary, but in mid-inspiration it is usually at the tenth vertebra posteriorly, at the eighth rib laterally, and at the sixth cartilage anteriorly. The normal diaphragmatic excursion averages about 3 cm in women and 5 or 6 cm in men.

When the diaphragms are lower than normal or when the mediastinum is narrower than normal, hyperinflation (such as occurs with emphysema) is suggested; when higher than normal, fibrosis or increased abdominal contents are suggested. Measured diaphragmatic excursion, when symmetrically reduced, may indicate generalized bronchial obstruction or muscular weakness. Unilateral limitation of motion implies paralysis or splinting.

The normal percussion note varies with the thickness of the chest wall and the force applied by the examiner. The clear, long, low-pitched sound elicited over the normal lung is termed *resonance*.

Dullness occurs when the air content of the underlying tissue is decreased and its solidity is increased. The sound is short, high-pitched, soft, and thudding, and lacks the vibratory quality of a resonant sound. It is heard normally over the heart and is accompanied by an increased sense of resistance in the pleximeter finger. Variations of the note intermediate between dullness and normal resonance are sometimes termed slight dullness or impaired resonance and are elicited normally over the scapulae, over thick musculature, and occasionally at the right apex. Asymmetry of apical resonance, however, is rarely elicited during the routine examination, and slight differences often require perusal of the roentgenogram to determine which side, if either, is normal or abnormal. When patients are examined while lying on the side, the dependent lung tends to have less resonance.

Flatness is absolute dullness. When no air is present in the underlying tissue the sound is very short, feeble, and high-pitched; flatness is found over the muscle of the arm or thigh.

Hyperresonance refers to a more vibrant, lower-pitched, louder, and longer sound heard normally over the lungs during maximum inspiration.

Tympany is difficult to describe but implies that the sound is moderately loud and fairly well sustained, with a musical quality in which a specific pitch is often noted. It is normally heard in the left upper quadrant of the abdomen over the air-filled stomach or over any hollow viscus. The pitch of tympany is variable, but it is usually high-pitched, clear, hollow, and drumlike.

The normal percussion note is resonant over all the lungs, except at the right apex, where occasionally slight dullness is detected (Fig. 11–14). Generalized hyperresonance not due to full-held inspiration may be found when the lung contains more than a normal amount of air (hyperinflation): however, unless the hyperresonance is pronounced, the considerable variations between observers, and be-

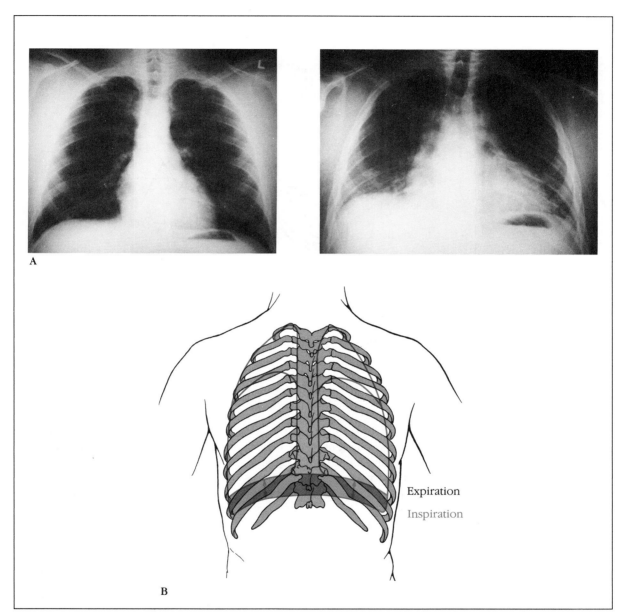

FIGURE 11–13
Normal diaphragmatic excursion. A. Full inspiration (*left*) and full expiration (*right*). B. Inspiration and expiration.

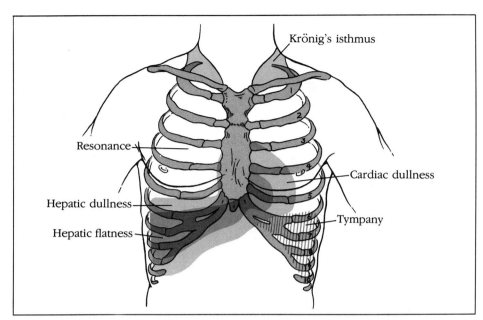

FIGURE 11–14
Percussion notes over the normal chest.

tween one observer's impressions at different times, impair the usefulness of this finding. Localized areas of hyperresonance are noted when pneumothorax is present, and occasionally over solitary bullae. Impaired resonance is difficult to evaluate but may be noted adjacent to areas of greater pathology and over lungs partially consolidated, as in diffuse bronchopneumonia. Dullness is elicited with pulmonary infiltration of almost any cause, regardless of the state of patency of the supplying bronchus, whenever the air content of the lung is partially or completely replaced by fluids or solids. When correlated with the character of the breath sounds on auscultation, and fremitus during palpation, the status of the underlying parenchyma in a dull area can be reliably predicted. Dullness also is noted when the pleurae and pleural cavity are thickened or filled with anything except air. (Rarely, air under great tension will give a dull rather than a hyperresonant note.) Extreme dullness, or flatness, is noted when no air at all underlies the pleximeter, as occurs, for practical purposes, only with pleural effusion. Tympany is rare over the lungs themselves. It occasionally occurs over a large pneumothorax.

AUSCULTATION

Auscultation begins within earshot of the patient. Listen to breathing as you walk into the room or even over the telephone. Breathing is silent in health, but heard at a distance with airways obstruction. Noisy inspiration is characterized by sound waves of random amplitude with an evenly spread frequency distribution between 200 and 2000 Hz (Hz is the frequency of oscillation in cycles/second). This is so-called "white noise." This inspiratory noise increases with increasing air flow obstruction. In contrast, inspiration is silent in emphysema with severe airways obstruction.

Musical sounds such as stridor or wheezing may also be heard. Stridor is a loud whooping or crowing musical sound caused by upper airways obstruction, e.g., trachea, larynx, and above. If the site is extrathoracic, the sound is louder in inspiration and may not be heard in expiration (Table 11–5).

A stethoscope fitted with a bell and a diaphragm is preferable. The bell is particularly helpful in very thin patients with deep intercostal spaces that do not permit the larger diaphragm to make full contact. Apply the stethoscope firmly to the chest wall and make certain that factitious sounds due to abnormal muscular movement, hair on the chest wall, and rubbing against the stethoscope do not occur. Cover systematically all portions of both lung fields posteriorly, laterally, and anteriorly, from above down, comparing areas side to side. Be certain that each bronchopulmonary segment is auscultated.

Instruct the patient to breathe, with his mouth open, a little deeper and faster than normal; demonstrate it to him yourself. Notice especially the character of the breath sounds and the presence of abnormal sounds. Notice any changes that occur during more rapid and deep respiration; in a normal person the breath sounds should increase in intensity with increasing flow rates (recruitment). Compare each area examined with the symmetric area of the opposite thorax and with other adjacent pulmonary zones. Direct the patient with instructions such as "a little deeper, please," "a little faster, please," "not quite so hard," until you are convinced that the abnormalities heard are not factitious. Ask him to phonate and to whisper a phrase such as "one, two, three" or "ninety-nine" and note the character of the vocal resonance perceived.

In recent years there have been renewed interest and major advances in understanding the generation of normal and abnormal breath sounds as well as adventitious sounds. This is due in large part to the availability of sophisticated sound recording equipment and the use of time-expanded wave-form analysis—an expansion of the time axis made by replaying recorded sounds from a computer memory at much slower speeds. The normal breath sounds heard at the chest wall are generated by turbulent flow in the large airways; the vibrations are transmitted through the airways and the airway walls to the chest wall. The sound is filtered, which increases the transmission of low frequencies or pitches, and attenuated. Whether a component of the sound is generated in small airways where laminar flow with its very low energy prevails is not clear. However, there is a general semiquantitative correlation with the intensity of regional breath sounds and regional ventilation shown in xenon-133 studies.

The importance of the character of normal or vesicular breath sounds is often inadequately emphasized. *Vesicular breath sounds* are breezy or swishy in character. The maximum frequency content is between 100 and 500 Hz. The inspiratory phase predominates, and the pitch is high. It is believed that the inspiratory component is primarily produced by turbulence in the mainstem, lobar, and segmental bronchi. However, there is information indicating that a portion of the sound originates in smaller airways, perhaps due to unstable vortices (whirlpools of gas flow).

TABLE 11–5. Classification of Common Lung Sounds

	Acoustic Characteristics	American Thoracic Society Nomenclature	Common Synonyms
Normal	200–600 Hz Decreasing Power with increasing Hz	Normal	Vesicular Pulmonary
	75–1600 Hz Flat until sharp decrease in power (900Hz)	Bronchial	Bronchial Tracheal
Adventitious		Bronchovesicular Adventitous	Bronchovesicular Abnormal
	Discontinuous, interrupted explosive sounds (loud, low in pitch), early inspiratory or expiratory	Coarse crackle	Coarse rale
	Discontinuous, interrupted explosive sounds (less loud than above and of shorter duration; higher in pitch than coarse crackles or rales), mid- to late inspiratory	Fine crackle	Fine rale, crepitation
	Continuous sounds (longer than 250 msec, high-pitched; dominant frequency of 400 Hz or more, a hissing sound)	Wheeze	Sibilant rhonchus
	Continuous sounds (longer than 250 msec, low-pitched; dominant frequency about 200 Hz or less, a snoring sound)	Rhonchus	Sonorous rhonchus

There is a silent pause between inspiration and expiration. Expiration is heard only as a short, fainter, lower-pitched puff less than one-fourth as long as inspiration. The expiratory sound is produced more centrally where rapidly moving airstreams converge. Vesicular breathing is normal over most of the lungs. *Bronchial breathing* is, for practical purposes, synonymous with *tracheal breathing* and is heard normally over the trachea and the main bronchi. It contains a wide band of frequencies from just audible to over 1000 Hz. In bronchial breathing, inspiration is louder and higher pitched, but the great change is in expiration, which is increased in duration so much that it actually is longer than inspiration; its pitch is high and its intensity greater. Its quality is hollow or tubular and rather harsh. *Bronchovesicular breath sounds* represent an intermediate stage; they are heard normally in the second interspaces anteriorly, in the interscapular area posteriorly, and often at the medial right apex. Inspiration is unchanged from vesicular breathing, but expiration is as loud, equal in length, and similar in pitch. Thus it is important to direct specific attention to this change in expiration, which may be heard over early

TABLE 11–5. (Continued)

Laennec's Original Term	Representation of Sound at Chest Wall	Time Expanded Waveforms
Bruit respiratoire pulmonaire ou respiration vesiculaire	Inspiration , Expiration	Inspiration
Bruit respiratoire bronchique		Inspiration
Bruits etrangers Rale muquex ou gargouillement	Inspiration / Expiration / Air Flow	
Rale humide ou crepitation	Inspiration / Expiration / Air Flow	
Rale sibilant sec ou sifflement		
Rale set sonore ou ronflement		

consolidation or atelectasis. Exaggerated vesicular breathing is heard normally at times in thin people and children, during exercise, and in unnecessarily loud and rapid respiration. Here the expiratory phase is more prominent than in vesicular breathing but is not of bronchovesicular character. The normal relationship of inspiration to expiration must be learned with respect to each area of the lung examined.

You must expect differences in vocal resonance due to thickness of the chest wall as well as the area to which the stethoscope is applied. Voice sounds are heard best near the trachea and major bronchi. Exaggerated voice sounds *(bronchophony)* are a normal finding over the trachea and right upper lobe posteriorly. Speech is heard only as indistinct noise.

Considerable auscultatory experience with the wide range of normal breath sounds is necessary before you can distinguish abnormal sounds with confidence. Breath sound amplitude may vary at comparable sites in normal individuals and between individuals. This is often due to differences in chest wall thickness, but amplitude may vary with no known explanation. Thus, when breath sounds differ at symmetric sites of the thorax, it may be impossible to know if pathological changes exist without the aid of a roentgenogram. Symmetric findings may be misleading; chronic bilateral apical tuberculosis may be present with symmetric bronchial or bronchovesicular breathing and may be misinterpreted as normal because of the symmetry. Nevertheless, comparing one side with the other and the upper lobe with the ipsilateral lower lobe are extremely helpful maneuvers during auscultation. Factitious sounds are confusing; every student should apply the stethoscope to the hairy chest and hear the varied sounds made by hair rubbing against the stethoscope. These can be minimized by wetting the skin. In addition, apply the stethoscope to the biceps muscle while it contracts and note the striking similarity to rales. For this reason, the room and the stethoscope must be warm and the patient relaxed so that involuntary muscular contractions of the chest wall will not occur and masquerade as pulmonary abnormalities.

Abnormalities of the breath sounds have great significance. What is normal in one area may be pathologic elsewhere. Bronchial and bronchovesicular breath sounds are due to increased transmission of sound through partially solidified lung, of any cause, provided the bronchus is patent. They are therefore heard with consolidation, compression, and fibrosis. Breath sounds are diminished with local or diffuse bronchial obstruction and with pleural disease. *Amphoric* and *cavernous breathing* are terms of little practical value that refer to exaggerated forms of bronchial breathing heard over large cavities.

When bronchial breathing is heard over the upper anterior chest, the finding may be due to increased transmission through consolidated lung or merely to normal tracheal breathing due to shift in tracheal position. This distinction (which may have great importance in differential diagnosis, as the upper lobe bronchus would then be interpreted as obstructed or patent) unfortunately is often difficult to make even after correlation with the roentgenogram. Transmitted tracheal sounds rather than bronchial breath sounds are probably present if the sounds are not heard in the axilla, if they are quite harsh, without a pause between inspiratory and expiratory phases, or if an area of vesicular breathing seems to be interposed between the trachea and the abnormal breath sounds. The presence of rales, of course, strongly favors bronchial breathing.

Continuous adventitial sounds are musical sounds of more than 250 msec in duration called *wheezes* or *rhonchi.* They have a recognizable and well-defined pitch. The pitch is determined by the frequency of the fundamental note; there may be harmonically related overtones. The pitch ranges from 60 to more than 2000 Hz. These sounds are generated when airway walls or intraluminal materials are set in rapid oscillation. This oscillation results from the Venturi effect of flow through a narrow lumen or from the dynamic compression of airways with raising intrathoracic pressure. The transmission of these sounds is better through airways than through the lung and chest wall, especially the high frequency components. Thus it is important to listen over the trachea or at the open mouth. Wheezes or rhonchi are categorized as: high- or low-pitched; monophonic or polyphonic; fixed or random; inspiratory, expiratory, or both; and by the timing in inspiration and expiration (Table 11–6).

TABLE 11–6. Some Causes of Wheezing and/or Rhonchi

Upper airway
   Tracheal stenosis
   Laryngeal obstruction
   Laryngeal spasm
   Laryngeal edema
   Vocal cord paralysis
   Epiglottis
Endobronchial obstruction
   Foreign body
   Bronchogenic carcincoma
   Bronchial adenoma
   Endobronchial granuloma
Endobronchial swelling, bronchospasm
   Asthma
      Allergic bronchopulmonary aspergillosis
      Toxic bronchospasm (Noxious fumes, gases, etc.)
      Occupational asthma
   Anaphylaxis
   Carcinoid
   Congestive heart failure
Loss of pulmonary architectural support
   Emphysema

High-pitched wheezes (formerly sibilant wheezes) are currently commonly referred to as simply *wheezes*. They have a frequency of 500 Hz or more. They are characteristic of asthma. They can be heard in inspiration, expiration, or both. They may be monophonic and occur randomly through the respiratory cycle or they may be polyphonic, i.e., notes with different pitches all starting at the same time and continuing to the end of expiration. These wheezes of asthma are often so loud that they can be heard without a stethoscope at some distance from the patient. They are so characteristic that once heard even lay people can reliably identify them. An ominous sign in the dyspneic, asthmatic patient with dyspnea and tachypnea is the absence of wheezing either generalized or localized; the latter suggests a pneumothorax or obstruction of an airway due to secretions, edema, and bronchospasm.

Paroxysmal monophonic wheezing in both inspiration and expiration originating from the larynx may simulate asthma. These wheezes are heard best at the larynx with some transmission to the chest but no wheezing from intrathoracic airways. It is caused by adduction of the vocal cords and narrowing of the glottis. Although a person with this condition may appear ill enough to require endotracheal intubation and mechanical ventilation, the arterial blood gases will be normal, and the chest roentgenograms will not show hyperinflation during an episode.

In individuals with diffuse interstitial fibrosis due to a variety of causes a series of short, late inspiratory wheezes of varying pitch and amplitude may be heard. With a maximum forced expiration, normal individuals can develop a wheeze at the end of the maneuver. This is due to dynamic compression of airways.

Low-pitched wheezes (formerly sonorous rhonchi) are currently commonly called *rhonchi*. They are characteristic of secretions in the airway. They can be heard in inspiration, expiration, or both. They are usually polyphonic and occur randomly throughout the respiratory cycle. They tend to be relatively short in duration. They frequently become partially or totally clear with coughing. A monophonic rhonchus, especially if localized, suggests endotracheal or endobronchial obstruction by a tumor, foreign body, scar, or granulomata. It may be in inspiration or expiration. It can often only be heard by having the patient assume several positions, e.g., lying on one side or the other, bending forward, supine or prone. The wheeze or sound of air moving may continue when the remainder of the lung ceases to generate sound at the end of a rapid deep inspiration or expiration.

Discontinuous adventitial sounds are short, intermittent explosive sounds of usually less than 20 msec called *crackles* or *rales*. These sounds are believed to be generated by the following mechanisms: (1) the sudden "explosive" opening of small airways with the rapid equalization of pressure producing a sequence of implosive sound waves (or perhaps with the release of tissue tensions)—*fine crackles;* (2) the intermittent passage of air through a closed airway when distal (upstream) pressure opens it—*coarse crackles;* or (3) the bubbling of air through secretions—coarse crackles. Fine crackles are shorter in duration and occur with approximately twice the frequency of coarse crackles. Crackles are further categorized as early or late inspiratory and expiratory. "Medium" crackles lie between fine and coarse. They can be identified using expanded wave forms and sophisticated statistical programs, but not reliably by auscultation (see Table 11–5).

Fine, late inspiratory crackles or rales are high-pitched. They have variable intensity and spacing. They have been described as Velcro rales, cellophane rales, dry rales, close to the ear, and similar to rubbing strands of hair together. They probably represent the sudden opening of a group of alveoli served by an individual small airway. They tend to recur at the same point in inspiration with the same amplitude from breath to breath. They are not altered by a cough. The pattern will vary with movement of the stethoscope over relatively small distances. They are usually not heard at the mouth. They tend to be more profuse at the bases or the dependent portion of the lung. They tend to "move" to an area made dependent, i.e., they will increase in the right lung when this is made dependent. These gravity-related phenomena disappear, and the rales may be heard throughout inspiration with increasing severity of disease. In mild ("early"), diffuse interstitial fibrosis they are more likely to be heard at the lateral bases; as the disease progresses they are heard at the posterior bases, and then are heard higher and higher up the chest. Fine crackles are also heard in "early" pulmonary edema, resolving pneumonia, and in areas of decreased ventilation (such as with diaphragmatic paralysis, pain after laparotomy, etc.)

Crackles occasionally may be heard in healthy individuals who are breathing normally. They can usually be heard in normal people who breathe with small tidal volumes, or breathe 100% oxygen at low lung volumes. They can also be heard over the lower anterior chest in a majority of individuals inspiring slowly from residual volume or following a cough at residual volume (post-tussive rales). Although post-tussive rales may be normal in dependent portions of the lung, they are abnormal in other areas.

Coarse, early inspiratory and expiratory crackles or rales are low-pitched, less frequent, and louder than fine rales. The frequency and loudness are usually variable. However, at the end of expiration they tend to be quite regular. They are not affected by changing position. They are characteristic of generalized air flow obstruction such as chronic bronchitis and emphysema.

An even more coarse, lower pitched, rattling or bubbling sound is associated with secretions in large airways especially during coughing. This sound is often recognized during a cough without a stethoscope; the cough is characterized as productive, wet or loose.

The simultaneous production of coarse crackles of varying pitch is characteristic of bronchiectasis of whatever cause, e.g., cystic fibrosis.

The *pleural rub* is a coarse, grating sound heard close to the ear in both inspiration and expiration. The inflamed pleural surfaces rubbing against each other produce usually low-pitched discontinuous sounds (crackles) that are very regularly spaced. If higher pitched crackles are produced, they may be extremely difficult to separate from coarse crackles.

The *mediastinal crunch* (Hamman's sign) is an extremely loud, knocking, crunching, or crackling sound heard synchronous with the heart beat along the lower left sternal border with a left pneumothorax or mediastinal emphysema; the latter may be associated with subcutaneous emphysema in the neck or over the anterior chest wall.

One can determine if a bronchopleural fistula remains open after a chest tube is inserted for a pneumothorax with the *bronchial leak squeak* sign. It is a high-pitched, continuous squeaking sound that can be produced by having the patient perform a Valsalva maneuver (after maximum inspiration, perform a forced expired volume maneuver against a closed glottis, "bearing down"). This will identify continued air leakage even if bubbling is not seen in the underwater drainage system. This squeak can also be heard with a broncho-pleural-cutaneous fistula. The pitch of the sound decreases as the size of the fistula increases. Two additional signs of bronchopleural fistula may be heard in patients being mechanically ventilated: (1) a continuous, loud, nonmusical whooshing sound in inspiration similar to that heard at the mouth in chronic bronchitis; and (2) a loud clicking sound at the end of inspiration.

Abnormal vocal resonance occurs for the same reasons as its tactile counterpart but is frequently more discriminating and reliable. The intensity of the voice sounds is decreased with pleural disease and when pulmonary ventilation is either diffusely or locally obstructed. Greater intensity and slightly increased clarity of the transmitted voice *(bronchophony)* is noted over areas of consolidation. Often a more sensitive way to define small, early, partial consolidation is to have the patient whisper while you listen with the stethoscope for distinctly heard, articulated syllables *(whispering pectoriloquy)*. *Egophony* refers to a change in the quality of the spoken voice, which is louder and sounds bleating or nasal. Check for egophony by asking the patient to say "ee," which will then sound like "ay." Egophony is rarely found except over an area of compressed lung above a pleural effusion.

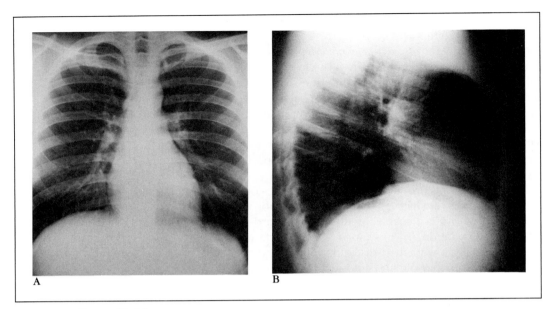

FIGURE 11–15
Normal chest roentgenograms. A. Posteroanterior. B. Lateral.

LABORATORY STUDIES

CHEST ROENTGENOGRAM

Careful examination of the patient is complemented by careful examination of the chest roentgenogram. Certain conditions present with abnormalities either on physical examination or roentgen examination alone; the roentgenogram almost always helps the evaluation of physical findings and cannot be properly interpreted itself without correlation with them. Figures 11–15 and 11–16 show normal and abnormal chest roentgenograms, respectively.

The patient is most often examined first, and the roentgenogram is seen subsequently. Some physicians prefer to see the roentgenogram first and then the patient; it can save valuable time to identify in advance the areas that require the most meticulous examination. The sequence is immaterial as long as the patient is reexamined following study of the roentgenogram, and the roentgenogram is rechecked following careful physical examination. This procedure permits both special attention to specific areas of the patient or film and a search for unusual physical findings when indicated. To fail to elicit abnormal physical findings over an area shown subsequently by the roentgenogram to be significantly diseased is unfortunate but not rare; to fail then to reexamine carefully and to ascertain the findings is deplorable.

The roentgenogram can be a valuable aid in learning physical diagnosis. The chest examination is incomplete without inspection of the chest roentgenogram. When a roentgenographic abnormality is found, every effort should be made to

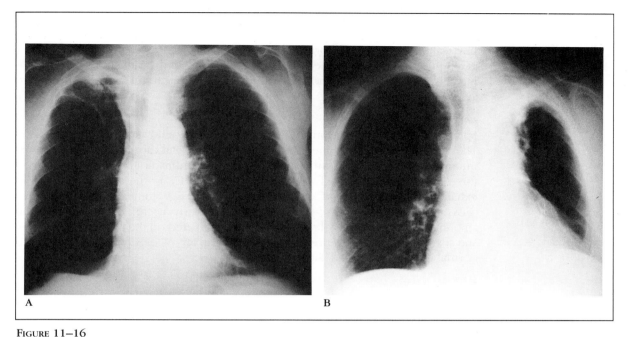

FIGURE 11−16

Abnormal chest roentgenograms. A. A 41-year-old man with laryngeal carcinoma. An infiltrate and marked atelectasis of the right upper lobe were noted. On physical examination, dullness, *bronchial breathing, fine inspiratory crackles, egophony,* and *pectoriloquy* were noted over the right upper chest; indicating an open bronchus. Patency of the bronchus was confirmed at bronchoscopy; transbronchial biopsy established the diagnosis of tuberculosis. B. A 63-year-old woman with a long history of cough and sputum production developed hemoptysis of approximately 60ml over last 24 hours. She had smoked two packages of cigarettes per day for over 40 years. On physical examination, there were dullness, absent breath sounds, and decreased voice transmission over the left upper chest. The chest roentgenogram showed marked atelectasis of the left upper lobe with elevation of the left hilum. At bronchoscopy, the left upper lobe bronchus was completely occluded by squamous cell carcinoma, which extended into the left mainstem bronchus.

obtain previous roentgenograms for comparison: *"an old chest roentgenogram is better than brains."* (Robert A. Green).

Examine the roentgenogram carefully. Be systematic, checking in order:

1. Soft tissues
2. Bones
3. Neck
4. Visible abdomen
5. Diaphragm
6. Mediastinum and heart
7. Lungs

Give special attention to areas over which physical abnormalities were elicited. If the film reveals an unsuspected abnormality, return to the patient and repeat the physical examination. Perform additional studies, such as changing the patient's position, shaking him, or checking for a tracheal tug, if the film suggests that these may be helpful. Go back and forth, if necessary, until careful correlation leads to accurate diagnosis.

SPIROMETRY

Spirometry provides a quantitative evaluation of the bellows function of the lung. The most helpful measurements are the: (1) forced vital capacity (FVC)—the maximum volume of air one can exhale from maximum inspiration with maximal effort; (2) the forced expired volume in 1 second (FEV_1)—the amount of the FVC exhaled in 1 second; and (3) the forced expired volume 1 second percent ($FEV_1\%$)—the FEV_1/FVC $\times$ 100. This is particularly useful in quantitating the amount of diffuse airways obstruction. FVC is predicted on the basis of age, height, and sex; 80 percent of that predicted is normal. An $FEV_1\%$ of 82 $\pm$ 9% is considered normal (see Fig. 11–7 and Table 11–12).

ARTERIAL BLOOD GASES

It is essential to evaluate arterial blood gases—the partial pressure of oxygen (PaO_2) and of carbon dioxide ($PaCO_2$), the pH, and the percent saturation of hemoglobin (SaO_2)—in patients with dyspnea, tachypnea (or other respiratory rate irregularities), or significant roentgenographic abnormality (Table 11–7). Adequate oxygenation cannot be determined accurately on a clinical basis; cyanosis may be seen only when the hemoglobin saturation is markedly reduced to about 75 percent with a PaO_2 of 40 mm Hg, e.g., equal to the normal mixed venous values. The clinical estimation of hypoventilation (retention of carbon dioxide) is also unsatisfactory because the signs and symptoms are late and nonspecific.

CLASSIC FINDINGS

A single abnormal finding is rarely diagnostic; correlation with other physical abnormalities and with the chest roentgenogram is necessary before the status of the underlying lung can be determined with confidence. Dullness and absent breath sounds, for example, occur with both pleural effusion and with an obstructed lobe

TABLE 11–7. Representative Normal Gas Pressures at Sea Level (mm Hg)

Partial Pressures	Air	Alveolus	Arterial Blood	Mixed Venous Blood
PO_2	159	104	100	40
PCO_2	0.3	40	40	46
pH	—	—	7.40	7.38

and often require the roentgenogram for differentiation; a small infiltrated lobe on the roentgenogram, however, may result from neoplasm or inflammatory fibrosis. Differentiation is made by the physical findings of dullness and diminished breath sounds in pleural effusion and dullness and bronchial breath sounds in an obstructed lobe.

In practice, the importance of one or another single finding may outweigh or be strengthened by others in correlative diagnosis. The following discussion describes the abnormalities that occur in various major pathologic states.

DIFFUSE DISEASES

AIRWAYS OBSTRUCTION (see Figure 11–7). *General:* The most sensitive measure of airways obstruction is the forced expired time (FET), which provides a semiquantitative estimate of the degree of obstruction: normal, 3 seconds or less; abnormal, 4 seconds or more. It is an essential component of the physical examination.

Breath sounds heard *over the chest* decrease in intensity with increasing airways obstruction. Indeed, one can estimate the $FEV_1\%$ quite accurately by systematically grading breath sounds during rapid inspirations, through the open mouth at six sites: the upper anterior chest, mid-axillae, and the posterior bases bilaterally. The sounds are graded as: 0, absent; 1, barely audible; 2, faint, but definitely audible; 3, normal; 4, louder than normal. The grades are added to give the breath sound intensity (BSI) score. The $FEV_1\%$ is normal with a score of 16 or greater: the FEV_1 approximates 40% with a score of 12. This analysis is less accurate if there is restrictive lung disease.

In contrast, inspiratory breath sounds heard *at the mouth* are loud, "noisy," and increase with increasing airways obstruction. These are nonmusical sounds having a wide spectrum of frequencies ("white noise"). Commonly, early inspiratory and expiratory coarse crackles are heard at the lung bases and at the mouth. Low-pitched, coarse, bubbling, or rattling crackles are heard with secretions in large airways. With increasing amounts of obstruction, wheezing, or rhonchi are heard. These can be precipitated by deep or forceful breathing. One may also find decreased fremitus, hyperresonance, and a barrel shape to the chest, but these signs are less sensitive and less specific.

The pathognomonic signs of this disease [emphysema] are furnished by a comparison of the indications derived from percussion and mediate auscultation. The respiratory sound is inaudible over the greater part of the chest, and is very feeble in the points where it is audible: at the same time, a very clear sound is produced by percussion.

RENÉ THÉOPHILE HYACINTHE LAËNNEC
(1781–1826)

Emphysema: Characteristic of emphysema is the absence of inspiratory breath sounds at the mouth and over the chest despite expiratory airflow obstruction. It should be noted that most (80 + %) individuals seeking medical care for obstructive airways disease have both chronic bronchitis and emphysema to varying degrees (Fig. 11–17).

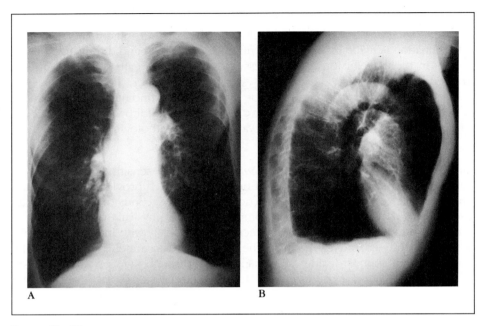

FIGURE 11—17
Roentgenograms of a man with extensive emphysema. A. Posteroanterior view. The diaphragms are markedly flattened and the vascular markings are irregularly distributed. There is marked hyperlucency at both lung bases, indicating bulla formation. B. Lateral view. The diaphragms are flattened as determined by an angle of greater than 90° between the sternum and diaphragm; and the anterior clear space—the distance between the sternum and the aorta—is greater than 3 cm (on original roentgenogram).

Asthma: A person with asthma may have a normal examination between episodes. With mild airways obstruction, only the FET may be prolonged. As the degree of obstruction increases, relatively low-pitched wheezing at end expiration becomes higher pitched and extends throughout expiration and inspiration; respirations increase. The symptomatic, tachypneic, actively wheezing person with asthma is likely to develop a paroxysm of coughing with the FET maneuver; thus, it is better to delay this until the patient improves.

In the presence of severe airways obstruction, an extremely high-pitched wheeze is heard at the very beginning of expiration, followed by silence. This almost silent or silent chest is an ominous sign in the obvious dyspneic and tachypneic person with asthma.

DIFFUSE INTERSTITIAL FIBROSIS (FIBROSING ALVEOLITIS). This disease is characterized by fine, late inspiratory crackles heard first at the lateral bases. As the disease progresses they are heard at the posterior bases, then higher and higher in the chest and over a greater portion of inspiration. With extensive disease, the diaphragms become elevated and the breaths are rapid and shallow (Fig. 11–18).

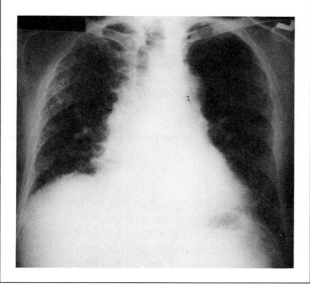

FIGURE 11–18
Chest roentgenogram of a 76-year-old physician with extensive diffuse interstitial fibrosis. Note the elevation of the diaphragms bilaterally and generalized cardiac enlargement—cor pulmonale (heart failure due to lung disease). Both lung fields have a diffuse reticulo-nodular infiltrate. There are multiple areas of hyperlucency which represent cyst formation and bronchiolectasis.

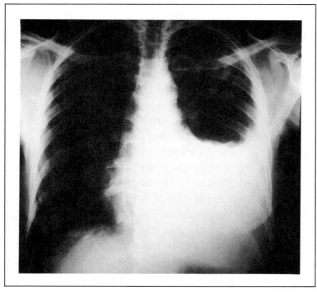

FIGURE 11–19
Large left pleural effusion. Note fluid extending upward along the lateral costal margin. There is also an infiltrate in the left upper lobe.

UPPER AIRWAYS OBSTRUCTION. Upper airways obstruction is defined as a narrowing of the airway from the trachea cephalad. It is characterized by monophonic, usually very loud, wheezing (stridor). It can be produced or accentuated by increasing the rate of air flow. If the obstruction is extrathoracic, the wheezing is usually limited to inspiration. The sound has been described as whooping or crowing. It can be heard at the open mouth or over the trachea and may be transmitted through the lung to the chest wall. Often it is loud enough to be heard at a considerable distance.

ACUTE RESPIRATORY FAILURE. Acute respiratory failure is generally defined according to arterial blood gas measurements: an arterial oxygen tension (PaO_2) 50 mm Hg or less; and/or an arterial carbon dioxide tension ($PaCO_2$) of 50 mm Hg or more with an appropriate decrease in pH. These criteria are used because of the great difficulties in clinically identifying hypoxemia and hypercarbia. However, the clinician must recognize the constellation of findings associated with respiratory failure.

The first most sensitive and quite specific sign of respiratory failure is an increase in respiratory rate ("the most vital of signs"). Normal people breathe in the range of 12 to 20 breaths/minute, perhaps to 24/minute. A rate of 35 is ominous. Observe the patient for breathing through an open mouth, with pursed lips on expiration with severe airways obstruction, flaring of the ala nasi, tensely lifting the head off the pillow, sitting bent forward with elbows on thighs, sweating, anxiety, and tachycardia. Look for use of the sternocleidomastoid muscles and intercostal retractions.

Carefully observe and palpate for evidence of *inspiratory muscle fatigue.* After the respiratory rate increases, the usual next sign of fatigue is *respiratory alternans,* a cyclic alternation between mostly abdominal breaths and then mostly rib cage breaths. We normally breathe predominantly with abdominal breathing when supine. This is characterized by the abdomen moving out and increased intraabdominal pressure. You should observe this and palpate it by placing one hand over the sternum and the other over the abdomen. Occasional short periods of respiratory alternans (with tachypnea) may precede overt respiratory failure by days. The most specific sign of inspiratory muscle fatigue is *abdominal paradox* or *paradoxical respiration,* that is, inward movement of the abdomen with a decrease of intraabdominal pressure during inspiration; the inspiration is thoracic or from the chest cage. This too can be seen and palpated. This is pathognomonic of diaphragmatic fatigue. However, one should exclude abdominal muscle contractions by palpation. It is also seen with bilateral diaphragmatic paralysis. This paradoxical breathing may precede or occur simultaneously with the development of hypercarbia. A later and most distressing sign is a reduction in rate (< 10/minute) and depth of respiration, a harbinger of death unless intubation and mechanical ventilation are instituted. These signs of inspiratory muscle fatigue accompany the previously described signs of the underlying disease process, such as asthma, chronic bronchitis, emphysema, and diffuse interstitial fibrosis.

LOCAL BRONCHIAL OBSTRUCTION

With obstruction of a large bronchus a lag may be present, the thorax may be contracted, and the trachea and mediastinal contents may be shifted toward the side of the obstruction. The shift may increase further with inspiration and decrease with expiration. Fremitus is decreased, percussion note is dull, and breath sounds are diminished or absent. No rales are heard. Bronchogenic carcinoma and, occasionally, other tumors, foreign bodies, or inflammatory stenosing lesions of the bronchi are responsible (see Fig. 11–16B).

LOCAL PARTIAL BRONCHIAL OBSTRUCTION

It is remarkable how rarely partial bronchial obstruction manifests itself clinically. In spite of the presence of air within the parenchyma of an obstructed lobe on the roentgenogram, the physical findings are often those of complete bronchial obstruction. At times, however, crackles may be present, and the breath sounds may still be heard, though diminished. A localized high-pitched or low-pitched inspiratory or expiratory wheeze or rhonchus may be present; the wheeze may persist after the patient abruptly stops a forced expiration or inspiration (i.e., when breath sounds have ceased elsewhere in the lung).

COMPRESSION

An otherwise normal compressed lung above a pleural effusion may be dull or tympanic to percussion. Fremitus is increased, and breath sounds are bronchovesicular or bronchial. Egophony is elicited. The findings of pleural effusion often merge gradually with those of a normal lung without the intervening abnormality of compressed lung.

CONSOLIDATION

The patient is usually ill, depending on the underlying condition. Ventilation is usually deep and rapid. Fremitus is increased, the percussion note is dull, and the breath sounds are loud and bronchovesicular or bronchial. Fine, late inspiratory crackles are heard. Bronchophony and pectoriloquy may be present. Consolidation occurs mainly in pulmonary infections and with large areas of pulmonary infarction (see Fig. 11–16A).

MEDIASTINAL LESIONS

The patient may be either asymptomatic or quite ill; he may be unable to lie on his back. The veins in the neck may be distended if the superior vena cava is compressed or occluded in the mediastinum. The distance from the sternum back toward the trachea is increased if the mass is in the anterior mediastinum. The lungs may be entirely normal. Percussion may reveal an increased width of dullness over the sternum. Table 11–8 presents some causes of mediastinal enlargement.

PLEURAL EFFUSION

The patient may or may not appear ill, depending on the cause of the effusion (Table 11–9) and the rapidity with which it has developed. The affected side of the hemithorax may bulge; ventilation may lag and be diminished. The trachea and mediastinum may be shifted to the opposite side. The percussion note is flat, frem-

TABLE 11–8. Some Causes of Mediastinal Enlargement

Enlarged lymph nodes
  Neoplasm
    Primary
    Secondary
  Sarcoidosis
  Tuberculosis
Esophageal
  Rupture
  Achalasia
  Diverticula
Vascular
  Pericardial cyst
  Aortic aneurysm
  Pulmonary hypertension
Tumors
  Dermoids, teratomas
  Neurofibromas, sarcomas
  Goiter
  Thymoma

itus is markedly decreased or absent, and breath sounds are absent. No rales are heard (Fig. 11–19).

With a moderate effusion, breath sounds may be heard underlying the effusion; physical findings of compression may be noted above it.

PNEUMOTHORAX

Whether the patient is symptomatic depends on both the extent, acuteness, and rapidity of progression of the pneumothorax and on the adequacy of the remainder of the lung. The scratch sign is most accurate in identifying a pneumothorax, especially if it is small. Place the stethoscope in the midline over either the sternum or the spine; then lightly scratch on the chest with a fingernail about 10 cm from the stethoscope. The transmitted sound will be louder and more harsh (lower frequency) on the side of the pneumothorax. The larger the pneumothorax, the more clear-cut the classic signs. Fremitus is diminished to absent, but the percussion note is hyperresonant. Breath sounds are also diminished to absent. When hydropneumothorax is present, a splash may sometimes be elicited by abruptly shaking the patient from side to side (a succussion splash); the dullness or flatness of the effusion shifts with change in position to a greater extent and more rapidly than in pleural effusion alone. Some causes of pneumothorax are shown in Table 11–10. A left pneumothorax is illustrated in Figure 11–20 (note the chest tube, placed to evacuate the air from the pleural space).

TENSION PNEUMOTHORAX

A tension pneumothorax is a true medical emergency. It results from a bronchopleural fistula with a ball valve mechanism that permits air to enter but not exit the pleural space. It is most commonly seen in intensive care units in patients being

TABLE 11-9. Definitions and Causes of Pleural Effusion*

I. Transudates
  A. Definition: Pleural fluid characterized by low protein content—<3gm%
  B. Causes
    1. Heart disease (congestive heart failure)
    2. Renal disease (sometimes acute glomerulonephritis; most common in nephrotic syndrome)
    3. Malnutrition with systemic edema
    4. Severe anemia of any cause
    5. Cirrhosis of the liver
    6. Myxedema
II. Exudates
  A. Definition: Pleural fluid characterized by high protein content—>3gm%
  B. Causes
    1. Infections
      a. Bacterial
      b. Mycobacterial
      c. Viral, rickettsial
      d. Fungal
      e. Parasitic
    2. Neoplasms
      a. Primary lung
      b. Metastatic
      c. Lymphoma
      d. Mesothelioma
      e. Meigs' syndrome
    3. Pulmonary infarction, embolism
    4. Vasculitis and immune disease
      a. Rheumatoid arthritis
      b. Systemic lupus erythematosis
    5. Pancreatic disease
    6. Drugs and toxins
      a. Allergy
      b. Toxicity
        1. Nitrofurantoin
        2. Heroin, other narcotics
        3. Asbestos
    7. Lymphatic obstruction
    8. Uremia
    9. Trauma (hemothorax)
    10. After abdominal surgery

---

*The divisions between transudates and exudates are not absolute. For example, long-standing heart failure may produce an exudative effusion. Specific diagnoses often require identification of an infecting organism or histologic confirmation. A very modest increase in specificity, sensitivity, and positive predictive value for an exudate can be obtained by measuring one or more of the following: (1) ratio of effusion protein to serum protein >0.5; (2) lactose dehydrogenase protein (LDH) > 200 IU/L; (3) effusion LDH/serum LDH >0.6. One should weigh the cost-benefit ratio of the increase in identification according to the clinical setting.

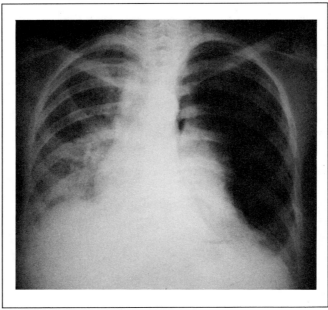

FIGURE 11–20
Chest roentgenogram showing left-sided *tension* pneumothroax. Note the *intrathoracic* tracheal air column: the heart and mediastinum are deviated to the right compressing the right lung. The left lung is completetly collapsed, and the left hemidiaphragm is low due to the increased intrathoracic pressure on the left.

mechanically ventilated and less commonly in association with trauma. The patient appears acutely ill, anxious, and diaphoretic. There is marked tachypnea and tachycardia. The patient may be hypotensive or without a palpable pulse because of a decreased return of venous blood to the heart. The most reliable sign is deviation of the trachea away from the side with decreased breath sounds and hyperresonance. Treatment consists of the immediate introduction of a needle into the affected side, which will result in a whoosh of air escaping through the needle and a return of the trachea to the midline and vital signs to normal (Fig. 11–20).

PULMONARY EDEMA (LEFT-SIDED HEART FAILURE)

If edema is acute and severe, the patient is in extreme distress; if edema is partial or chronic, minimal or no dyspnea may be present at rest. The respiratory rate and use of accessory musculature reflect this difference. Fremitus may be normal or slightly decreased. Associated signs of pleural effusion may be present at the base. Breath sounds are of fair quality, and resonance is normal or only slightly impaired. Fine, late inspiratory crackles are heard when the edema is primarily interstitial (mild or "early"). As the disease progresses, coarse rales early in inspiration and throughout expiration are heard. Search for other signs of failure: jugular venous distention, a third heart sound, an enlarged and tender liver, edema, etc. In patients

TABLE 11–10. Some Causes of Pneumothorax

Spontaneous
   Primary
      Rupture of subpleural bleb
         After severe coughing, parturition, etc.
         Without a precipitating event
   Secondary
      Chronic obstructive pulmonary disease
      Cystic fibrosis
      Diffuse interstitial fibrosis of lung and related vasculitides and granulomatous disease
      Suppurative pneumonias
      Lung abscess
      Asthma
      Neoplasm with necrosis
      Pulmonary infarction with necrosis
      Tuberculosis
      Marfan's syndrome
      Tuberous sclerosis
      Ecchinococcosis
      Lymphangioleiomyomatosis
      Biliary cirrhosis
Traumatic
   Iatrogenic ("complications")
      Mechanical ventilation
         ↑ Peak ventilating pressures
         ↑ Positive end expiratory pressure
      Thoracentesis or pleural biopsy
      Transbronchial or percutaneous lung biopsy
      Insertion of central lines (through subclavicular or neck approaches)
   Noniatrogenic
      Penetrating
         Stab wounds
         Gunshot wounds
      Nonpenetrating
         Chest wall compression (e.g., by steering wheel, with sudden deacceleration)
         Rib fractures
         Rapid decompression (e.g., scuba divers)

with emphysema, who develop left-sided heart failure, breath sounds may increase in intensity toward normal.

SPECIAL MANEUVERS

Compare the abnormal findings on physical and roentgenographic examination and correlate them (Table 11–11). Recheck the physical examination carefully if any discrepancy between physical and roentgenographic findings is noted. If the roentgenogram alone was abnormal, additional physical abnormalities may be elicited; for example, the post-tussive inspiration may be rewarding in the demonstration of crackles in nondependent areas of the lung. If only abnormal physical findings were present, and if they persist on repeat examination, recheck the roentgenogram more carefully.

TABLE 11–11. Correlation of Abnormal Physical Findings to Localized Disease

Disease	Tracheal Deviation[a]	Percussion	Vibration[b]	Rales
Pneumothorax	Away or N	Hyperresonant	↓ or 0	0
Obstructed bronchus				
With atelectasis	Toward or N	Dull	↓ or 0	0
With consolidation	N	Dull	↓ or 0	0
Open bronchus				
With atelectasis	Toward or N	Dull	↑	0
With consolidation	N	Dull	↑	+
Pleural effusion	Away or N	Flat	↓ or 0	0

N = normal; + = present; 0 = absent; ↑ = increased; ↓ = decreased. The presence of the findings will vary with the extent of involvement.
[a]Toward or away from side of lesion.
[b]Vibration includes both fremitus and breath sounds, which vary in the same way.

TABLE 11–12. Some Pulmonary Function Values*

Lung volumes (ml)
Vital capacity (VC)	5,000
Residual volume (RV)	1,500
Functional residual capacity (FRC)	3,500
Total lung capacity (TLC)	6,500

Ventilation
Tidal volume (VT)	500 ml
Respiratory frequency (f)	12–16/min
Minute ventilation (VE)	5,000 ml/min
Alveolar ventilation (VA)	3,500 ml/min

Ventilatory function tests
Forced expired volume in 1 second (FEV_1)	4,100 ml
FEV_1/forced vital capacity (FVC) × 100 (FEV_1%)	
% in 1 sec	83
% in 3 sec	97
Forced expired flow during middle half of forced expiratory vital capacity (FEF_{25-75})	4.6 L/sec

*For a normal 20-year-old man, 170 cm in height. Normal values are predicted according to age, sex, and height.

A change in the patient's position is a helpful special maneuver. It is often difficult to distinguish the crackles of inflammatory and fibrosing conditions from those of chronic pulmonary congestion. Note carefully the distribution of the crackles. If they are posterior and basal, place the patient flat on his stomach and instruct him to remain stationary for at least a half hour. Recheck the examination. Congestive crackles will often disappear posteriorly and appear anteriorly, whereas inflammatory crackles will not be affected. Certain wheezes due to extrabronchial compression or intrabronchial polypoid lesions appear only with change in position. Dullness and absent breath sounds at one lung base may indicate either fluid or obstruction; if the patient lies on the same side for a half hour, dullness will now extend high into the axilla if free fluid is present. Obtain a roentgenogram in the lateral decubitus position to confirm the finding. The physical findings of pleural effusion change slowly with positioning; rapid change suggests combined pneumothorax and effusion. Place the patient on the contralateral side. Dullness should now be rapidly replaced with hyperresonance or tympany. A shifting linear fluid level on the roentgenogram confirms these findings. Shaking such a patient vigorously may demonstrate a succussion splash.

If a mediastinal mass is noted in the film, check for a tracheal tug. Place your fingers on the thyroid cartilage and attempt to raise it cephalad. A pulsatile resistance suggests aortic aneurysm.

If a nodular shadow connected to the hilum with broad vascular bands is seen and an arteriovenous malformation is suspected, listen over the proper anatomic area for a bruit with the patient holding his breath. Note whether it increases with inspiration; it may disappear completely with a held forced expiration (Valsalva maneuver).

If the differential diagnosis between pneumothorax and a large bulla is unclear from the roentgenogram and physical examination, perform the coin test. Have an aide place one coin flat against the anterior chest wall and tap it with another while you listen with the stethoscope posteriorly, or vice versa. Normally, and with bulla, you will hear only a dull thudding sound, but with pneumothorax the note will have a distinct metallic ringing quality.

CHAPTER 12

CARDIOVASCULAR SYSTEM

The heart is the root of life and causes the versatility of the spiritual faculties. The heart influences the face and fills the pulse with blood.

HUANG TI
(2697–2597 B.C.)

The clinical examination of the cardiovascular system has been significantly modified by information made available with the advent of cardiac catheterization and advances in noninvasive techniques. A sound modern interpretation of both normal and pathologic cardiovascular phenomena requires a clear understanding of the anatomy and physiology that underlie their genesis. The unique aspect of clinical cardiovascular observation has to do with its transient nature. Phenomena pass by relatively rapidly (though recurrently) on a time axis that is constantly moving. It is understandable, then, that the cardiovascular examination presents a challenge to our perceptive ability that is unrivaled by other systems. The examiner must frequently use two or more senses simultaneously: one for identification of a finding, the other for timing purposes. This correlation of vision, touch, and sound requires patience and practice. It is, in a sense, the essence of bedside observation.

Complete evaluation of the cardiovascular system extends beyond the examination of the heart itself. It must include a careful analysis of the peripheral arterial and venous circulations. Occlusion of a coronary artery may produce alarming signs and symptoms that are easily recognized by the physician; occlusion of a deep femoral vein, on the other hand, frequently results in more subtle clinical findings that may go unnoticed but are nevertheless equally threatening to the life of the patient. In this discussion the circulatory system will be considered comprehensively.

As elsewhere in medicine, the "diagnostic negative" may be of great significance in the assessment of the circulatory system. Subtle or transient cardiovascular phenomena too often escape the casual observer. Your strategy must therefore be directed toward the conscious exclusion of certain diagnostic possibilities as you progress through a systematic evaluation. Is the arterial pulse increased? Is there an A wave? Is there a presystolic extra sound? A *No* answer to this type of inquiry is justified only if you have actively excluded the possibilities. To begin with, then, you must guard against undue preoccupation with auscultation and particularly with listening only for murmurs. This common trap most frequently awaits the inexperienced observer. Rushing for the stethoscope prematurely will certainly result in an inadequate examination. A detailed history coupled with careful preliminary observations (particularly inspection and palpation) often permits you to predict the auscultatory findings with remarkable accuracy. More importantly, when you place your stethoscope on the chest you know what you are looking for and why.

To recognize and to understand the signs of vascular disease, you must first develop an appreciation of the enormous variability of the so-called normal range. The circulatory system, perhaps more than any other, is constantly adapting to internal and external factors, with changes in cardiac rate, intravascular pressure, and stroke volume. Keep in mind that while the cardiac output may triple with heavy exercise, it may also double with excitement. If the patient is angry or fearful, if he has just smoked a cigarette or finished a large meal, if he has had to hurry to his appointment, if he is chilled or overheated, his cardiovascular system will respond accordingly. Even the simple act of standing or of lying down on the examining table calls into play several major hemodynamic mechanisms. Thus, it is difficult for the physician to be certain of a basal or steady state at the time of examination. You must learn to recognize the physiologic variables, so as not to confuse them with signs of disease. The young conditioned athlete, the overweight businessman, and the slightly anemic young housewife must be expected to present very different patterns of blood pressure, pulse rate, and heart sounds.

ANATOMY AND PHYSIOLOGY

A sound heart is the life of the flesh.
                         PROVERBS 14:30

The normal relationships of the cardiac valves and the great vessels must be appreciated in order to interpret the clinical examination. As demonstrated in Figure 12–1, the mitral and tricuspid valves share a common fibrous ring, and the aortic valve also is part of this fibrous "cardiac skeleton." The projection of the normal relationship on the plain chest roentgenogram is also shown as an aid in visualizing the internal anatomy when observing the body surface.

In normal circulation, unoxygenated blood is returned by way of the systemic veins to the right atrium and then to the right ventricle. The left atrium and left ventricle receive fully oxygenated blood from the pulmonary veins. Figure 12–2 portrays diagrammatically both the normal circulation and typical oxygen saturations and fluid pressures.

The physiology of human circulation has two very different divisions—the *systemic* and *pulmonary* (Fig. 12–3). These circuits are obviously integrally related but vary from one another in several characteristics. The pulmonary circuit is a low-pressure, low-resistance system. Although resistance vessels are found in the pulmonary circuit, they probably do not play a significant role in normal pulmonary circulation. In addition, the lung contains many potential arteriovenous shunts that, when opened, can further serve to lower pulmonary pressure. Both its distensibility and the presence of potential arteriovenous shunts allow the pulmonary circuit to permit increases in blood flow without significant increases in pressure—a property termed **capacitance**. The pulmonary circulation is therefore termed a high-capacitance circuit in the normal state. The usual pressures seen in this portion of the circulation are noted in Figure 12–2.

In contrast to pulmonary circulation, the systemic circuit has been considered a high-pressure, high-resistance system. Indeed, the arterial portion of the systemic circulation does offer variable, active resistance to blood flow from the left ventri-

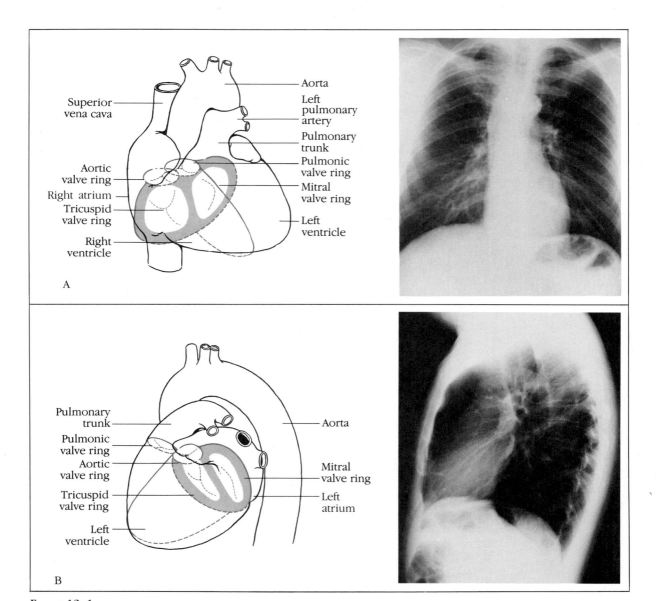

FIGURE 12–1

Normal anatomy of the heart. Anteroposterior (A) and left lateral projections (B), compared with their cardiac silhouette on chest roentgenogram.

cle. The term **afterload** is used to refer to the strain placed on the left ventricle by this resistance or impedance to outflow. The venous portion of the systemic circulation, however, is (like the pulmonary system) a low-resistance, high-capacitance circuit. If intravascular volume is increased, the systemic veins can act as a reservoir and thereby decrease the effect of volume overload on the rest of the

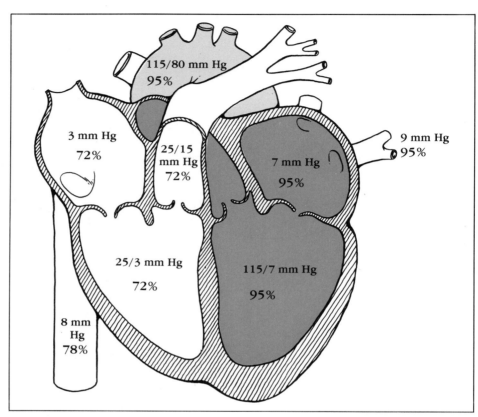

Figure 12–2
The normal central circulation. Oxygenated blood is depicted in red. Pressures (in mm Hg) and oxygen saturations (in %) are average normal values.

circulatory system. Ultimately, any major increase in intravascular volume will be reflected in increased blood return to the left heart. The volume filling the left ventricle during diastole as a result of this venous return is termed **preload** and is reflected by the left ventricular end-diastolic pressure. Examples of normal pressures in the systemic circuit are seen in Figure 12–2.

Many of the findings related to the circulatory system, which are noted in the history and physical examination in succeeding pages, result directly from these anatomic and physiologic principles. For example, evaluation of systemic blood pressure and cutaneous perfusion will reflect with reasonable accuracy the state of systemic resistance and afterload. Observation of the venous pressure will give information related to preload and systemic capacitance vessels. The state of the pulmonary vascular resistance may be suggested by findings related to the pulmonic component of the second heart sound. As you proceed through the subsequent sections, the various findings in the history and physical examination will be better understood and remembered if they are correlated with the anatomy and physiology of the circulatory system (Fig. 12–4).

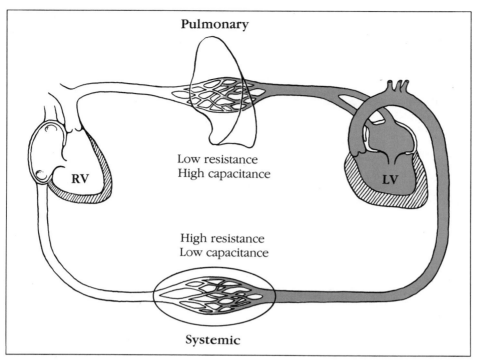

FIGURE 12–3
Normal pulmonary and systemic circuits. Oxygenated blood is shown in red.

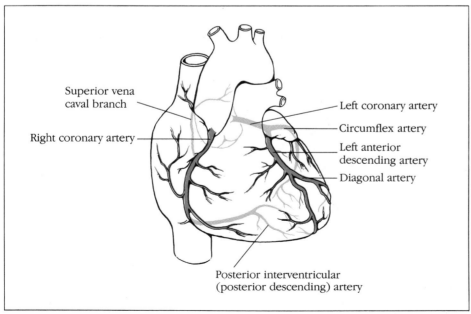

FIGURE 12–4
Anatomy of the coronary arteries.

HISTORY

The seat of it, and sense of strangling, and anxiety with which it is attended, may make it not improperly be called angina pectoris.

They who are afflicted with it, are seized while they are walking (more especially if it be up hill, and soon after eating), with a painful and most disagreeable sensation in the breast . . .

WILLIAM HEBREDEN
(1710–1801)

In the cardiovascular system a carefully taken, meticulously explored, and logically ordered history is extremely important to correct diagnosis and therapy.

Major cardiac disease may be present in an asymptomatic patient, but far more frequently the patient's history will establish the direction of both the physical examination and special studies of cardiovascular function. In certain circumstances the history will give the diagnosis even in the face of an unremarkable physical examination (e.g., as frequently occurs in angina pectoris). Characteristic symptoms of cardiovascular disease are discussed below.

DYSPNEA

Dyspnea of cardiac origin is characteristically related to effort until the advanced stages of heart disease, when it may become present even at rest. The labored respirations result from the increased work of breathing caused by decreased compliance of the lungs and decreased diffusing capacity due to an abnormal increase in pulmonary venous pressure. Because we all experience breathlessness with heavy exertion, mild dyspnea early in the course of cardiac disability requires careful, detailed assessment. Any unexplained reduction in exercise tolerance should arouse suspicion. The patient's inability to keep up with associates of the same age is noteworthy. The level of activity that brings on the symptom must be explicitly determined and quantitated; for example, the number of flights of stairs resulting in distress. Is the complaint abnormal for the patient's age, build, and apparent physical condition? Has there been a slow progression, rapid progression, or sudden onset of the present state? How long does it take to restore natural breathing with rest? To what extent does it interfere with daily activity? Are there associated symptoms, such as pain, palpitation, or cough? (See also Chaps. 5 and 11.)

PAROXYSMAL NOCTURNAL DYSPNEA

This describes the onset of breathlessness at night, which usually awakens the patient with an alarming smothering sensation. This invariably prompts him to assume the sitting position or to get up from bed. There may be associated wheezing and cough. It generally occurs 2 to 4 hours after lying down and infrequently occurs more than once nightly. Occasionally, non-effort-related paroxysmal dyspnea occurs during the waking hours. It is sometimes precipitated by a disturbance in cardiac rhythm with an excessively rapid or slow heart rate.

ORTHOPNEA

Dyspnea precipitated by assuming the recumbent position is referred to as orthopnea. It is a symptom of relatively late onset and is frequently relieved or improved when the thorax is again elevated. In clinical practice, orthopnea is referred to as two-, three-, or four-pillow (or more) orthopnea, depending on the extent of elevation. It may disappear with improvement that follows therapy. It is a useful index of the patient's status.

PAIN

It is not the delicate neurotic person who is prone to angina, but the robust, the vigorous in mind and body, the keen and ambitious man, the indicator of whose engine is always at "full speed ahead."

SIR WILLIAM OSLER
(1849–1919)

Pain is an important symptom of circulatory disease. Most commonly it is a consequence of ischemia, but it may arise from the pericardium or aorta, or from elevation of the pulmonary arterial pressure.

Angina pectoris is a common manifestation of coronary artery disease and is the symptom of inadequate oxygen delivery to the myocardium. It is usually located in the retrosternal area and may radiate into the neck or into either or both arms (usually the left). It is characteristically constrictive or oppressive (from the Latin *angere,* "to strangle"), although patients will describe anginal discomfort quite variably (e.g., burning, aching, squeezing), and many will refuse to call the sensation *pain.* Factors that increase cardiac work (myocardial oxygen demand) such as exercise, excitement, cold weather, and meals, tend to provoke angina. Anginal discomfort is not infrequently associated with transient dyspnea, diaphoresis, or nausea. The essence of the diagnosis of angina pectoris centers on distress that occurs in the substernal area, is related to effort, and is relieved within minutes by rest. Fleeting stabs or jolts of pain, or pain lasting for hours or days, is not angina pectoris. Angina pectoris is seldom restricted to the left anterior chest or inframammary region—a common site for noncardiac chest pain. While most angina results from an increase in cardiac work, spasm of a normal or diseased coronary artery, or thrombus formation at the site of an arteriosclerotic lesion, may decrease myocardial oxygen delivery enough to cause ischemic pain. The term *variant angina* describes discomfort associated with spasm of a normal coronary artery; *mixed angina* describes pain due to the spasm of a coronary vessel already narrowed by arteriosclerosis. *Unstable angina* is a syndrome probably resulting from thrombus formation in coronary arteries.

The *Levine sign* (a clenched fist over the sternum or even subtle flexion of the fingers or pressing on the anterior chest with the flat of the hand) suggests an ischemic cause for the chest discomfort being described by the patient. *Claudication* refers to ischemic pain caused by an inadequate arterial circulation to a muscle group, usually the legs (from the Latin *claudicare,* "to limp"). It is similar to angina in that it is precipitated by exercise and relieved by rest. *Pericardial* pain may be retrosternal and may mimic the pain of myocardial ischemia in many respects. It is persistent and, unlike angina, is often intensified by inspiration (pleuritic) and relieved by changes in body position, such as sitting up.

PALPITATION

This is a general term that describes an awareness of the heartbeat that may occur with increased stroke volume, irregularity of rhythm, tachycardia, or bradycardia. The precise identification of the underlying disturbance requires electrocardiographic confirmation. Nonetheless, a close clinical estimate may at times be possible by tapping out various cadences on the back of the hand and asking the patient to select the one that most closely simulates what he felt. Palpitation often is of no consequence, but its importance must be judged in the context of associated symptoms.

COUGH

Cough, especially while recumbent, is a common complaint with pulmonary congestion. It may be a dry hack or may produce clear, thin sputum. **Hemoptysis** may accompany cough when pulmonary venous pressures are greatly elevated, as in mitral stenosis or severe left ventricular failure (see Chap. 11). Dyspnea is usually associated with cough of cardiac origin.

SYNCOPE

Syncope of cardiac origin has two general causes: (1) inability of the heart to maintain an adequate cardiac output for a given level of activity or (2) cardiac arrhythmia resulting in sudden loss of cardiac output. Both of these mechanisms result in decreased perfusion of the central nervous system, causing loss of consciousness, occasionally seizure activity, and loss of motor control. Abnormalities that prevent the maintenance of an adequate cardiac output include left ventricular outflow obstruction (aortic stenosis, obstructive hypertrophic cardiomyopathy), obstruction to flow at the mitral orifice (mitral stenosis [rare], atrial myxoma), and pulmonary hypertension (severe). Syncope caused by these conditions generally occurs during physical exertion (when cardiac output cannot keep up with increased demand) and rarely happens at rest.

Either tachyarrhythmias (especially ventricular tachycardia or fibrillation) or bradyarrhythmias (e.g., complete heart block) can result in sufficient reduction in cerebral blood flow to cause syncope. Syncopal episodes due to bradyarrhythmia (often termed *Stokes-Adams attacks*) can occur with the patient either at rest or performing activity. A history of palpitations or fatigue may also be obtained in some patients.

While syncope has many causes in association with other cardiac symptoms, including the simple faint (Table 12–1), it should alert the clinician to a limited spectrum of disorders such as those mentioned above.

TABLE 12–1. Some Causes of Syncope

I. Volume deficit
  A. Blood loss
  B. Dehydration
    1. Addison's disease
    2. High fever
    3. Salt-wasting renal disease   ↓ Intravascular volume
    4. Diabetes insipidus
    5. Diuretics
      a. Exogenous
      b. Glycosuria
  C. Heat or erythroderma
  D. Vasodilatory drugs and toxins   ↑ Vascular capacitance
  E. Tussive syncope } Maldistribution of volume
II. Neurogenic
  A. Decreased cardiac output (vasovagal syncope)
  B. Some intracranial lesions
  C. Hypoxemia
  D. Hypoglycemia
  E. Seizures
  F. Autonomic insufficiency
  G. Pain
  H. Hysteria
III. Cardiogenic
  A. Mechanical or obstructive
    1. Aortic stenosis
    2. Hypertrophic, obstructive cardiomyopathy (IHSS)
    3. Myxoma
    4. Mitral stenosis
    5. Massive pulmonary embolism
    6. Pulmonary hypertension
  B. Arrhythmias

PHYSICAL EXAMINATION

1. With patient sitting, note the general appearance (respiratory pattern, vital signs, color—cyanosis or pallor).

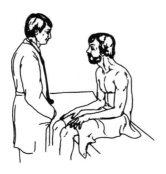

2. With patient recumbent and head elevated 30 degrees, examine the following:
   a. Upper and lower extremities (arterial pulses, venous pattern, color, nails, hair, temperature, edema).
   b. Neck (carotid pulses, jugular venous pressure, jugular venous pulse, thyroid).
   c. Precordium (inspection, direct percussion, palpation, auscultation).

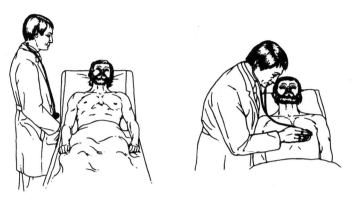

3. With patient in left decubitus position, repeat palpation and auscultation.

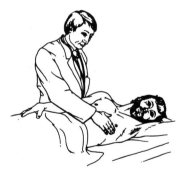

4. With patient sitting (again), repeat palpation and auscultation (precordium and neck).

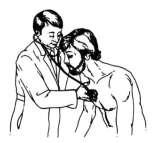

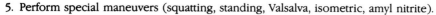

5. Perform special maneuvers (squatting, standing, Valsalva, isometric, amyl nitrite).

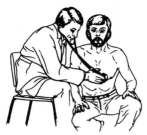

Begin with the patient sitting. Your initial observations, including examination of the fundi and lungs, have been performed earlier in the physical examination. Then have the patient recline with arms at sides. Station yourself on the right. You may wish to retake the blood pressure. Then examine the extremities, neck, and precordium, in that order. The male patient will be disrobed to the waist. A towel or examination gown is very satisfactory for draping the female chest; it can be manipulated to allow all necessary observations without causing undue embarrassment. Have adequate light and a quiet room, and eliminate all distractions as much as possible. Position the examining table or bed, which preferably has an adjustable head, at a comfortable height.

GENERAL OBSERVATION

Preliminary inspection begins during history taking (see Chaps. 3 and 4). Facies, body build, character of respiration (supine and sitting), general color, obvious pulsations, and signs of emotional tension may all be casually observed at this time.

The *face* may give clues to cardiovascular disease. In addition to the anxious expression of the patient suffering from chest pain, facial features may give clues to the discrete kind of heart disease. Patients with *mitral stenosis* may have either a malar flush or a slight cyanosis of lips and cheeks, which often is so distinctive that the valve disease can be promptly diagnosed by the experienced observer before auscultation. The protuberant eyes of Graves' disease may alert the physician to the thyrotoxic etiology of a rapid irregular heart rhythm and congestive failure. Malar telangiectasia and alopecia in a young woman with cardiac complaints require consideration of the myopericarditis of lupus erythematosus. The head nodding of severe aortic regurgitation should alert you to consider this diagnosis.

Cyanosis is a bluish skin color caused by a relative decrease in oxygen saturation (or increase in desaturated hemoglobin) of the cutaneous capillary blood. Normal arterial blood is about 95 percent saturated (venous blood is about 70 percent saturated). When the arterial saturation falls below 85 percent, cyanosis usually becomes manifest (unless anemia is so severe that less than the 5 gm of desaturated hemoglobin required to produce cyanosis is present).

Cyanosis may be central or peripheral (Table 12–2). *Central cyanosis* has three major causes: (1) congenital heart diseases with right-to-left shunts, (2) pulmonary arteriovenous fistulas, and (3) advanced pulmonary disease with hypoxemia. Cen-

TABLE 12–2. Some Causes of Cyanosis

I. General cyanosis
    A. Decreased oxygenation of blood
        1. Lung disease
        2. Arteriovenous pulmonary shunts
          a. Congenital
          b. Acquired
        3. Right-to-left intracardiac shunts
    B. Increased desaturated hemoglobin (>5 gm)
        1. Erythrocytosis
        2. Abnormal hemoglobins
II. Peripheral cyanosis (due to increased tissue oxygen extraction with slow flow)
    A. Congestive heart failure
    B. Hyperviscosity
    C. Veno-occlusive disease
    D. Hypotension
    E. Distal vasoconstriction
        1. Drugs
        2. Cold
        3. Anxiety

tral cyanosis is generalized and is associated with arterial oxygen desaturation. Polycythemia and clubbing are frequently present. *Peripheral cyanosis* (sometimes called acrocyanosis) is limited to the hands, feet, tip of the nose, ear lobes, and lips. It results from a critical reduction in systemic blood flow that usually is due to diminished cardiac output (heart failure shock) or obstructive peripheral arterial disease. The extremities are usually cold and mottled. Clubbing is not a consequence of these disorders alone. Light pressure will produce a sustained white print in the bluish background, which fades slowly.

Severe anxiety or pain may cause diaphoresis (sweating). Marked diaphoresis—a cold, "clammy" sweat—may be associated with an acutely decreased cardiac output, as in acute myocardial infarction. Pallor can be a component of shock as well, and is due to intense cutaneous vasoconstriction in the face of decreased cardiac output.

EXTREMITIES

GENERAL

First examine the arms and legs, paying particular attention to the hands and feet. Make your observations in the following order: (1) fingernails and toenails, (2) skin color, (3) hair distribution, (4) venous pattern, (5) presence of swelling or atrophy, and (6) obvious pulsations. Develop the habit of comparing sides. Estimate skin temperature by light, quick palpation with the tips of the fingers or with the back of the middle phalanges of the clenched fist. Compare identical sites on both sides and the gradation of temperature along the limb. The level of vascular tone in the extremities is under sympathetic control. Vasodilation results in rubor, warmth, throbbing of the distal digits, and capillary pulsations of the nailbeds, with distention of the superficial veins. Vasoconstriction results in pallor, coldness, and collapsed superficial veins. Smoking cigarettes, chilling, or apprehension may cause vasoconstriction. In the dependent position the superficial veins become distended, and the venous valves may be identified as nodular bulges; with elevation of the limb the veins collapse. These changes in caliber are at times a cause of undue concern to patients.

CLUBBING

Clubbing of the digits has been previously mentioned, in Chapter 4. Three cardiovascular causes of clubbing are cyanotic congenital heart disease, infective endocarditis, and pulmonary disease often associated with cor pulmonale.

ARTERIES

Arterial occlusion may be complete or partial; it may occur acutely or gradually. Chronic arterial insufficiency results from gradual reduction in vessel caliber, which may be due to degenerative or inflammatory processes of the vascular wall. Examination of a limb with chronic arterial insufficiency may show some or all of the following:

1. Diminished or absent pulses.
2. Audible systolic bruits, especially those extending into early diastole, heard over major arteries (femoral or subclavian).
3. Reduced or absent hair peripherally (over the digits and dorsum of the hands or feet).
4. Atrophy of muscles and soft tissues.
5. Thin, shiny, taut skin.
6. Thickened nails with rough transverse ridges and longitudinal curving.
7. Mild brawny edema.
8. Coldness on palpation.
9. Intense grayish pallor on elevation of the extremity. Dependency after a minute or two of elevation produces a dusky, plum-colored rubor that develops very gradually (30 seconds to 1 minute).
10. Flat, collapsed superficial veins.
11. Delayed venous filling time. Empty the superficial veins by elevating the extremity. Prompt filling (less than 10 seconds) occurs normally with lowering.

In examining an upper or lower extremity for suspected underlying arterial insufficiency, it is particularly important to assess the effects of exercise in order to identify early disease. Three important changes may be elicited with exercise.

1. Pallor of the skin may occur over the distal limb.
2. Arterial pulses may disappear.
3. Systolic bruits not present at rest may become apparent over the major arteries.

These important diagnostic signs may become apparent only following exercise.

Advanced arterial insufficiency shows all the above features, and in addition there may be (1) a bluish gray mottling of the skin unchanged by position, (2) early ulceration between or on the tips of the digits, (3) tenderness to pressure, (4) stocking or glove distribution anesthesia. These signs indicate that gangrene is imminent.

Chronic occlusion of the aortic bifurcation is associated with (1) absent femoral pulses, (2) intermittent claudication extending into the buttocks, and (3) sexual impotence. These together comprise Leriche's syndrome.

Acute arterial occlusion usually begins with agonizing pain in the affected extremity, which below the occlusion site is pale, cyanotic, and pulseless. It may also be tender and exhibit stocking distribution anesthesia. This is a serious emergency.

Figure 12–5 illustrates several maneuvers for examining the peripheral arterial pulses. Use the three middle fingers (not simply a single finger) and vary the pressure. Occlude the vessel completely at first and release gradually. Bimanual palpation of the abdominal aorta in the epigastric and periumbilical areas should also be performed to evaluate possible aneurysmal dilation. Examination of the peripheral arterial system should include auscultation over the femoral arteries, abdominal aorta, and carotid and subclavian arteries for bruits that might indicate occlusive disease.

ARTERIAL PULSE

When a patient affected by this disease [aortic regurgitation] is stripped, the arterial trunks of the head, neck, and superior extremities immediately catch the eye by their singular pulsation.

SIR DOMINIC JOHN CORRIGAN
(1802–1880)

The pulse examination is done both in assessment of vital signs (rate and rhythm, as discussed in Chap. 5) and as part of the cardiovascular examination, in which all pulses listed in the red box are examined for (1) pulse rate, (2) rhythm, (3) amplitude, (4) any special quality, and (5) elasticity of the vessel wall. Amplitude may be classified as increased, normal, diminished or absent; or a numerical system of 0 to 4+ may be used, with 2+ being normal. The following diagrammatic representation is often used in recording pulses:

		Carotid	Brachial	Radial	Aorta	Femoral	Dorsalis pedis	Posterior tibial
	(R)	2+	2+	2+	0	1+	1+	1+
Normal = 2+								
	(L)	2+	2+	2+	0	1+	1+	1+

The ulnar and popliteal arteries are often included.

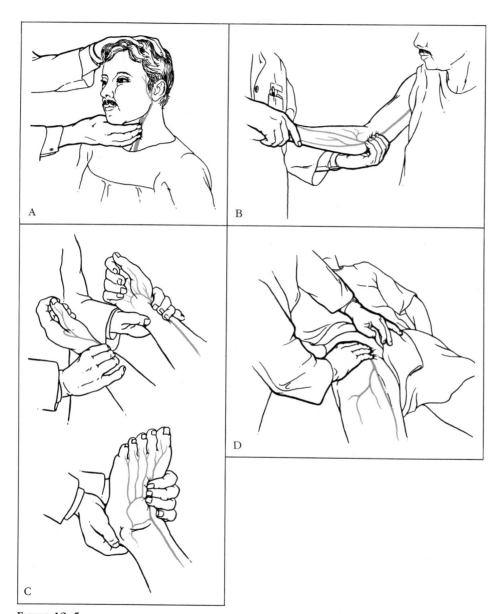

FIGURE 12–5
Examination of the pulses. A. Carotid pulse. B. Epitrochler pulse. C. Radial and dorsalis pedis.
D. Femoral pulse.

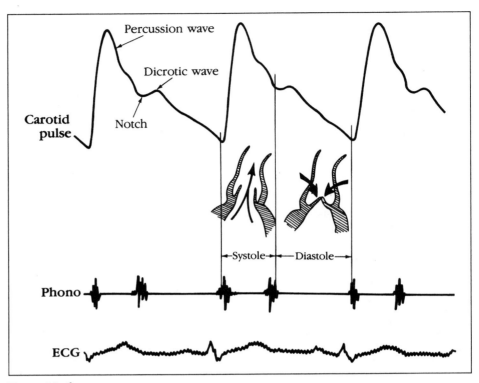

FIGURE 12–6
Normal carotid pulse. Pulse contour is shown as related to the timing of aortic valve motion, phonocardiogram, and electrocardiogram.

In addition to rate and regularity, the arterial pulse should be examined for its amplitude and contour. The amplitude of the pulse is largely a function of the pulse pressure, which is related to stroke volume, elasticity of the arterial circulation, and peak velocity of the ejection of blood from the left ventricle. If the stroke volume increases—as with excitement, heat, alcohol ingestion, exercise, or slowing of the heart rate—the pulse pressure widens, resulting in a bounding quality on palpation.

The amplitude of the pulse obviously contributes to its contour. However, important information about the characteristics of left ventricular ejection can be learned from assessing the rate of rise and the shape of the arterial pulse wave. Because of the distortion that occurs when the pulse wave is transmitted distally, the carotid arteries must be used for accurate evaluation of pulse contour. An excellent way of analyzing pulse contour is to correlate it with a graphic record. Figure 12–6 shows such a tracing that was recorded from a normal carotid artery. The initial percussion wave is separated from the dicrotic wave (not palpated in the normal state) by a dicrotic notch caused by aortic valve closure. A second systolic wave (tidal wave) usually follows the percussion wave but is not often palpable. The record is qualitative, but it helps the beginner to understand better what

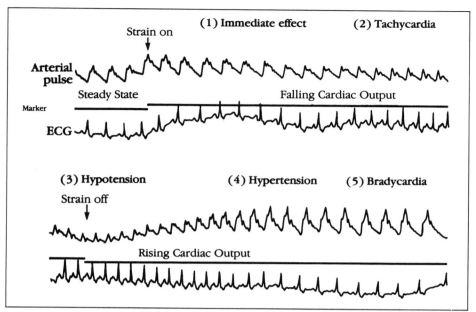

FIGURE 12–7
Normal response to Valsalva maneuver (see text).

he feels. The upstroke normally takes no more than 0.10 second, and the rounded crest takes another 0.08 to 0.12 second. The brachial and femoral pulses are usually synchronous.

The *Valsalva maneuver* is a test that you can perform on yourself right at this moment. It will challenge your ability to observe and to interpret a rather complex series of physiologic variations. Close your glottis and strain down hard for several seconds while palpating your carotid or radial pulse. What happens?

The normal response to the Valsalva maneuver is shown in Figure 12–7. The explanation is as follows: (1) The high intrathoracic pressure decreases venous return, causing an abrupt drop in cardiac output after several seconds. (2) The normal response to the decreased output is twofold: peripheral vasoconstriction and tachycardia. (3) Despite this compensatory mechanism, the pulse pressure dwindles; that decrease causes the pulse to become feeble. (4) After release the cardiac output is suddenly restored, causing an abrupt increase in blood pressure due to the temporary increase in peripheral vascular resistance. (5) Increased blood pressure in turn triggers a reflex bradycardia (slowing), which is transient and somewhat delayed. Finally, the normal state returns. Responses (4) and (5) disappear with many forms of heart disease.

The quality of the arterial pulse may provide clues to many circulatory disorders other than peripheral vascular disease.

Water-hammer pulse (Table 12–3) is characterized by a wide pulse pressure, a low diastolic pressure, and a dicrotic notch that is absent or displaced downward

TABLE 12–3. Some Characteristic Arterial Pulse Wave Forms

Normal	

Water-hammer pulse
    Occurs in aortic insufficiency and other
        abnormalities associated with wide
        pulse pressure
    A bounding pulse	

Anacrotic pulse (pulsus tardus) Occurs in aortic stenosis	
Bifid pulse (pulsus bisferiens) Occurs in aortic insufficiency	

Spike-and-dome pulse
    Occurs in obstructive hypertrophic
        cardiomyopathy	

Pulsus alternans Occurs in left ventricular failure	

on the descending limb of the tidal wave. The pulse has a collapsing, bounding quality that is reinforced by elevating the arm above the head. It is a classic sign of aortic regurgitation but is seen in other conditions in which there is a low-resistance runoff due to a leak in the arterial system—for example, patent ductus arteriosus and peripheral arteriovenous fistula. It is the basis for other peripheral signs of aortic regurgitation, including hopping carotids, pistol-shot sounds, Duroziez's sign, de Musset's sign, and others. Although interesting, these signs add little of diagnostic importance.

Bounding pulses of lesser degree, which are characterized by a wide pulse pressure with a normal or slightly lower diastolic pressure, also occur. Fever, anemia, hepatic failure, thyrotoxicosis, and complete heart block are all capable of producing a bounding pulse. They have in common an increased stroke volume and frequently a diminished peripheral resistance.

Weak pulse (pulsus parvus) has a normal contour but a low amplitude. It feels weak and thready. The pulse pressure is narrowed by a low stroke volume and associated peripheral vasoconstriction. It is present with low-output failures of all types. Common causes include mitral stenosis, acute myocardial infarction, shock, and constrictive pericarditis.

Anacrotic pulse (pulsus tardus) (see Table 12–3) is associated with valvular aortic stenosis. The ascending limb is delayed and the summit is broad. The pulse pressure may be narrowed (pulsus parvus). The slow rise and delayed peak can often be appreciated with careful practice.

Bifid pulse (pulsus bisferiens) (see Table 12–3) is characterized by double systolic peaks that can usually be felt with the palpating finger. Bifid pulse is found with aortic regurgitation, which may be isolated or, more frequently, may be associated with some degree of aortic stenosis.

Another type of pulse with two systolic waves is the *spike-and-dome pulse* of dynamic aortic outflow tract obstruction (obstructive hypertrophic cardiomyopathy) (see Table 12–3). This pulse is characterized by an extremely brisk initial wave (spike) followed by a rounded dome that occurs after the muscular obstruction to left ventricular outflow develops. The rounded dome is not as easily felt as the second peak of the bifid pulse of aortic regurgitation, and consequently the two waves of this pulse may be difficult to appreciate. However, the abrupt rise and fall of the spike may be a significant clue to the presence of this disorder.

The *dicrotic pulse* has two waves but only one is systolic, and the second is a very prominent dicrotic wave occurring in diastole. This pulse is best appreciated in a more peripheral artery (brachial or femoral) and is usually seen in younger patients with myocardial disease and in hypovolemic states.

In *pulsus alternans* (see Table 12–3) the regular consecutive beats are of alternating large and small amplitude. It can be detected by palpation (best appreciated in a peripheral vessel) or by use of a blood pressure cuff. Alternate systolic pressures may vary by as much as 25 mm Hg. It is an important sign of left ventricular failure.

Bigeminal pulse (bigeminy) is a coupling of two beats separated by a pause. It results most often from alternating normal and premature beats. The second beat is weak due to reduced diastolic filling time.

Pulsus paradoxus is an important sign of cardiac tamponade. It is found with tense pericardial effusions and less frequently with chronic constrictive pericarditis. The term refers to a weakening of the pulse during normal inspiration. It is really a misnomer, however, because this is an exaggeration of the normal (up to 10 mm Hg) inspiratory decline in systolic blood pressure. Multiple mechanisms for pulsus paradoxus have been postulated. The observed fall in systolic blood pressure with inspiration is thought to be caused by normal inspiratory augmentation of venous return to the right heart chambers in a heart with restricted capacity for diastolic filling. As a result, there is a reciprocal decrease in left ventricular filling and a fall in systolic blood pressure. Increased capacitance of the pulmonary vasculature in inspiration (with less of the right heart output entering the left ventricle from the lungs, therefore) may also play a role. Although pulsus paradoxus may be detected by palpation, it is more reliably quantitated by using the sphygmomanometer. As the pressure in the cuff is slowly reduced, the first Korotkoff sounds will appear only during expiration (upper systolic level). As one lowers the pressure, the sounds begin to occur in both inspiration and expiration (lower systolic level). A difference of greater than 10 mm Hg between these two points is abnormal. A common noncardiac cause of pulsus paradoxus is the labored respiration of the patient with obstructive pulmonary disease (asthma, emphysema).

Abdominal bruits may be a sign of intra-abdominal disease. Because such bruits commonly occur in young healthy individuals, it is important to be cautious about overinterpretation of such a bruit as an isolated finding. In the presence of hypertension, however, a bruit heard in the epigastrium or subcostal region may be an important sign of renal artery stenosis. Abdominal bruits are best heard using the diaphragm of the stethoscope. They are commonly very soft and of medium or low pitch. Similar systolic bruits have been observed in patients with mesenteric arterial disease as well as over greatly enlarged spleens. Venous hums are at times identified over the cirrhotic liver due to torrential flow through venous collaterals. In addition, neoplasms of the pancreas, stomach, and liver may rarely produce abdominal systolic bruits due to arterial involvement or an increase in local blood flow.

There is no disease more conductive to humility than aneurysm of the aorta.

SIR WILLIAM OSLER
(1849–1919)

Aneurysm of an artery produces a pulsatile swelling along the course of the vessel. The aorta and the popliteal artery are the vessels most often involved. A systolic thrill may be felt over the aneurysm. The aorta should always be carefully palpated for the presence of an aneurysm. This is usually felt as an expansile mass in the epigastrium and midabdomen (Fig. 12–8). Rupture of an aortic aneurysm is usually indicated by severe, constant back pain and is often associated with pain in one or both groins and a mass in the flank. It constitutes a serious surgical emergency and is an important consideration in any patient with an acute abdomen (see Chap. 14). If the thrill noted over such a mass is continuous, one should suspect an arteriovenous fistula.

DISORDERS OF RHYTHM

When the heart slowed down after partial recovery, I found that the jugular and liver pulses were of the ventricular form, that the presystolic murmur had disappeared, and that the heart was irregular; in other words, all evidence of auricular activity had disappeared. [*Atrial fibrillation*]

SIR JAMES MACKENZIE
(1853–1925)

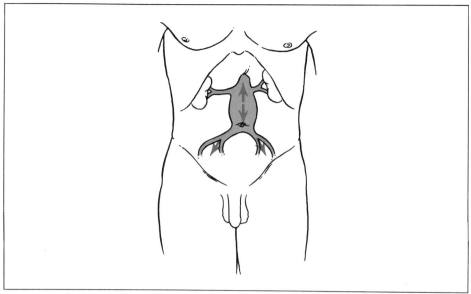

FIGURE 12–8
Abdominal aortic aneurysm. Note the radiation of the murmur, indicated by arrows.

The electrocardiogram is indispensable for the precise recognition and identification of arrhythmias, but much can be learned by careful examination at the bedside. Some of the common arrhythmias and their associated physical findings are listed in Table 12–4. Observations regarding the pulse rate and regularity of the rhythm should be made. Hints regarding the presence or absence of synchronized atrial and ventricular activity can be found in the jugular venous wave form (see following section). The presence of premature beats can be noted, as well as their efficacy in maintaining stroke volume.

VEINS

That the blood in the veins therefore proceeds from inferior or more remote to superior parts, and towards the heart moving in this and not in the contrary direction, appears most obviously.

WILLIAM HARVEY
(1578–1657)

Varicose veins is the term usually applied to dilation of the superficial leg veins. *Varicose* means "dilated, swollen." The rate of blood flow through these vessels is diminished, and the intraluminal pressure is increased. There are two types of varicose veins: primary, due to an inherent weakness of the vessel wall and venous valves; and secondary, due to proximal obstruction in the vena cava, pelvic veins, or iliofemoral veins. Both the greater and lesser saphenous system may be in-

TABLE 12-4. Some Common Arrhythmias and Their Associated Physical Findings

ECG	Jugular Venous Pulse	Arterial Pulse	Cardiac Examination
Long PR interval	Prolonged AV wave interval	No effect	Diminished intensity S_1
Short PR interval	Decreased AV wave interval	No effect	Increased intensity S_1
Left bundle-branch block	No effect	No effect	Reversed split S_2 (paradoxical split)
Right bundle-branch block	No effect	No effect	Persistently split S_2
2nd degree AV block	"Extra" A waves	Slow rate	"Extra" S_4
3rd degree AV block	Intermittent cannon A waves	Slow rate	Variable intensity S_1; intermittent S_4
Atrial fibrillation	Absent A waves	Irregularly irregular rate	Variable intensity S_1
Premature atrial contraction	Early A waves	Irregular rate	Premature cardiac cycle
Paroxysmal atrial tachycardia	Rapid venous pulsations	Rapid, often diminished	"Bouncing precordium" (loud S_1)
Premature ventricular contraction	Possible cannon A wave	Irregular	Premature cardiac cycle
Ventricular tachycardia	Intermittent cannon A waves	Rapid, usually diminished	Variable intensities, "cascade" rhythm

volved. The greater saphenous vein lies superficially on the anteromedial aspect of the thigh and lower leg. It drains into the common femoral vein on the groin. The lesser saphenous vein lies superficially on the posterolateral aspect of the calf from the ankle to the popliteal space. Both saphenous veins communicate with the deep femoral venous system by means of multiple communicating or perforating veins that pierce the fascia. When the valves in the perforating veins are incompetent, the superficial saphenous varicosities may fill from the deep venous system.

Diagnosis, usually simple, is made by inspection of the dependent limb. In severe cases, pigmentation, edema, and even ulceration of the skin in the region of the medial malleolus point to significant venostasis. It is important to determine two additional facts in patients with varicose veins: Are the valves incompetent in the communicating veins between the superficial and deep systems? Are the deep veins patent?

The presence of incompetent communicating or perforating veins can be demonstrated simply. Lift the leg to empty the veins. Apply a tourniquet around the thigh with the patient in the recumbent position. When the patient assumes an erect position, the incompetent valves in the communicating veins permit the varicosities to fill rapidly from above *(Trendelenburg's test)*.

Patency of the deep veins may be established by the use of the *Perthes' test*. A tourniquet is used to occlude the subcutaneous veins at knee or thigh level. This tourniquet must be at or below the lowest significant incompetent perforator. Filling of the superficial varicosities from above is prevented by the tourniquet. As the patient walks, the muscles exert a pumping action on the deep veins and drain the dilated superficial varicosities. Failure of the varicosities to empty means either that the tourniquet is placed too high and a large incompetent communicating vein permits the varices to fill, or that the deep veins have been damaged by an inflammatory process, disturbing their normal function.

Venous thrombosis may be acute (thrombophlebitis) or silent (formerly termed phlebothrombosis), deep or superficial. Superficial thrombophlebitis produces redness, induration, and tenderness adjacent to the involved venous segment, which is thickened and cordlike. Diagnosis is easily made, but remember that there may be associated deep thrombosis.

Acute inflammatory thrombosis of a major vein (deep thrombophlebitis) results in rather striking pain, tenderness, warmth, and swelling of the involved limb. Sensation is preserved, and superficial veins may be distended. There may be considerable reflex arteriospasm, which at times may cause the extremity to become pale and the peripheral pulses to be reduced or even absent (phlegmasia cerulea dolens). This must be differentiated from acute arterial occlusion, which usually occurs without swelling of the extremity.

Deep venous thrombosis involving the deep femoral and pelvic veins may be entirely asymptomatic, and fatal pulmonary embolism may occur without warning. It is worthwhile for the physician to become "thrombosis conscious" and constantly to watch for minor suggestive signs in his bedfast patients. These include (1) tenderness along the iliac vessels and below the inguinal ligament, along the femoral canal, in the popliteal space, over the deep calf veins, and over the plantar veins; (2) minimal swelling detectable only by measuring and comparing the circumference of both calves and both thighs at several levels; (3) unexplained low-grade fever and tachycardia; and (4) a trace of ankle edema.

EDEMA

Edema has many causes (Table 12–5). It is graded 1 + through 4 + on the basis of pitting produced by sustained, light pressure with the thumb over the medial malleolus or pretibial area (Fig. 12–9). Cardiac edema is usually dependent (feet and ankles, or back and flanks if the patient is supine). It is a common though not reliable sign of congestive heart failure. Unilateral edema occurs following the occlusion of a major vein. Chronic peripheral arterial occlusion may cause mild "brawny" (nonpitting) edema.

NECK

In the assessment of cardiovascular status the physician should make four separate observations in the neck: (1) carotid pulse (2) jugular venous pressure, (3) jugular venous pulse (wave form), and (4) venous and arterial auscultation.

CAROTID PULSE

With the patient supine, palpate each carotid medial to the sternocleidomastoid muscle just below the angle of the jaw. The three-finger method may be used, although some examiners prefer to use the thumb (Fig. 12–10). Auscultation of the carotid arteries to detect bruits is advisable prior to carotid palpation (Fig. 12–10).

Carotid pulsations may be striking in hyperkinetic states and particularly with aortic regurgitation *(Corrigan's sign)*. A carotid thrill is commonly felt with aortic stenosis but may result from increased flow associated with aortic regurgitation. It also occurs with partial occlusion of the orifice of the common carotid artery. A bruit may be heard over a partially occluded carotid artery but may also be related to a nonobstructive plaque, carotid tortuosity, or transmission of an aortic murmur.

Diminished or absent carotid and brachial pulsations may result from a diffuse process involving the aortic arch and its major branches. This is called the aortic arch syndrome. It may be due to arteriosclerosis, aortitis, aortic dissection, or congenital anomalies. Isolated occlusion of the common carotid artery may cause neurologic symptoms and signs. Internal carotid pulsation may be estimated by palpating the vessel in the tonsillar fossa.

Carotid sinus pressure increases vagal tone and results in slowing of the heart rate. On occasion this response may be exaggerated, and carotid sinus pressure will result in extreme bradycardia (even cardiac standstill) or hypotension (the carotid sinus syndrome). The Valsalva maneuver, combined with carotid sinus pressure, results in more pronounced vagal tone. Carotid sinus pressure is frequently used in the diagnosis and treatment of certain arrhythmias. It is also helpful in transiently slowing the heart rate to aid in auscultation. Carotid sinus pressure should be applied cautiously (if at all) in the elderly, who are prone to have carotid artery atherosclerosis. The carotid pulse may be palpated from behind or anteriorly.

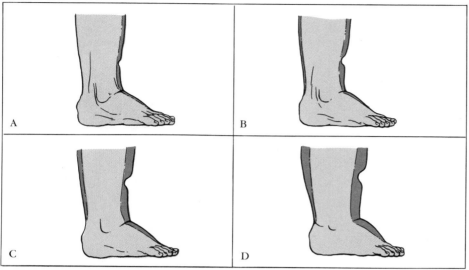

FIGURE 12–9
Grading of edema. A. 1+: slight pit, normal contours. B. 2+: deeper pit, fairly normal contours. C. 3+: deep pit, puffy appearance. D. 4+: deep pit, frankly swollen.

TABLE 12–5. Some Causes of Edema

I. Increased hydrostatic pressure in the vascular space
  A. Increased volume
    1. Congestive heart failure
    2. Renal failure
    3. Certain hormones (estrogens, corticosteroids)
    4. Certain drugs (indomethacin, sodium-rich compounds)
  B. Increased mechanical pressure (total volume normal or low)
    1. Venous thrombosis
    2. Compression of veins (tumor, scar, fibrosis, gravid uterus, etc.)
    3. Pericardial constriction
    4. Portal hypertension
    5. Prolonged standing
II. Decreased oncotic pressure in the vascular space—hypoproteinemia ($\downarrow$ albumin)
  A. Nephrotic syndrome
  B. Starvation
  C. Protein-losing enteropathy
III. Tissue or vascular damage
  A. Vasculitis
  B. Allergy
  C. Trauma
  D. Burns
  E. Ischemia
  F. Infection
IV. Other
  A. Myxedema
  B. Lymphedema

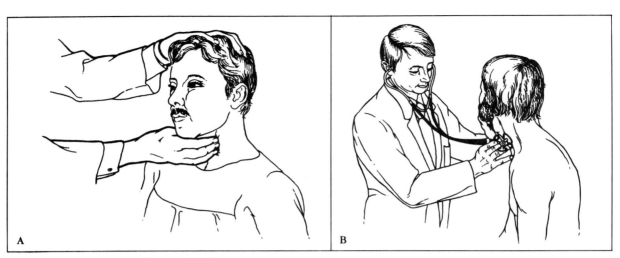

FIGURE 12–10
A. Palpation of the carotid pulse. Some examiners prefer palpating the carotid pulse with the patient in the sitting position. B. Auscultation of the carotid artery.

JUGULAR VENOUS PRESSURE

The first of the two sudden elevations (venous pulse) immediately precedes ventricular systole, while the second coincides nearly exactly with it; . . . in the third place and finally, a light pressure suitably applied to the lower portion of the neck can impede them or suppress them entirely, while the pulsations of the carotid persist with all their intensity.

PIERRE CARL EDOUARD POTAIN
(1825–1901)

Satisfactory examination of the neck veins requires a bed or table that will allow the patient's head and trunk to be elevated to various heights. Clothing should be removed from the neck and upper thorax, and good illumination should be available. If pillows are removed and the head is turned slightly away from the examiner (without putting a marked stretch on the neck), the neck veins can be visualized in the majority of patients. The head of the bed should be raised and lowered to bring the patient to the position where venous pulsations and the meniscus of the internal jugular vein (marking the height of the venous pressure) can be easily seen.

Maximum information can be gained only with proper technique. A finger is placed on the opposite carotid artery for timing purposes. Occasionally, tangential lighting with a pocket flashlight is helpful. The neck veins are frequently distended when the patient is supine, tending to collapse with inspiration and to refill during expiration. Light pressure over the jugular bulb causes them to distend further, and release is followed by collapse to the previous level. Because of the effects of gravity, distention usually disappears when the head of the bed is elevated 30 to 45 degrees. This position is satisfactory for determining jugular venous pressure in

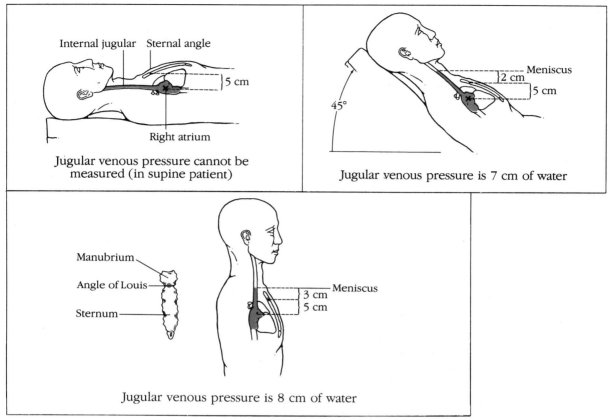

FIGURE 12–11

Measuring the jugular venous pressure. The sternal angle (angle of Louis) is a bony ridge palpable between the manubrium and the body of the sternum at the level of the second intercostal space. It is always 5 cm vertically above the mid-right atrium. In any position, therefore, one may measure the distance from the sternal angle to the meniscus of the internal jugular vein and add 5 cm to obtain the jugular venous pressure.

the majority of instances. With severe elevation of jugular venous pressure, greater degrees of elevation of the bed may be needed.

Observe the base of the neck for venous pulsations. Four simple maneuvers should be followed in order: (1) note the general character of the pulse, which is normally diffuse and undulant; (2) observe any variation produced by respiration; (3) apply light pressure to the root of the neck, observing the effect on the pulsations; and (4) gradually elevate the head of the bed or the examining table in increments and note the overall effect. Lastly, the jugular venous pressure (JVP) is estimated by thinking of the neck veins as manometer tubes directly attached to the heart (right atrium). The internal jugular vein is more reliable than the external for this purpose. Both will collapse, however, at the point at which the intraluminal

TABLE 12–6. Estimating the Jugular Venous Pressure

Height of Meniscus above Sternal Angle	Degree of Venous Elevation
2–4 cm	Mild
4–8 cm	Moderate
>8 cm	Severe

pressure falls below the level of atmospheric pressure. With practice, this point can be identified, and its level above a reference point, such as the sternal angle (angle of Louis), can be estimated while the head of the bed is adjusted gradually upward. The sternal angle has been chosen for this purpose since its distance above the midpoint of the right atrium remains relatively constant (about 5 cm) in all positions (Fig. 12–11). Although a reasonable estimate of the jugular venous pressure in centimeters above the sternal angle can usually be achieved, a simpler scale of normal, mildly, and markedly increased will often suffice (Table 12–6).

Jugular venous pressure elevation is an important sign of congestive heart failure, although elevations of venous pressure may result from mechanical obstruction to venous inflow by intrathoracic, neoplastic, inflammatory, or vascular masses. The presence of jugular venous hypertension may escape notice in obese or bull-necked individuals. Also, extreme venous hypertension may go unnoticed because the veins may be distended all the way to the angle of the jaw and pulsations are not seen. Pregnancy invariably increases jugular pressure. Exertion, anxiety, premenstrual increases in blood volume, and abdominal pressure (caused by corsets and binders) may produce mild elevations.

JUGULAR VENOUS PULSES (WAVE FORM)
The bedside examination of the neck veins is a noninvasive method of assessing right atrial hemodynamics. The internal jugular vein connects without valves to the right atrium and accurately displays right atrial wave form and pressure to the careful observer. Two major waves occur in the normal right atrium during each cardiac cycle (Fig. 12–12). The larger of these is the A wave, which is generated as the atrium contracts to fill the ventricle just prior to systole. As the atrium relaxes and its pressure falls, the x descent is seen while ventricular systole begins and the tricupsid valve is closed. The right atrial pressure rises as the atrium is filled from the periphery, and the V wave, which is smaller than the A wave, is generated. As the atrium empties during early diastole, a fall of the V wave or y descent is seen. (The C wave, a positive deflection on the x descent, can sometimes be recorded on pulse tracings. It probably reflects displacement of the tricuspid valve apparatus into the right atrium during ventricular systole and is of little clinical significance.)

It is important to differentiate venous from arterial pulsations. The venous pulse is diffuse and undulant and usually disappears or markedly decreases in the sitting position. Venous waves can usually be obliterated by moderate pressure at the base of the neck. Venous *pressure* decreases with inspiration, although the venous *waves* may become more prominent during inspiration. Arterial pulsations in the neck are localized and brisk and are usually best seen high and medial to the sterno-

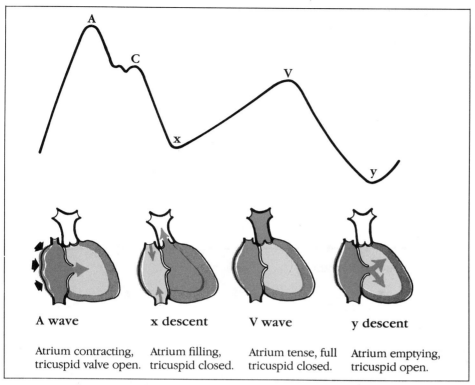

A wave   **x descent**   **V wave**   **y descent**

Atrium contracting,   Atrium filling,   Atrium tense, full   Atrium emptying,
tricuspid valve open.   tricuspid closed.   tricuspid closed.   tricuspid open.

FIGURE 12–12
Venous pulse. Events occurring in the right atrium are reflected in the jugular venous wave form.

cleidomastoid muscle, while venous pulsations are seen lower and more laterally, either under or just behind the sternocleidomastoid muscle. Arterial pulsations are unaffected by position and do not vary with respiration, nor can they be obliterated by pressure at the base of the neck as the venous pulse can.

To time the jugular pulse, you must use two senses in order to answer the question, "Is this wave occurring before or after the first sound?" Perhaps the simplest method is to use vision and touch, observing the venous pattern while palpating the opposite carotid pulse. If the wave precedes the arterial pulsation, it must be an A wave; if it is synchronous or a little delayed, it is a V wave. A second method is to use vision and hearing. Listen to the heart while making similar observations. Exceptions to this rule are caused by the occasional rhythm disturbance which superimposes atrial and ventricular contraction.

Giant A waves result from very forceful right atrial contraction. They are seen with tricuspid stenosis. More commonly they result from the loss of diastolic compliance that accompanies right ventricular hypertrophy, as in pulmonic stenosis or pulmonary hypertension. Figure 12–13 shows the venous waves seen with marked

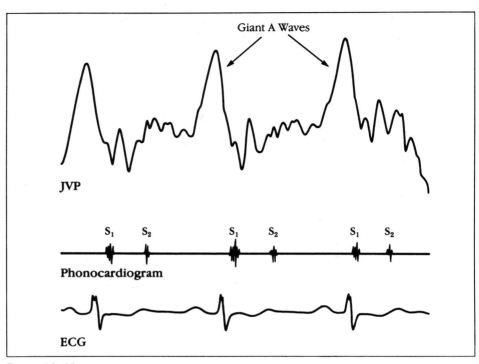

FIGURE 12–13
Giant A waves. Jugular venous pulse (JVP) tracing demonstrating giant A waves with marked pulmonary hypertension.

pulmonary hypertension. The right atrium contracts vigorously to fill the poorly compliant right ventricle, and a large A wave is seen in the neck veins. With the onset of atrial fibrillation and the loss of the effective atrial contraction, giant A waves as well as normal A waves are no longer seen in the jugular venous pulse.

Cannon waves occur with certain arrhythmias characterized by atrioventricular dissociation (complete atrioventricular block, ventricular and junctional tachycardia, artificially paced ventricular rhythm, and premature ventricular beats). When atrial contraction occurs during ventricular systole, cannon waves result. The origin is the same in all these, namely, contraction of the right atrium against a closed tricuspid valve due to synchronous atrial and ventricular systole. Since the blood cannot move forward there is striking backward regurgitation into the jugular system, resulting in these sporadic, prominent A waves (Fig. 12–14).

Large V waves are transmitted to the neck with tricuspid regurgitation, which reflects abnormal right atrial filling through an incompetent tricuspid valve during systole. The jugular venous pulse tracing in Figure 12–15 shows V waves from a patient with rheumatic tricuspid regurgitation. Atrial fibrillation is often present with this condition. With the loss of organized atrial contractions, no A wave is seen. The large positive V wave occurs during ventricular systole (but slightly ear-

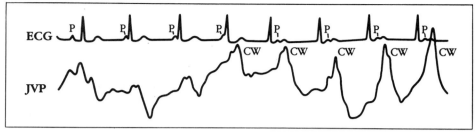

Figure 12–14
Cannon waves. Jugular venous pulse (JVP) tracing demonstrating cannon waves (CW). P waves on the ECG give the timing for atrial contractions.

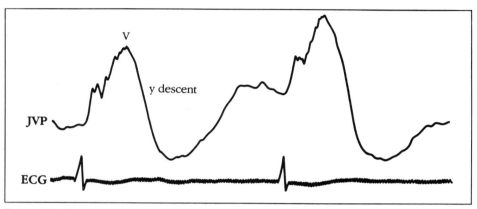

Figure 12–15
Large V waves. Jugular venous pulse (JVP) tracing demonstrating large V waves in a patient with rheumatic tricuspid regurgitation.

lier than the normal V wave) and can be timed by observation of the neck veins with simultaneous palpation of the carotid pulse or auscultation of the heart.

Sharp y descent is associated with an elevated mean pressure and is seen with chronic pericardial constriction and occasionally in acute pericardial effusion with tamponade. It may be seen in severe right heart failure of any cause. In these conditions the pressure drops only briefly following tricuspid opening and remains elevated during the rest of the cardiac cycle. The sharp descents result in a characteristic **M**-shape in the jugular venous wave form (Fig. 12–16).

JUGULAR VENOUS AUSCULTATION
Venous hum refers to a phasic roaring heard in about 25 percent of normal adults (and almost always in children) at the lower border of the sternocleidomastoid muscle in the sitting position. It is accentuated in diastole and may be transmitted to the upper precordium. Hums are attenuated by compression over the jugular vein, the Valsalva maneuver, and recumbency. They are generally an innocent finding of no consequence, although they may be confused with cardiac murmur.

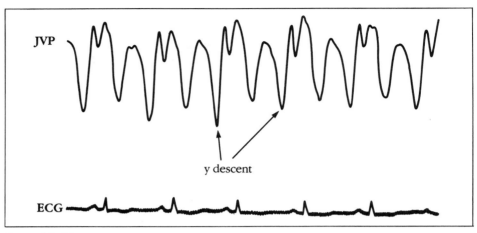

FIGURE 12–16
Sharp y descent. Jugular venous pulse (JVP) tracing demonstrating rapid y descent.

HEART EXAMINATION

INSPECTION AND PALPATION OF THE PRECORDIUM

Move toward the foot of the bed and observe the precordium from the level of the anterior chest. The character and location of any visible cardiac impulses should be noted. Minor precordial movements can be amplified by observing during expiratory apnea. The commands "Now take in a breath, let it all out, hold it" will provide the optimal setting for detecting these pulsations. At times it may be helpful to place a tongue blade or stiff card over the precordial impulse, observing the movement of the free edge. This simply acts as a mechanical amplifier (Fig. 12–17). Now palpate the precordium carefully with the hand lightly applied, using primarily the middle and ring fingers.

Palpation of the precordium to discern movement is usually best performed using the pads of the distal and middle phalanges. Detection of thrills (palpable murmurs), however, is usually best accomplished using the sensitive area just proximal to metacarpophalangeal joints. Often, the sensation in this area is greater in one hand or the other. Trial and practice of palpation using different areas of the hand as well as alternating hands will soon allow the examiner to determine which portion of which hand will yield the most information.

The four major areas that are explored are the apex, left sternal border, pulmonic area, and aortic area (Fig. 12–18). The value of palpation lies in the estimation of heart size, ventricular hypertrophy, identification of low frequency (and sometimes inaudible) vibrations, and ectopic impulses.

What is seen and felt over the precordium varies markedly with position, phase of respiration, amount and distribution of muscle and fat, and thoracic cage configuration. In normal people the cardiac apex is usually the most lateral impulse of cardiac origin that can be felt on the chest wall. It is often referred to as the point

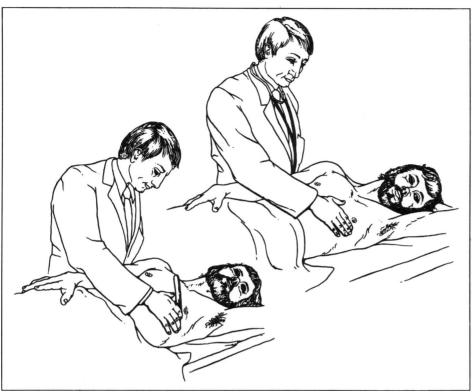

FIGURE 12–17
Palpation of the precordium. The morphology of the apical impulse can often be appreciated best in the left decubitus position. The impulse may be amplified by placing a tongue blade over the impulse.

of maximum impulse (PMI). In some patients with cardiac disease, however, the cardiac apex may not be the point of maximum impulse.

In order to appreciate the distinction between right- and left-sided events, as well as to note areas of paradoxical impulse, it is frequently helpful to palpate the precordium with two hands simultaneously. In this way, nonsynchronous movements can be distinguished from each other.

The normal apical impulse is in the fourth or fifth interspace, should not be felt in more than one interspace, usually occupies less than the first one-half of systole, and should not be felt farther to the left than halfway between the midsternal line and the lateral thoracic border. Placing the patient in the left lateral decubitus position (see Fig. 12–17) brings the cardiac apex closer to the chest wall. For purposes of auscultation and analysis of the configuration of the apical impulse, this is a useful maneuver, but assessment as to location and duration of the apical impulse should be made with the patient supine. A graphic recording of the normal apex impulse is shown in Figure 12–19. Medial to the apical impulse one can often

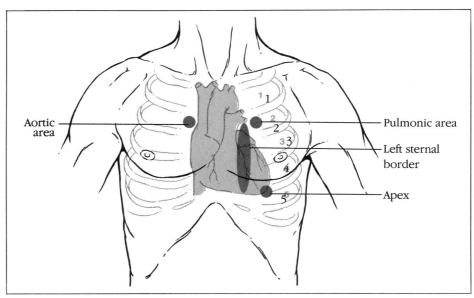

FIGURE 12–18
Areas of routine palpation of the precordium.

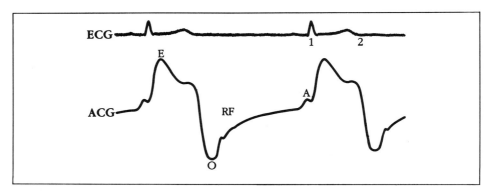

FIGURE 12–19
Normal apexcardiogram. The sharp outward movement (E) corresponds to ventricular systole and may be easily palpated at the cardiac apex. (O = end systole; RF = rapid filling.)

appreciate an inward motion that corresponds to retraction of the interventricular groove (septal retraction).

An outward systolic movement along the left sternal border is usually thought to be indicative of right ventricular pressure or volume overload; however, young, normal subjects frequently have a palpable impulse along the left sternal border, and this sign must be carefully interpreted in light of other findings. Similarly, pulmonary closure may be palpable in this group of patients without reflecting an increase in pulmonary artery pressure.

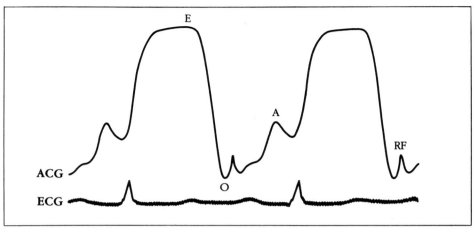

FIGURE 12–20
Apexcardiogram of left ventricular hypertrophy. Note the prolonged outward systolic motion and the exaggerated A wave, both of which are often palpable. Rapid filling (RF) in early diastole may, as here illustrated, produce a palpable impulse.

Abnormal precordial movements are of prime diagnostic importance. They may be systolic or diastolic, outward or inward. Sustained low-frequency movements are usually visible and palpable; high-frequency vibrations are palpable only. Sustained high-frequency vibrations are called thrills, which are simply palpable murmurs. Short, high-frequency vibrations are known as shocks, which are palpable heart sounds.

Left ventricular hypertrophy produces a sustained systolic apex impulse (greater than one-half systole) that may be displaced laterally and downward. A graphic record of this movement is shown in Figure 12–20. Atrial contraction in the setting of a poorly compliant, thick-walled left ventricle may result in a palpable presystolic component to the apical impulse of left ventricular hypertrophy. This presystolic distention can usually be felt with the palpating hand, especially with the patient in the left lateral decubitus position. A tongue blade held lightly over the apex will amplify this double impulse, making it easily demonstrable at the bedside without special equipment. The excursions may be timed by simultaneously listening to the heart, which usually discloses the presence of a presystolic sound or fourth heart sound in these patients. This finding is commonly associated with hypertension, aortic stenosis, and coronary disease.

Left ventricular dilatation due to heart failure also produces displaced dynamic apex impulse. This movement may be double for yet another reason: the effect of rapid passive filling in early diastole. An early diastolic extra sound (S_3) usually accompanies this abnormality. Advanced coronary disease, cardiomyopathies, and certain valvular diseases resulting in left ventricular failure are major causes of this abnormality. In some patients this early diastolic filling wave may be seen more easily than it can be felt or heard.

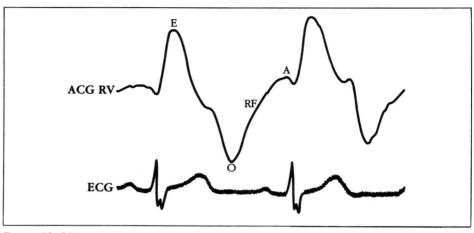

FIGURE 12–21
Apexcardiogram of right ventricular hypertrophy. Apexcardiogram was recorded at the left sternal border in a patient with right ventricular (RV) overload. The outward movement, which occupies only the early part of the systole, is characteristic of right ventricular volume overload. (Courtesy of the Division of Cardiology, Georgetown University Hospital.)

Right ventricular hypertrophy and dilatation produce similar movements that are usually more diffuse and can be felt along the left sternal edge (Fig. 12–21). The impulse of the volume- or pressure-loaded right ventricle frequently can be felt with a finger placed under the xyphoid process while the patient gently inhales. Right ventricular impulses are often single but may exhibit presystolic distention or a rapid filling wave just as the left ventricle does. The impulse of the pressure-loaded right ventricle is more sustained than the rapid outward early systolic movement found in patients with atrial septal defect (a lesion that results in selective volume overload of the right ventricle). Pulmonary artery dilatation produces a localized systolic lift in the second or third left intercostal space.

Constrictive pericarditis may produce a typical early diastolic out-thrust along the sternal border or over the midprecordium. This sometimes is associated with a short inward movement during systole. The diastolic movement is often misinterpreted as a systolic event, but when unquestionably present it is pathognomonic of this one condition. Palpate and listen at the same time!

Maneuvers that bring the heart closer to the chest wall will accentuate most of the precordial movements. Having the patient hold his breath in full expiration and/or rolling him a quarter of a turn to the left, or having him lean forward in the sitting position, may be very helpful. Longstanding cardiac enlargement, when present during childhood, may cause a visible precordial bulge.

PERCUSSION

The methods of direct and indirect percussion described in Chapter 11 are occasionally applicable to the estimation of heart size. When the left border of cardiac dullness falls outside the midclavicular line, the heart is usually enlarged. However, as more detailed knowledge of normal and abnormal precordial movements has been accumulated, palpation has largely replaced percussion in cardiac examination. The superiority of the echocardiogram and roentgenogram for evaluation of overall heart size and chamber enlargement has relegated percussion of the heart largely to a place of historical interest.

AUSCULTATION

Immediately, on this suggestion, I rolled a quire of paper into a kind of cylinder and applied one end of it to the region of the heart and the other to my ear, and was not a little surprised and pleased to find that I could thereby perceive the action of the heart in a manner much more clear and distinct than I had ever been able to do by the immediate application of the ear.

RENÉ THÉOPHILE HYACINTHE LAËNNEC
(1781–1826)

GENERAL

Cardiac auscultation must be learned at the bedside. Diagrams, tape recordings, and phonocardiograms are of great help to the student but are no substitute for personal experience. Proficiency requires years of studied practice coupled with a clear understanding of the origin of normal and abnormal cardiac sounds. Certain frustrations are inevitable at first, but do not be disheartened.

STETHOSCOPE

In order for the stethoscope to function, two things have to happen. There has to be, by God, a sick man at one end of it and a doctor at the other! *The doctor has to be within thirty inches of his patient.*

DICKINSON W. RICHARDS
(1895–1973)

There is a frequently quoted saying that what you put in your ears is of less importance than what lies between them. While this is true to a great extent, a well-designed efficient stethoscope is indispensable. Several crucial factors must be considered in its selection; therefore, it is wise to try a variety of instruments before selecting your own. It will be a very close friend for a long time.

Earpieces must fit snugly. An earpiece that is too small or too tight may partially or completely occlude itself against the anterior wall of your external auditory canal. The earpieces should be comfortable and parallel to the long axis of your external auditory canal (Fig. 12–22).

Tubing with an inner diameter of less than ⅛ inch will attenuate high frequencies. Thick-walled tubing, particularly plastic, will reject outside noise better than the thin, flexible rubber variety. Double tubing extending all the way to the endpiece is slightly superior to the Y configuration. Tubing length should not exceed 12 to 15 inches so that the overall distance from ear to chestpiece is no greater than 21 inches.

Endpieces are of two standard types, the bell and the diaphragm. They are available in many sizes; the 1-inch bell and the 1½-inch diaphragm are generally selected for examining adults (Figure 12–22B). The rigid diaphragm has a natural

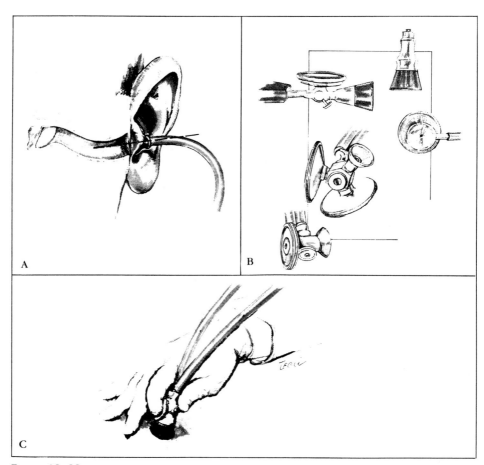

FIGURE 12–22
The stethoscope. A. Correct fit in external auditory meatus. B. Common types of stethoscope endpieces. C. Correct method for holding stethoscope endpiece, permitting variable pressure against chest wall.

frequency of around 300 cps. It therefore acts as a filter, eliminating low-pitched sounds. High-pitched sounds, such as the second heart sound, and high-pitched murmurs are best heard with the diaphragm. The vaulted trumpet bell has been shown to have a slight advantage over the more shallow varieties. With the bell, the skin becomes the diaphragm, and the natural frequency varies depending on the amount of pressure exerted, much as the timpani player varies the pitch of his instrument by tensing the drumhead. It probably ranges from 40 cps with light pressure to 150 to 200 cps with firm pressure. When you try to detect low-pitched sounds and murmurs, therefore, the bell should be applied as lightly as possible (Figure 12–22C). Alternating firm and light pressure may aid in detecting low frequency sounds, which become more obvious "by their absence" when firmer pressure is applied.

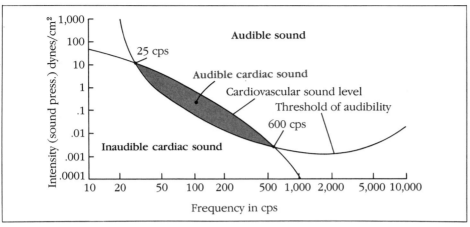

FIGURE 12–23
Ranges of audible and inaudible sound. Only a narrow range of sound generated in the heart may be heard on auscultation.

CARDIAC SOUND

Sound intensity is objective; loudness therefore depends on both the intensity of the sound at its origin and the sensitivity of the ear. Needless to say, people vary greatly in auditory acuity, particularly at the upper and lower limits of audibility. Although the human ear at times may perceive frequencies from 20 to 16,000 cps and higher under special conditions, its maximal sensitivity is in the range of 1000 to 2000 cps. Figure 12–23 compares the average hearing threshold with the average intensity of cardiovascular sounds. Notice that only vibrations ranging from 25 to 600 cps achieve intensity levels that are high enough to become audible by the average listener, although the heart produces vibrations ranging from 1 to 1000 cps.

In simple terms this means that vibrations originating in the heart with frequencies below 25 cps (and there are many) are entirely inaudible. This reinforces the importance of palpation, since with experience much information from the inaudible range can be derived by this method. Additionally, a sound of 500 cps will be perceived to be louder to the ear than one of 60 cps, even when each sound has the same intensity at the stethoscope earpiece. This means that great care must be taken to train the ear to perceive low-pitched sounds, as they are easily overlooked.

The ear adjusts itself to the intensity of sound. A loud sound causes the ear to protect itself by decreasing its receptive ability. This produces the phenomenon called "masking": if a faint sound follows a loud one, it may actually be entirely inaudible. High levels of ambient noise may also mask faint sounds and murmurs.

Four reference points are used for localization of sounds on the surface of the chest as shown in Figure 12–24. Because the pulmonic and tricuspid valves are located near the chest wall, their sounds are transmitted to auscultatory areas close by. The aortic and mitral valves, however, are situated deep in the chest, and their

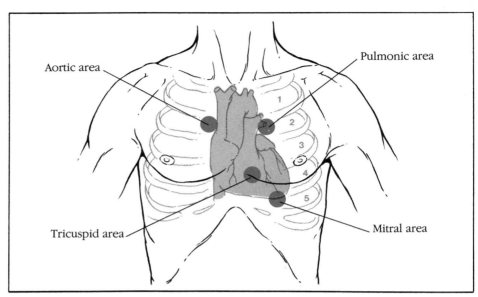

FIGURE 12–24
Areas of routine auscultation of the precordium.

sounds are transmitted in the direction of blood flow to points closer to the chest wall. The mitral sounds are referred to the apex; the aortic sounds follow the ascending aorta as it curves forward and are well heard in the second right intercostal space, where the aorta is closer to the anterior chest wall. However, sounds generated at the mitral and aortic valves are usually heard over much of the precordium.

HEART SOUNDS

The gallop stroke is diastolic and is due to the beginning of sudden tension in the ventricular wall as a result of blood flow into the cavity.
  It is more pronounced if the wall is not distensible . . .

PIERRE CARL EDOUARD POTAIN
(1825–1901)

GENERAL

You should clearly understand the physiologic origin of normal cardiovascular sound. Individual differences in loudness, quality, and pitch occur in patients of varying age and build. Sounds may be remarkably loud and clear in young, thin-chested patients and in patients with tachycardia due to exercise or excitement. They may be quite muffled and practically inaudible in obese or barrel-chested individuals. The heart may sound very different as the stethoscope position is changed from point to point in the same patient. This is partially due to the relative proximity of the various valves. The first sound as heard at the apex may not only become softer at the base but may also seem shorter and have a different quality due to the damping effect of the interposed soft tissues. Similarly, the second sound

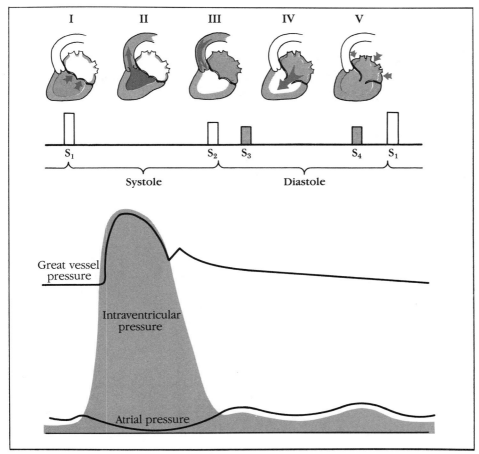

FIGURE 12–25
Heart sounds in relation to cardiac events and pulse wave forms. I. Atrioventricular valve closure corresponds in time to the first heart sound. II. Systolic ejection period begins with opening of the aortic and pulmonic valves. III. With ventricular emptying, aortic and pulmonic valve closure corresponds in time to the second heart sound (S_2). IV. With atrioventricular valve opening, the rush of blood from atria to ventricles may be associated with an early ventricular filling sound (S_3). V. Atrial contraction, causing increased ventricular filling, corresponds to tensing of the ventricular myocardium and a late ventricular filling sound (S_4).

loses intensity and changes quality as the stethoscope is moved downward toward the apex.

The cardiac cycle is schematically represented in Figure 12–25. The sounds of greatest importance are the first and second heart sounds, which divide the cardiac cycle into systole and diastole (technically, ventricular systole and diastole). Although there is controversy concerning the origin of the first sound, it may be considered here to be related to closure of the mitral and tricuspid valves and to the related phenomena of tensing of the myocardium, atrioventricular valve (tricuspid, mitral), supporting structures (papillary muscle, chordal apparatus), as well as to changes in blood velocity. The second sound results from aortic and pulmonary valve closure. A physiologic third sound is at times audible during the period of rapid filling of the ventricles. The normal first and second heart sounds range in frequency from 60 to 200 cps. The physiologic third sound is low-pitched, usually around 40 cps or less. In Figure 12–25 these events are correlated with their corresponding systemic or left-sided pressure relationships.

TECHNIQUE OF AUSCULTATION

In order to derive the maximum benefit from cardiac auscultation, you must develop a systematic approach that is repeated in the examination of each patient. Begin by listening at the apex, but do not simply skip from one major valve area to another. Such skipping is a common mistake that results in missing much important information. Many intermediate points and satellite areas must be scrutinized as the stethoscope is moved slowly and systematically from the apex to the tricuspid area, up along the left sternal border to the pulmonic area, and thence to the aortic area. Maneuvers that bring the heart closer to the chest wall will increase the loudness of certain sounds. Two standard accessory positions should always be used: the left lateral position, which usually makes louder sounds at the apex; and the sitting position, which may bring out otherwise inaudible murmurs at the base and along the left sternal border. In emphysematous patients, heart sounds, usually faint over the precordium, may be well heard over the epigastrium and in the suprasternal notch. Always notice the effects of position changes and of respiration on the quality of the sounds. Exercising the patient may be of great help, but it is not necessarily routine. Listening to the heart as the patient squats may also be useful in special instances.

The key to successful auscultation lies in listening to one thing at a time. It is frequently worthwhile to close your eyes and take a relaxed, comfortable position while focusing all your attention on listening. The following routine will eliminate many errors of omission:

1. **Observe and time the rate and rhythm.** Is the rate unusually fast or slow? Are there any irregularities of rhythm?
2. **Identify the first and second sounds and listen to them separately.** Is the first sound normal, accentuated, diminished? Next, listen solely to the second sound and establish its characteristics, intensity, and splitting. Compare the first and second sounds in the various areas.
3. **Now that the sounds are familiar, focus first on systole and then on diastole.** Listen specifically for extra sounds only (not murmurs).
4. **Listen now for the presence of murmurs—first in systole, then in diastole— scanning all major areas.** Notice the point of maximum intensity and the transmission of any murmurs heard.

At times it is difficult even for the experienced clinician to identify systole and diastole. This is particularly true with rapid heart rates in which the systolic and diastolic intervals tend to become equal in duration. Two techniques may be of value. One is to correlate the heart sounds with the apex impulse or the carotid pulse, both of which are systolic in timing. The first sound should just precede these phenomena. Because of the time required for the mechanical transmission of the pulse wave, peripheral arteries such as the radial or femoral are not suitable for timing heart sounds. The second technique is to familiarize yourself with the second sound at the base, which is invariably the loudest, and to inch the stethoscope downward toward the apex, keeping this sound clearly in your ear.

FIRST HEART SOUND

The first sound is louder, longer, and lower pitched than the second sound at the apex. Since the tricuspid component is usually not well heard at the apex, a single component first sound (mitral valve) is heard there,

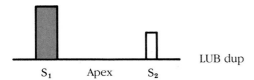

S_1 Apex S_2 LUB dup

but because the mitral valve closes from 0.02 to 0.03 second before the tricuspid, splitting of the first sound is actually common normally, and is particularly well heard in the fourth left intercostal space at the left sternal border (tricuspid area).

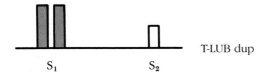

S_1 S_2 T-LUB dup

The first heart sound is accentuated in many conditions, some of which are not abnormal. Sinus tachycardia in a healthy young person may result in a prominent first sound. Anemia, hyperthyroidism, and other disorders that result in a hyperkinetic circulation cause a similar change. The increased left atrial pressure of mitral stenosis, or a short PR interval that causes the mitral and tricuspid valves to close from a relatively open position, will also increase the intensity of the first sound.

S_1 S_2 LUB dup

Low-output states or delayed atrioventricular conduction (long PR interval) may result in a quiet first sound. Atrioventricular dissociation (complete heart block) with ventricular systole being variably related to atrial contraction, as well as atrial fibrillation with its variable diastolic filling periods, is associated with marked changes in intensity of the first sound.

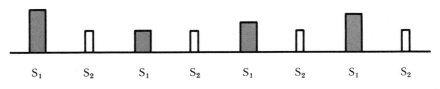

LUB dup lub dup LUB dup

SECOND HEART SOUND

The second sound results from combined aortic and pulmonary valve closure. It is almost always louder than the first sound at the base. The aortic component is widely transmitted to the neck and over the precordium and usually is the only component of the second sound heard at the apex.

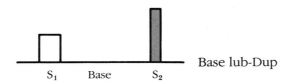

Base lub-Dup

The pulmonary component of the second sound is softer and normally is heard only along the high left sternal border. Although the second left intercostal space is called the pulmonic area, analysis of the second sound and its splitting is frequently best accomplished in the third interspace.

Respiratory variations in the timing of the two components of the second sound occur in most patients. Physiologic splitting of the second sound may be demonstrated in most normal people during inspiration. Closure of the aortic and pulmonic valves during expiration is synchronous or nearly so because right and left ventricular systole are approximately equal in duration. With inspiration, venous blood rushes into the thorax from the large systemic venous reservoirs. This increases venous return and prolongs right ventricular systole by temporarily increasing right ventricular stroke volume, with resultant delay in pulmonic valve closure. At the same time venous return to the left heart diminishes due to the increased pulmonary capacity during inspiration. This shortens left ventricular systole and permits earlier aortic closure. The two factors combine to produce transient "physiologic splitting" of the pulmonic second sound during inspiration.

Analysis of the respiratory variation of the second sound should take place during normal quiet respiration and not with forced or held inspiration or expiration. In some patients, complete fusion of the two components of the second heart sound may only occur in the sitting position.

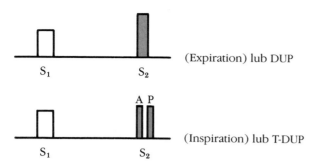

The aortic or pulmonic components of the second sound may be accentuated with elevation of the pressure in either of the respective circuits (i.e., systemic or pulmonary artery hypertension). With aortic or pulmonary stenosis they may become diminished or inaudible due to decreased mobility of the diseased cusps. Delayed pulmonic valve closure results in persistent splitting of the second sound, which may not vary at all with respiration (fixed splitting) or may vary with it in the usual manner (i.e., not fusing in expiration but widening during inspiration). Atrial septal defect with volume overload causing prolonged right ventricular ejection is the most frequent cause of fixed splitting of the second sound. Pulmonary stenosis and ventricular septal defects often cause wide splitting of the second sound with retention of normal respiratory variation. Delayed electrical activation of the right ventricle (i.e., right bundle-branch block), causes persistent splitting of the second sound with normal respiratory movements.

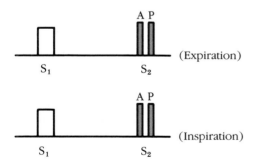

Reversed or paradoxic splitting of the second sound results from delayed left ventricular activation (left bundle-branch block or artificial pacing from the right ventricle) or prolonged emptying time of the left ventricle for mechanical reasons (aortic stenosis, marked hypertension, or poor contractility as seen in cardiomyopathy or myocardial ischemia).

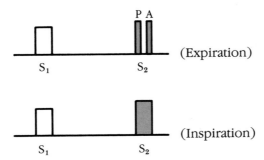

The basic cause of reversed splitting of the second sound is late aortic valve closure resulting from prolonged or delayed left ventricular ejection. Thus, in expiration right ventricular ejection is shortest and pulmonic valve closure precedes aortic valve closure. When prolonged right ventricular systole and shortened left ventricular systole occur with inspiration, the two valve sounds become superimposed. Examination for paradoxic splitting is best accomplished during normal quiet respiration or minimally exaggerated breathing with the mouth open.

EXTRA HEART SOUNDS

THIRD SOUND. Early diastolic extra sounds (S_3, ventricular gallop, or protodiastolic extra sound) occur during the period of rapid ventricular filling. They may be normal (physiologic) or abnormal (commonly heard in mitral regurgitation and ventricular failure of variable cause).

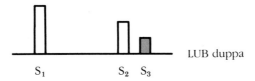

The S_3 is low pitched and is often difficult to detect. Careful location of the cardiac apex in the left lateral decubitus position with light application of the bell of the stethoscope is imperative for detection of this sound.

The physiologic third sound is a low-pitched sound that is audible at or near the apex. It is best heard with the patient in the left decubitus position, and it frequently disappears when he sits erect. It varies in intensity with respiration, usually becoming louder with expiration. It is extremely common in children and young adults but is seldom heard in normal persons over 30 years of age.

In contradistinction to the physiologic S_3 of younger people, the occurrence of a third heart sound at an older age is related to cardiomyopathy, ischemic heart disease, or valvular disease. Pathologic third heart sounds generally connote ventricular failure but may be seen in patients with mitral regurgitation or myocardial infarction before significant ventricular dysfunction develops.

An S_3 may arise from the right ventricle as well as the left ventricle. Right-sided third sounds tend to exhibit respiratory variation in intensity. Right ventricular S_3's occur with tricuspid regurgitation or right ventricular failure. They are usually best heard at the lower left sternal border or in the epigastrium.

PERICARDIAL KNOCK. This is a sharp sound heard in early diastole. It occurs in patients with constrictive pericarditis and is associated with the early, rapid filling phase of ventricular diastole. Its timing is earlier than a third heard sound.

OPENING SNAP. This sound, associated with rheumatic involvement of the mitral (or tricuspid) valve, occurs early in ventricular diastole prior to the rapid filling phase. It results from the opening movement of the stiffened atrioventricular valve leaflets (a silent occurrence in the normal heart) and occurs earlier when atrial pressure is higher (usually connoting greater obstruction to ventricular inflow).

TUMOR PLOP. This sound, which is generated by the movement of atrial masses (most notably left atrial myxomas) into the atrioventricular orifice, also occurs in conjunction with the early rapid filling phase of the ventricles. Its characteristic quality gives rise to the term *plop*.

Each of these early diastolic sounds has a slightly different quality and timing that only repeated actual auscultatory experience will allow you to distinguish.

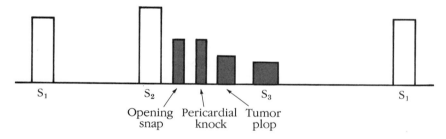

FOURTH SOUND. Presystolic extra sounds (S_4, atrial gallop) are dull and low-pitched. They are best heard at the apex with the patient rolled onto his left side and the bell of the stethoscope lightly applied precisely over the apex impulse. At times they are more easily felt than heard. The fourth heart sound is caused by vigorous atrial contraction in patients with decreased left ventricular compliance, which may be caused by left ventricular hypertrophy or myocardial ischemia. With pulmonary hypertension or pulmonary stenosis, a fourth heart sound originating in the right ventricle may be heard along the left sternal border. As with most right-sided auscultatory events, a right ventricular fourth sound increases with inspiration. Fourth heart sounds are so frequent over the age of 50 that their presence may not necessarily imply cardiac disease in that age group.

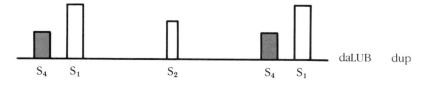

GALLOPS. When an S_3 and/or an S_4 is associated with a rapid heart rate, the heart sounds assume the cadence of a galloping horse. Gallop rhythm is regarded as a sign of congestive heart failure. With more rapid rates, the third and fourth sounds are superimposed and result in a single loud prolonged "summation" gallop.

EJECTION SOUNDS. Ejection sounds occur in early systole. They may originate in either of the great vessels or their valves. They are generated by abrupt distention of a dilated great vessel during early ventricular ejection or by upward movement of stiffened deformed valve leaflets. Ejection sounds heard in congenital valvular pulmonary stenosis increase in intensity with expiration and decrease with inspiration (as opposed to most other right-sided events). The ejection sound of pulmonary hypertension is not as apt to vary with respiration. Pulmonic ejection sounds are best heard at the base and high left sternal border. Aortic ejection sounds do not vary with respiration and are heard equally well at the apex and base.

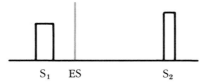

S_1 ES S_2

SYSTOLIC CLICKS. A systolic click is usually single, but two or more clicks may be heard. They are usually midsystolic, high-pitched, and sharp. They are extremely variable, changing with respiration or position or spontaneously. Clicks are heard best along the left sternal border or just inside the apex. Previously these clicks were felt to be extracardiac in origin and were regarded as benign. Now they are most often associated with prolapse of the mitral valve (or, occasionally, the tricuspid valve). Their origin is thought to be the sudden tensing of the redundant valve leaflets and chordal structures associated with prolapse. With sitting or standing they tend to move earlier in systole, and with lying and squatting they are somewhat delayed (see Table 12–12).

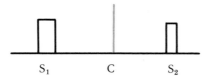

S_1 C S_2

CRUNCHES. A systolic crunch or knock (Hammon's crunch) may be heard in patients with mediastinal emphysema or a small left-sided pneumothorax. In the latter case it has been referred to as "noisy pneumothorax"; it is frequently audible to the patient and at times to the physician at some distance from the bedside.

RUBS. The pericardial friction rub is a sign of pericardial irritation. It may be heard anywhere over the precordium but is often loudest along the left sternal border or directly over the sternum. Sometimes it is quite loud, but frequently it is faint, high-pitched, and evanescent. Firm pressure with the diaphragm of the stethoscope, and/or auscultation with the patient sitting up and leaning forward with breath held in expiration, are maneuvers that will bring out a friction rub. Friction rubs have a superficial, scratchy, to-and-fro quality, often suggesting squeaky leather. They lag somewhat, giving the effect of being slightly out of step with the heart sounds. A fully developed friction rub has three components that correspond with the systolic, early diastolic, and presystolic phases of the cardiac cycle. One should hear at least two components before diagnosing a rub. The intensity of the rub may vary with respiration, but a true pericardial rub should be audible with respiration halted. Friction rubs may be simulated by movements of the stethoscope's end-piece on the surface of the skin, and particularly by hair.

Atrial contraction   Ventricular systole   Ventricular diastole

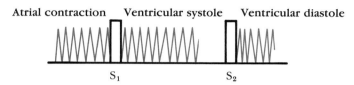

S_1 S_2

MURMURS. Heart murmurs are immensely important in cardiac diagnosis. In order to interpret them intelligently, however, you must understand the factors that govern their production and transmission. Furthermore, you must be able to describe them in precise and appropriate terms. The phonocardiogram, though of limited diagnostic value, is helpful as a teaching tool, since it allows time for study and correlation of events that ordinarily are passed by rapidly.

Blood flow within the circulation may be laminar or turbulent. Ideally flow is silent because of its laminar character. With laminar flow through any tube, the layer of fluid adjacent to the wall is stationary while the velocity of flow increases progressively within the inner layers and is maximal at the center. As this velocity exceeds a critical level, turbulence develops and in turn produces vortices or swirls. These in turn emit high-frequency sound vibrations termed *murmurs* when heard in and around the heart and *bruits* when heard over peripheral vessels.

Production of murmurs is favored by a number of basic factors that tend to promote turbulence, including (1) lowering the viscosity of the fluid, (2) increasing the diameter of a tube, (3) changing the caliber of a tube abruptly, and (4) increasing the velocity of flow. The velocity of blood flow is vitally important in governing two important characteristics of a murmur: intensity and pitch. The intensity of a murmur is directly proportional to the velocity cubed. The faster the flow, the louder the murmur. Thus, exercise, when it speeds blood flow, causes most murmurs to become louder. Pitch is also directly proportional to velocity. The faster the flow, the higher the pitch; the slower the flow, the lower the pitch. There are other causes of murmur production that are of lesser importance and will not be included here.

Transmission of murmurs also has a profound effect on both pitch and loudness. Sound intensity diminishes in direct proportion to the square of the distance that it must travel. Obviously the closer the murmur source to the chest wall, the louder it will sound. The natural damping effect of interposed tissues is compounded by the tendency of sound to be reflected backward at the interface between media of

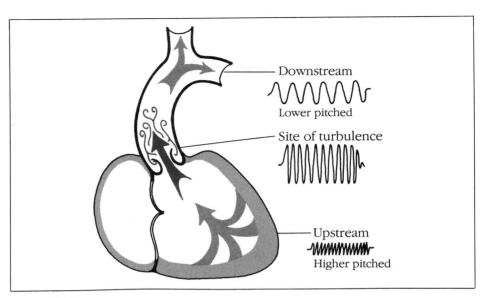

FIGURE 12–26
Differential radiation of various pitches of a murmur. Higher frequencies preferentially radiate upstream and lower frequencies preferentially radiate downstream.

different densities, such as muscle, lung, bone, skin, and air. In fact, high frequencies tend to be dampened preferentially by this phenomenon; in other words, the pitch will become lower due to the effects of transmission across these interfaces. Another important factor that governs pitch is related to the transmission of a murmur within the cardiovascular system itself. As one moves backward against the stream, high frequencies tend to be preserved and lows tend to be dampened out. In moving downstream (or forward), high frequencies tend to be lost and lows tend to be preserved. This phenomenon is shown in Figure 12–26. It is not surprising, then, that many murmurs sound quite different as the stethoscope is moved over the precordium.

TYPES AND CAUSES OF MURMURS
Description of murmurs is divided into six categories: timing, location and radiation, loudness, pitch, duration, and quality. They are defined as follows:

1. **Timing:** Systolic, diastolic, continuous.
2. **Location and radiation:** Point of maximum intensity described in terms of anatomic landmarks: apex, left sternal border; left base (pulmonic area); right base (aortic area); intermediate zones by exact intercostal space. Areas to which the murmur radiates over the precordium.
3. **Loudness:** Graded on a six-point scale, described in Table 12–7.
4. **Pitch:** Low (25–150 cps); medium (150–350 cps); high (350–600 cps) (see Fig. 12–26).
5. **Duration:** Classified and illustrated in Table 12–8.

TABLE 12–7. Grading of Heart Murmurs

Grade	Description
I/VI	Heard only after special maneuvers and "tuning in"
II/VI	Faint, but readily heard
III/VI	Loud, but without a thrill
IV/VI	Associated with a thrill, but stethoscope must be fully on chest to be heard
V/VI	Heard with stethoscope partly off the chest Palpable thrill
VI/VI	Heard with stethoscope entirely off the chest Palpable thrill

TABLE 12–8. Duration of Heart Murmurs

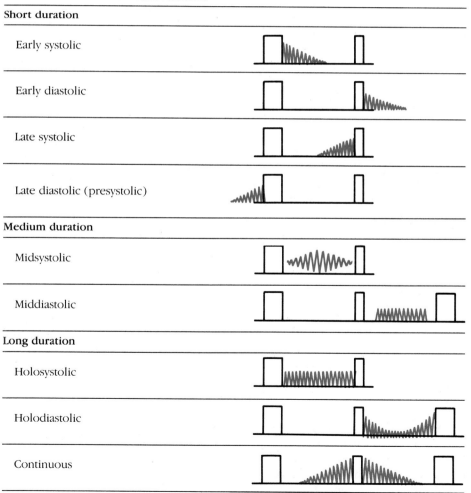

Short duration

Early systolic

Early diastolic

Late systolic

Late diastolic (presystolic)

Medium duration

Midsystolic

Middiastolic

Long duration

Holosystolic

Holodiastolic

Continuous

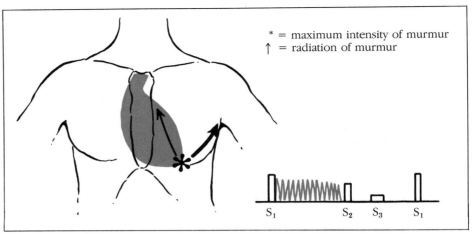

* = maximum intensity of murmur
↑ = radiation of murmur

S_1 S_2 S_3 S_1

FIGURE 12–27
Diagram of the heart sounds as it might appear in the written workup.

6. **Quality:** Crescendo (increasing in loudness) or decrescendo (decreasing in loudness). Descriptive terms include blowing, harsh, rumbling, musical, cooing, whooping, honking, regurgitant, ejection.

On your written workup it is often useful to diagram what you hear through the stethoscope as illustrated in Figure 12–27. Note that not only duration but timing and quality (crescendo or decrescendo) are represented.

SYSTOLIC MURMURS

I found among such children, most of them quite young, a murmur of remarkable intensity, but with other characteristics which I thought unusual; what surprised me was that the murmur was almost the only sign of cardiopathy and that it was accompanied by no other physical signs (save only the purring thrill) . . . [ventricular septal defect]

HENRI ROGER
(1809–1891)

For the sake of simplicity most systolic murmurs may be grouped into one of two categories: midsystolic (often ejection) murmurs and holosystolic (regurgitant) murmurs. This subtyping of systolic murmurs correlates their quality with the underlying pathophysiologic mode of origin and eliminates errors produced by overdependence on the geographic site of maximum intensity, which may be unreliable. Table 12–9 lists causes of systolic murmurs.

MIDSYSTOLIC MURMURS. These murmurs are usually produced by the forward outflow of blood through the pulmonary or aortic valves. Because of their hemodynamic basis, ejection murmurs have a characteristic personality in that they occur in midsystole, are medium-pitched, and rise and fall in a crescendo fashion, ending before the second sound. The four principal causes are (1) valvular or subvalvular

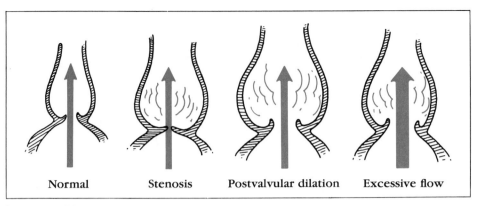

FIGURE 12–28
Various mechanisms of generation of murmurs. Turbulent flow resulting from any of these mechanisms may result in cardiac sound.

TABLE 12–9. Some Causes of Systolic Murmurs

Aortic outflow obstruction
   Valvular aortic stenosis
   Subvalvular aortic stenosis
   Supravalvular aortic stenosis

Pulmonic outflow obstruction
   Valvular pulmonic stenosis
   Subvalvular (infundibular) pulmonic stenosis

Functional
   Youth
   Anemia
   Hyperthyroidism

Great vessel dilatation
   Aortic root dilatation of aging
   Idiopathic dilatation of the pulmonary arteries

Mitral regurgitation

Tricuspid regurgitation

Congenital
   Ventricular septal defect
   Atrial septal defect

---

stenosis; (2) high-velocity rate of ejection through the valves, which may themselves be normal (increased stroke volume); (3) dilation of the vessel beyond the valve; or (4) a combination of these factors (Fig. 12–28).

   Aortic murmurs.   Aortic systolic ejection murmurs occur with valvular and subvalvular stenosis (Fig. 12–29), primary dilation of the ascending aorta, and increased left ventricular stroke output. The latter may be due simply to hyperkinetic states or may be a compensatory increase in forward flow through the valve because of diastolic backflow due to aortic regurgitation. Aortic systolic murmurs are usually best heard in the aortic area, but they are frequently transmitted to the

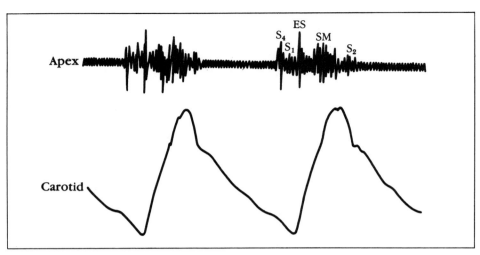

FIGURE 12–29
Systolic murmur (SM), with ejection sound (ES), generated in a patient with valvular aortic stenosis.

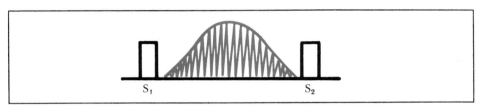

FIGURE 12–30
Representation of a functional systolic murmur.

entire precordium and sometimes are maximal at or inside the apex, where their pitch may seem higher or their sound musical while maintaining their characteristic ejection quality. They are often transmitted to the carotid arteries. They may be accompanied by a thrill in the second right intercostal space. Because of an increase in stroke volume following a longer diastolic filling period, the intensity of the murmur is increased during the systole following a premature beat (postextrasystolic accentuation).

Pulmonic murmurs.   Pulmonic systolic ejection murmurs occur with pulmonary valvular and subvalvular stenosis, dilation of the pulmonary artery, and increased pulmonary flow, as with atrial septal defect. They are usually best heard in the second and third intercostal spaces and may radiate to the left upper chest.

Innocent murmurs.   The functional or innocent systolic murmur is commonly heard in children and young adults, especially women. It is characteristically soft, early, short, and variable (Fig. 12–30). It is usually heard best at the pulmonic area or along the left sternal border but at times is audible only at or medial to the apex. Functional murmurs vary with position and respiration and frequently have

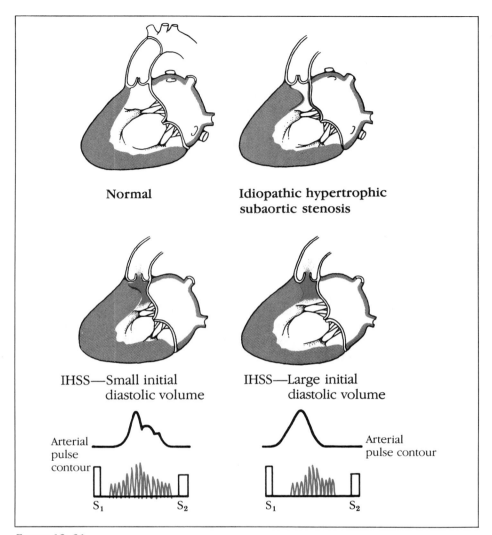

FIGURE 12–31
Idiopathic hypertrophic subaortic stenosis (IHSS) (hypertrophic cardiomyopathy with obstruction). With a small diastolic volume, the obstruction of the hypertrophic septum narrows the left ventricular outflow tract to a relatively greater degree than occurs with a larger initial diastolic volume.

a peculiar vibratory quality. They are not associated with any structural abnormality or recognizable heart disease. The "hemic" systolic murmur commonly heard with anemia and the basal systolic murmurs frequently associated with thyrotoxicosis, fever, and exercise are functional murmurs, but in these instances the cardiac output is elevated.

Occasionally it may be difficult to determine whether an ejection murmur is being generated from the right or left side of the heart. This distinction may be made by having the patient perform a Valsalva maneuver. Following release, the original intensity returns within the next two or three beats when the murmur is generated at the pulmonic valve, but may take five to seven cycles to return if generated at the aortic orifice.

Subaortic murmurs. The murmur resulting from dynamic left ventricular outflow tract obstruction (asymmetric septal hypertrophy [ASH] with obstruction, hypertrophic cardiomyopathy with obstruction) has characteristics common to both mitral regurgitation and aortic stenosis (Fig. 12–31). It is usually best heard at the cardiac apex but is readily transmitted to the base (it is rarely heard well in the neck). The murmur is usually midsystolic but sometimes has a holosystolic configuration. With increases in left ventricular diastolic volume or peripheral resistance, the murmur decreases in intensity. Maneuvers that decrease left ventricular volume or peripheral resistance will enhance the intensity of the murmur. A nearly pathognomonic finding is the response of the murmur to squatting and standing—usually the murmur decreases (at least one grade) with prompt squatting (during which venous return and afterload are acutely increased) followed by an increase in intensity with standing.

HOLOSYSTOLIC MURMURS. These are produced by backflow of blood from the ventricle to the atrium through an incompetent mitral or tricuspid valve, or by flow through a ventricular septal defect. Because they are due to the escape of blood from a chamber of relatively high pressure into one of relatively low pressure, and since this pressure differential lasts throughout systole, regurgitant murmurs differ from ejection murmurs. They are longer in duration, usually holosystolic, and may engulf the first or second sound or both. They are often of constant intensity, but they may increase or decrease in late systole. They are less apt to rise and fall in intensity as an ejection murmur does. Figure 12–32 illustrates the mode of origin of holosystolic murmurs.

Mitral regurgitation. This is the commonest cause of a holosystolic murmur. It tends to be loudest at the apex and is transmitted toward the axilla. There may be an associated thrill. The murmur of mitral regurgitation does not change in intensity during the cycle following an extrasystole.

In those cases in which mitral regurgitation has occurred precipitously, the murmur tends to decrescendo in late systole as left atrial pressure rises rapidly and decreases regurgitant flow (Fig. 12–33). When regurgitation takes place because of posterior mitral leaflet dysfunction, the anteriorly directed regurgitant stream may cause the murmur to radiate to the aortic root (the posterior wall of which is contiguous with the anterior left atrial wall).

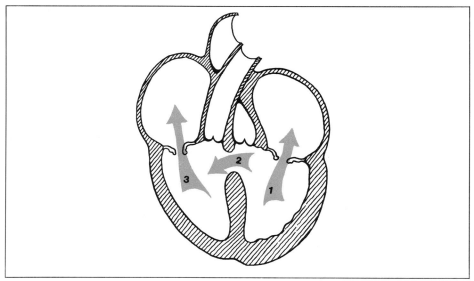

FIGURE 12–32
Mode of origin of holosystolic murmurs. 1. Mitral regurgitation. 2. Interventricular septal defect with left-to-right shunt. 3. Tricuspid regurgitation.

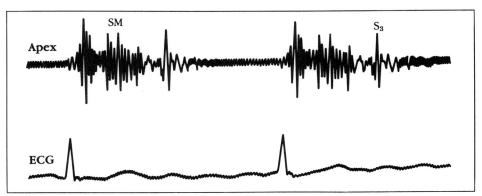

FIGURE 12–33
Decrescendo systolic murmur (SM) of acute mitral regurgitation. While caused by mitral regurgitation, the murmur tapers toward end systole as left atrial pressure rises abruptly and regurgitant flow diminishes.

Tricuspid regurgitation.   Tricuspid regurgitation causes a murmur, similar to that of mitral insufficiency, that is best heard over the tricuspid area. It can also be distinguished by the fact that it may become louder with inspiration (Carvallos sign), or with sustained pressure of the examiner's hand on the right upper quadrant of the abdomen.

Ventricular septal defect.   The murmur of ventricular septal defect is heard best in the third and fourth left intercostal spaces. It frequently causes a thrill and has a loud, coarse quality that is practically pathognomonic. It tends to radiate like the spokes of a wheel about its loudest point.

LATE SYSTOLIC MURMURS. A murmur beginning in midsystole, often initiated by one or more systolic clicks, is characteristic of prolapse of the mitral valve (Fig. 12–34). The murmur tends to crescendo in late systole and responds in characteristic fashion to various maneuvers. When relative volume depletion occurs (as with sitting or standing), the murmur begins earlier in systole. With squatting or elevation of the legs (causing volume expansion) the murmur tends to begin later in systole. Unfortunately, the murmur of mitral valve prolapse is not always characteristic (see Table 12–12).

PAPILLARY MUSCLE DYSFUNCTION. When ischemia or myocardial infarction involves the papillary muscles or the portion of the left ventricle from which they arise, mitral regurgitation may occur as a result of a decrease in the support of the mitral valve apparatus. The resulting murmur is then said to be due to papillary muscle dysfunction. It is characteristically a nonholosystolic murmur, which may radiate to the axilla (if the anterior mitral leaflet is affected) or to the base (if the regurgitant jet is primarily due to posterior leaflet incompetence). Increases in left ventricular volume tend to be associated with increases in the murmur. This is thought to be due to increases in the left ventricular size with further displacement of the mitral valve apparatus, holding the leaflet partially open.

DIASTOLIC MURMURS

Mitral stenosis may be concealed under a quarter of a dollar. It is the most difficult of all heart diseases to diagnose.

SIR WILLIAM OSLER
(1849–1919)

Diastolic murmurs may also be divided into two categories: early murmurs of aortic and pulmonic regurgitation, and mid- to late diastolic murmurs of mitral and tricuspid stenosis.

Aortic regurgitation results in a high-pitched murmur that begins immediately with aortic closure and diminishes progressively with diastole. Its intensity varies roughly with the size of the leak (Fig. 12–35). It is heard best along the left sternal border with the patient sitting and holding his breath in expiration. Because of its high pitch, this murmur is best heard using the diaphragm endpiece firmly applied. A low-pitched diastolic murmur may be heard at the apex in patients with aortic regurgitation without associated mitral stenosis. This murmur, which sounds like the murmur of mitral stenosis, is referred to as an Austin Flint murmur.

Pulmonic regurgitation causes a diastolic murmur that at times cannot be distinguished from the aortic counterpart simply by auscultation alone. Its pitch, timing, quality, and location are similar, although it tends to be more localized to the pulmonic area. When pulmonic regurgitation is found in the setting of severe pulmonary arterial hypertension, the resulting sound is called a Graham Steell murmur. Congenital pulmonic regurgitation occurs with normal pressures in the

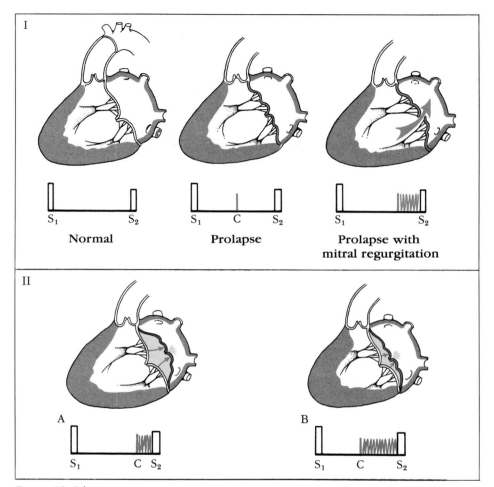

FIGURE 12–34

Spectrum of mitral valve prolapse. I. The typical findings in mitral valve prolapse. Prolapse without mitral regurgitation may result in a systolic click (C) without a murmur being heard. If mitral regurgitation is present, a late systolic murmur may be heard. II. The changes in the findings of prolapse with changes in left ventricular volume. A. Larger left ventricular volume results in a later click (C) and murmur. With increased ventricular volume, more time is taken than with decreased volume for mitral leaflets to move from the position of first closure (S_1) to the point at which they are checked on their prolapse (C). B. Smaller left ventricular volume causes the click and murmur to move earlier in systole. With decreased ventricular volume, less time is taken than with increased volume for mitral leaflets to move from their position of first closure (S_1) to the end of their prolapse (C). In either case, if mitral regurgitation is present, a systolic murmur follows the click.

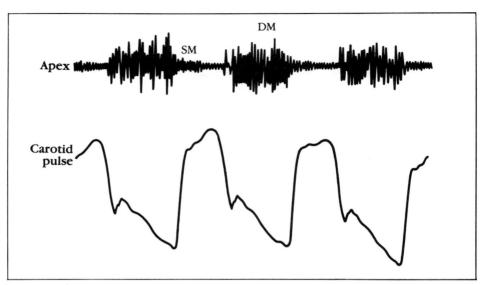

FIGURE 12–35
Diastolic murmur (DM) of aortic regurgitation. This phonocardiogram, recorded at the apex and shown with the carotid pulse tracing, also shows an early systolic murmur.

pulmonary artery and results in a diastolic murmur that is low- to medium-pitched and begins at an interval after the second sound.

Mitral stenosis characteristically produces a low-pitched, localized, apical rumble. Often it can be heard only with the bell and with the patient rolled onto his left side. As is the case with the third and fourth heart sounds, the low-pitched rumble of mitral stenosis must be sought precisely over the apical impulse.

The murmur often has presystolic and early diastolic components. The early diastolic component is related to the rapid, passive filling phase. The presystolic component results from rapid flow during atrial systole and disappears with the onset of atrial fibrillation. The murmur of mitral stenosis may be enhanced by increasing blood flow through the valve, such as by having the patient cough or exercise.

Figure 12–36 illustrates the hemodynamic basis for the mitral diastolic murmur. The murmur is loudest in early and late diastole, at which time the pressure gradient is greatest across the narrowed mitral valve. The early diastolic component is frequently initiated by a sharp click called a mitral opening snap. The opening snap can usually be heard at the apex but often is more easily discerned medial to the apex or along the left sternal border. Its separation from the second sound is related to the left atrial pressure; the higher the left atrial pressure, the closer the opening snap is to the second sound, and vice versa. This "2-OS" interval (the time between S_2 and the opening snap) may be used to estimate roughly the severity of the stenosis.

The murmur has a decrescendo quality through early and middiastole. During the latter third of diastole the gradient increases sharply due to atrial contraction,

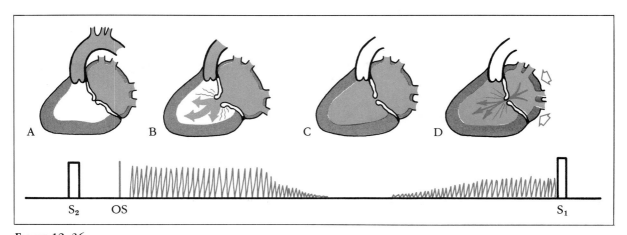

FIGURE 12–36
Hemodynamic basis for the auscultatory findings of mitral stenosis. A. Aortic valve closes; second heart sound (S_2) is generated. B. Mitral valve opens and opening snap (OS) occurs; early diastolic component is generated. C. Flow from left atrium to left ventricle diminishes, and murmur decreases in middiastole. D. Atrial systole increases flow across mitral valve, resulting in presystolic increase in intensity of murmur. Ventricular systole then causes closure of thickened mitral valve, resulting in loud first heart sound (S_1).

causing a presystolic accentuation of the murmur. With atrial fibrillation, effective contraction is lost, and the presystolic accentuation usually disappears. The murmur of mitral stenosis may be distinguished from the Austin Flint murmur of aortic regurgitation by altering peripheral resistance. Increases in peripheral resistance (as with isometric exercise) will increase the intensity of the Austin Flint murmur, but will decrease the intensity of the diastolic rumble of mitral stenosis. Decreases in peripheral resistance (as with amyl nitrite inhalation) have the opposite effect, decreasing the intensity of the Austin Flint murmur but increasing the rumble of mitral stenosis.

The diastolic murmur of tricuspid stenosis is similar in timing and quality to the mitral murmur but is frequently higher pitched and localized near the tricuspid area or along the left sternal border. Inspiration usually makes it louder. A tricuspid opening snap may also occur. Some causes of diastolic murmurs are listed in Table 12–10.

CONTINUOUS MURMURS
Continuous murmurs begin in systole and continue into diastole without interruption. Although it is called continuous, such a murmur may not occupy the entire cardiac cycle. Continuous murmurs are found in those situations in which there is a flow from a high- to a lower pressure chamber that is uninterrupted by the opening or closing of cardiac valves. The prototype of a continuous murmur is the Gibson murmur of patent ductus arteriosus (Fig. 12–37). This murmur begins in systole, peaks around the second sound, and then spills over into diastole, but it may not continue through to the first sound. It is heard maximally under the left

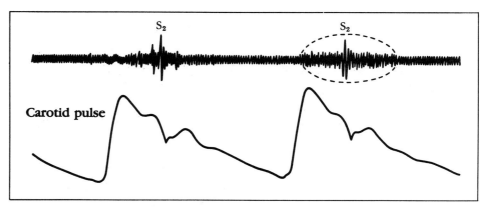

Figure 12–37
Continuous murmur of patent ductus arteriosus. Murmur peaks around second heart sound
(S₂).

Table 12–10. Some Causes of Diastolic Murmurs

Mitral stenosis
    Valvular disease
    Increased flow (relative)
    Left atrial myxoma
Tricuspid stenosis
    Valvular disease
    Increased flow (relative)
    Right atrial myxoma
Austin Flint
Pulmonic regurgitation
    Valvular disease
    Pulmonary hypertension (Graham Steell)
Aortic regurgitation

---

clavicle and in the pulmonic area. Other causes of continuous murmurs are listed
in Table 12–11.

Enhancing Diagnostic Acumen

*... we give the name of observer to the man who applies methods of
investigation, whether simple or complex, to the study of phenomena which he
does not vary and which he therefore gathers as nature offers them. We give the
name experimenter to the man who applies methods of investigation, whether
simple or complex, so as to make natural phenomena vary, or so as to alter
them with some purpose or other ...*

                                     Claude Bernard
                                     (1813–1878)

SIMPLE MANEUVERS

Several simple bedside maneuvers that will often enhance diagnostic accuracy can
be used as adjuncts to routine cardiac examination (Table 12–12).

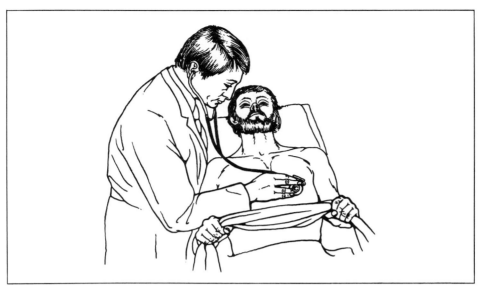

FIGURE 12–38
Isometric exercise. Patient grips towel tightly with both hands and pulls. Caution must be taken that patient does not perform the Valsalva maneuver during isometric exercise.

TABLE 12–11. Some Causes of Continuous Murmurs*

Surgical or traumatic AV fistula
Patent ductus arteriosus
Pulmonary AV fistula
Coronary AV fistula
Intercostal AV fistula
Rupture of the sinus of Valsalva

*The combined murmurs of aortic stenosis and aortic regurgitation, or of mitral stenosis and mitral regurgitation, may fill the entire cardiac cycle, but by definition they are *not* continuous murmurs. They are combinations of separate systolic and diastolic murmurs.

ISOMETRIC (HANDGRIP) EXERCISE. Isometric exercises (simply done by having the patient squeeze tightly with both hands) results in tachycardia and an increase in peripheral resistance and cardiac output (Fig. 12–38). These hemodynamic alterations cause the murmurs of aortic regurgitation and mitral regurgitation to intensify and the murmurs of left ventricular outflow obstruction to diminish.

AMYL NITRITE. The inhalation of amyl nitrite over a period of 15 to 20 seconds results in a prompt fall in peripheral resistance and mean arterial pressure with a reflex increase in heart rate, cardiac output, and stroke volume. Characteristic alterations of the auscultatory findings ensue. The lower systemic resistance produces either

TABLE 12–12. Effect of Some Physical Maneuvers on Cardiovascular Dynamics and Heart Sounds

Maneuver	Peripheral Resistance (Afterload)	Left Ventricular Volume (Preload)	Effect: Murmur of Aortic Stenosis	Murmur of Hypertrophic Obstructive Cardiomyopathy	Murmur of Mitral Regurgitation	Click Murmur of Mitral Valve Prolapse	Murmur of Mitral Stenosis	Murmur of Aortic Insufficiency and Austin Flint
Supine with passive leg raising	— or ↑	↑	↑	↓	—	↑	↑	—
Sitting or standing	↓	↓	—	↑	—	↓	—	↑ or —
Prompt squatting	↑	↑	— (early) ↓ (late)	↓	↑	↑	↓	↑
Isometric exercise (e.g., handgrip)	↑	↑	↓	↓	↑	↑	↓	↑
Valsalva maneuver	↑	↓	↓	↑ or ↓ or —	↓	↓	↓	↓
Exercise	↓	↓	↑	↑	—	↓	↑	↑
Amyl nitrite	↓	↓	↑	↑	↓	↓	↑	↑

↑ = increased; ↓ = decreased; — = no change; → = later in systole; ← = earlier in systole.

TABLE 12–13. Classic Physical Findings in Some Cardiac Disorders

Description	Phonocardiogram (inspiration unless noted)
MITRAL STENOSIS Small pulse; tapping apex impulse, parasternal lift; presystolic apical thrill; accentuated S_1 and P_2; mitral opening snap (OS); mitral diastolic rumble, with presystolic accentuation. Cold hands and feet. Atrial fibrillation (late).	
MITRAL REGURGITATION *Chronic,* Normal or small, brisk, arterial pulse; apical systolic thrill; sustained apical lift displaced to left: normal or soft S_1, apical regurgitant systolic murmur (SM); early diastolic extra sound (S_3). Mild forms may show murmur only.	
Acute, severe Usually caused by disruption of supporting structure apparatus. Varying degrees of congestive heart failure, loud S_1; harsh decrescendo systolic murmur, S_3 and S_4; right ventricular lift; increased P_2; right-sided filling sounds.	
Mitral valve prolapse Normal S_1 and S_2; one or more midsystolic clicks, and/or a late systolic murmur; frequent arrhythmias; often associated with slender body habitus and minor musculoskeletal deformities.	
AORTIC STENOSIS Small, slow-rising pulse; narrow pulse pressure (in severe cases); sustained apical lift displaced to the left; systolic thrill in aortic area; decreased or absent A_2; systolic ejection murmur at base and over carotids; systolic ejection sound (ES); carotid thrill. Cold hands and feet.	

TABLE 12–13. Classic Physical Findings in Some Cardiac Disorders

Description	Phonocardiogram (inspiration unless noted)
IDIOPATHIC HYPERTROPHIC SUBAORTIC STENOSIS (IHSS)	
Brisk carotid pulse, often with two waves; prominent A wave in jugular venous pulse; thrill at apex or left sternal border; triple apical impulse (presystolic and two systolic waves); fourth heart sound; crescendo-decrescendo systolic murmur at apex and left sternal border.	S_4 S_1 SM A_2 P_2 S_3
PULMONARY STENOSIS	
Normal pulse; jugular A wave; parasternal lift; pulmonic thrill; pulmonary component of second sound absent or soft and delayed, causing widely split S_2; systolic ejection murmur in pulmonic area; right-sided presystolic extra sound in tricuspid area (S_4) (severe); pulmonary ejection sound (mild).	S_4 S_1 ES SM A_2 P_2
AORTIC REGURGITATION	
Prominent carotid pulsations; water-hammer or bisferiens pulse. Capillary pulsations of the nail-beds; diffuse, sustained apex impulse displaced down and left; loud M_1, accentuated A_2; decrescendo diastolic murmur (DM) along left sternal border; low-pitched rumbling diastolic murmur at apex (Austin Flint).	S_1 SM A_2 P_2 DM
SYSTEMIC HYPERTENSION	
Elevated blood pressure; carotid tortuous and usually full; hypertensive funduscopic changes; sustained double apical lift displaced to the left; normal or accentuated S_1, accentuated A_2; presystolic extra sound; aortic systolic ejection murmur.	S_4 S_1 SM A_2 P_2
PULMONARY HYPERTENSION	
Cyanosis (at times); small pulse; narrow pulse pressure; cold extremities; atrial fibrillation (late); giant jugular A wave; parasternal lift; systolic lift in the pulmonic area; pulmonary ejection sound; pulmonic diastolic murmur (Graham Steell); systolic ejection murmur in pulmonic area; right-sided S_3 and S_4.	S_4 S_1 ES SM A_2 P_2

TRICUSPID STENOSIS

Small pulse; giant A wave in jugular pulse; elevated jugular pressure; quiet precordium, tricuspid diastolic murmur (DM) accentuated with inspiration (*Note:* Tricuspid stenosis is usually associated with mitral stenosis.)

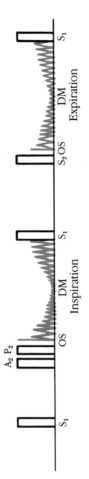

TRICUSPID REGURGITATION

Jugular V wave; elevated venous pressure; right ventricular parasternal lift; systolic thrill at tricuspid area; tricuspid regurgitant systolic murmur louder with inspiration; atrial fibrillation; early diastolic extra sound (over right ventricle).

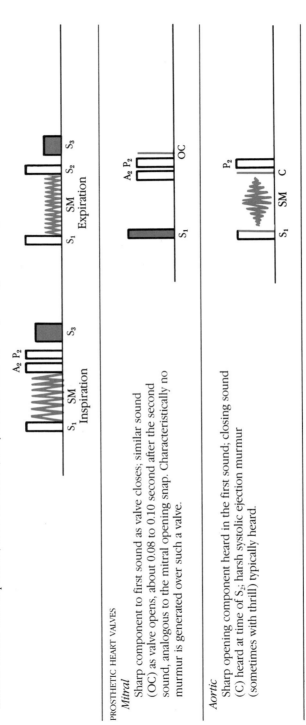

PROSTHETIC HEART VALVES

Mitral

Sharp component to first sound as valve closes; similar sound (OC) as valve opens, about 0.08 to 0.10 second after the second sound, analogous to the mitral opening snap. Characteristically no murmur is generated over such a valve.

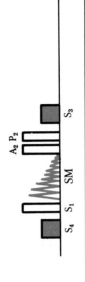

Aortic

Sharp opening component heard in the first sound; closing sound (C) heard at time of S_2; harsh systolic ejection murmur (sometimes with thrill) typically heard.

MYOCARDIAL INFARCTION

Tachycardia; pallor; small arterial pulse; narrow pulse pressure; apical late systolic bulge of ischemic myocardium; soft heart sounds; presystolic or early diastolic extra sounds; pericardial friction rub; apical systolic murmur (papillary muscle dysfunction); any of the arrhythmias.

TABLE 12–13. (*Continued*)

Description	Phonocardiogram (inspiration unless noted)

ATRIAL SEPTAL DEFECT

Normal pulse; brisk parasternal lift; lift over pulmonary artery; normal jugular pulse; systolic ejection murmur in pulmonic area; low-pitched diastolic rumble over tricuspid area (at times); persistent wide splitting of S_2.

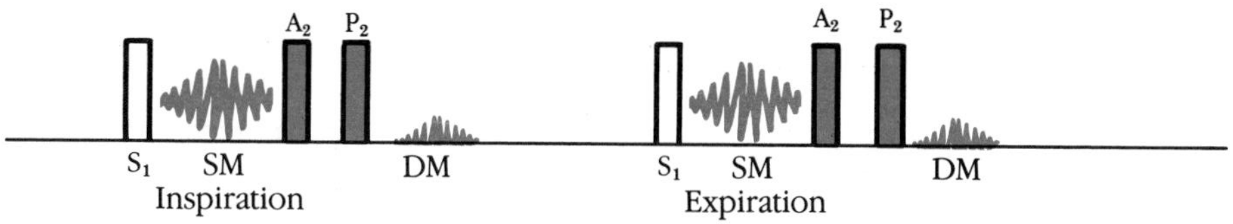

S_1 SM A_2 P_2 DM — Inspiration

S_1 SM A_2 P_2 DM — Expiration

VENTRICULAR SEPTAL DEFECT

Small pulse; normal jugular pulse; parasternal lift and left ventricular apical lift; systolic thrill and loud systolic regurgitant murmur in third and fourth interspaces along left sternal border; apical diastolic rumble.

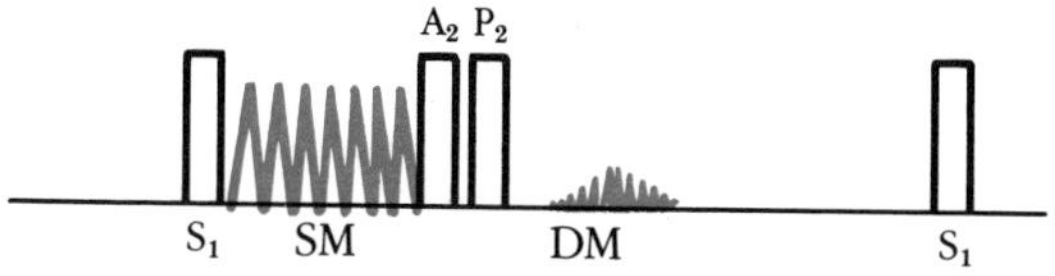

S_1 SM A_2 P_2 DM S_1

PERICARDITIS

Tachycardia; friction rub; diminished heart sounds and enlarged heart to percussion (with effusion); pulsus paradoxus; neck vein distension, narrow pulse pressure and hypotension (with tamponade).

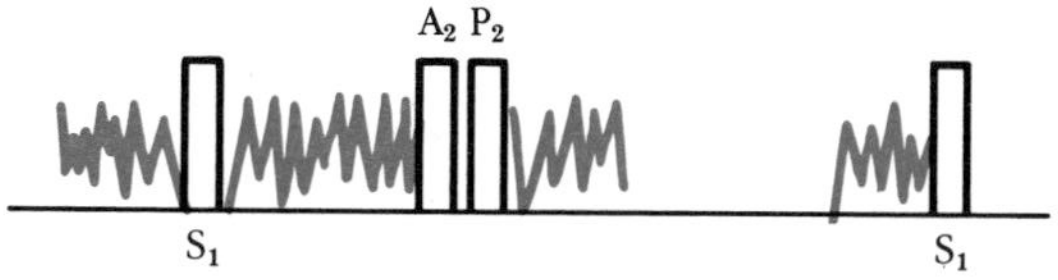

S_1 A_2 P_2 S_1

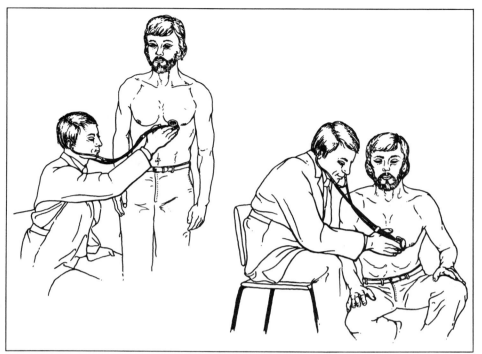

FIGURE 12–39
Prompt squatting. With the examiner auscultating from the sitting position, the patient moves
quickly from standing to squatting.

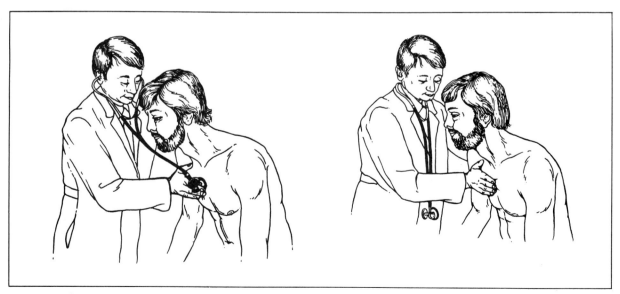

FIGURE 12–40
Palpation and auscultation with the patient in the sitting position and leaning forward. Thrills
associated with aortic outflow murmurs and the diastolic murmur of aortic insufficiency
may at times be appreciated only in this position.

no change or a decrease in regurgitant murmurs (i.e., those of mitral regurgitation, aortic regurgitation, and ventricular septal defect). The increased flow causes increased intensity of outflow murmurs (i.e., aortic stenosis, pulmonic stenosis, and mitral stenosis). This intervention will help distinguish outflow from regurgitant murmurs. The murmur of organic mitral stenosis increases while the Austin Flint murmur of aortic regurgitation decreases.

PROMPT SQUATTING. Rapid squatting causes an increase in afterload and venous return (Fig. 12–39). This results in a decrease in the dynamic obstruction associated with obstructive hypertrophic cardiomyopathy, or IHSS, and a resultant decrease in the systolic murmur. The murmur of valvular aortic stenosis does not change.

LEANING FORWARD. In order for the examiner to appreciate better the findings at the cardiac base, the patient should be asked to lean forward in the sitting position (Fig. 12–40). Thrills may be better palpated in this position, and soft diastolic murmurs may at times be appreciated only in this way.

CHAPTER 13

BREAST

This thy stature is like to a palm tree and thy breasts to clusters of grapes.
SONG OF SOLOMON 7:7

Careful examination of the breast should be part of every complete physical examination regardless of whether or not the patient has noted any particular signs or symptoms. Breast cancer is one of the most common malignancies occurring in women. It is a tumor that offers reasonable chance of a cure if it is recognized early and adequate therapy is carried out. Early detection is the key to successful treatment, and an important aspect of early detection of breast carcinoma is the careful performance of this routine part of the physical examination.

ANATOMY

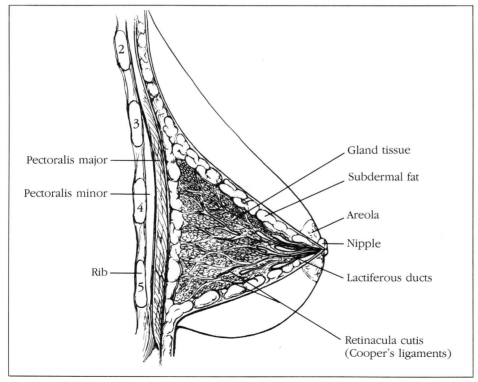

FIGURE 13–1
Cross-sectional anatomy of the breast.

311

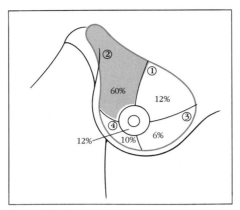

FIGURE 13–2
Clinical quadrants of the breast, with the percentage of all cancers of the breast found in each.

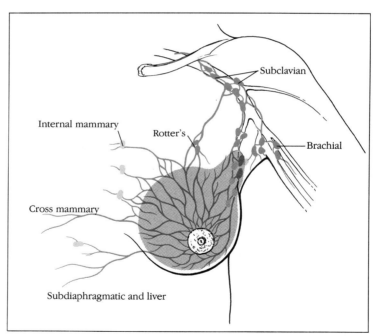

FIGURE 13–3
Nodal drainage of the breast.

HISTORY

Approximately 90 percent of breast cancers are first detected by patients themselves prior to seeking medical advice. They usually have noticed a lump or mass during bathing. Other complaints may include breast dimpling or retraction, nipple discharge, inflammation of the skin, and breast or bone pain. A family history of carcinoma of the breast in mother, maternal aunts, or sisters is a strong predisposing feature of this malignancy. To have breast-fed children is considered by some epidemiologists to lessen a woman's chance of breast cancer. Trauma to the breast probably functions more to call attention to a mass than to induce carcinomatous change.

Most breast masses are benign in origin and are associated with cyclic changes in the breast accompanying the menses. However, any mass of concern to the patient must be of equal concern to the physician. The woman complaining of such a lesion is likely to be apprehensive (with reason) about cancer and must be assured by a compassionate and thorough investigation.

PHYSICAL EXAMINATION

1. With patient sitting, inspect for asymmetry, retraction, skin change. Inspect with patient in three positions:
   a. Arms at side
   b. Arms on hips
   c. Arms overhead

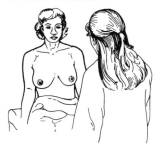
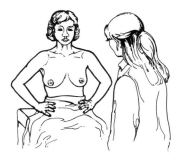
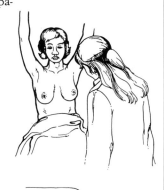

2. With patient sitting, palpate breasts with arms at side and overhead. Palpate axillary nodes.
3. With patient supine, palpate breasts and regional nodes.

GENERAL

Complete examination of the male or female breast demands a thorough and systematic approach. Adequate exposure is important. The patient should disrobe to the waist, although the female breasts should be kept covered by a towel except during the actual examination (Fig. 13–4). The patient should be examined in both the seated position and while supine.

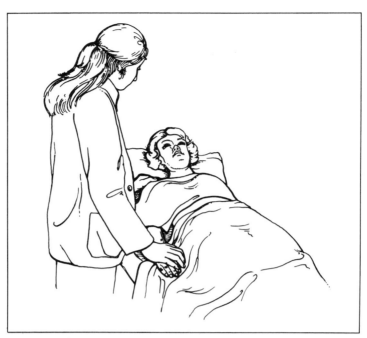

FIGURE 13–4
Woman draped for examination.

On the basis of a physical examination the examiner should be able to note the following diagnostic points:

1. Where is any lesion located? (Using the quadrants illustrated in Fig. 13–2, draw the lesion on your workup.)
2. Is the lesion single or multiple?
3. What is the consistency of the mass?
4. What is the size of the mass (in cm or mm)?
5. Is the mass tender?
6. Is the mass mobile or is it fixed to the chest wall?
7. Is the nipple displaced or retracted?
8. Is there retraction, dimpling, or erythema of the skin overlying the mass? Are there skin nodules?
9. Are there any regional lymph nodes, axillary or supraclavicular, palpable?

The normal female breast shows considerable variation in size, shape, and consistency. In the obese patient the breast may be large and pendulous; in the slender person it may be thin and small. In young patients the breast tends to be firm, somewhat elastic in consistency, and cone-shaped. The borders of the breast tissue are clearly delineated, and it is possible to move the entire breast freely over the anterior chest wall. It is often very sensitive to palpation. This may be particularly marked just prior to the menstrual period. In older patients the breast develops an

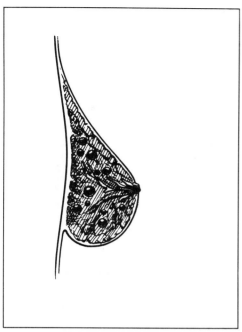

FIGURE 13–5
Fibrocystic changes.

irregular consistency and the sharply delineated border tends to be obscured. This is particularly true after pregnancy and lactation.

The breasts tend to undergo cyclic changes that are reflected in alterations in fullness and thickness of the normal breast tissue. These changes accompany menstruation and are associated with epithelial hyperplasia and lobular edema. When such alterations are marked, the patient may experience a degree of discomfort and the breast may be somewhat nodular (Fig. 13–5). Normal breast tissue may be characterized by a faint but distinct generalized nodularity. In some individuals this may be pronounced. This may make the recognition of a distinct tumor difficult.

INSPECTION

Some degree of asymmetry is not uncommon and is usually the result of a difference in breast development. Increased size of one breast may, however, indicate the development of cyst, inflammation, or tumor. Asymmetry is most easily observed while the patient is in the sitting position.

The skin overlying the breast should be carefully observed. The edema associated with inflammatory carcinoma or the ulcerative involvement of the nipple seen in Paget's disease should be noted. Local areas of redness may indicate underlying inflammation and are important in the detection of early breast infection.

The nipple should be carefully examined for evidence of bleeding, discharge, retraction, or ulceration (Table 13–1).

TABLE 13–1. Some Lesions of the Nipple

Lesion	Associations		Appearance
Inversion	Normality or, if of recent onset, malignancy		
Discharge	Type of nipple discharge		
	Serous	Bloody	
Adenosis	−	+	
Fibrocystic disease	+	+	
Duct ectasia	+	+	
Intraductal papilloma	+	+	
Intraductal papillary carcinoma	+	+	
Paget's disease	Malignancy		
Hyperpigmentation	Adrenal insufficiency		
Retention cysts	Normality		
Ulceration	Infection, neoplasm		
Inflammation	Infection, neoplasm		

Skin retraction is usually an indication of carcinoma, although it may result from traumatic fat necrosis. It is, however, a sign of malignancy and should be carefully searched for. The examination is best done by having the patient assume a position that will exert a pull on the suspensory ligaments of the breast. She should be examined while sitting erect and with her arms raised directly overhead. Elevating the arms should result in equal elevation of both breasts. A lesion producing shortening of the suspensory ligaments is likely to produce some retraction or deviation of the nipple. Another method of bringing out retraction is to produce contraction of the pectoral muscles, which in turn results in general traction on the breast tissue and tends to exaggerate any retraction that may be present. The patient should place the palms of both hands together and on command push the hands against each other. This may also be accomplished by placing her hands on her hips and pushing forcibly against them (Fig. 13–6A). It may be necessary to repeat these maneuvers several times so that all parts of the breasts can be adequately inspected. Another method of demonstrating retraction is to have the patient lean forward at the waist with her hands placed on the back of a chair. This demonstrates whether the breasts, as they fall away from the thorax, produce equal traction on the suspensory ligaments bilaterally. These maneuvers must be employed to detect early lesions. Obviously, with a grossly detectable lesion these steps are unnecessary (Table 13–2).

Inspection of the breasts should include careful observation of axillary and supraclavicular regions for evidence of bulging, retraction, discoloration, or edema, because these are the important lymphatic drainage areas from the breasts.

PALPATION

The consistency of normal breast tissue varies widely. This variation will depend on such factors as age, obesity, stage of the menstrual cycle, and pregnancy. As you gain experience in the art of physical examination, the range of normal condition will become apparent.

Palpation of the breast is best carried out by means of a definite system of examination. Regardless of the patient's presenting complaint it is important to examine completely both breasts and their lymphatic drainage areas lest some serious lesion be overlooked. It is convenient to begin the examination in the upper lateral aspect of each breast. The right breast is usually examined first, and palpation is carried out using the fingertips (Fig. 13–7). Gentle, light palpation should first be used; deeper exploration may be indicated if there is considerable breast substance. Palpation should be carried out in a clockwise direction until the entire breast has been examined. The nipple should be palpated for the presence of induration or a subareolar mass, and gentle pressure or a stripping action should be used to see whether discharge can be detected. Upon completion of examination of the right breast, the left breast is examined in a similar manner, again beginning in the upper lateral area and proceeding in a clockwise direction.

Palpation should be performed with the patient in both supine and seated positions. With the patient in the supine position, the patient's arms should be placed overhead. This spreads the breast tissue out over the pectoralis major muscle.

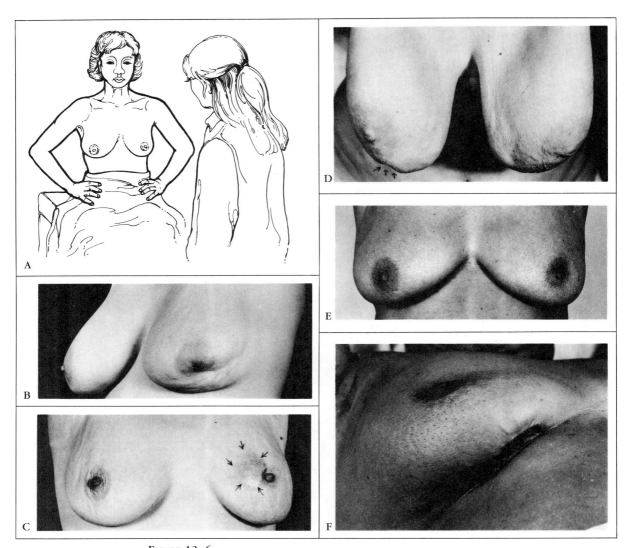

FIGURE 13–6

Some techniques of breast observation. A. Hands-on-hips technique may bring out retraction. B. Accentuation of nipple retraction and retraction of the skin, with deformity of breast contour accentuated by elevation of the arms. C. Large tumor of the medial aspect of the left breast and evidence of skin invasion as indicated by arrows. Despite its location adjacent to the nipple, there is very little evidence of nipple retraction. D. The indentation of the contour of the right breast, as indicated by arrows, is demonstrated by having the patient lean forward, thereby revealing an underlying breast tumor. E. Patient viewed from the front with both arms elevated. Both breasts are deceptively innocent. F. With the patient observed in the recumbent position, a large, ulcerative breast cancer is obvious in the costal mammary fold.

TABLE 13–2. Some Visible Signs of Breast Cancer

Lesion	Cause
Peau d'orange	Lymphedema due to obstruction of lymphatic drainage by tumor

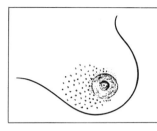 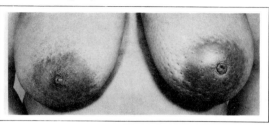

Retraction of the skin	Tumor involvement of Cooper's ligaments

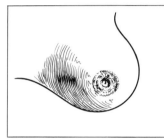 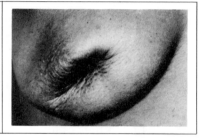

Increased venous pattern	Tumor obstruction of normal venous drainage

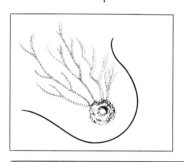

Erythema	Inflammatory tumor infiltrating skin or infection secondary to tumor

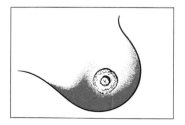

TABLE 13-2. (*Continued*)

Lesion	Cause
Paget's disease	Tumor originating in nipple

The examiner should note the texture of the skin and the consistency and elasticity of the breast tissue. An increase in firmness may suggest infiltration or neoplasia. Tenderness to palpation usually indicates a cyst. Malignant lesions by themselves are seldom tender but may coincide with widespread chronic cystic mastitis, in which case tenderness may be present.

If a mass is palpated, its size and location should be carefully recorded. This is usually done by considering the breast as the face of a clock with the nipple at the central point. The mass may be precisely located in regard to its distance from the nipple, and its size should be carefully estimated and recorded. It is often helpful to make a sketch of the area, describing the exact location and consistency (Fig. 13–8). The surface of the mass should be described; malignant tumors may have irregular infiltrating margins, whereas benign tumors may be sharply demarcated and smooth. The consistency of the mass may be helpful: soft cystic lesions are more likely to be benign; firm and irregular masses are more likely to be malignant.

The examiner should observe whether the lesion is freely movable or is fixed in position. Benign tumors are usually movable. Inflammatory lesions may be moderately fixed; advanced malignant lesions are often fixed to other structures as they become invasive. In general, benign lesions tend to have discrete margins, whereas malignancies tend to have boundaries that are difficult to define.

Both axillae should be systematically examined. This is best performed by examination with one hand while the examiner's opposite hand holds the patient's arm (Fig. 13–9). The boundaries of the axilla should be carefully palpated, and it is helpful to have the patient's arm go through a full range of motion during the examination in order to uncover any lesions that might otherwise be hidden beneath the pectoral muscle or subcutaneous fat.

The supraclavicular areas should be examined in a similar fashion; the neck should be palpated since the deep jugular nodes may be involved in metastatic spread. Because hepatic metastases are commonly found in patients with the advanced disease, the position and character of the liver edge should be noted.

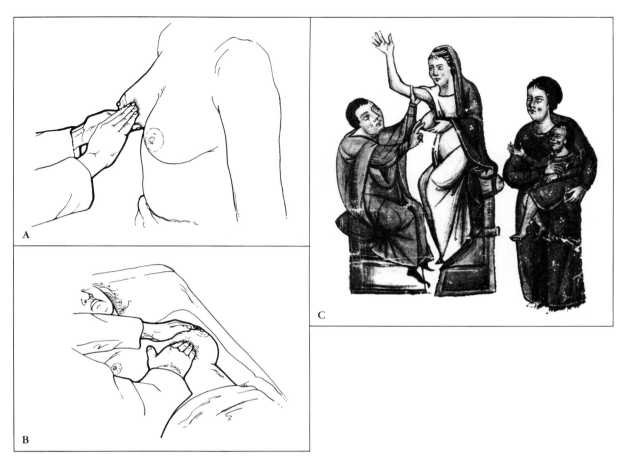

FIGURE 13–7
Technique of palpation of the breast. A. Patient seated. B. Patient supine. C. Breast palpation, from a late thirteenth century herbal.

If abnormalities are discovered, they are best documented in the written workup by careful description and mapping as illustrated. Figure 13–10 shows xeromammographic features of several common breast findings, both normal and abnormal.

Breast carcinomas are extremely variable in appearance, and a high index of suspicion is necessary if early diagnosis is to be achieved. Accurate diagnosis may only be obtained by biopsy, and this procedure should be promptly suggested if any question exists in the mind of the examiner. This may be accomplished by fine needle aspiration (FNA).

Some general features of **carcinoma** include a firm or hard consistency and lack of tenderness on palpation. Lesions of moderate size shorten the supporting ligaments of the breast, producing dimpling of the skin or nipple. A bloody or whitish discharge from the nipple may occur if there is neoplastic involvement of the ducts

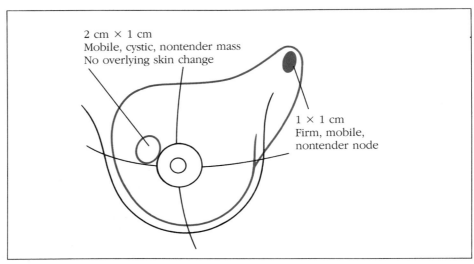

2 cm × 1 cm
Mobile, cystic, nontender mass
No overlying skin change

1 × 1 cm
Firm, mobile,
nontender node

FIGURE 13–8
Sample sketch of a cystic lesion of the left breast, such as may be recorded in the written workup.

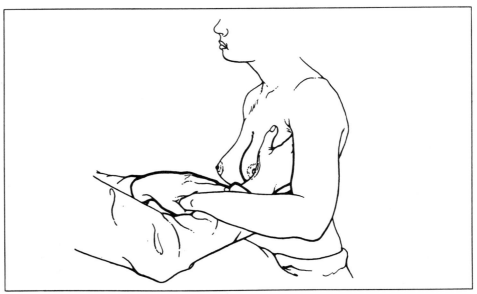

FIGURE 13–9
Technique of examination of the axilla.

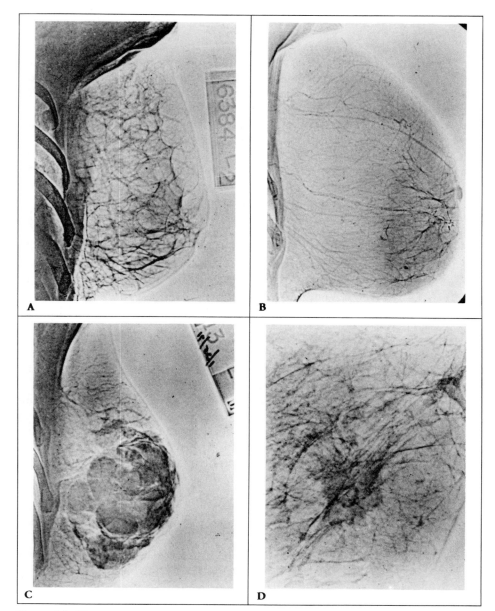

FIGURE 13–10

Xeromammography: a sensitive diagnostic study in breast disease. A. Xeromammogram of a premenopausal woman showing normal breast architecture and suspensory ligaments. B. Xeromammogram of a postmenopausal woman showing thinning and atrophy of the breast tissue and supporting structures. C. Xeromammogram of a 19-year-old woman with a firm lobulated mass within the breast. This is a typical appearance of a fibroadenoma. D. Xeromammogram of a portion of breast tissue in a postmenopausal woman with a firm but indistinct mass palpable within the left breast. The appearance is typical of scirrhous carcinoma, showing its infiltrating nature and retraction of the nipple.

or if the carcinoma is intraductal in origin. Advanced lesions may interfere with lymphatic drainage, producing an edematous thickening of the skin termed *peau d'orange* (like the skin of an orange). Advanced carcinomas may also be associated with palpable regional lymph nodes.

Inflammatory carcinoma is a special variety of cancer characterized by edema and erythema of the skin that produce a red, raised margin resembling acute cellulitis. This may simulate an inflammatory lesion and be associated with pain, fever, and tenderness. This type of carcinoma is usually produced by extensive lymphatic spread of neoplasm. It is more common in premenopausal women, is sometimes seen during pregnancy, and has a poor prognostic outlook.

Intraductal papilloma is characterized by a bloody or dark discharge from the nipple. Gentle pressure in the quadrants of the breast will often permit one to identify the involved duct system. Careful palpation or stripping in this region will often result in production of the characteristic discharge.

Fibroadenoma (adenofibroma) is a nontender, firm lesion that is often multilobulated. It is most often found in young women and is smooth-walled.

Fibrocystic changes are exceedingly common and are characterized by multiple nodules diffusely located in both breasts. The breast tissue is usually thickened and is often tender to palpation. The breasts frequently vary in size and degree of tenderness in association with the menstrual cycle. Occasionally the process may be fairly localized, or discrete nodules may be located in the presence of diffuse cystic changes. In either event biopsy is required for diagnosis.

Traumatic fat necrosis is a lesion that may simulate carcinoma, producing dimpling of the skin and retraction of the nipple. The consistency of the lesion is often firm, adding to the confusion. In some instances no history of trauma will be elicited. This lesion is more often encountered in large breasts containing increased amounts of fatty tissue. Absolute diagnosis can be established only by biopsy.

Paget's disease of the nipple is characterized by an excoriation or dry scaling lesion of the nipple. It may extend to involve the entire areola, tends to bleed easily on contact, and is always associated with an underlying carcinoma. It should be noted, however, that the underlying malignancy may not be palpable. Diagnosis may be achieved only by biopsy.

Mastitis is generalized inflammation of breast tissue, usually occurring during lactation. It is often associated with chills and fever. The involved breast tends to be red, edematous, and tender. Axillary lymphadenitis may occur, but fluctuation develops late or not at all. The soft, fatty nature of breast tissue tends to produce a spreading infection with little tendency to localization and abscess formation. This condition is usually associated with pyogenic infection.

Carcinoma of the male breast usually occurs as an irregular hard nodule underlying the areola. Because of the relative paucity of breast tissue, fixation to the chest wall occurs early. Metastasis is common by the time the carcinoma is detected. In general the prognosis is poor.

Gynecomastia is, by definition, a female type of breast occurring in a male patient. It is usually but not always unilateral. It must be distinguished from fatty breast occurring in a normal male. In the young patient the breast tends to assume a conical shape and be glandular in consistency, resembling the breast of a pubertal

TABLE 13–3. Some Causes of Gynecomastia

Physiologic
    Neonatal
    Pubertal
    Involutional, male climacteric

Endocrine
    Testicular failure
    Testicular tumors
    Hyperthyroidism
    Adrenocortical tumors
    Hermaphroditism
    Pituitary tumors

Liver disease
    Alcoholic
    Non alcoholic

Malnutrition and renutrition

Bronchogenic carcinoma

Drugs

Estrogens	Cimetidine
Chorionic	Isoniazid
gonadotropins	Amphetamines
Digitalis	Diethylpropion
Phenothiazines	Marijuana
Reserpine	Tricyclic antidepressants
Aldactone	Diazepam
Androgens	Cytotoxic agents
Methyldopa	Busulfan
	Vincristine
	Nitrosoureas
	Combination chemotherapy

Combination of two or more drugs
Combination of drugs and other illnesses noted above
Idiopathic

female. In elderly men the nodularity may be more irregular, and it may be difficult to rule out neoplasm. Biopsy, of course, is required under these circumstances. When gynecomastia is bilateral, it may be related to some systemic disease. For example, in patients with cirrhosis of the liver, altered metabolism of estrogens may lead to gynecomastia. Certain testicular tumors may cause gynecomastia, as may certain drugs. Other causes of gynecomastia are noted in Table 13–3. Sophisticated biochemical studies may be necessary to complete the diagnostic workup in these patients.

SELF-EXAMINATION

The technique of self-examination of the breast has been widely advocated as a means of early detection of malignant disease. Patients frequently seek advice regarding the method and frequency of its use. This brief description may be of help in advising patients on this matter.

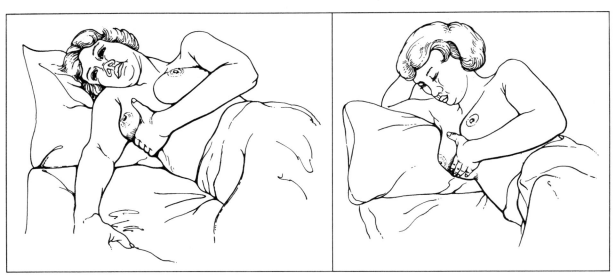

FIGURE 13–11
Self-examination of the breasts.

The patient should establish a regular schedule for monthly breast examination. This is ideally carried out immediately following the end of her menstrual period. An examination during the period may be unsatisfactory because of the temporary changes in consistency and tenderness that so often occur. The woman, however, may use the menstrual period as a reminder to inspect her breasts. After the menopause, monthly examination should, of course, be continued. The patient should be instructed to consult her physician immediately upon detecting a lump of any kind. The judgment and course of action should then be her physician's responsibility. She should also be warned to be alert for dimpling or puckering of the skin, retraction of either nipple, any thickening or change in consistency, or any alteration in symmetry, size, contour, or position. A discharge from the nipple may be significant. Pain, swelling, or inflammation may indicate advanced cancer, although more often they are associated with nonmalignant conditions. Having thus been advised of what to look for, she should be instructed in the following techniques:

1. **Observation**. The patient should place herself before a mirror with her arms at her sides. She should carefully examine her breasts in the mirror for symmetry, size, and shape, searching for any evidence of puckering, dimpling of the skin, or retraction of the nipple. She should then raise her arms above her head and again study her breasts in the mirror, looking for the same physical signs. She should also be alert for any evidence of fixation of the breast tissue to the chest wall. This may be displayed as she moves her arms and shoulders.

2. **Palpation**. This should be performed in the reclining position. This position permits the breasts to spread over a greater area and thins the breast tissue, making accurate palpation easier. A small pillow or folded towel should be placed beneath the shoulder on the side of the breast to be examined (Fig. 13–11). This raises that

side of the body and distributes the weight of the breast tissue more evenly over the chest wall. The arm on the side to be first examined is placed at her side, and the breast is gently examined with the flat surface of the fingers of her opposite hand. The technique calls for gentle palpation of the breast tissue against the chest wall, usually beginning on the outer half of the breast, paying particular attention to the upper outer quadrant where the axillary tail of breast tissue is thickest and where most tumors occur.

She should then raise the arm above her head and thoroughly examine the inner half of the breast beginning at the sternum. When the entire breast has been carefully palpated, the pillow is placed beneath the opposite shoulder and the woman investigates the second breast in exactly the same manner.

Palpation of the breast should be thorough and unhurried. Every portion of the breast must be deliberately and carefully examined if small lesions are to be detected.

The patient should be instructed to place the greatest emphasis on the regions where most breast cancers develop, namely in the upper outer quadrant, including the axillary tail of the breast and beneath the nipple. If the technique is to be effective, she must establish a definite habit pattern and conduct a thorough examination at monthly intervals. The method will only be effective if it is used regularly.

SECTION V

ABDOMEN AND PELVIS

14. GASTROINTESTINAL SYSTEM
   Richard D. Judge
   George D. Zuidema
15. MALE GENITOURINARY SYSTEM
   AND HERNIA
   Edward J. McGuire
   George D. Zuidema
16. FEMALE GENITOURINARY SYSTEM
   Theodore M. King

Abdominal pain is one of the most common conditions which call for speedy diagnosis and treatment. Usually, though by no means always, there are other symptoms which accompany the pain, but in the majority of cases of acute abdominal disease, pain is the main symptom and complaint.

SIR ZACHARY COPE
(1881–1974)

Abdominal Examination*
1. Inspect position, general appearance, abdominal wall, flanks, and back.

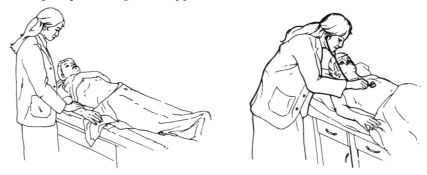

2. Auscultate abdomen for bowel sounds, rubs, hums, and bruits.
3. Percuss abdomen for organ size, masses, and tympany.

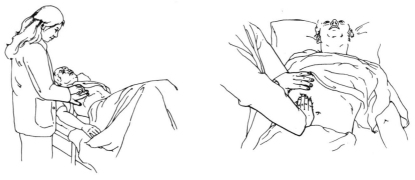

4. Palpate for tenderness, masses, and organ size.

In acute abdomen or limited physical examination proceed now to:

1. *Rectal examination* for appearance, sphincter tone, masses, and blood in stool.
2a. In men—*genitourinary examination* for hernia, testicular masses, and tenderness.
2b. In women—*pelvic examination* for tenderness, discharge, and masses.

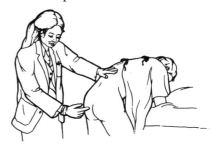

* The male genitourinary, the female pelvic, and the rectal examinations in both sexes are often done at the end of the physical examination for convenience. They are, however, logically associated with the gastrointestinal system and are an essential part of the immediate physical examination done in evaluation of an acute abdomen.

CHAPTER 14

GASTROINTESTINAL SYSTEM

A good eater must be a good man; for a good eater must have a good digestion, and good digestion depends upon a good conscience.

BENJAMIN DISRAELI, LORD BEACONSFIELD
(1804–1881)

Evaluation of the gastrointestinal system is a blend of meticulous history, careful physical examination, and judicious use of radiologic and endoscopic studies. Although proper diagnosis can frequently be obtained by history and physical, confirmation may mandate a contrast study of the bowel, selected endoscopy, or biopsy. With increased skill and experience the examiner should be able to predict confidently the findings of these special studies in the majority of circumstances.

ANATOMY

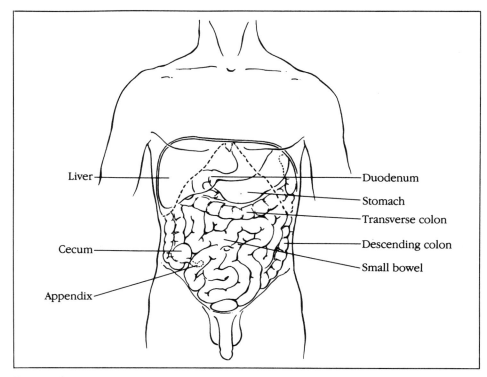

FIGURE 14–1
Schematic abdominal contents.

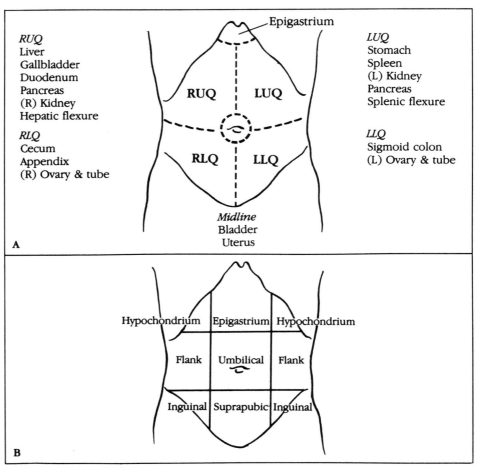

RUQ
Liver
Gallbladder
Duodenum
Pancreas
(R) Kidney
Hepatic flexure

RLQ
Cecum
Appendix
(R) Ovary & tube

LUQ
Stomach
Spleen
(L) Kidney
Pancreas
Splenic flexure

LLQ
Sigmoid colon
(L) Ovary & tube

Midline
Bladder
Uterus

FIGURE 14–2
Superficial topography of the abdomen. A. Four-quadrant system. B. Nine-region system.

HISTORY

In the evaluation of chronic gastrointestinal complaints, a careful analysis and description of the symptoms, how they developed, the order in which they appeared and changed, are usually far more informative than the physical examination.

HOWARD M. SPIRO
(1924–   )

Gastrointestinal complaints are among the most common given by patients to their physicians.

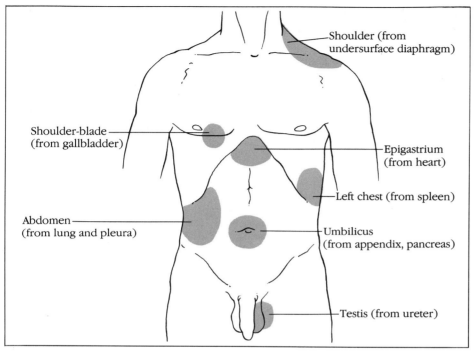

FIGURE 14–3
Common sites of referred pain.

PAIN

Pain of gastrointestinal origin varies greatly, depending on its underlying cause (Fig. 14–3). The major pain mechanisms include:

1. Capsular stretching—as in liver congestion due to heart failure
2. Irritation of the mucosa—as in acute gastritis
3. Severe smooth muscle spasm—as in acute enterocolitis
4. Peritoneal inflammation—as in acute appendicitis
5. Direct splanchnic nerve stimulation—as in retroperitoneal extension of a neoplasm, such as carcinoma of the pancreas

The *character, duration,* and *frequency* of gastrointestinal pain are functions of their mechanism of production; the *location* and *distribution* of referred pain are related to the anatomic site of origin. *Time of occurrence* and elements that *aggravate* and *relieve* the discomfort, such as meals, defecation, and sleep, also have special significance directly related to the underlying cause.

An outline of major sites of localization of pain usually includes the following:

Esophageal: Midline retrosternal; radiation to the back at the level of the lesion
Gastric: Epigastric; radiation occasionally to back, particularly left subscapular

Duodenal: Epigastric, radiation to back, particularly right subscapular

Gallbladder: Right upper quadrant or epigastric; radiation to right subscapular or midback

Pancreatic: Epigastric; radiation to midback or left lumbar area

Small intestinal: Periumbilical

Appendiceal: Periumbilical, migrating later to right lower quadrant

Colonic: Hypogastrium, right or left lower quadrant, depending on site of lesion; sigmoid pain with possible radiation to the sacral region

Rectal: Deep pelvic localization

ACUTE ABDOMEN

It is a curious but well known fact that many who are taken with abdominal pain in the daytime endure till evening until feeling compelled to send for the doctor. It follows that important diagnoses often have to be made at night . . . when the physician, weary with the day's work, is both physically and mentally below his best.

SIR ZACHARY COPE
(1881–1974)

There is no arena of clinical diagnosis in which the need for a rapid and complete history and physical examination is more dramatically urgent than in the assessment of the patient with catastrophic abdominal disease. For that reason we have taken the unconventional approach of presenting the evaluation of the patient with the "acute abdomen" prior to describing the more routine abdominal examination. You should note that the history surrounding the abdominal event is key to accurate diagnosis. Physical examination and further diagnostic studies are based on clues elicited during the carefully taken history.

The term *acute abdomen* suggests the importance and urgency which often accompanies acute intra-abdominal disease. Because of this urgency one should attempt to clarify the problem and arrive at a precise diagnosis when the patient is seen for the first time. The success of the examiner will depend on the thoroughness of his examination and his ability to pursue an orderly approach to the problem. Carelessness will be accompanied by a marked decline in accuracy. Early diagnosis is of crucial importance; the delay of even a few hours may permit peritonitis to develop or perforation of a viscus to occur. Delay also almost inevitably results in unnecessary morbidity and the likelihood of an increased mortality rate. The temptation to temporize is often strong in order to observe the course of the patient. While this may sometimes be justified, in many instances it will only result in the loss of a golden opportunity to treat surgical emergencies early and achieve superior results. It is often stated that abdominal pain that develops in a patient who has previously been well and persists for over 6 hours is caused by a condition requiring surgical attention. The practice of consistently performing a thorough examination of the acute abdomen will result in making a correct diagnosis early in the course of the disease, permitting prompt surgical treatment, if indicated.

Although the patient with acute abdominal distress is usually in pain, it is important to withhold the use of sedative or analgesic drugs until a satisfactory diagnosis has been made and one can ascertain whether surgical intervention will be required. Analgesics alter physical signs and symptoms to such an extent that accurate diagnosis often becomes impossible following their administration.

The patient who is suffering from acute, severe pain is not likely to be able to cooperate by furnishing a complete narrative history. In fact, under the urgency of the situation it may be important to depart from the routine and ask direct questions. Historical information derived from the patient himself should be supplemented whenever possible by detailed questions asked of his family and friends. The relatives or friends who accompany the patient to the hospital should be consulted regarding significant points before they are permitted to leave.

Whenever possible, a complete and detailed history and physical examination should be performed. Under some circumstances the severity of the illness may make prompt emergency treatment imperative. Under these circumstances the diagnostic approach will require abbreviation. It is still necessary, however, to obtain sufficient information to provide an adequate working diagnosis. Shortcuts are likely to be expensive in time, accuracy, and human life. Each symptom must be carefully and thoroughly evaluated in terms of its relationship to physical findings and other symptoms.

The **patient's age** is pertinent. The occurrence of certain disease processes is often limited to certain age groups. Recognition of this factor makes it possible to improve diagnostic accuracy.

A clear **description of the disease process** is of utmost importance. The patient should be asked to fix the exact time at which the pain began and the manner of its beginning. For example, pain of gradual onset may be associated with appendicitis, while the sudden onset of acute abdominal pain, awakening the patient from sleep, may be associated with perforation of a duodenal ulcer. It should also be noted whether the onset of the pain is related to some injury or exertion, no matter how trivial. The severity of the condition may be estimated by asking whether the patient collapsed or lost consciousness at the onset of the symptoms. Severe symptoms are more likely to be associated with such intra-abdominal catastrophes as acute pancreatitis, perforated ulcer, ruptured ectopic pregnancy, or strangulation obstruction of the bowel.

The character, distribution, and mode of onset of the pain should be carefully evaluated. Even the generalized pain associated with perforated ulcer or hemorrhage from a tubal pregnancy usually begins in a specific location, later spreading and becoming generalized. With perforated duodenal ulcer, for example, pain characteristically originates in the epigastrium with severe intensity but rapidly becomes generalized. For a time the pain may be more acute in the right flank and right lower quadrant, as the irritating gastric fluid passes down the gutter on the right side of the abdomen.

Pain that arises from the small intestine is usually felt primarily in the epigastrium and periumbilical areas. This is true whether it is simple mechanical intestinal obstruction or strangulation obstruction, since the innervation of the small bowel corresponds to the distribution of the ninth through the eleventh thoracic nerves. Because the innervation of the appendix is derived from the same source, this also explains why appendicitis usually begins with onset of pain in the epigastrium, followed by radiation to the right lower quadrant as the peritoneum and the psoas muscle become secondarily involved. Pain associated with large-bowel conditions is usually referred to the hypogastrium or to the actual site of the lesion.

In addition to noting the origin of the pain, it is also significant to follow its change in **localization**. The shifting of pain from the upper abdomen to the lower abdomen may be associated with the accumulation of irritating or infected peritoneal fluid in the pelvis. This may occur with a perforated ulcer or acute pancreatitis.

The **nature of the pain** is often a help in diagnosis. Crampy, constricting pain is characteristic of biliary colic, whereas burning pain is more likely associated with peptic ulceration. Back pain that is severe and constant may be associated with pancreatitis. Appendicitis is usually associated with a constant aching pain, except when a fecalith is present, in which case it may be colicky in nature.

The **radiation of the pain** is often significant. This is particularly true of colic associated with obstruction of hollow viscera, for the pain radiates to the area of distribution of the nerves coming from that segment of spinal cord supplying the affected viscus. For this reason biliary colic is frequently referred to the area beneath the right scapula, and renal colic is frequently referred to the testis.

The **relationship of pain to respiration** should always be noted. With intra-abdominal sepsis, such as peritonitis or abscess, deep inspiration may cause pain. On the other hand, pleuritic pain is made worse by inspiration but often disappears when the patient holds his breath.

A complete history inquires into the possible **relationship of pain to urination**. In addition to the many urinary conditions that may produce this, peritonitis or an abscess lying adjacent to the bladder may cause pain on urination and may even be associated with hematuria.

Vomiting may be associated with the following intra-abdominal conditions: acute gastritis; irritation of the peritoneum or mesentery (e.g., vomiting may appear early in the course of peritonitis associated with appendicitis or perforated ulcer); obstruction of hollow viscera producing smooth muscle spasm (e.g., biliary or ureteral colic or intestinal obstruction may be associated with vomiting); bacterial toxins or certain tissue metabolites may have a direct central action and may produce vomiting on a reflex basis. This is often seen in cases of septic peritonitis.

It is important to note the time relationship between the onset of pain and the exact time of vomiting. With biliary-tract calculus or sudden, severe peritoneal irritation, vomiting occurs early in the course of the disease and is likely to be violent. Low small-bowel obstruction may be associated with delayed vomiting, whereas vomiting occurs promptly with high small-bowel lesions. With large-bowel obstruction, vomiting may be a very late feature or may not occur at all. With appendicitis the onset of pain almost always antedates vomiting by several hours.

Not all intra-abdominal emergencies are associated with vomiting. Massive intraperitoneal hemorrhage may occur in absence of vomiting, and intussusception may be deceptive because vomiting may occur late or not at all.

The physical characteristics of the vomitus should be noted. In acute gastritis the vomitus consists largely of gastric contents occasionally flecked with small amounts of blood. With intestinal obstruction the characteristics of the vomitus show considerable variation. As the condition progresses, the character changes from gastric contents to bilious material, becoming yellowish green and finally consisting of brown, feculent-smelling fluid. Feculent vomiting may occur in either dynamic or adynamic intestinal obstruction.

If the patient denies vomiting, it is worthwhile to ask him about nausea or anorexia. There is considerable variation in the ease with which people vomit, and the presence of nausea or loss of appetite may in some individuals carry the same significance as vomiting does in others.

The condition of the **bowels** and nature of the **stool** should be investigated. An estimate of the patient's normal bowel habits should be obtained as well as careful analysis of how the acute illness may cause departure from his normal routine. The presence of gross or occult blood should be noted. The combination of blood and mucus in the stool is suggestive of intussusception. Pelvic infections may alter bowel habits and produce lower abdominal pain, diarrhea, and in some instances, tenesmus.

In women a careful **menstrual history** should be recorded, noting the characteristics of the period, including the last date of onset and the nature of the flow. Those data are necessary if one is to consider the diagnosis of threatened abortion, tubal pregnancy, and other gynecologic problems.

Vascular catastrophes, such as abdominal aortic aneurysm undergoing rupture, can produce severe pain and profound constitutional symptoms. They also require rapid diagnosis and surgical intervention.

Past history of the pain involved may be extremely valuable in making a diagnosis of such conditions as hiatus hernia, duodenal ulcer, and gastric carcinoma. The possible relationship to previous attacks of jaundice, hematemesis, melena, and so on may also contribute important information (Table 14–1).

It is obviously necessary to exclude medical diseases before deciding on the need for surgical intervention. A number of medical conditions may mimic intraabdominal emergencies. Examples are typhoid fever, pericarditis, lower lobe pneumonia, pyelonephritis, black widow spider bites, and porphyria. These possibilities emphasize the need for a thorough, objective, and systematic approach to examining entirely the patient who presents with abdominal pain.

The general rule can be laid down that the majority of severe abdominal pains which ensue in patients who have been previously fairly well, and which last as long as six hours, are caused by condition of surgical import.

SIR ZACHARY COPE
(1881–1974)

OTHER GASTROINTESTINAL SYMPTOMS
Illness isn't the only thing that spoils the appetite.

IVAN TURGENEV
(1818–1883)

The less acutely ill patient may present with a history of dysphagia, vomiting, and bowel dysfunction, which are discussed below.

TABLE 14–1. Some Causes of Acute Abdominal Pain

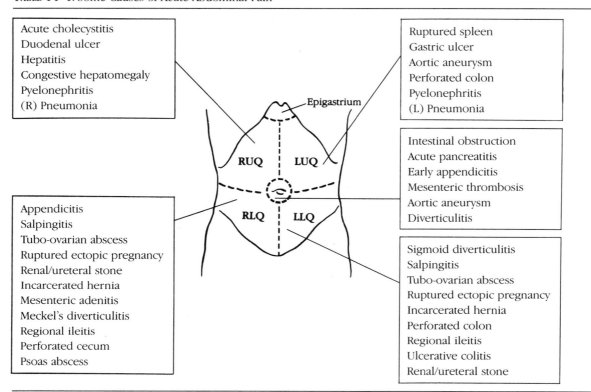

Acute cholecystitis
Duodenal ulcer
Hepatitis
Congestive hepatomegaly
Pyelonephritis
(R) Pneumonia

Ruptured spleen
Gastric ulcer
Aortic aneurysm
Perforated colon
Pyelonephritis
(L) Pneumonia

Intestinal obstruction
Acute pancreatitis
Early appendicitis
Mesenteric thrombosis
Aortic aneurysm
Diverticulitis

Appendicitis
Salpingitis
Tubo-ovarian abscess
Ruptured ectopic pregnancy
Renal/ureteral stone
Incarcerated hernia
Mesenteric adenitis
Meckel's diverticulitis
Regional ileitis
Perforated cecum
Psoas abscess

Sigmoid diverticulitis
Salpingitis
Tubo-ovarian abscess
Ruptured ectopic pregnancy
Incarcerated hernia
Perforated colon
Regional ileitis
Ulcerative colitis
Renal/ureteral stone

Dysphagia is usually more prominent and severe with solid food than liquids. The sensation is generally localized by the patient to the approximate level of obstruction. It is an important symptom and must never be ignored. Table 14–2 presents some causes of dysphagia.

Vomiting is often associated with upper gastrointestinal disorders. The patient should be questioned regarding the frequency, time of occurrence, and aggravating factors, as well as the quantity, color, odor, and taste of the vomited material.

Bowel function varies greatly among individuals. Direct observation of a stool specimen by the physician is far more accurate than a patient's description. Normal frequency of bowel action varies from several times daily to once every 3 to 5 days. Diarrhea or constipation of recent onset requires detailed description. The former is particularly important when it occurs mostly at night and suggests diabetes mellitus.

Additional gastrointestinal symptoms of importance include hematemesis, melena, anorexia, a sense of abdominal fullness, heartburn (pyrosis), regurgitation, flatulence, and belching.

TABLE 14–2. Some Causes of Dysphagia

Mechanical obstruction of the esophagus
  Congenital stricture
  Stricture due to corrosives
  Foreign bodies
  Carcinoma of the esophagus or stomach
  Extrinsic compression, as with aortic aneurysm
  Esophageal diverticula/pouches
  Reflux esophagitis with stricture

Dysphagia secondary to pain
  Pharyngitis
  Laryngitis

Neurologic dysfunction of the esophagus
  Bulbar paralysis
  Syphilis
  Lead poisoning
  Rabies
  Tetanus
  Parkinson's disease
  Botulism
  Myasthenia gravis
  Poliomyelitis
  Achalasia of the esophagus
  Plummer-Vinson syndrome (iron deficiency anemia and esophageal webs)
  Hysteria

There is no substitute for seeing the patient while he is having pain.

HOWARD M. SPIRO
(1924–   )

PHYSICAL EXAMINATION

1. Inspection of facial expression, respirations, position, skin (jaundice, pallor, pigmentation, etc.), nutrition, hydration, hands and nails, mouth, abdominal contour—masses, bulges, peristalsis, venous pattern
2. Auscultation for bowel sounds, rubs, bruits

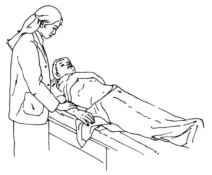
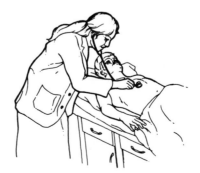

3. Palpation and percussion for tenderness, rigidity, masses, visceromegaly, rebound, fluid
4. Special maneuvers for psoas sign, obturator sign, etc. (if indicated)

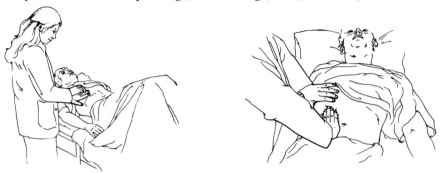

5. Rectal/vaginal examination to be considered now in acute abdominal disease

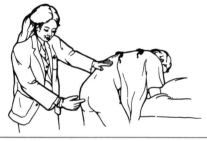

GENERAL

Jaundice is the disease that your friends diagnose.

SIR WILLIAM OSLER
(1849–1919)

As the first step in the examination of the abdomen, make sure that the patient is completely relaxed and properly positioned. His head should lie comfortably on one or two pillows, and his arms should be at his sides. The knees should be raised slightly in order to relax the abdominal musculature. Draw aside the bedclothes to make sure there is adequate exposure from the costal margin to the symphysis pubis. It is helpful to have the bed or examining table high enough to permit you to work in comfort and to have the patient close enough to the edge to permit access to the entire abdomen. Both the room and your hands should be warm, since chilling produces involuntary muscle spasm that hampers satisfactory examination. Lighting, of course, must be adequate.

A systematic plan for abdominal examination follows this sequence: inspection, auscultation, percussion, and palpation. By closely following this method the examiner may avoid omissions.

Because the gastrointestinal tract is highly sensitive to emotional state, a logical first step is to assess the patient's **face** and demeanor for signs of depression, agitation, exhaustion, hostility, and fear. A pale face with beads of perspiration may be associated with the shock accompanying acute pancreatitis or strangulation obstruction of the intestine. Pallor may be associated with massive intraperitoneal hemorrhage from a ruptured spleen or may reflect the anemia associated with acute and chronic blood loss. It should be remembered, however, that intra-abdominal catastrophes may occur without producing characteristic changes in the facies. In the late stages of many acute intra-abdominal processes, profound changes in facial expression may be accompanied by dulling of the eyes, shrinking of the tongue, and a cool skin, reflecting loss of circulating blood volume and impending failure of the circulation.

The **position** assumed by the patient is worth noting. With biliary or intestinal colic he may be unable to lie quietly; intraperitoneal hemorrhage may produce profound restlessness. This is contrasted with the patient suffering from generalized peritonitis who lies quietly with his knees drawn up to relax his abdominal muscles and relieve intra-abdominal tension.

The **respiration rate** should be noted, for a rapid rate may be associated with intrathoracic disease. Tachypnea may also be associated with generalized peritonitis, intestinal obstruction, intra-abdominal hemorrhage, or anxiety. The movement of the abdominal wall with respiration should be observed. Limitation of movement may be associated with abdominal distention, rigidity of the abdominal musculature, or limited mobility of the diaphragm.

Briefly note the tate of **skin** and **nails** and the **hair distribution**. Patients with gallbladder or liver disease may show evidence of jaundice. The yellow discoloration of the sclera and skin is frequently more obvious in daylight than in artificial light, where it may pass unnoticed, even when moderately severe. Other important skin changes include (1) pigmentation that may reflect malabsorption, regional enteritis, adenomatous polyps of the bowel, or hemochromatosis; (2) xanthomas associated with biliary cirrhosis; (3) erythema nodosum from ulcerative colitis; (4) a flush suggesting carcinoid neoplasm; (5) generalized edema caused by intestinal malabsorption; and (6) spider angiomata or petechiae, palmar erythema, ecchymoses, and hair loss, which separately or together indicate chronic liver disease.

Outward signs of the patient's **nutritional state** indirectly reflect gastrointestinal function. Weight loss and emaciation need little emphasis here because of their obvious importance. Nail changes include (1) koilonychia (spooning) with chronic iron deficiency, and (2) clubbing with intestinal malabsorption, regional enteritis, ulcerative colitis, and hepatic cirrhosis. Dehydration may cause reduction of ocular tension, xerostomia, and persistent ridging of the skin on the dorsum of the hand when lightly pinched. Serious fluid loss frequently accompanies gastrointestinal disease.

Fever is not a constant companion of intra-abdominal disease. In the presence of shock, septicemia, acute pancreatitis, strangulating intestinal obstruction, or perforated ulcer, the temperature may be normal or subnormal at onset. A low-grade fever may accompany the early stages of acute appendicitis; higher temperatures occur with peritonitis. High fever is not often associated with the early stages of acute abdominal disease.

The **pulse rate** and its character should be carefully noted. It is true that a normal

TABLE 14–3. Some Characteristic Mouth Odors in Disease

Name	Description	Condition
Acetone breath	Smells of acetone—sweet, like fruity chewing gum	Diabetic ketoacidosis
Fetor hepaticus	"Mousy" odor, sickly sweet	Hepatic failure
Acid breath	Acrid, acid smell	Peptic disease
Fetid breath	Sickening odor of decay	Lung abscess Esophageal diverticulum
Feculent breath	Odor like feces	Lung abscess Severe bowel obstruction
Bitter almonds	Can be detected by only some examiners (perception is a genetic trait)	Cyanide toxicity
Uriniferous breath	Odor like urine	Renal failure

pulse does not necessarily mean a normal condition within the abdomen, although it may indicate that the patient is reacting well to his disease. It is worthwhile to follow the pulse rate at intervals, for it is likely to increase in rate as the intra-abdominal infection or hemorrhage progresses. As peritonitis advances, the pulse may show slight irregularity or be somewhat bounding. In advanced peritonitis the pulse is rapid and thready. This is a bad prognostic sign.

MOUTH

A detailed examination of the mouth is considered in Chapter 9, but it should be emphasized that inspection of the oral cavity is an important part of the gastrointestinal examination. Observe the lips, oral mucosa, teeth and gingivae, and tongue. Is salivation adequate? Although some nutritional deficiencies are reflected in the oral cavity, many nonpathologic changes may be observed. Some of these include (1) cracking of the lips due to exposure to weather and cold; (2) angular stomatitis from poorly fitting dentures; (3) mild gingivitis, a very common finding in otherwise healthy people; (4) prominent fungiform papillae, usually along the midline, giving an appearance called "geographic tongue"; and (6) normal furring or coating of the tongue, which is merely dead epithelium combined with yeast and saprophytes. The well-known "coated tongue" may be of some concern to a patient, but it is common in healthy people. Severe halitosis may occur with chronic gastroesophageal disease, particularly neoplasm (Table 14–3). Fetor hepaticus is a term describing a characteristic odor associated with severe liver failure; at times it is apparent at some distance from the patient's bed. In peptic disease of the stomach and duodenum the patient's breath often has an acid odor.

Glossitis and stomatitis often accompany deficiency states caused by chronic gastrointestinal disorders, such as sprue, with associated malabsorption and depleted body stores of iron, vitamin B_{12}, folic acid, niacin, thiamine, and riboflavin. Melanin spots about the face and mouth are a sign of intestinal polyposis. They are frequently drab brown or dark bluish black and may be mistaken for simple freckles.

ABDOMEN

Drink a glass of wine after your soup, and you steal a ruble from the doctor.

RUSSIAN PROVERB

INSPECTION

For convenience, we divide the abdomen into topographic segments. This division permits precise localization of physical signs and symptoms and makes it possible to correlate physical signs with the anatomic location of viscera within the abdomen. A number of systems for describing topographic anatomy have been advocated, as illustrated under "Anatomy." In describing historical location or physical findings, refer to one of these systems.

As you inspect the abdomen, first observe the skin, its color, and its texture. Are there any unusual lesions, striae, or surgical scars (Fig. 14–4)?

Usually the venous pattern is barely perceptible, and the drainage of the lower two-thirds of the abdomen is downward (Fig. 14–5). Superficial abdominal veins may be dilated and tortuous because of vena caval obstruction. With portal hypertension of hepatic cirrhosis, the veins may appear to radiate from the umbilicus as a result of backflow through the collateral veins within the falciform ligament. This pattern is termed *caput medusae.*

Next, observe the general contour of the abdomen. Is it symmetrical? Is there any localized bulging or prominence? A scaphoid abdomen often accompanies cachexia; protuberance may result from gaseous distention, ascites, or neoplasm. Observe specifically for hernia.

An *umbilical hernia* protrudes through the umbilical ring. In the newborn a congenital umbilical hernia may result from improper closure of the abdominal wall; a hernia of the umbilical cord, also termed an *omphalocele,* is produced. The peritoneal sac is not covered by the skin of the abdominal wall.

True umbilical hernias are common during the first year of life. In this type the peritoneal sac is covered by skin. Increased intra-abdominal pressure due to trauma, cough, or constipation may contribute to their formation.

Umbilical hernias in adults are more common in women. Obesity, pregnancy, ascites, or congenital defect may be contributing factors. Umbilical hernias may show wide variation in size, but the neck of the sac is often small. This type of hernia usually contains omentum but may contain large or small bowel and other viscera as well. Strangulation is a frequent occurrence. Diastasis or separation of the rectus muscles is often associated.

An *epigastric hernia* occurs through a weakness in the linea alba between the xiphoid and the umbilicus, usually due to a developmental defect. Pregnancy, obesity, trauma, or constipation may be contributing factors. These hernias are most common in young adult males. The hernial sac is usually small and may contain omentum but rarely intestine. Strangulation rarely occurs.

Incisional hernias, as the name indicates, occur through surgical incisions. Infection, poor wound healing, faulty wound closure, postoperative vomiting, ileus, partial wound disruption, and obesity may be contributing factors. This type of hernia often reaches large size, and the intestines are usually adherent to the underside of the peritoneum. Strangulation is uncommon but may occasionally occur.

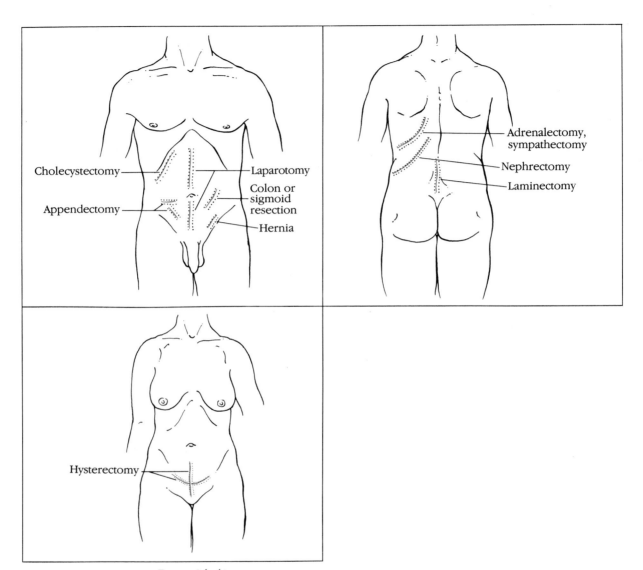

FIGURE 14–4
Common surgical scars.

A *spigelian hernia* occurs at some point in the semilunar line at the lateral margin of the rectus muscle, usually in the lower abdomen at the linea semicircularis where the posterior rectus sheath is absent.

Is the umbilicus in the midline and normal? Instruct the patient to cough or bear down, and notice whether this produces any bulging. Does this maneuver cause any pain? Normally it does not. Note any unusual movement causing a slight protrusion with inspiration due to descent of the diaphragm. A decrease in respiratory

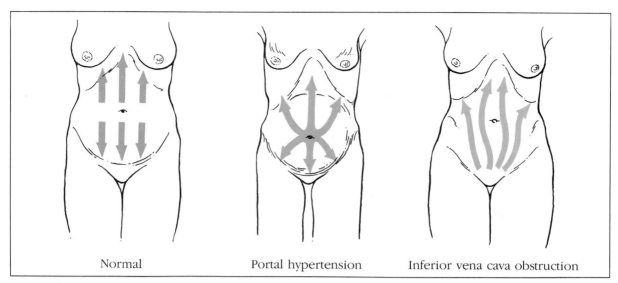

FIGURE 14—5
Abdominal venous patterns.

movements of the abdomen may suggest intraperitoneal fluid, or it may be associated with acute abdominal pain, such as with peritonitis. Are there any visible
peristaltic waves? With intestinal obstruction, peristaltic waves may be visible passing across the abdomen.

Finally, are there any vascular pulsations? Occasionally in the thin individual with
a flat or scaphoid abdomen, the normal aortic pulsation may be evident in the
epigastrium.

AUSCULTATION

Many experienced examiners will auscultate the abdomen before percussion or
palpation are begun (as opposed to the classic order). In the presence of abdominal disease, percussion and palpation may cause slowing of the bowel and diminution of peristaltic sounds. Moreover, the stethoscope itself may be used, concurrent with careful auscultation, as the first instrument of light palpation. It is useful
to warm the stethoscopic head (often done by simply holding it in your hand or
under your armpit) before placing it on the abdomen.

Most intestinal sounds originate from the small bowel and have a high-pitched,
gurgling quality, better sensed than described. Frequency of intestinal sounds varies in relation to meals, but usually five or more sounds occur each minute. The
examiner should be accustomed to hearing the sounds that accompany normal
peristalsis.

Abnormal bowel sounds are distinguishable only when you have developed a
clear appreciation of the normal variation in peristaltic sound. Peristalsis may be

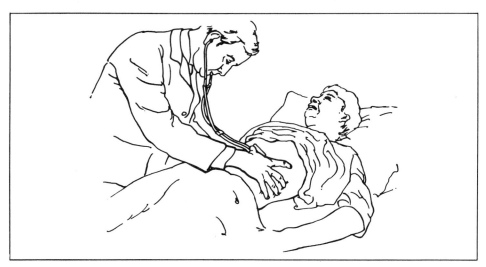

FIGURE 14–6
Checking for succussion splash.

increased, diminished, or absent in the presence of intra-abdominal disease. Absence of bowel sounds suggests **paralytic ileus** due to diffuse peritoneal irritation. Before bowel sounds can be said to be absent, however, it is necessary to listen for periods of at least 1 minute in all portions of the abdomen. Increased peristalsis will usually be audible in patients with acute intestinal obstruction. In these patients the abdomen tends to be silent between bouts of colic. As the cramps occur, the bowel sounds gradually increase in intensity, rise to a crescendo, then pass away. The patient will often complain of crampy abdominal pain that coincides with the onset of the peristaltic activity. As paralytic ileus subsides, or in the presence of chronic partial small-bowel obstruction, a variety of gurgling and tinkling sounds may be detected. These sounds are produced by peristaltic activity in dilated, fluid-filled loops of bowel. In general, no specific rhythm may be present, and it may or may not be accompanied by cramping pain.

With outlet obstruction of the stomach, a **succussion splash** is at times detectable because of the presence of fluid and gas in the distended organ. This is easily appreciated by placing the stethoscope diaphragm over the epigastrium and shaking the patient vigorously from side to side (Fig. 14–6). A characteristic sloshing and gurgling sound is readily identified. It is important to determine the interval since the previous meal, as it is possible to elicit this sign in a normal person immediately after ingestion of a large quantity of fluid.

Rubs may be heard over the liver in patients with hepatic tumor or infection, and over the spleen in splenic infarction, neoplasia, and infection. **Bruits** over these organs suggest a vascular tumor, intense extramedullary hematopoiesis (e.g., as in myelofibrosis), or arteriovenous malformation. Other vascular bruits in the abdomen are discussed in Chapter 12.

PERCUSSION AND PALPATION

Generally speaking, the looser the texture, and more tender the fibre, of animal food, the easier it is of digestion.

WILLIAM BEAUMONT
(1785–1853)

Percussion and palpation are performed together. No two physicians follow exactly the same approach, and in time you will develop your own method. Whatever it is, adhere to it strictly, for this is the surest way of avoiding damaging omissions.

Right-handed examiners nearly always prefer to approach the abdomen from the patient's right side. Because the area is sensitive and frequently ticklish, some preparation against the shock of first contact with the examining hand is helpful. Chat with the patient. Touch the patient first on the forearm, very lightly, and do not try to elicit information until he settles down. If he absolutely cannot relax, have him palpate his own epigastrium, then place your hand on top of his, and finally beneath his. Finally, ask him to withdraw his own hand. This maneuver, though rarely necessary, can be helpful with very tense patients and with children.

Keep in mind that this will be one of the most difficult parts of the routine examination. Proceed slowly: do not rush. When difficulty is encountered, have the patient breathe with his mouth open. This automatically causes some relaxation. Such suggestions as "Now, relax as if you were falling asleep" may be valuable under certain circumstances. If the bed is low, do not hesitate to kneel down beside it or sit down on the edge. The rule that prohibits sitting on the patient's bed can be violated under special circumstances if done tactfully. Finally, concentrate all your senses on the examination. In particular, watch the patient's facial expression. A slight wince or almost inaudible gasp may be of major importance as you proceed.

Consider next your objectives, which are simple and limited. You must try to determine the presence or absence of (1) tenderness (superficial or deep), (2) organ enlargement, (3) abdominal mass, (4) spasm or rigidity of the abdominal muscles, (5) ascites, or (6) exaggerated tympanites. There is no universally accepted sequence for routine abdominal examination, and you may begin in any one of the quadrants and proceed in a clockwise manner until all four have been examined.

Before beginning active palpation, ask the patient to cough. If peritoneal irritation is present, coughing will elicit a sharp twinge of pain that may then be localized to the involved area. This permits you to carry out the major portion of the abdominal examination without touching the area of maximal tenderness. You should try to begin your examination of the abdomen at the site most distant from any pain, so that the patient does not instantly tighten the abdominal musculature to protect himself, thus obscuring your examination.

Hyperesthesia should be tested for routinely. This may be done by lightly stroking the abdomen with the point of a pin, stroking the abdomen from above downward. The patient is requested to note if the pin stroke feels sharper at a given location. Hyperesthesia suggests the presence of visceral or parietal peritoneal ir-

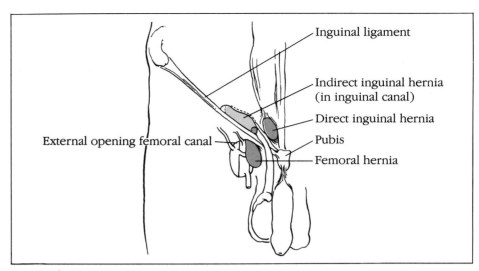

FIGURE 14–7
Common hernia sites.

ritation. It may be detected in the segmental distribution of that portion of the spinal cord from which the affected viscus is innervated or along the distribution of the peripheral nerves that may be involved directly by the inflammatory process. This physical sign is helpful when present, but it should certainly not be considered a constant finding in acute abdominal conditions, and its absence does not rule out intra-abdominal disease.

It is important to examine the sites of possible external herniation as a routine measure (Fig. 14–7). Particular attention should be paid to the femoral canal to rule out the presence of a small hernia or Richter's hernia. Incarcerated or strangulated hernias are so often the cause of or associated with intra-abdominal processes that this observation should be performed without fail in all cases. The femoral artery should be palpated during this part of the examination, since absence of its pulsations or inequality between the two sides may suggest embolic disease or the presence of a ruptured or dissecting aneurysm.

Test for muscular spasm of the abdominal wall. All areas of the abdomen should be palpated to evaluate the extent of the muscular spasm present. It is helpful to ask the patient to breathe deeply during this part of the examination, for voluntary rectus muscular spasm will give way as the patient exhales. True muscular spasm will not change, and the abdomen will remain rigid and tense during expiration. Extensive rigidity involving both rectus muscles is suggestive of diffuse peritoneal irritation. With localized or early peritonitis the spasm may be limited to a portion of the abdomen. It is helpful to palpate both recti simultaneously in order to evaluate the extent and severity of the muscle spasm.

Palpation of the abdomen includes examination of the costovertebral angles bilaterally. This may be easily accomplished using the index finger. It is also helpful to palpate with one finger to outline gently the areas of tenderness within the

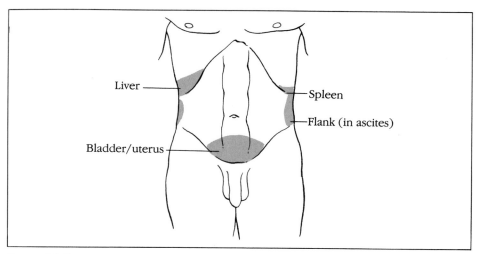

FIGURE 14–8
Areas of dullness on abdominal percussion.

abdomen. This serves the dual purpose of achieving accurate localization while producing minimal discomfort to the patient.

Light palpation is aimed primarily at eliciting minor degrees of tenderness and guarding. It is performed with the flat of the hand, not the fingertips, and sudden increases in pressure should be avoided. When changing position, remove the hand rather than drag it across the surface; the latter produces a disagreeable sensation resulting in undue muscle spasm. Such voluntary guarding may be suspected when tightness follows temporary relaxation during the first phase of expiration. It usually passes away gradually as the examination progresses.

Areas of tenderness should be localized as accurately as possible without producing undue discomfort. It may be necessary to cause additional discomfort during palpation of the abdomen. The need for this should be explained to the patient in advance so that he understands its importance.

A clear understanding of anatomic relationships and their variations is indispensable for the interpretation of tenderness of visceral origin. Sometimes, however, abdominal pain and tenderness do not actually arise from abdominal organs. This condition, referred to as parietal tenderness, is identified by having the patient, in the supine position, contract the abdominal muscles (by raising his head or feet) so as to prevent the transmission of pressure to the underlying viscera. Under these circumstances persistent tenderness on light palpation or gentle pinching probably arises in the abdominal wall itself. Similarly a mass that remains palpable under these conditions is probably situated superficially within the abdominal wall.

Percussion is of relatively limited diagnostic value, but it is a simple method of relaxing abdominal tension. Percuss the four quadrants briefly while noting the degree of resonance (Fig. 14–8 shows areas of dullness on abdominal percussion). Next, delineate the upper and lower borders of the liver in the midclavicular line. They should be no more than 10 cm apart, but liver dullness along the lower

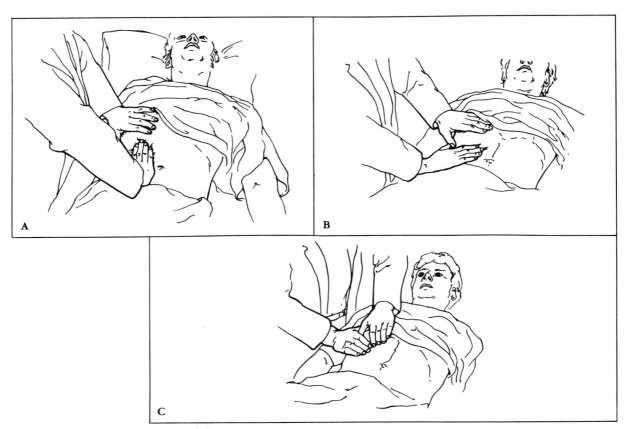

FIGURE 14–9
Palpation of the liver. A. Proper position of the hands. B. Incorrect (horizontal) positioning (see text). C. Hooking.

border may be partially obliterated by gas in the overlying bowel, making the overall dimension less than 10 cm. Next, outline Traube's space (the gastric air bubble) in the left upper quadrant; then, if possible, find the area of splenic dullness lateral to this, remembering that percussion has very limited value in delineating enlargement of the spleen.

Move to the suprapubic area and outline the upper border of the urinary bladder if possible. Watch carefully for evidence of tenderness while percussing. Percussible enlargement of the urinary bladder may or may not be of pathologic significance, depending on other factors. Remembering always that in the premenopausal woman, an enlarged uterus may simply reflect pregnancy. A resonant note obtained in what should normally be a dull area anteriorly is suggestive evidence of free air within the peritoneal cavity. In the presence of intestinal obstruction, a gas-filled bowel may be pushed up anteriorly; in that situation percussion is of no value.

In some instances it may be possible to demonstrate the presence of shifting **dullness** by means of percussion in patients with acute abdominal disease. This test alone may be of little help, since no information is obtained regarding the character of the fluid present, and it is seldom that this would alter the decision to operate. Needle paracentesis of the abdominal cavity may be of help in obtaining a sample of the free fluid present, permitting its culture and microscopic examination prior to laparotomy. This procedure is of little or no value in the presence of intestinal obstruction where loops of fluid-filled and gas-filled bowel predominate.

The next step in the examination consists of *deep palpation* of the abdomen in an effort to determine the size of liver, kidneys, and spleen, and to discover the presence of any abnormal intra-abdominal masses. Deep palpation requires great experience and skill. The flat of the right hand is usually used, and at times the left is placed over it for reinforcement. Pressure is very gradual and steady; special care is necessary at this point in order not to cause undue discomfort to the patient.

SPECIFIC ORGAN EXAMINATIONS

PALPATION OF THE LIVER. The bimanual technique (Fig. 14–9) is always helpful for deep palpation, particularly of the liver and kidneys. The posterior hand is placed between the twelfth rib and the iliac crest, just lateral to the paraspinous muscles. In palpating the liver, place the anterior hand firmly inward and upward in the right upper quadrant and instruct the patient to take a deep breath and hold it. You will want to release your pressure slightly at the height of inspiration, at the same time moving the fingertips gently upward toward the costal margin. When palpable, the liver edge is felt to slip over the fingertips at this moment. Proper placement of the anterior hand is important, as shown in Figure 14–9A. Horizontal placement of the hand (Fig. 14–9B) tends to force the whole liver backward, making the edge less accessible. Another common error concerns the level of placement of the palpating hand. Begin low, below the percussed border of dullness. Liver enlargement can be missed by palpating too close to the costal margin, so that the whole organ is beneath the hand and the edge is not palpated. At times, palpation can be better accomplished by the hooking technique (Fig. 14–9C).

The anterior hand should parallel the rectus muscle, not the costal margin. The hooking technique is occasionally preferable. The liver edge may be normally felt, particularly in women and children. At times the liver may extend 4 or 5 cm below the right costal margin without actually being enlarged. Delineation of the overall size by percussion may help to differentiate this ptosis (dropping down) from true enlargement. Overall size in the midclavicular line is usually less than 15 cm, but the patient's size, habitus, and pulmonary status are important considerations.

The principal causes of hepatic enlargement are congestion, cirrhosis, neoplasm, and hepatitis. Tenderness is more likely with congestion and inflammation; irregular nodularity, with neoplasm; a very hard consistency, with cirrhosis. There are also other causes for liver enlargement that are beyond the scope of this discussion.

The sign of inspiratory arrest (Murphy's sign) may be seen in the presence of acute cholecystitis. This is elicited by having the patient take a deep breath while the examiner maintains pressure against the abdominal wall in the region of the gallbladder. As the liver descends with inspiration, the gallbladder comes in contact with the examining hand and the patient experiences a sharp pain and inspiration is arrested.

Inflammatory processes involving the liver or gallbladder may be elicited as tenderness in the right upper quadrant on fist percussion of the lower anterior chest wall. When this test is negative, one should hesitate to diagnose right upper quadrant inflammation.

SPLEEN. The spleen, though not physiologically part of the gastrointestinal system is, because of its location in the abdomen, examined here. The patient is supine, arms at side, and knees flexed slightly. Outline the area of splenic dullness as a first step. This should be done not so much to delineate the splenic size but rather to loosen the abdomen. Percussion may outline a greatly enlarged spleen, directing initial palpation to the left lower portion of the abdomen. Figure 14–10A shows the position of the examiner's hands. Note that pressure is light. Press the tips of the index and middle fingers of the right hand to a point just beneath the costal margin. Then ask the patient to turn his head to the side away from you and take a long, deep breath through his mouth. Do not move the hand as the patient inhales. The edge of an enlarged spleen will then brush against the fingers, lifting them slightly upward. As the patient exhales, probe the left upper quadrant more deeply, moving the fingertips in a slightly rotary motion. If nothing is felt, drop the hand about 1 cm and repeat. Do not dig. This will cause spasm of the muscles, making palpation difficult. Furthermore, slight splenic enlargement can be missed because the fingertips may be below the splenic edge, which will glide over the backs of the fingers.

Two special maneuvers may be helpful. First, have the patient slip his left forearm under the small of his back (Fig. 14–10B); this position will tend to thrust the spleen upward. Second, roll the patient on his right side with the right leg straight and the left knee flexed (Fig. 14–10C). The tips of the palpating fingers should be placed 1 or 2 cm below the costal margin with this maneuver. The keys to satisfactory splenic palpation are proper instructions to the patient with respect to breathing and gentleness by the examiner.

Normally the spleen is not palpable in the adult. It must be two or three times normal size before it becomes palpable.

Splenomegaly is common to many different and unrelated types of disease. It may be due to hyperplasia, congestion, or infiltrative replacement of the splenic pulp by neoplasm, myeloid elements, lipid, or amyloid.

Splenic hyperplasia occurs as a response to many systemic bacterial, parasitic, viral, or mycotic infections. Acute enlargement occurs with hematogenous dissemination of the infectious organisms as, for example, in bacterial endocarditis, septicemia, or miliary tuberculosis. Chronic enlargement of the spleen occurs with malaria, rheumatoid arthritis, and other relapsing or progressive inflammatory diseases. Splenic hyperplasia is common to many of the chronic anemias, whether due to conditioned deficiencies, hemolysis, or inherited defects in erythropoiesis. It is also the cause of splenomegaly in polycythemia vera.

Splenic congestion as a consequence of portal hypertension may be secondary to chronic hepatic disease, chronic congestive heart failure, or occlusion of the

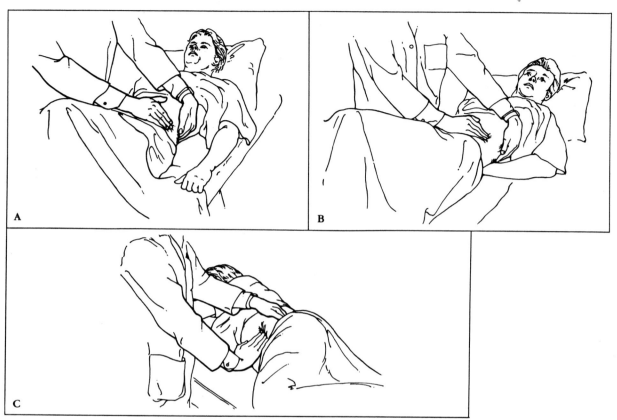

FIGURE 14–10
Palpation of the spleen. A. Positioning of examiner's hands. B. Patient's hand under his back.
C. Patient rolled to right side.

splenic or portal veins. The most common cause of congestive splenomegaly is
cirrhosis of the liver.

Splenic infiltration by neoplastic cells results in the marked enlargement associated with the leukemias and lymphomas. Occasionally splenomegaly may also be
produced by replacement of the splenic pulp by amyloid, lipid-filled reticuloen-
dothelial cells (e.g., Gaucher's disease), or myeloid elements (extramedullary hematopoiesis).

A classification of splenomegaly according to the degree of enlargement is listed
in Table 14–4. The designations depend on the distance (in centimeters) of the
splenic edge below the left costal margin, on deep inspiration, as follows: slight
enlargement, 1 to 4 cm; moderate enlargement, 4 to 8 cm; great enlargement, more
than 8 cm.

If the spleen is greatly enlarged it may be missed on routine palpation. This
pitfall can be avoided by (1) careful preliminary inspection during which the
splenic edge may actually be visible in the abdomen with respiration, (2) prelimi-

TABLE 14–4. Some Causes of Splenomegaly

Slight enlargement
  Subacute bacterial endocarditis
  Miliary tuberculosis
  Septicemia
  Rheumatoid arthritis
  Syphilis
  Typhoid
  Brucellosis
  Congestive heart failure
  Acute hepatitis
  Acute malaria
  Pernicious anemia

Moderate enlargement
  Cirrhosis of the liver
  Acute anemia
  Chronic lymphocytic leukemia
  Lymphoma
  Infectious mononucleosis
  Polycythemia vera
  Hemolytic anemia
  Sarcoidosis
  Rickets

Great enlargement
  Chronic granulocytic leukemia
  Chronic malaria
  Congenital syphilis in the infant
  Amyloidosis
  Agnogenic myeloid metaplasia
  Sarcoidosis
  Rare diseases
    Gaucher's disease, Niemann-Pick disease, kala-azar, tropical eosinophilia

nary percussion of the area of splenic dullness, and (3) repeated palpation at ever lower levels of the abdomen until the pelvic brim is reached. When it is suspected that the splenic capsule has been acutely distended by rapid enlargement of the spleen, such as can occur in infectious mononucleosis, splenic infarction, or intrasplenic hemorrhage, great caution must be exercised lest excessive examination or manipulation lead to splenic rupture.

KIDNEYS. The kidneys are assessed as part of the abdominal examination by deep palpation below the costal margins in the supine patient, using the nonpalpating hand to lift upward from below. Because the right kidney is lower than the left, it is occasionally normally palpable, especially in very thin patients. Flank masses or tenderness in the area of the kidneys is otherwise abnormal. A full description of renal examination and associated historical and physical findings is given in Chapter 15.

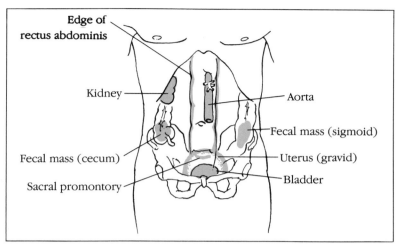

FIGURE 14-11
Some *normal* abdominal "masses."

URINARY BLADDER. Occasionally, a distended bladder may extend as high as the level of the umbilicus and be mistaken for a tumor. Tenderness over the bladder suggests intravesicular inflammation. As with the kidneys, a more complete description of bladder examination is presented in Chapter 15.

UTERUS. In women of childbearing age, a lower abdominal mass may be a gravid uterus. Full exploration of this possibility, including gynecologic examination (Chap. 16) and urine pregnancy test, must precede any radiologic studies.

OTHER FINDINGS
Normal findings on palpation and percussion are highly variable and depend largely on the degree of obesity and general body build, as well as on the patient's ability to cooperate (Fig. 14–11). The aorta is often palpable in the epigastrium and may be slightly tender. The normal aorta in the elderly, asthenic patient is easily mistaken for an aneurysm. The descending colon and cecum are commonly felt with considerable ease, particularly when they contain feces, and this normal finding may be misinterpreted as neoplasm unless roentgenographic studies are available.

Palpable masses should always be localized with respect to the previously described landmarks, and they should, if possible, be described in terms of consistency and contour. Frequently, however, they are only vaguely outlined, particularly when they are associated with tenderness or fluid or when the abdomen is obese and tense. Gastric, pancreatic, and colonic neoplasms, pancreatic cysts, and distended gallbladders may be palpable, usually at advanced stages of the disease.

Evaluation of the greatly distended abdomen is conducted by palpation and percussion. When the percussion note is high-pitched and tympanitic (drumlike), there is probably an obstruction that has produced gaseous distention of the un-

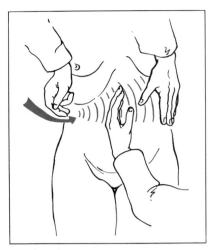

FIGURE 14–12
Demonstration of the fluid wave.

derlying small intestine, stomach, or colon. A flat or dull percussion note suggests either the presence of fluid in the peritoneal cavity or abdominal fullness associated with ovarian cyst or obesity. The usual method for demonstrating intra-abdominal fluid requires two examiners (Fig. 14–12). The assistant places the edge of his hand on the middle of the abdomen in order to limit the transmission of the impulse by the abdominal wall. The examiner then taps one flank while palpating the opposite flank, in order to detect the transmission of a fluid wave.

A false-positive sign may result if the patient is very obese or if there is a large ovarian cyst containing a sizable volume of encapsulated fluid. With ascites the distention is symmetrical and the flanks are particularly full. A tympanitic note detected in the midline, anteriorly, reflects associated gaseous distention of the bowel (the gas-containing bowel floats). The area of dullness is localized to the flanks and may be noted to shift with a change of position. In contrast, ovarian cysts may produce asymmetrical abdominal swelling; the dullness is located anteriorly with the tympanitic note in the flanks as the gas-containing bowel is displaced laterally. Shifting dullness on change of position is usually not present.

A fluid wave may not be obtained if the volume of ascites is only moderate and abdominal distention is slight. In such a case it may be possible to elicit a fluid wave if the examination is performed during the expiratory phase of a cough or during a Valsalva maneuver. This produces contraction of the abdominal muscles, reduces the volume of the abdominal cavity, and temporarily puts the ascites under enough tension to elicit a wave. This sign may be obtained in the presence of intra-abdominal cysts of fluid-filled intestines, although under these circumstances "shifting dullness" in the flanks will not be obtained.

Ascites may be associated with intra-abdominal masses, which are obscured by the presence of the fluid and therefore are difficult to palpate. Under these circumstances it is sometimes possible to detect such a mass by ballottement. This technique calls for lightly thrusting the fingers into the abdomen in the region of the suspected mass. The thrust will tend to displace the fluid, permitting the mass to bound upward, producing a characteristic tapping sensation against palpating fingers.

The recognition of masses may be made easier by repeating the abdominal examination after analgesics have been administered or the patient has been anesthetized prior to operation.

Rebound tenderness is elicited by exerting deep pressure into the abdomen in an area away from the suspected acute inflammatory process and then quickly releasing the pressure. If peritoneal irritation is present the patient experiences a twinge of pain either at the site of pressure or in the area of inflammation. This test is more reliable than cough tenderness. If the peritoneal irritation is localized to an area of inflammation, the rebound tenderness will be referred to that area. If generalized peritoneal irritation is present, rebound tenderness will be referred to the area of pressure. This test may be of particular value in obese patients. It is often accompanied by marked discomfort to the patient and should not be employed in the presence of obvious diffuse generalized peritonitis.

Intra-abdominal inflammation that secondarily involves the iliopsoas muscle may be detected by the iliopsoas test. The patient is asked to flex his thigh against the resistance of the examiner's hand. If inflammation is present in this location, contraction of the psoas muscle will be accompanied by pain. An alternative way of testing this function is to have the patient lie on the unaffected side and extend his thigh toward the affected side (Fig. 14–13). This test is not likely to be positive in the presence of subacute infection or if the abdominal wall is rigid.

If the inflammatory process lies adjacent to the obturator internus muscle, as in the presence of pelvic abscess, lower abdominal pain may be elicited by flexing the thigh to a 90-degree angle and rotating it internally and externally. This is known as the obturator test (Fig. 14–14).

It is sometimes difficult to differentiate an acute upper abdominal process from intrathoracic disease. In this situation, deep pressure on the opposite side of the abdomen directed toward the affected side will produce pain if the basic process is intra-abdominal; however, it will not elicit pain if the disease is intrathoracic.

The chest should be examined routinely in order to rule out diaphragmatic pleurisy, lower lobe pneumonia, pericarditis, or pleural effusion. Any of these conditions may be confused with intra-abdominal disease.

No examination of the abdomen is complete without examination of the back, conveniently done just before or at the time of the rectal examination. An episode of acute abdominal pain caused by pyelonephritis may reveal itself in costovertebral angle tenderness. Ecchymoses of the flanks (Grey Turner's sign) suggest retroperitoneal bleeding, which may occur with hemorrhagic pancreatitis. The intergluteal crease must be carefully examined for lesions. It is a favorite site for the occurrence of psoriasis. The pilonidal cyst is found overlying the sacrum and is seen as a punctuate lesion just above or in the intergluteal crease which may have a tuft of hair, erythema, or both surrounding it. It can become infected, forming an abscess. The pilonidal cyst is particularly likely to occur in hirsute men.

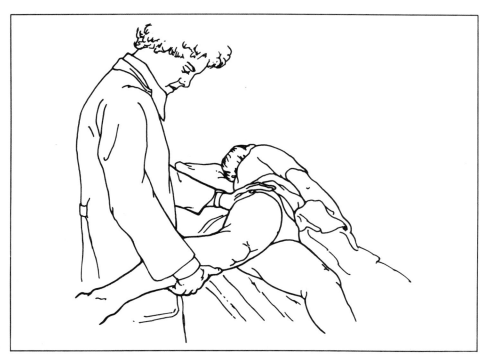

FIGURE 14–13
Psoas maneuver.

RECTUM

An important part of the examination in acute abdominal disease includes digital examination of the rectum. It is desirable in acute situations to have the patient lying on his back, permitting the rectum to be examined anteriorly, posteriorly, and on both sides with the examining finger. This maneuver may be helpful in detecting such conditions as prostatitis, seminal vesiculitis, pelvic abscess, appendicitis, and tubo-ovarian abscess. Bimanual examination of the rectum and vagina permits careful evaluation of the contents of the pelvis and the cul-de-sac. This is an important part of the examination of female patients and should be included as an integral part of all examinations of such patients with acute abdominal distress.

In any patient, it is impossible to overemphasize the importance of the rectal examination. This simple and vital procedure is too often passed by because it entails extra effort on the part of the physician and tends to be somewhat disagreeable to the patient. No gastrointestinal evaluation is complete without it.

The skin surrounding the anus should be carefully inspected for signs of inflammation or excoriation.

Local infections such as perianal and perirectal abscesses will appear as an area of swelling, with variable degrees of erythema about the anus. Local pain and tenderness are usually prominent, and the patient will usually show systemic signs of sepsis such as fever and tachycardia.

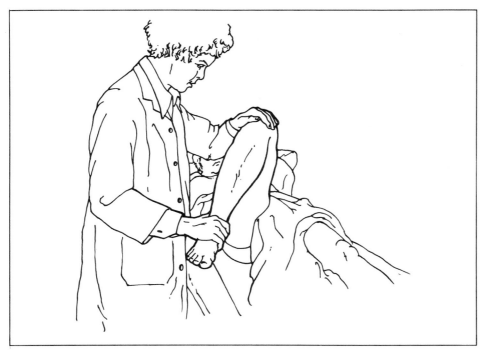

FIGURE 14–14
Obturator maneuver.

An anorectal fistula is a tract that has an external opening, often visible on inspection of the anal skin, and an internal opening into the anus or rectum. Less often it may enter the urethra or even the urinary bladder. The anorectal fistula is caused by drainage of a perianal or perirectal abscess.

External hemorrhoids are varicose veins that originate below the anorectal line and are covered by anal skin. They appear as bluish, shiny masses at the anus. They may not be visible when the patient is at rest, but will usually protrude after standing or straining at stool. If not reduced, they become edematous and may thrombose. When thrombosis occurs, local pain may be intense, and removal of the thrombus may be necessary to obtain relief. Internal hemorrhoids arise above the anorectal junction and are therefore covered by rectal mucosa. Because of their soft consistency they are not palpable by rectal examination.

The examination itself consists of digital and endoscopic study. Digital examination (described in further detail in Chaps. 15 and 16) is performed with the patient in the supine or knee-chest position, or flexed at the hips and bending over. On occasion it is helpful to examine the patient in the squatting position, for this may bring a high-lying rectal lesion within reach of the examining finger. Insertion of the examining finger should be gentle and gradual, and sufficient time should be allowed for the patient to relax after insertion has been accomplished. Excessive resistance at the anal ring is commonly due to simple spasm caused by

TABLE 14–5. Examinations of the Anus, Rectum, and Large Bowel

Lesions often visible by external examination	Lesions (above the rectum) often demonstrable by barium enema
Dermatitis	Inflammatory bowel disease
Pilonidal cyst	Diverticula
Perianal cyst	Megacolon
External hemorrhoids	Irritable bowel
Rectal prolapse	Neoplasm
Carcinoma of the anus	Polyps
Anal fissures and fistulas	Strictures
Palpable lesion	Ischemia
Cancer of the rectum	Foreign bodies
Polyps	
Cancer of the prostate	
Fibroids of the uterus	
Rectal shelf	
Abscess	
Foreign body	
Stricture	
Endometriosis (palpable during bimanual pelvic examination)	
Lesions visualized by proctoscopy	
Inflammation of the bowel	
Internal fistulous openings	
Cancers of the rectum and bowel	
Polyps	
Villous adenoma	
Internal hemorrhoids	
Strictures	
Spasm	
Bowel ischemia	
Foreign bodies	
Lacerations of the bowel	

nervousness, and this can at times be overcome by asking the patient to strain a little before palpation is begun. If there is considerable spasm and local pain due to anal pathologic changes, a local anesthetic suppository may be used to minimize discomfort.

Lesions detectable on rectal examination include anal fissure. It is a superficial linear ulcer, usually found in the posterior midline. It is tender, and patients may report pain and slight bleeding with bowel movements. The anal sphincter will usually be in spasm, and a suppository with local anesthesia may be necessary to permit examination. The fissure may be visualized directly by anoscopy.

Polyps of the rectum are a relatively common finding. They may be pedunculated or sessile, and some (villous adenomas) are so soft that they are difficult to palpate. Direct visualization and biopsy are necessary to distinguish them from rectal carcinoma. The latter lesion is usually felt as a sessile polypoid mass with nodular. raised edges and areas of ulceration. It usually has a hard consistency.

Rectal prolapse can be diagnosed by asking the patient to strain and by observing the appearance of rectal mucosa emerging from the anus. The prolapse involves the entire circumference of the bowel and may range in size from only a few centimeters to a very extensive prolapse involving a major portion of rectum.

Intraperitoneal metastases from any of several malignant sources may develop in the pelvis anterior to the rectum. These metastases may be felt as a hard, nodular area at the tip of the examining finger; this finding is referred to as a rectal shelf.

PROCTOSCOPY

Proctoscopy is a general term used for direct visualization of the terminal portion of the bowel. Anoscopy is performed with a short instrument using an external light source and is useful for seeing such lesions as fissure in ano, cryptitis, internal hemorrhoids, and the opening of a fistulous tract.

The sigmoidoscope is used for examination of the rectum and lower sigmoid. It is 25 cm in length and has a light source at its tip. It is passed to its full length and the mucosa is carefully viewed as the instrument is removed. Sigmoidoscopy is helpful in the diagnosis of various types of polyps, inflammatory lesions, and rectal cancer. Biopsy can be performed easily. The bowel must be cleansed by enema in order for this examination to be conducted.

The fiberoptic colonoscope is used to study higher levels of the colon. A 60-cm model can be used to examine the rectum or sigmoid; 100-cm models can visualize the transverse and right colon as well. Successful use of these instruments requires special endoscopic expertise and careful preparation of the patient's bowel in advance.

Radiologic studies are useful in establishing the diagnosis of various lesions above the rectum. Barium enema and air-contrast barium enema require careful preparation of the patient by laxatives and enemas if one is to visualize mucosal detail. Lesions that can be detected by barium and other studies are listed in Table 14–5.

CHAPTER 15

MALE GENITOURINARY SYSTEM AND HERNIA

I have never yet examined the body of a patient dying with dropsy attended by coagulable urine, in whom some obvious derangement was not discovered in the kidneys.

RICHARD BRIGHT
(1789–1858)

Though classically recorded on the written record *before* the musculoskeletal and neurologic examinations, examination of the male and female genitalia, as well as the rectal examination, are generally done *last* in the sequence of the actual physical. These are sometimes embarrassing and uncomfortable, though essential, examinations, and the understanding sympathy and deftness of the examiner will contribute considerably to the ease of the patient.

Examination for hernia is generally done as part of the examination of external genitalia in men; the rectal is a logical part of the internal genital examination in both men and women.

ANATOMY

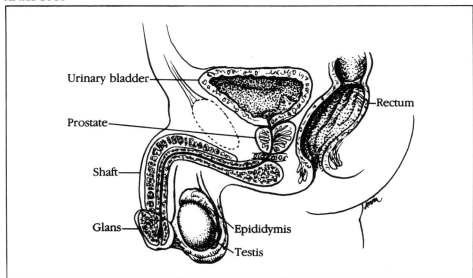

FIGURE 15–1
Cross-section of male genitalia.

363

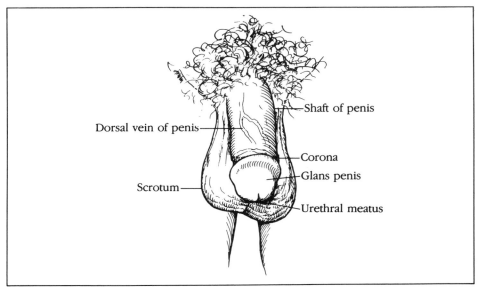

FIGURE 15–2
External male genitalia.

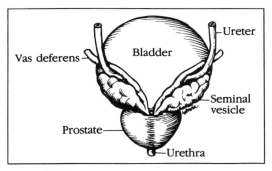

FIGURE 15–3
Prostate and seminal vesicles.

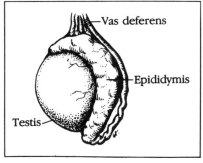

FIGURE 15–4
Testis and epididymis.

HISTORY

Pain in the testicle is met with in renal colic and in a few cases of appendicitis.

SIR ZACHARY COPE
(1881–1974)

Though difficult for many students initially, candid inquiry into excretory and sexual function is essential for their patients' well-being. If shyness or prudery allows a cancer of the prostate gland to go undetected, the price of modesty has been too high. Ask questions about the genitourinary system with the same professional objective interest you show in the rest of the history. While you should avoid embarrassing a reluctant patient, an understanding, tactful questioning will allow you to gather the necessary information.

Genitourinary symptoms may be divided into several general categories.

TABLE 15–1. Some Causes of Frequency

Large Volume	Small Volume
Polydipsia	Cystitis
Renal tubular disease	Urethritis
Diuretics	Neurogenic bladder
Glycosuria	Extrinsic mass to the bladder
Diabetes insipidus	Bladder tumor
Adrenal insufficiency	Structural defects of bladder and urethra
Alcohol	(including prostatism)

IRRITATIVE BLADDER AND URETHRAL SYMPTOMS

Frequency, urgency, and *dysuria* are symptoms that often occur together and are usually secondary to inflammatory disease of the bladder, the prostate, and the urethra. They may also signal carcinoma of the bladder or prostatic obstruction.

Cystitis is the most common disorder of the bladder. It is far more frequent in women than in men. Infection of the bladder in men can occur, however, with obstruction (as with a large prostate gland), foreign body (such as a Foley catheter), neurologic disease affecting bladder emptying, or other predisposing states.

Acute prostatitis may result in fever, urethral discharge, and irritative bladder symptoms. *Chronic prostatitis* is usually asymptomatic.

Urethritis, not infrequently of gonococcal origin (though other organisms may cause urethral inflammation), presents with irritation and urethral discharge.

INCONTINENCE

Careful history taking will identify the type of incontinence and lead to the appropriate treatment. *Stress incontinence,* or the involuntary loss of urine caused by straining, coughing, or lifting, occurs most frequently in the multiparous woman and often is associated with cystourethrocele. This incontinence can be corrected surgically. *Urge incontinence* (precipitous micturition) is the involuntary loss of urine associated with the sudden urge to void. It may occur with inflammatory disease of the bladder and urethra but also with a neurogenic bladder with uninhibited contractions and may be idiopathic. *Dribbling incontinence* is the constant loss of urine in varying amounts with or without stress. It may be produced by a vesicovaginal fistula, ectopic ureter, or after prostatectomy when the sphincters of the bladder have been damaged. *Paradoxical incontinence,* the involuntary dribbling of urine, is due to chronic urinary retention. This may be produced either by obstruction of the urethra in the male, as in benign prostatic hypertrophy, or secondary to a neurogenic bladder, as in sensory paralytic bladder produced by diabetes (Table 15–1).

PAIN

Renal pain usually is present in the costovertebral angle and may radiate anteriorly. Afferent nerves carrying sensation from the kidneys reach the spinal cord through the tenth, eleventh, and twelfth thoracic nerves. Referred pain of renal origin is therefore interpreted by the patient over the somatic distribution of these nerves in the abdominal wall. The fibers supplying the ureter enter the spinal cord from the twelfth thoracic nerve and the first three lumbar nerves. Pain referred from the ureter is distributed over the somatic distribution of the subcostal, iliohypogastric, ilioinguinal, and genitofemoral nerves, depending on the portion of the ureter that is diseased. Since both the ilioinguinal nerve and the genital branch of the genitofemoral nerves supply the scrotum, pain from the ureter often radiates into the testicle or scrotum. Renal pain may be due to pyelonephritis, calculi, perinephric abscess, tumor, glomerulonephritis, or intermittent hydronephrosis. *Vesical pain* is usually present in the suprapubic region. Pain may be severe, with bladder distention, and it may be relieved by voiding, as occurs with interstitial cystitis; or pain may be continuous when associated with urinary retention or acute cystitis. *Testicular pain* usually is due to neoplasm, infection, or local trauma, but pain may occasionally be referred to this region. *Prostatic* and *urethral pain* may be referred on occasion to the low back area.

MASS

A perceptible mass in the *renal area* is rarely noted by the patient but may occur with neoplasm. A *suprapubic mass* may signal bladder distention or neoplasm. A *scrotal mass* may be inflammatory, neoplastic, traumatic, cystic (spermatocele, hydrocele, varicocele), or a hernia.

URINARY CHANGES

CLOUDY URINE

A patient complaint of cloudy urine may suggest pus in the urine (as with infection), but is most often due simply to phosphate precipitation in an alkaline urine, a normal event.

PNEUMATURIA

Pneumaturia, usually described as "bubbles in the urine as it comes out," may develop with urinary tract infection due to gas-forming bacteria, or it may signal an enterovesical fistula caused by inflammatory or neoplastic disease of the gastrointestinal tract.

HEMATURIA

Blood in the urine must be considered to be due to neoplasm until proved otherwise. Initial or terminal hematuria is usually associated with disease of the lower urinary tract. Blood present throughout urination may come from kidneys, ureters, or bladder. Calculi, infection, trauma, and acute glomerulonephritis are frequently associated with hematuria (Table 15–2).

NOCTURIA

Nocturia is usually a significant symptom and is seen in association with benign prostatic hypertrophy, diabetes mellitus, urinary tract infections, and with reversed diurnal rhythm such as occurs with renal and cardiac insufficiency.

TABLE 15–2. Some Causes of Hematuria

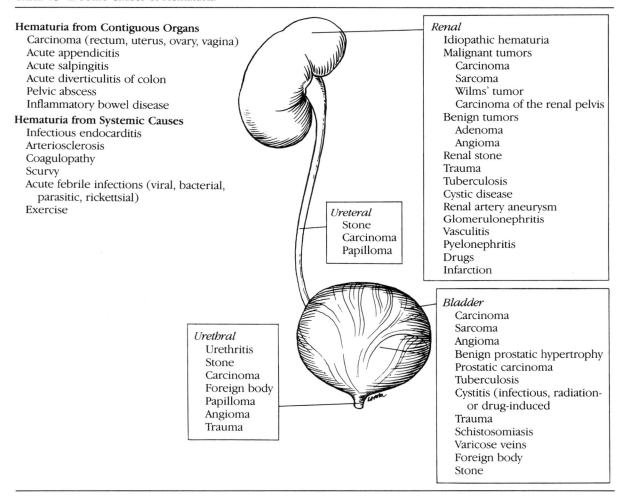

Hematuria from Contiguous Organs
  Carcinoma (rectum, uterus, ovary, vagina)
  Acute appendicitis
  Acute salpingitis
  Acute diverticulitis of colon
  Pelvic abscess
  Inflammatory bowel disease
Hematuria from Systemic Causes
  Infectious endocarditis
  Arteriosclerosis
  Coagulopathy
  Scurvy
  Acute febrile infections (viral, bacterial,
    parasitic, rickettsial)
  Exercise

Renal
  Idiopathic hematuria
  Malignant tumors
    Carcinoma
    Sarcoma
    Wilms' tumor
    Carcinoma of the renal pelvis
  Benign tumors
    Adenoma
    Angioma
  Renal stone
  Trauma
  Tuberculosis
  Cystic disease
  Renal artery aneurysm
  Glomerulonephritis
  Vasculitis
  Pyelonephritis
  Drugs
  Infarction

Ureteral
  Stone
  Carcinoma
  Papilloma

Urethral
  Urethritis
  Stone
  Carcinoma
  Foreign body
  Papilloma
  Angioma
  Trauma

Bladder
  Carcinoma
  Sarcoma
  Angioma
  Benign prostatic hypertrophy
  Prostatic carcinoma
  Tuberculosis
  Cystitis (infectious, radiation-
    or drug-induced
  Trauma
  Schistosomiasis
  Varicose veins
  Foreign body
  Stone

GASTROINTESTINAL SYMPTOMS

Nausea, vomiting, and abdominal distention may be associated with renal or ureteral calculi. Hydronephrosis is frequently a silent lesion that may produce symptoms that suggest gallbladder disease or duodenal ulcer when the right kidney is affected, and a lesion of the colon when the left kidney is affected. The presenting symptoms of chronic renal insufficiency (azotemia) frequently are nausea and vomiting.

LOCAL LESIONS

"Sores" of the external genitalia may bring a patient to the physician. Infection (especially venereal infection) and neoplastic disease are the leading causes.

TABLE 15–3. Some Clinical Features of Uremia

General	**Stomach and intestines**
Cachexia	Abdominal pain
Fatigue	Enteritis
Weakness	Ascites
Edema	**Nerves and muscles**
Vital signs	Confusion, obtundation
Tachycardia	Asterixis
Tachypnea	Parasthesias
Hypertension	Osteoporosis, pathologic fractures
Hypothermia (occasionally)	**Skin**
Head, ears, eyes, nose, throat	Easy bruising
Band keratopathy	Itching
Conjunctivitis	Hyperpigmentation
Conjunctival pallor	Pallor
Uremic breath	Uremic frost
Heart	
Pericarditis	
Congestive heart failure	
Chest	
Gynecomastia	
Pleuritis, pleural effusion	
Pneumonitis	
Dyspnea	

SEXUAL DYSFUNCTION

Although some men will openly admit to having sexual difficulty (or to having "lost their nature"), others will be so ashamed that they will disguise this complaint as "prostate trouble" or "fatigue," hoping that the doctor will understand and direct attention to their sexual function. Primary sexual problems include impotence, loss of libido, premature ejaculation, and loss of erection. These symptoms are probably most commonly due to small vessel disease although psychologic causes and a number of common antihypertensive drugs and diseases (e.g., diabetes mellitus) may also induce impotence. A thorough medical and psychologic investigation is indicated for these most significant symptoms.

PROSTATISM

The symptomatic manifestations of prostatic enlargement are called, collectively, "prostatism." Symptoms produced by an enlarged prostate gland are of two major types: (1) irritative bladder symptoms as described above, and (2) obstructive symptoms characterized by a urinary stream decreased in size and force, with hesitancy and interruption of the stream during voiding. Obstructive symptoms may also be produced by a urethral stricture, a urethral valve, or a bladder neck contracture.

HYPERTENSION

Many patients will have been told that they have high blood pressure. Increased blood pressure may occur as both cause and consequence of chronic renal disease.

Hypertension, therefore, calls for a careful historical and physical assessment of the urinary system.

UREMIA

The symptoms (and signs) that may occur in uremia are given in Table 15–3.

PHYSICAL EXAMINATION

1. Palpate kidneys and urinary bladder as part of abdominal examination.

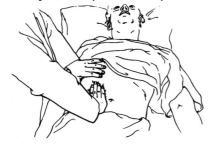 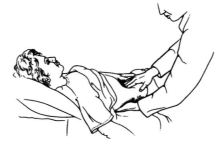

2. Inspect external genitalia: hair distribution, scrotum, and penis.
3. Palpate regional nodes, penis, testes, and epididymis.
4. Check for hernia bilaterally.

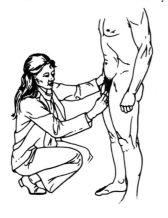 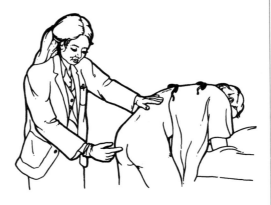

5. Consider doing rectal examination now if not done as part of gastrointestinal examination: sphincter tone, prostate, ampulla, stool for occult blood.

The examination of the urine is the most essential part of the physical examination of any patient with Bright's disease.

THOMAS ADDIS
(1881–1949)

KIDNEYS, URETERS, AND URINARY BLADDER

The upper urinary tract is assessed as part of the abdominal examination. The patient is supine with knees slightly raised. Begin by scrutinizing the upper abdo-

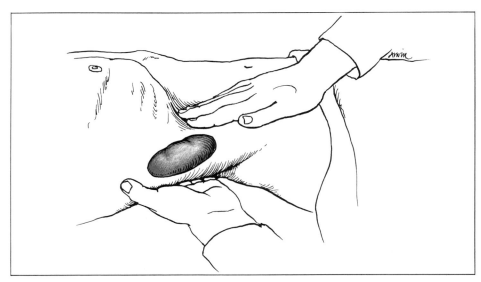

FIGURE 15–5
Palpation of the kidney.

men for obvious symmetry or bulging, particularly in the flanks. Close observation during the patient's deep inspiration and expiration may give important clues as to the site of pathologic change.

KIDNEYS

In palpating the **renal areas**, place one hand posteriorly beneath the costal margin and press directly upward (Fig. 15–5). The other hand palpates for the kidney and is placed below the costal margin at about the midclavicular line. The patient is then asked to take a deep breath, a maneuver that depresses the diaphragm and pushes the kidney downward. As the patient inhales, the hand is pressed inward and upward toward the costal margin. The technique is similar to that used for palpation of the liver and spleen except that the hand is gradually pressed more deeply into the abdomen. The right kidney is palpated from the right side, while the left kidney is examined by reaching across the abdomen or preferably by moving around the patient to his left side. When pathology is suspected, it may be valuable to have the patient lie on his side. The uppermost kidney tends to fall downward and medially in this position, making it somewhat more accessible to palpation.

Percussion is not used routinely, but it may be valuable at times in generally outlining masses in the renal areas that are unusually large. Auscultation is valuable for detecting bruits that may originate in the renal arteries. It is carried out over the costovertebral angles posteriorly and in both upper quadrants of the abdomen. Auscultation is particularly important in the hypertensive patient, because renal-vascular disease causing an elevated blood pressure may be surgically remediable. Transillumination is a particularly valuable technique in children. The room is

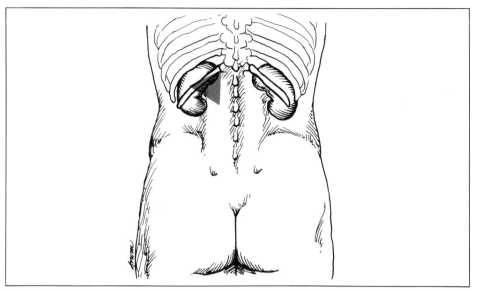

FIGURE 15–6
Costovertebral angle.

darkened and the light source is pressed into the costovertebral angle posteriorly. A hydronephrosis will transmit light; a solid tumor will not.

Since the right kidney normally is somewhat lower than the left, it is occasionally palpable, particularly in asthenic patients.

The usual causes of renal enlargement are infection, tumor, hydronephrosis, and polycystic kidneys. (In dramatic circumstances of polycystic disease, the palpating hand may detect a crepitant—"crackling"—sensation over the kidney as the multiple cysts are compressed.) Masses in the area of the kidney may also be due to bowel lesions (tumors, abscesses), retroperitoneal tumor, gallbladder, or spleen.

The examiner should look also for possible tenderness originating in and around the kidney. Renal pain is elicited by pressure at the costovertebral angle—the angle formed by the junction of the twelfth rib and the paraspinous muscles (Fig. 15–6). In this region the kidney is nearest to the skin surface, and deep pressure by the examiner's fingers may elicit pain due to intrinsic renal parenchymal disease. Costovertebral angle pain must be differentiated from pain produced by muscular spasm. Muscle pain can be demonstrated by deep palpation directly over the back muscles that lie medial to the costovertebral angle.

Acute pyelonephritis usually produces fever, and the patient may be extremely ill. There is tenderness to deep palpation or percussion in the costovertebral angle, and the entire flank region may be tender. When the peritoneum overlying the kidneys is affected by the inflammatory reaction, signs of peritonitis are present, with abdominal distention, muscle spasm, rebound tenderness, and hypoactive bowel sounds.

Perinephric abscess may be associated with a low-grade or septic elevation in temperature. There usually is exquisite tenderness on the affected side, and rarely a bulging mass may be felt in the flank. Scoliosis of the spine with the concavity pointed toward the affected side occurs because of irritation of the psoas major and quadratus lumborum muscles. The diaphragm is elevated and somewhat fixed on the affected side; because of inflammatory reaction, basilar rales may be present. Edema of the skin may occur over the abscess.

Hydronephrosis (or pyohydronephrosis) occurs when there is obstruction to the flow of urine from the intrarenal collecting system. Initially there is hypertrophy of the musculature of the renal pelvis, but as the obstruction persists or progresses, decompensation and dilation occur. The resultant enlarged kidney may be palpated on bimanual examination. In small children, transillumination of the renal areas may help to differentiate cystic mass from solid tumor. As the back pressure increases, the hydronephrotic process progresses; the renal blood supply is compromised, producing ischemia. Eventually the renal parenchyma is destroyed, leaving a thin-walled cystic mass.

Benign tumor of the kidney is rare and usually is too small to be palpated.

The *embryoma* (Wilms' tumor) is malignant. It usually occurs in children under the age of 5 years. The presenting sign often is a palpable mass in one or both renal areas. Renal cell carcinoma (hypernephroma), the most common renal malignant neoplasm, may produce a palpable mass in the flank. Extension of the tumor into the renal vein and inferior vena cava will produce dilated veins in the abdominal wall. The left spermatic vein empties into the left renal vein and may be obstructed by a tumor growing into the renal vein. This obstruction produces a varicocele on the left side of the scrotum that does not decompress when the patient is supine.

> *Gout produces calculus in the kidney. . . . The patient has frequently to entertain the painful speculation as to whether gout or stone be the worst disease.*
>
> THOMAS SYDENHAM
> (1624–1689)

Renal stone disease is very common and can present with excruciating pain (renal colic) in the back, flank, or radiating to testis, thigh, or penis. On physical examination, marked costovertebral angle tenderness may be present, especially if there is an associated pyelonephritis. Acute renal colic frequently produces abdominal distention and either hypoactive or absent bowel sounds. A history of predisposition to stone should be sought (Table 15–4) when the diagnosis is suspected, and a urine analysis (which often shows microscopic blood) and abdominal film (showing calcium stones) should be obtained (Fig. 15–8). If the diagnosis is still in doubt, an intravenous urogram should be obtained (Fig. 15–9).

Renal ectopia will produce a palpable mass in the lower part of the abdomen (Fig. 15–7). In crossed renal ectopia, both kidneys are on the same side and are often fused, giving rise to a rather large mass that suggests neoplasm. A *horseshoe kidney* is due to the fusion of the lower pole of each kidney, producing an isthmus of renal tissue across the midline, which may be palpable in a thin patient. *Poly-*

TABLE 15–4. Renal Stones

Type of Stone and Incidence	Causes	X-Ray Appearance

Calcium oxalate
Calcium phosphate
Calcium oxalate and phosphate } (74%)
	Hypercalciuria
	  Most common cause—idiopathic
	    hypercalciuria
	  Common cause—primary
	    hyperparathyroidism
	  Rarer causes
	    Renal tubular acidosis
	    Vitamin D excess
	    Vitamin A excess
	    Calcium carbonate excess
	    Sarcoidosis
	    Hyperthyroidism
	    Paget's disease of bone
	    Prolonged immobilization
		Radiopaque

	Hyperoxaluria
	  Most common cause—small bowel disease,
	    malabsorption
	  Uncommon causes
	    Genetic hyperoxaluria
	    Vitamin B_6 deficiency
	    Ethylene glycol (antifreeze ingestion)
	    Vitamin C excess
	    Dietary excess of oxalate
	      (rhubarb,spinach)
	    Methoxyfluorine anesthesia
		Radiopaque

Magnesium-ammonium phosphate (15%)	Recurrent urinary tract infection with urea splitters giving increased urinary pH	Radiopaque

Uric acid stone (8%)	Excess uric acid excretion
	  Idiopathic
	  Associated with myeloproliferative disease
		Radiolucent

Cystine, xanthine (3%)	Genetic—rare	

cystic kidneys are usually bilateral and contain multiple cysts. As the cysts enlarge, palpable masses are produced in the renal areas. Unless infected, the renal masses are usually not tender. In this progressive genetic disease, renal failure ultimately occurs.

Ultrasonography of the kidneys has, in recent years, proven itself to be a superb noninvasive diagnostic method of visualizing many of these renal abnormalities.

URETERS

The ureters are not accessible to physical examination. Ureteral obstructions and strictures, however, may produce hydronephrosis on the involved side. Ureteral obstruction may result from stones as they pass from the kidney. The stones commonly are arrested in their passage at the three narrowest areas of the renal-ureteral-vesicular pathway: the ureteropelvic junction, the pelvic brim where the ureter crosses the iliac vessels, and the ureteral-vesical junction. The passage of the

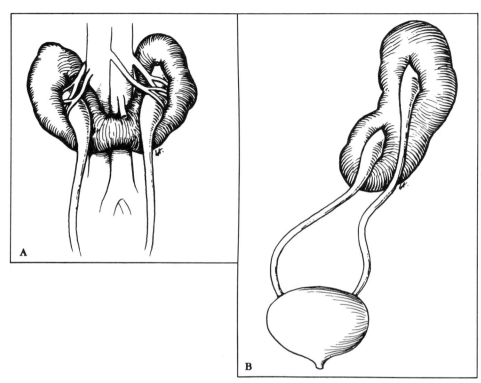

FIGURE 15–7
Renal ectopia. A. Horseshoe kidney. B. Fused kidney.

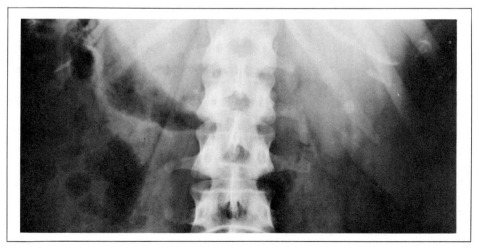

FIGURE 15–8
Nephrolithiasis on plain film (radiopaque stone).

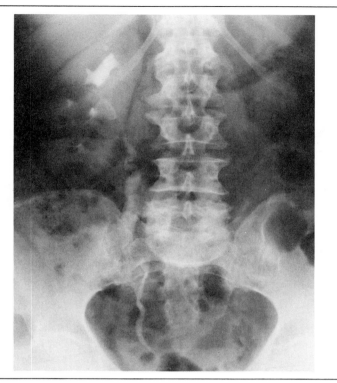

FIGURE 15–9
Nephrolithiasis on intravenous pyelography with hydroureter (radiolucent stone).

stone, or its arrest in the ureter, may be associated with the violent pain and other findings described as renal colic.

Ureteral stricture may occur congenitally or as a result of inflammation, fibrosis, surgical accident, or tumor in the retroperitoneum.

URINARY BLADDER

The **bladder** is examined by inspection, percussion, and palpation. When distended it produces a bulging mass in the lower part of the abdomen over which dullness may be elicited by percussion. At times this dullness may extend up as far as the umbilicus. The region of the symphysis should be carefully palpated. Bladder pain is usually elicited by direct palpation over the suprapubic area. Bimanual examination may be performed at the time of rectal examination with the man in the lithotomy position; the examiner places one finger in the rectum pressing upward, the opposite hand on the lower abdominal wall (Fig. 15–10). The best results are obtained with the patient under anesthesia. In women, the bladder is easily palpated bimanually at the time of pelvic examination.

The empty bladder is not accessible to physical examination, but when distended with urine it can be mistaken for a lower abdominal tumor unless this possibility

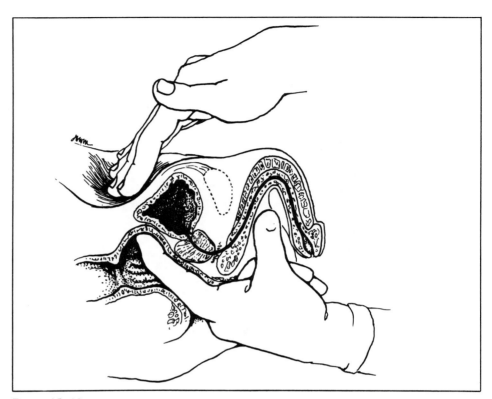

FIGURE 15–10
Bimanual palpation of the urinary bladder.

is kept in mind. On bimanual examination the empty bladder feels much like a thick-walled, collapsed balloon. It is not tender and is freely movable, with no lateral extensions or palpable discrete masses.

Cystitis, which occurs particularly in women, is the most common disorder of the bladder. Tenderness is often elicited by palpation over the suprapubic region (Table 15–5). Obstruction below the bladder may be due to vesicle neck contraction or hypertrophy of the prostate. Chronic obstruction causes trabeculation, cellules, and diverticula of the bladder. As residual urine increases, bladder capacity may increase, and the bladder may finally decompensate. The bladder may then be palpable in the suprapubic region as a midline mass. When large diverticula occur, these may also be palpated. *Tumors* and *calculi* of the bladder are common, particularly in men, but usually produce no physical findings unless the lesions are large.

In those cases where there is a sandy sediment in the urine, there is calculus in the bladder or kidneys.

HIPPOCRATES
(460?–377? B.C.)

TABLE 15–5. Some Causes of Cystitis

In women
   Short urethra
   Postcoital ("honeymoon") cystitis
Recent urinary catheterization
Incomplete emptying of the bladder
   Obstruction (prostatic disease)
   Cystocele
   Neurogenic bladder
Urethritis
Pyelonephritis
Intravesicular disease
   Foreign body
   Stone
   Tumor
   Parasites
Some systemic immunosuppressive diseases (e.g., diabetes mellitus)
Radiation to bladder
Drugs and chemicals

A *neurogenic bladder* is one in which neurologic disease leads to bladder dysfunction. Physical findings may be pathognomonic of the various types of neurogenic bladder (Fig. 15–11).

1. *Sensory paralytic bladder* is produced by a lesion on the sensory side of the sacral reflex as in tabes dorsalis. Saddle anesthesia may be present. When the bladder becomes decompensated, a suprapubic mass may be palpated.

2. *Motor paralytic bladder* results from a lesion affecting the motor side of the reflex arch, as in poliomyelitis. Saddle anesthesia may also be present. The patient is unable to initiate micturition, and a distended bladder is palpable in the suprapubic region.

3. *Autonomous neurogenic bladder* is produced by a lesion affecting sacral segments 2, 3, and 4, such as occurs in myelomeningocele. Saddle anesthesia is present. Urine can be forced from the bladder by pressure in the suprapubic region.

4. *Reflex neurogenic bladder* due to a transverse myelitis of the spinal cord, as in trauma, characteristically produces a hyperactive bulbocavernosus reflex. Associated neurologic findings due to the paraplegia facilitate this diagnosis.

5. *Uninhibited neurogenic bladder* is seen in normal infants and after cerebrovascular accidents. The bulbocavernosus reflex is normal or hyperactive.

EXTERNAL GENITALIA

In the normal uncircumcised man the foreskin should be easily retractable. At the time of retraction the external meatus is examined by separating it with the thumbs placed on either side of the distal glans penis. The shaft is then carefully palpated while searching for areas of tenderness or induration, and the urethra is milked

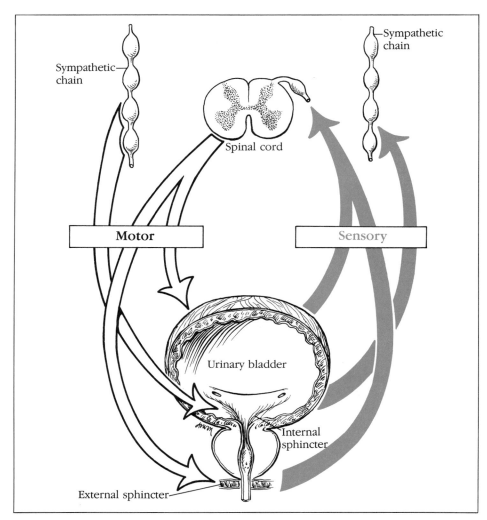

FIGURE 15–11
Simplified scheme of the neurologic control of the bladder. Both sensory and motor components of normal bladder function depend on autonomic and somatic neurologic integrity.

downward to express any secretions present. Congenital anomalies of the penis are uncommon. *Balanoposthitis* is seen in uncircumcised men, because of recurrent infection of the prepuce and glans penis. There is erythema, local discomfort, and sometimes a purulent discharge. *Phimosis* occurs when it is impossible to retract the prepuce and is usually secondary to recurrent balanoposthitis (Fig. 15–12). There may be local signs of infection. *Paraphimosis* results when the prepuce is retracted behind the glans penis and cannot be returned to its normal position. Impairment of local circulation to the glans in this circumstance may lead to edema and, if not relieved, gangrene.

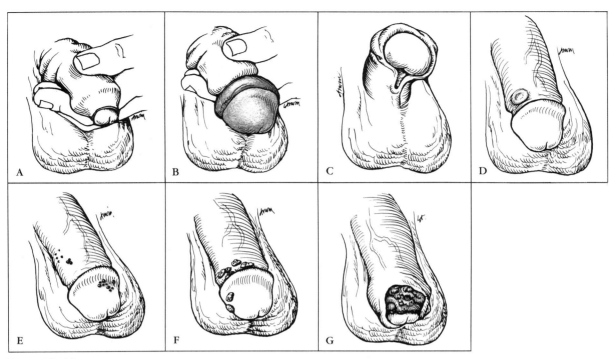

FIGURE 15–12
Some lesions of the penis. A. Phimosis. B. Paraphimosis. C. Hypospadias. D. Syphilitic chancre. E. Herpes progenitalis. F. Condylomata acuminata. G. Epidermoid carcinoma.

Stenosis of the external urethral meatus produces a serious obstructive lesion. There is often meatal ulceration and crusting. *Hypospadias* may be discovered on close inspection of the ventral surface of the penis. Its classification is dependent on the location of the external urethral meatus. An associated chordee is produced by fibrosis in the area of the malformed urethra, producing a downward curvature of the penis on erection. *Epispadias,* in which the urethra opens in the dorsum of the penis, is less common than hypospadias and is often associated with exstrophy of the bladder. Urinary incontinence is often an associated finding. Urethritis produces a few abnormal physical findings. The urethra may be tender to palpation, and often there is a purulent urethral discharge.

The *primary lesion of syphilis,* which appears 2 to 4 weeks after infected sexual contact, is a painless ulcer with indurated borders and a relatively clean base. Palpable inguinal lymph nodes are often present. *Lymphopathia venereum* begins with a small penile lesion that may be papular or vesicular. Painful enlarged inguinal lymph nodes called buboes may ulcerate and drain. *Granuloma inguinale* results in a painful superficial ulceration that is erythematous and velvety in appearance.

Herpes progenitalis, a viral infection, produces multiple superficial vesicles on the foreskin or glans. These may be indistinguishable from the chancre of primary syphilis—except that they are very painful.

Epidermoid carcinoma is usually found in uncircumcised men as a painless ulceration that fails to heal. Growth frequently begins beneath the prepuce. Palpable lymph nodes may indicate metastatic extension of the neoplasm.

The skin of the scrotum is inspected, and each testis is palpated between the thumb and the first two fingers. The comma-shaped structure bulging on the posterolateral surface of each testis is the epididymis, and it is palpated in the same manner. The spermatic cord extends upward from the epididymis to the external ring. The vas deferens can be easily palpated as a small solid cord between the thumb and index finger, using the opposite hand to exert gentle downward traction on the testis.

The testes lie freely in the scrotum. In the average man they are 3 or 4 cm by 2.5 cm in size, being correspondingly smaller in boys. The epididymis and vas deferens are discretely palpable but not tender. Transillumination is a commonly employed technique for examining the scrotal contents. It is performed in a darkened room. Transillumination helps to differentiate a hydrocele from a solid lesion. A scrotal mass that transilluminates freely can be presumed to be a hydrocele. If doubt still exists, ultrasonography of the testes can be employed. This technique allows the examiner to differentiate a solid lesion from cystic lesion and can be used to "visualize" areas of atypical sonodensity in the testicle itself.

Acute epididymitis results in a painful mass in the scrotum (Fig. 15–13). Initially it may be possible to distinguish the enlarged tender epididymis from the testis, but later the testis and epididymis become an inseparable mass. The spermatic cord is often thickened and indurated. *Chronic epididymitis* results from recurrent bouts of epididymitis. The epididymis is enlarged and indurated. Tuberculous epididymitis may mimic acute and chronic epididymitis. The vas deferens often contains a group of enlargements that resembles a string of beads, giving rise to the term *beading of the vas deferens*.

Acute orchitis may occur from any infectious disease process but most often is associated with mumps parotitis. The testis is enlarged and painful, and the overlying scrotal skin is erythematous.

A *testicular tumor* usually results in an enlarged testis that is not translucent. Any hard or firm nodular area in the testis must be regarded as a tumor. *Hydroceles* may obscure tumors. When the testis cannot be palpated because of a hydrocele, aspiration of the fluid will facilitate palpation. Testicular ultrasound will detect hydroceles and identify suspicious areas in the testicle.

Torsion of the spermatic cord occurs spontaneously, most often in prepubertal boys, resulting in acute ischemia to the epididymis and testis. Examination of the scrotum reveals a painful mass that is usually elevated. In this condition, elevating the testis may increase the pain, in contradistinction to epididymitis, in which elevation of the testis will somewhat relieve the pain. Epididymitis is often associated with pyuria, whereas torsion usually is not. However, this differential diagnosis is difficult on the basis of physical examination alone, and both epididymitis and torsion can be confused with torsion of the appendix testis and vice versa. A localized tender area on the superior aspect of the testes is typical of a torted testicular appendix. Once any of these processes have been present for several hours, phys-

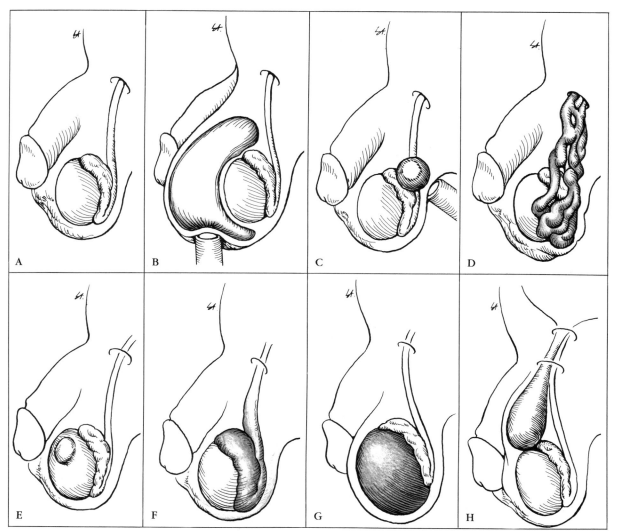

FIGURE 15–13
Some scrotal lesions. A. Normal. B. Hydrocele. C. Spermatocele. D. Varicocele. E. Testicular tumor. F. Epididymitis. G. Orchitis. H. Hernia.

ical examination does not provide sufficient information for diagnosis, and scrotal exploration is usually required.

When no testis is palpable in the scrotum, three possible abnormalities exist. The testes may be absent, ectopic, or undescended. Ectopic testes are not abnormal, but are extrascrotal, located distal to the external ring. Ectopic testes can be in the suprapubic fat, in the thigh, or even perineum. Undescended testes are almost always abnormal and can be located anywhere in the retroperitoneum or

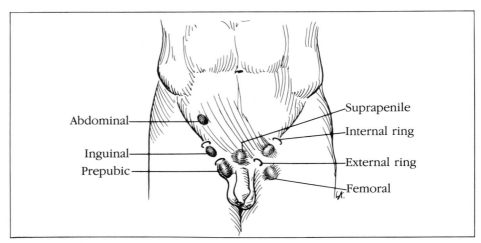

FIGURE 15–14
Common sites of testicular ectopia and cryptorchidism.

inguinal canal (Fig. 15–14). Fertility in an undescended testis can probably be enhanced by scrotal placement prior to age 2. Undescended testes have 40 times the incidence of testicular carcinoma as compared to normal testes, which is probably not influenced by orchiopexy.

HERNIA

Abdominal hernias have in common a sac lined with peritoneum that protrudes through some defect in the abdominal wall. The contents of inguinal and femoral hernias are variable. Omentum, small bowel, large bowel, or bladder may be encountered within the hernial sac (Fig. 15–15).

Examination of the inguinal canal is not difficult (Fig. 15–16). The examining finger is inserted in the lower part of the scrotum, and the scrotum is inverted so that the finger passes along the inguinal canal to palpate the external ring. When performed slowly and carefully this examination causes minimum discomfort to the patient. The examining finger should always identify the following normal structures: the extent of the os pubis, the spermatic cord as it lies within the inguinal canal, the size and perimeter of the external inguinal ring, and the area of Hesselbach's triangle medial to the deep epigastric vessels.

The indirect inguinal hernial sac emerges through the internal ring, traverses the inguinal canal with the contents of the cord, and appears at the external ring. If it extends into the scrotum it is termed a scrotal hernia (Fig. 15–17). The neck of the indirect hernial sac lies lateral to the deep epigastric artery.

Indirect hernias are the most common inguinal hernias. They are thought to be congenital and may result from failure of the processus vaginalis to obliterate. Hernias in children and young adults are usually of the indirect type. Hernias limited to the inguinal canal are termed incomplete, while those that emerge from the external ring are complete. In the female a complete hernia may enter the labium majus as a labial hernia.

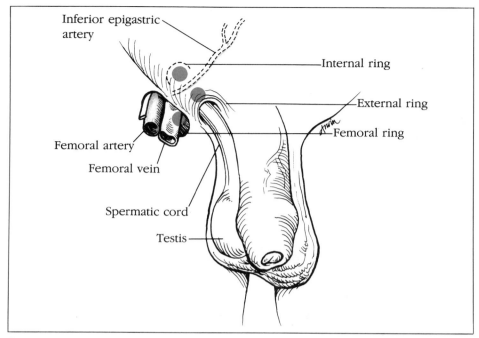

FIGURE 15–15
Common sites of hernias.

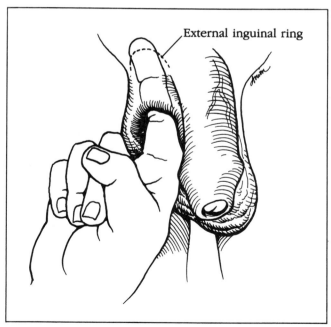

FIGURE 15–16
Technique of examination for inguinal hernia.

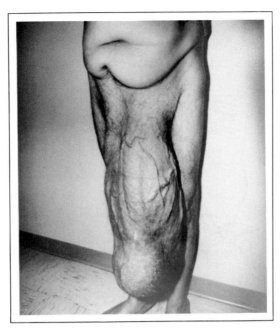

FIGURE 15–17
Massive inguinal hernia.

The direct inguinal hernial sac protrudes through Hesselbach's triangle medial to the deep epigastric artery and appears at the external ring without passing through the inguinal canal. It is apparent, therefore, that the direct hernial sac does not lie in close relationship with the spermatic cord. *Direct hernias* usually result from weakness of the fascia transversalis in the region of Hesselbach's triangle and present as a rounded swelling. They are almost always reducible and rarely enter the scrotum. Most direct hernias occur in individuals over 40 years of age.

On physical examination the external ring may sometimes appear to be enlarged. Relaxation of the external ring, however, is insufficient evidence on which to make a diagnosis of indirect inguinal hernia. If the examining finger encounters a mass in the inguinal canal, the presumptive diagnosis of hernia may be made. This may be confirmed by palpating an impulse in the external ring when the patient coughs. The differentiation between an indirect inguinal and a direct inguinal hernia should not be difficult. If the hernia can be completely reduced, the examining finger may be inserted into the external inguinal ring, and, when the patient coughs, the leading edge of the hernia may be palpated with the tip of the finger. On the other hand, if the finger is inserted into Hesselbach's triangle, the sac of an indirect hernia will be felt striking the side of the finger.

It may sometimes be difficult to establish the diagnosis of inguinal hernia in a woman. It should be possible to identify the inguinal ligament and os pubis and from these anatomic points to locate the external inguinal ring. If a sac is palpated when the patient coughs, the diagnosis of inguinal hernia may be made. It may help to place the palmar surface of the hand over the area of the internal inguinal ring in an effort to feel an impulse with cough. It is occasionally possible to see a small indirect inguinal hernia as a bulge that appears on coughing. Examination in both standing and supine positions may help to bring these points out.

Examination of the femoral region is more difficult than is the study of the inguinal area. The external opening of the femoral canal may be located anatomically just medial to the femoral artery and deep to the inguinal ligament. A simple precept to remember in examining the patient's right femoral area is that when the examiner's right index finger is placed on the patient's right femoral artery, the middle finger will overlie the femoral vein and the ring finger will overlie the femoral canal. A swelling lying within the femoral canal that transmits an impulse on coughing may be diagnosed as a *femoral hernia*. It must be distinguished from psoas abscess, lymphadenitis, and saphenous varix.

Femoral hernia is the most common hernia in women, and the points raised in the above discussion of examination of the femoral region are applicable in examining the female patient as well.

As a general rule, the incidence of strangulation is high in femoral hernias. Consequently, early operation is desirable.

A *sliding hernia* is a special type that deserves mention. The large bowel (or bladder) slips retroperitoneally between the leaves of its mesentery to herniate or protrude through the defect in the abdominal wall. On the right side the cecum may be the presenting part, while on the left the presenting part may be the sigmoid colon. In either event it is important to recognize this entity, since the wall of the bowel or bladder rather than a peritoneal sac makes up the leading edge of the hernia. Failure to make the proper diagnosis may lead the surgeon to open the bowel accidentally, thinking he is incising a hernial sac. It is often difficult to reduce a sliding hernia, and irreducibility should raise the examiner's suspicions as to this possibility.

When a hernia can no longer be reduced and the contents of the hernial sac cannot be returned to the peritoneal cavity, it is said to be *incarcerated*. If the blood supply to the viscera lying within the hernial sac has been cut off, it is said to be a *strangulated hernia*. It is often difficult and sometimes impossible to tell with certainty whether a hernia is simply incarcerated or whether it is strangulated. It is reasonable to attempt to reduce an incarcerated hernia if the incarceration is recent and one can be certain that the contents are completely viable. Strangulated hernias usually show local signs of inflammation, although this is not invariable. When inflammatory signs are present it is unwise to attempt vigorous reduction lest strangulated bowel be returned to the peritoneal cavity.

If it is decided to attempt nonoperative reduction of an incarcerated hernia, this should be performed with the patient in the recumbent position. This may be accomplished by exerting constant gentle pressure over the sac. The patient will often be experienced in reducing the hernia himself and may be able to accomplish this with ease. In difficult cases it may be necessary to lower the head of the bed, flex the leg on the affected side to relax the abdominal muscles, and attempt to gently guide the contents of the hernial sac through the inguinal ring. If local pain and tenderness are present, presumptive diagnosis of strangulation may be made and operative reduction and repair of the hernia is the procedure of choice. It should be noted that it is sometimes possible to reduce the entire hernia, together with the internal ring, into the abdominal cavity without actually freeing the contents of the hernial sac from the constricting internal ring. Under these circumstances, continued pain or tenderness in the region indicates the need for urgent surgical attention.

Large femoral hernias may be difficult to diagnose correctly because of their tendency to leave the abdominal cavity by way of the femoral canal and then be directed upward to overlie the inguinal ligament. They may be differentiated from inguinal hernias, however, if it is remembered that the sac of the femoral hernia lies lateral to and below the level of the symphysis pubis, while the sac of the inguinal hernia lies medial to it and above.

It is sometimes difficult to detect early strangulation in femoral hernias, since such local signs as pain or tenderness may be minimal. The femoral canal is the most likely site for the development of a *Richter's hernia*. The systemic signs of strangulation—such as tachypnea, leukocytosis, and fever—should invariably lead one to inspect this area with great care. The localized gangrene of the bowel wall without intestinal obstruction may lead to perforation and abscess formation just below the inguinal ligament. This should be differentiated from psoas abscess and femoral lymphadenitis.

Hydrocele of the canal of Nuck may occur in women. In the course of embryologic development, the round ligament leaves the retroperitoneal area to traverse the inguinal canal and insert itself on the labium majus. A processus vaginalis of peritoneum descends with the round ligament, and if the process is incompletely fused and obliterated, a hydrocele may result. A hydrocele may lie anywhere between the internal inguinal ring and the labium majus. Hydrocele of the canal of Nuck may be difficult to demonstrate but is characterized by its cystic, irreducible, translucent appearance.

Occasionally a patient will have indirect and direct hernias simultaneously. These are termed *saddlebag hernias*.

PROSTATE GLAND

As explained previously, the prostate is assessed during rectal examination. The technique of digital examination of the rectum is considered in Chapter 14. The prostate gland is best examined while the patient is standing and bending over the examining table (Fig. 15–18) or, when he is unable to stand or is in bed, in the Sims' position. Ample lubrication of the examining finger and perianal region facilitates the procedure. The index finger is introduced pointing toward the umbilicus, as this approximates the direction of the anal canal. The patient is asked to bear down slightly, which helps to relax the anal sphincter, and with gentle pressure the finger is easily introduced into the anal canal.

The muscle tone of the anal sphincter is estimated and the bulbocavernosus reflex is tested. The patient is asked to relax the sphincter as much as possible, and

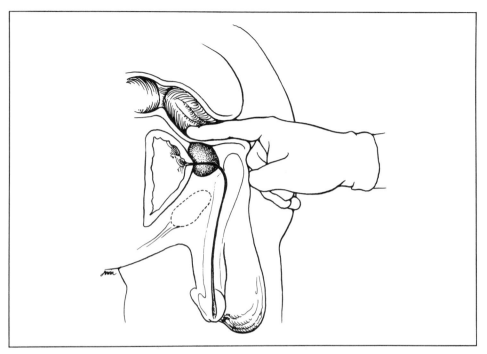

FIGURE 15–18
Examination of the prostate.

the glans penis is squeezed with the opposite hand. Normally this produces involuntary contraction of the anal sphincter. Voluntary contraction may produce a false-positive test. The presence of a bulbocavernosus reflex signifies an intact reflex arc in the region of the sacral cord, which also innervates the urinary bladder.

The prostate gland is examined by gentle palpation of the anterior wall of the rectum. The upper limits, lateral margins, and medial sulcus should be outlined. Each lobe is carefully palpated while the examiner searches for areas of irregularity or enlargement. The region of the seminal vesicles extends upward and laterally along the upper margin of the prostate gland.

Normally the sphincter tone is good, and the bulbocavernosus reflex is present. The prostate varies greatly in size, usually increasing with age. It is smooth and rubbery in consistency and normally not tender. The lateral borders are usually well defined (Fig. 15–19). The seminal vesicles are normally not palpable.

Acute prostatitis results in fever, urethral discharge, and an exceedingly tender, enlarged prostate gland on rectal examination. An abscess may develop and can be demonstrated as a fluctuant mass in the prostate gland. The seminal vesicles often are involved in inflammatory reaction and may be dilated and extremely tender. *Chronic prostatitis* is usually asymptomatic. At times rectal examination shows the prostate to be boggy or irregular. Areas of fibrous tissue may be palpated, thus

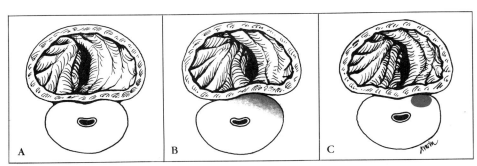

FIGURE 15—19
Diagnosis of some prostatic lesions. A. Normal. An approximately 2.5-cm, firm, smooth, heart-shaped gland. The medial sulcus can be felt as a depression between the two lateral lobes. B. Inflammatory nodule. The area of inflammation is raised above the surface of the gland, with induration decreasing at the periphery of the nodule. C. Cancerous nodule. The cancer is not raised. There is an abrupt demarcation of induration at the periphery of the lesion.

simulating neoplasm. *Prostatic calculi* are seldom of clinical importance. They may often be palpated at rectal examination and mistaken for carcinoma.

Benign prostatic hypertrophy is extremely common in men over 50 years of age. The prostate is of variable size. Small glands may be as obstructive as the large glands because it is the intraurethral protrusion that produces obstruction, not extraurethral enlargement. The gland is usually symmetric and has a smooth, rubbery consistency. The medial sulcus can be identified, and the lateral borders are well defined.

Carcinoma of the prostate occurs in approximately 20 percent of men over 60 years of age. The initial lesion usually involves the peripheral zone and when posterior is readily palpable at rectal examination. The early lesion feels like a small nodule on the posterior surface of the gland. Similar nodules can also be caused by calculi, chronic infection, or benign adenoma. More advanced malignant lesions usually are stony hard, irregular, and painless on palpation.

FEMALE GENITOURINARY SYSTEM

CHAPTER 16

There is only one way to be born and a thousand ways to die.

SERBIAN PROVERB

The objective of this portion of the physical examination is to assure normality or to diagnose abnormalities of the reproductive organs of the woman. More specifically the objective is to determine the size, shape, and mobility of the reproductive organs and to locate any source of intrapelvic pain and evidence of inflammation, discharge, or structural abnormality in the genitalia.

In view of this objective, the student should refer to the procedure as a pelvic examination rather than as a vaginal examination. The latter, of course, implies an examination only of the vagina itself rather than of the entire pelvic contents.

The pelvic examination is an essential part of the total evaluation of female patients. Although there is a natural reluctance on the part of both patient and physician about this portion of the physical examination, such reluctance must not interfere with prompt and thorough evaluation of the pelvic area. A physical examination in which the pelvic examination is deferred is as incomplete as one in which the cardiac examination is deferred.

ANATOMY

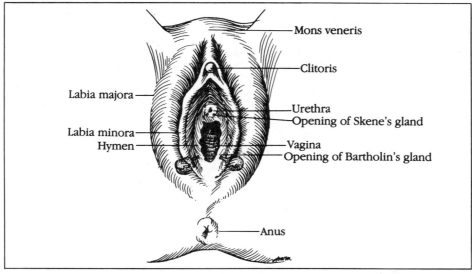

FIGURE 16–1
External female genitalia.

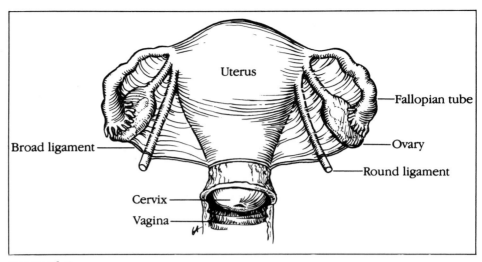

FIGURE 16–2
Internal female genitalia.

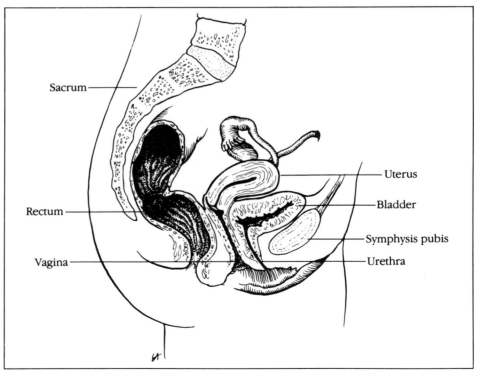

FIGURE 16–3
Cross-sectional anatomy of the female pelvis.

HISTORY

No one who is not female can be in a position to make accurate statements about women.

OTTO WEININGER
(1880–1903)

Gynecologic symptoms may point to local disease (infections, tumors) or signal systemic disorders (menstrual irregularities with thyroid disease and the vulvovaginitis of diabetes, for example). Moreover, gynecologic disorders may be associated with generalized symptoms resulting from a primary pelvic disease.

Menstrual symptoms are common. Specific inquiry should always be directed to the following:

1. Age of onset of menses (menarche)
2. Amount of discharge per period (small vs. large)
3. Duration of period
4. Interval between periods
5. Character of menstrual discharge (clots, odor)
6. Menstrual symptoms—especially pain
7. Intermenstrual period.

Endocrine disorders may precipitate an early menarche or delay puberty and menstruation. A delay in sexual maturation may occur with any debilitating disease (starvation, inflammatory bowel disease, juvenile arthritis) around the time of puberty. Vigorous continuous exercise (as in gymnasts or ballet dancers) may also delay menarche.

The amount of menstrual blood lost at each period varies from woman to woman. In an individual woman, however, marked decrease or increase in flow may be the hallmark of systemic (especially endocrine) or local (e.g., tumor) disease (Table 16–1).

A normal flow can last anywhere from 2 to 6 days. However, this is extremely variable. Similarly the interval between periods—a traditional 25 to 28 days—is not fixed, even in individual women. However, marked variations in interval may also suggest gynecologic disease.

Menstrual blood is generally dark and is normally without clots. With excessive menstrual bleeding, however, the menstrual flow may be redder and clots may form.

Menstrual pain *(dysmenorrhea)* is not always abnormal. It may begin a day or two before flow and continue well into the menstrual period. Some women are so afflicted that they must take to their beds for the duration of their period. Constitutional, psychologic, and local factors may all produce dysmenorrhea.

Bleeding between periods (spotting) may occur as the menopause approaches but is also a cardinal signal of gynecologic malignancy. It should be thoroughly investigated.

The date of the last menstrual period should be ascertained, particularly since delay—while potentially due to a variety of emotional, structural, or metabolic up-

TABLE 16–1. Some Causes of Excessive Menstrual Bleeding

Endocrine	**Vascular**
Puberty (anovulatory)	Chronic right heart failure
Maturity (anovulatory, progesterone deficiency)	Arteriosclerosis
Menopause	**Hematologic**
Hypothyroidism	Coagulation defects
Genital	Leukemia
Fibromyoma	
Chronic salpingo-oophoritis	
Endometriosis	
Malignancy of the uterus	
Acute infectious systemic disease	

sets—may also be due to pregnancy. Other symptoms of pregnancy include weight gain, morning sickness, and breast swelling and tenderness.

Vaginal discharge worries many women. Leukorrhea, a white discharge, may suggest bacterial, fungal, or parasitic infection. The duration, character, odor, and irritation caused by the discharge should be recorded in the history.

Gastrointestinal symptoms may be the hallmark of gynecologic disease or pregnancy. Nausea and vomiting may hint at pregnancy. Loss of appetite, weight loss, constipation, and abdominal pain and distention can be symptomatic of gynecologic malignancy.

Urinary symptoms, as discussed in Chapter 15, may be associated with vaginal or uterine disease as well as disorders primary to the urinary system.

Sexual dysfunction and *infertility* in women are serious complaints that may require extensive evaluation, beginning with a careful and complete history and physical and including pelvic examination.

PHYSICAL EXAMINATION

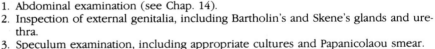

1. Abdominal examination (see Chap. 14).
2. Inspection of external genitalia, including Bartholin's and Skene's glands and urethra.
3. Speculum examination, including appropriate cultures and Papanicolaou smear.
4. Bimanual examination of internal genitalia.
5. Rectovaginal examination.

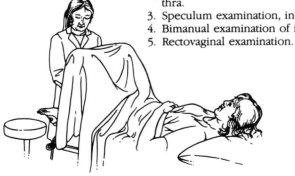
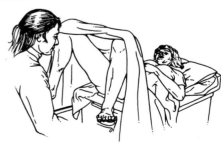

*Rupture of a tubal gestation is one of the causes of sudden death in young
women who have previously been in perfect health.*

Sir Zachary Cope
(1881–1974)

GENERAL

To understand the importance of acquiring competence in this particular aspect of
physical diagnosis, one should consider two questions: (1) Who should have such
an examination? and (2) who should carry out the examination?

First, of course, all hospitalized women should have the benefit of careful pelvic
examination. In addition, any woman coming to the physician because of pelvic
complaints (or with the request for routine prophylactic pelvic checkup) should
be examined, as well as women with systemic complaints of any kind.

There is often a great reluctance on the part of physicians (and parents) to examine the very young. This attitude can be very detrimental. In a series of cases of
ovarian malignancy, those patients who were teen-aged or younger had a significantly worsened prognosis, chiefly because of the much greater amount of time
lost through postponement of the examination necessary to make a correct diagnosis. Actually, gentle rectal examination in even very young girls can yield a great
deal of helpful information; and if there is any suspicion of a pelvic lesion, examination under light anesthesia should be carried out. Youth does not convey an
immunity to pelvic disease, and the physician should not deny his patients the best
possible care simply because they are young. In general, if a mother thinks the
problem is serious enough to bring her daughter to the doctor, the doctor should
consider the complaints to be serious enough to examine the patient.

Second, who should carry out the examination? Pelvic examination of the female
patient is a specialized gynecologic procedure only in the sense that auscultation
of the heart is a specialized procedure reserved for the cardiologist. In other words,
any physician who retains among his or her basic skills the ability to percuss the
cardiac border or listen to the heart sounds should also retain the ability to use
the vaginal speculum and carry out a careful bimanual pelvic examination.

In either instance—for either the noncardiologist or the nongynecologist—the
purpose of such examinations is to identify those patients who should be referred
for specialized diagnosis and treatment. Such referral is also an obligation when
the examination has been unsatisfactory or incomplete. Thus, to reassure a woman
that "everything is all right" when both ovaries have not been clearly felt could be
signing her death warrant. All physicians—internists, surgeons, pediatricians, as
well as gynecologists—should perform pelvic examination on their patients. If the
examination is inadequate or the results are inconclusive, careful referral, not
bland reassurance, is required.

None of us considers our reproductive organs in the same sense that we regard
other parts of our anatomy. Thus, the embarrassment that some women anticipate
in relation to this type of examination may cause them to postpone it. Similarly, in
their personal hygiene, some women will often fail to inspect or palpate lesions
that, on other parts of the body, they would examine minutely. As a physician,

therefore, one must proceed with this embarrassment clearly in mind and do one's best to place the patient at ease. This has practical as well as humane aspects—the more relaxed the patient, the more easily the examination will be accomplished. Patient cooperation is essential, and an undue tightening of the abdominal muscles or the levator ani sling can effectively bar the physician from accomplishing the objective of this examination.

The examination is best conducted in a room designed and equipped for that specific purpose. Ideally, separate toilet and dressing facilities should be part of the room. A curtained cubicle is no substitute for four walls and a solid door. If the physician is male, a female nurse or aide should be present.

The patient should empty her bladder and rectum immediately before the examination and should disrobe completely.

Draping the patient is important. The most satisfactory draping is a square sheet. The patient holds one corner over her xiphoid, the corners adjacent to this are placed one over each knee, and the fourth corner hangs between her legs and over her perineum. Draping in this manner minimizes embarrassment to the woman while permitting adequate exposure for the examination.

The routine nature of the office ritual helps put the patient at ease. The relative impersonality of the physician's behavior and the manner of arranging the draped sheet all heighten the reassuring effect. In elevating the corner of the sheet which hangs over the perineum and tucking it under the sheet on her abdomen, one is well advised to be looking not at her perineum but directly into her eyes, and to be commenting on something far afield from the complaints of the moment.

The perineum is as tender and sensitive as any area examined in the course of physical diagnosis. The doctor who hurts a patient instantly makes her an opponent rather than an ally in the job of accomplishing a satisfactory examination.

Anyone—man or woman—placed in the lithotomy position and then touched abruptly on the perineum will experience the anal sphincter reflex. The external anal sphincter (and portions of the levator ani) will involuntary contract, creating a barrier to a comfortable examination. Accordingly the examiner's initial contact with the perineum should be at some distance from the labia and should be firm but gentle.

All the tender areas of the introitus are anterior (clitoris, labia minora, and urethral meatus), and insertion of the intravaginal fingers should be posterior, with adequate lubrication. Jamming or shoving motions should be avoided. Although subsequent portions of the examination are inevitably somewhat uncomfortable, the entire initiation of the procedure can be such that optimum patient comfort is achieved and maintained.

EXTERNAL GENITALIA

Inspection precedes palpation here as in other realms of physical examination. However, the inspection can be brief and unembarrassing to the patient. One is seeking superficial skin lesions of the groin and perineum, evidence of erythema on the labia, and signs of an abnormal vaginal discharge.

Palpation also can be effected briefly and can yield evidence of the strength of the pelvic floor, the presence of Bartholin's cysts (Fig. 16–4), or the presence of

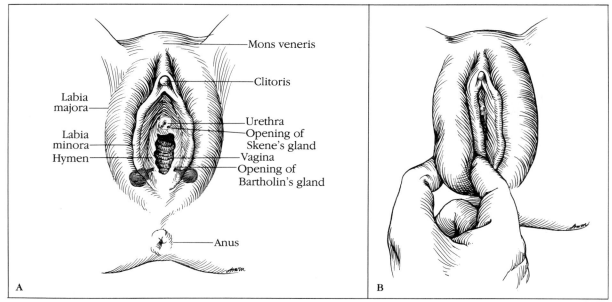

FIGURE 16–4
A. Bartholin's glands. B. Technique of palpation of Bartholin's glands.

pus in Skene's glands. Evaluate the general strength of perineal support by asking the patient to bear down and then observing any ballooning that may develop anteriorly (cystocele) and posteriorly (rectocele) (Fig. 16–5). The perineal body may be assayed by depressing the posterior fourchette with two fingers of the gloved hand and testing the general resistance. The presence of pus in Skene's glands can be determined by gently stripping these areas upward and watching for the appearance of purulent material at the urethral meatus.

With the exception of instances in which you must pause for an unexpected finding (e.g., vulvar or labial lesions), the inspection and palpation of the external genitalia can be expertly completed in 1 to 2 minutes.

SALINE DROP
Before introduction of the intravaginal fingers, obtain material for microscopic examination. Insert a saline-moistened swab into the vagina to collect a specimen and then place the swab in a small test tube containing 1 ml or at most 2 ml of physiologic saline solution. Keep the solution slightly warm, perhaps by having the attendant hold the test tube in her clenched fist until the rest of the pelvic examination is completed. Then examine the specimen (while the patient is dressing, for example). A drop on a regular slide without stain or fixation of any kind, will yield considerable information.

Under most circumstances the principal cellular element noted will be the vaginal epithelial cells. A significant number of leukocytes imply inflammation, and a significant number of erythrocytes indicate a bleeding lesion. The *Trichomonas*

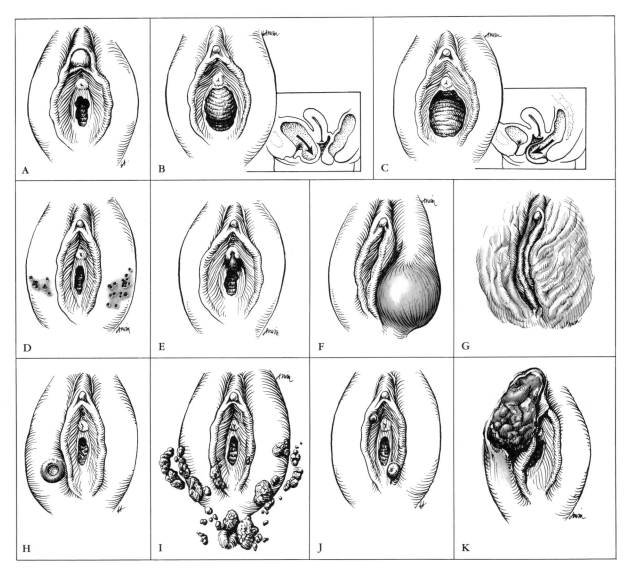

FIGURE 16–5

Some lesions of the external female genitalia. A. Clitoral enlargement. B. Cystocele. C. Rectocele. D. Herpes of vulva. E. Urethral caruncle. F. Bartholin's gland cyst. G. Labial varicosities. H. Syphilitic chancre. I. Condylomata acuminata. J. Hidradenoma of vulva. K. Carcinoma of vulva.

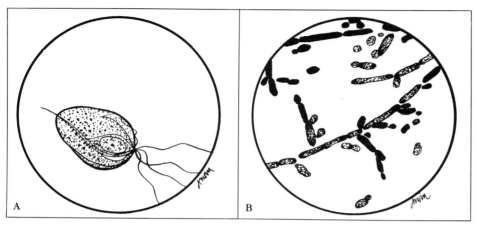

FIGURE 16–6
Saline drop. A. *Trichomonas vaginalis.* B. *Candida albicans.*

vaginalis parasite is recognized by its flagellate motion; *Candida albicans,* by its configuration (Fig. 16–6).

SPECULUM EXAMINATION

Inspection of the cervix and upper vagina precedes internal palpation and is done with the vaginal speculum. This is perhaps the most valuable single diagnostic instrument in gynecology, and the student should spend a few moments learning its simple mechanism.

The Graves or duck-billed speculum is made up of two blades. The posterior blade is fixed and the anterior is movable. The two blades are held together by a thumbscrew on the handle that can be loosened to separate the blades. The thumbscrew should always be tightly fastened and the blades in close approximation when the speculum is in ordinary use, or the chances of pinching the labia are increased.

The anterior blade is hinged and carries the thumbpiece on the side, which permits it to be elevated, separating the two blades when the speculum is assembled. The thumbscrew here should be all the way back, permitting the blades to be in close approximation on introduction of the speculum into the vagina.

To avoid interference with cytologic studies and to minimize the discomfort, the speculum should have no lubrication other than warm water. It is best held with the handle grasped loosely and the blades firmly held between the index and middle fingers. On introduction of the speculum, the pressure should be largely against the posterior fourchette and the blades should be oblique. If the flat surfaces of the blades are horizontal, the introitus is often overly stretched; if the blades are vertical, the suburethral area can be hurt.

As soon as the broad portions of the blades have passed the introitus, the spe-

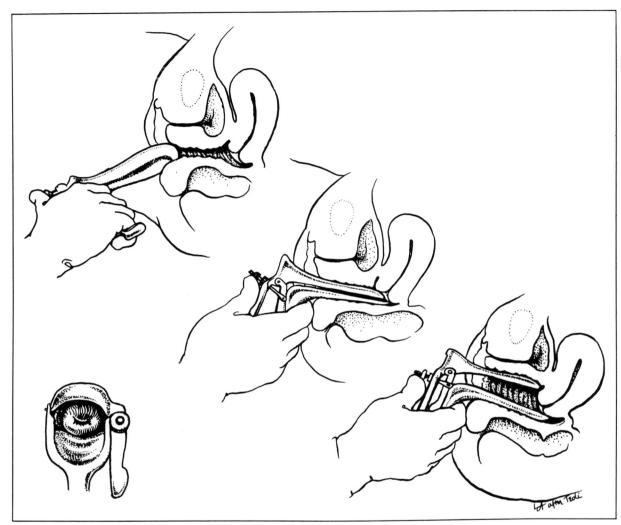

FIGURE 16–7
Insertion of the vaginal speculum (see text).

culum is rotated so that the blades are horizontal, and the handle is elevated so that the speculum is advancing at a 45-degree angle toward the examining table. The blades should not be separated until the speculum is fully inserted. As the thumb presses the lateral thumbpiece to elevate the top blade, the hand should lift on the handle to lower the fixed posterior blade. In this way the two blades move away from each other, and the cervix and vaginal walls are exposed (Fig. 16–7).

Inspect the vaginal wall and cervix carefully under a good light (Table 16–2, Figs. 16–8, 16–9).

SPECIAL TESTS

CULTURES

In any sexually active woman, it is wise to obtain a sample of vaginal secretions for gonorrhea cultures. Women with *Neisseria gonorrhoeae* vaginitis, cervicitis, or proctitis need *not* have *any* symptoms.

PAPANICOLAOU SMEAR

There are many ways to obtain cells for cytodiagnosis. Perhaps the most important single requirement is to obtain an adequate representation of the endocervical sample. The procedure described here is the Fast technique, which is designed to combine samples from the posterior vaginal pool and from the cervical canal and cervical face (Fig. 16–10). Since this test is for the identification of epithelial lesions, the specimen should be obtained before the upper vagina and cervical face are wiped off.

The slide and the bottle of ether-alcohol fixative should be labeled and prepared in advance to facilitate prompt fixing after spreading the cellular specimen. By using the handle of the Ayres spatula or a similar spatula, a thick sample of cells from the posterior cul-de-sac is obtained and placed on the slide at the frosted end. The spatula is immediately reversed, the longer arm of the tip is placed in the cervical os, and the blade is rotated a full circle. This portion of the sample is spread the length of the slide, catching and distributing some of the original cul-de-sac specimen. Then, with the tip of the spatula the entire specimen is spread evenly and the slide dropped immediately into the ether-alcohol.

A Papanicolaou ("Pap") smear should be part of the routine pelvic examination in every woman. The frequency with which a Pap smear is taken is determined by the patient's sexual activity, family history, age, use of contraceptive drugs, past cytologic diagnoses, and other considerations.

CERVICAL BIOPSY

The cervix is insensitive to cutting, and a liberal biopsy can be taken without discomfort to the patient. Various punch biopsy forceps are available that will obtain samples from the cervical face and endocervix without distortion.

Remember that cervical cytology has not replaced the biopsy. Cytologic study has its greatest value for the normal-appearing cervix, as an aid in screening, and in raising the examiner's index of suspicion. Where there is an evident lesion, the examiner's suspicion should already have been alerted and a biopsy should be taken. A negative cytologic report in the presence of a lesion does not remove the need for biopsy. Table 16–3 presents the classification of cervical carcinoma.

BIMANUAL PELVIC EXAMINATION

After the specimens are obtained and the speculum removed, bimanual pelvic examination is done. The abdominal hand brings the pelvic structures within reach of the intravaginal fingers for palpation. Remember that the area that can be covered depends largely on the position of the abdominal hand. The beginner tends to place the abdominal hand too close to the pubic bone, and should move it at least three-quarters of the way toward the umbilicus (Fig. 16–11).

TABLE 16—2. Some Vaginal Lesions

Lesion	History	Physical Signs	Appearance
Bacterial or chlamydial vaginitis (gonococcus chlamydia)	Leukorrhea, yellow discharge; dyspareunia, burning discharge	Vaginal wall inflammation Cervix inflamed; pooled pus from os cervix	
Senile vaginitis	Postmenopausal bleeding, discharge, itching, burning, dyspareunia	Friable mucosa, small, shrunken introitus; small cervix	
Candida vaginitis	Discharge (thin to purulent); irritation and redness of vulva	Mucosal redness Whitish or grayish patches	

Trichomonas vaginitis	Leukorrhea, soreness, burning, itching	"Strawberry" punctate erosions of cervix and mucosa Foamy pus pooled in fornix
Gartner's duct cyst	If large, possible bulging from vaginal outlet	Cyst on anterolateral vaginal wall

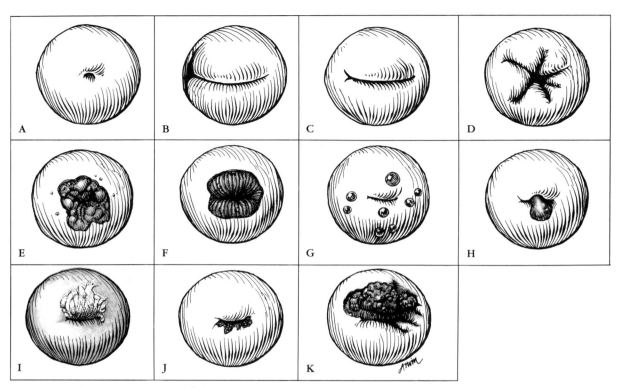

FIGURE 16–8
Some cervical lesions. A. Virgin. B. Parous. C. Minor tear. D. Stellate tear. E. Erosion. F. Eversion. G. Cysts. H. Polyp. I. Leukoplakia. J. Early cancer. K. Advanced cancer.

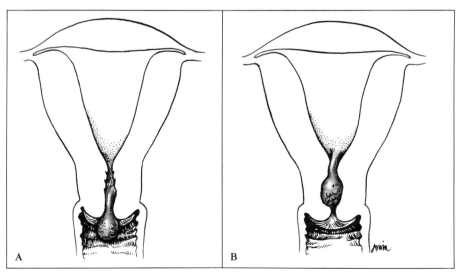

FIGURE 16–9
Cervical polyps. A. Exocervical. B. Endocervical.

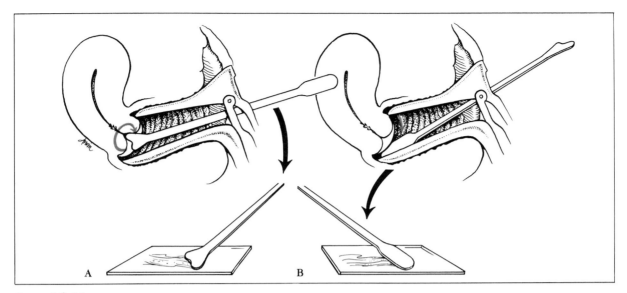

FIGURE 16–10
Technique of the Papanicolaou smear. A. Cervical scraping. B. Vaginal pool sampling.

The examining fingers should be well lubricated and gently inserted over the posterior fourchette. It is often most comfortable to rest one foot on a low stool, with the elbow of the intrapelvic hand resting on the knee.

CERVIX
The cervix will be most easily palpated, and as a general rule it points the opposite way from the fundus. If the cervix points posteriorly, the fundus of the uterus will usually be found anteriorly; if the cervix is in the axis of the vagina, the fundus will more often be retroverted and found in the cul-de-sac (Fig. 16–12). Motion of the cervix should not produce pain. In ectopic pregnancy or adnexal inflammation the pain on cervical motion is severe enough that the patient will usually indicate its presence without specific questioning.

UTERUS
The body of the uterus is then held between the examining hands, and its size, contour, and mobility are determined. Irregularities in its surface (as with myomata) can usually be determined with ease (Fig. 16–13). The cul-de-sac area should also be examined for bulging, tenderness, and masses. A uterine mass always requires further investigation, but x-ray films should not be ordered until you are certain that your patient is not pregnant.

The broad ligament structures beside the uterus do not generally yield palpable findings. The vaginal fingers go posteriorly under the broad ligament, and the abdominal fingers beside the uterus approach them so that the tissues of the broad ligament and the fallopian tube can be run between the fingers from bottom to top. In a normal patient no masses should be encountered.

TABLE 16–3. Classification of Cervical Carcinoma

Stage	Extent	Stage	Extent
0	Carcinoma in situ (preinvasive)	I	Carcinoma is confined to cervix
II	Carcinoma extends beyond cervix but has not yet reached pelvic wall It may involve vagina but not lower third	III	Carcinoma has reached pelvic wall, involves lower third of vagina, or is associated with lymph node metastases on pelvic wall
IV	Carcinoma involves bladder or rectum or has extended outside true pelvis (e.g., metastases to vulva, abdomen, lungs, bones, distant nodes)		

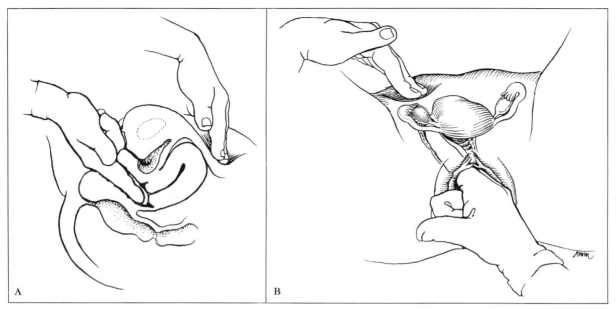

FIGURE 16–11
Technique of bimanual pelvic examination. A. Lateral view. B. Perineal view.

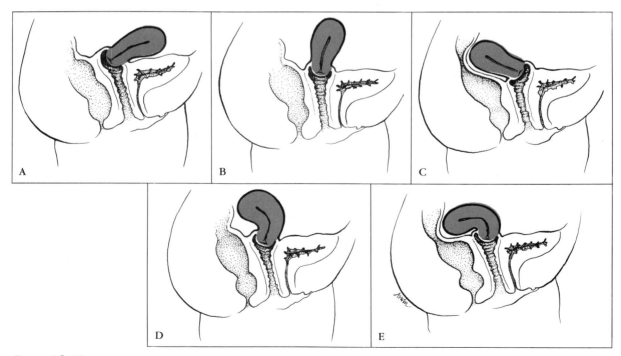

FIGURE 16 -12
Some malpositions of the uterus. A. Normal position. B. Slight retroversion. C. Marked retroversion. D. Slight retroflexion. E. Marked retroflexion.

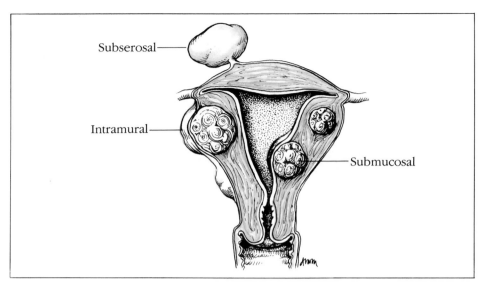

FIGURE 16–13
Uterine fibroids (myomata). These are truly benign smooth muscle tumors and are the most common of pelvic tumors.

OVARIES

The intravaginal fingers now move downward and backward again at the lateral wall, the abdominal hand moves over just inside the anterior superior spine of the ileum, and the same process is repeated. Here the examiner should encounter the ovary, and size, shape, and mobility can be determined. (Tables 16–4 and 16–5 describe some important ovarian lesions.) The gonads of women are as sensitive to pressure as the gonads of men; gentleness is imperative.

RECTOVAGINAL EXAMINATION

The examination is completed by rectovaginal abdominal palpation (Fig. 16–14). Entry into the rectum is facilitated by liberal use of lubrication and having the patient bear down. The middle finger is gently inserted in the rectum and the index finger in the vagina. This immediately gives much greater access to the adnexal regions and the posterior surface of the broad ligament and also reveals the presence or absence of rectal lesions.

Hard, fixed nodules in uretrosacral ligaments, cul-de-sac, or rectovaginal septum may respresent *endometriosis*—the deposition of functional endometrial tissue in areas outside the uterus (Fig. 16–15). Multiple sites usually are involved. The patient is commonly a young, nulliparous woman with dysmenorrhea, infertility, dyspareunia, bowel dysfunction (including rectal bleeding), hematuria (if the bladder is involved), or other symptoms, depending on the site of implantation of the endometrium, which goes through cyclic menstrual proliferation and bleeding much as does endouterine tissue. Almost one-fifth of patients with endometriosis will have no symptoms at all.

TABLE 16–4. Benign Ovarian Cysts and Tumors*

Lesion	Discussion	Appearance
Cystic Non-neoplastic	Follicle, lutein cysts, etc.—functional retention cysts arising in follicles or corpora lutea Usually no symptoms, but may undergo spontaneous rupture, bleeding, torsion Also includes inflammatory and endometrial cysts	 *Follicle cyst*
Neoplastic	Pseudomucinous, serous, and dermoid cysts May grow to huge size	 *Dermoid cysts (containing hair, teeth)*
Solid	Fibroma (of fibrous muscle tissue); Brenner tumor of epithelial cells (rarely malignant)	 *Solid mass, though cystic degeneration may occur*

*On physical examination, all tumors may be felt as abdominal or pelvic masses, depending on size.

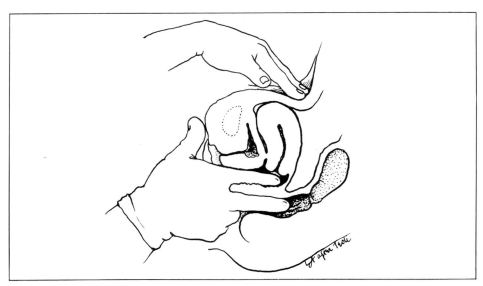

FIGURE 16–14
Technique of rectovaginal examination.

TABLE 16–5. Clinical Manifestations of Ovarian Tumors

Benign	Malignant
1. May be totally asymptomatic	1. May be totally asymptomatic
2. Rupture or hemorrhage may mimic an acute abdomen	2. Necrosis or rupture may mimic acute abdomen
3. May undergo torsion, with or without infarction	3. Torsion is rare
4. Infection is rare	4. Symptoms of vague abdominal distress, bladder and bowel irritability 2° pressure
5. Symptoms and signs are those of intrapelvic or intra-abdominal mass	5. Abdominal swelling
	6. Irregular vaginal bleeding
	7. May cause ascites, weight loss, intestinal obstruction, metastatic disease

INFECTIONS OF THE FEMALE GENITALIA

The label "pelvic inflammatory disease" has been used to the detriment of patients as a diagnostic term for pelvic pain of unknown causes. Its use should be limited to the occurrence of pelvic peritonitis as a result of an infection involving the uterus, tubes, or ovaries, caused by pathogenic organisms (Fig. 16–16).

The clinical diagnosis of acute pelvic inflammatory disease has an accuracy of less than 75 percent. The remainder of the individuals with the commonly accepted clinical signs and symptoms of acute pelvic infection have either other surgical problems or no discernible pelvic abnormalities.

The increasing incidence of gonorrheal infection combined with recognition of asymptomatic male carriers of gonorrhea and the frequency of chlamydial venereal

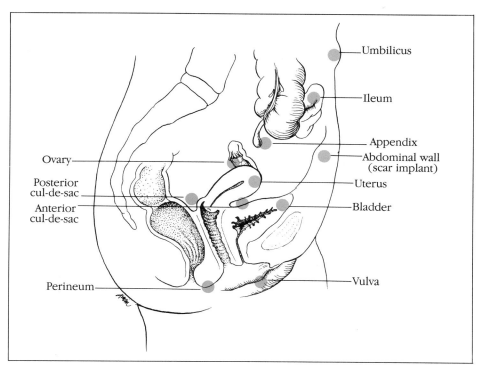

FIGURE 16–15
Some sites of endometrial implants.

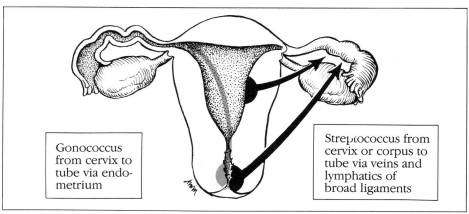

FIGURE 16–16
Routes of pelvic infection.

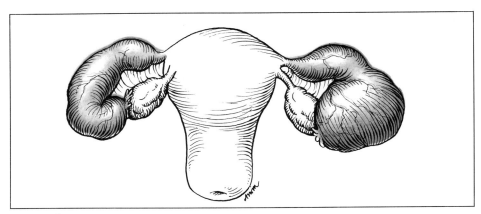

FIGURE 16–17
Chronic pelvic gonorrheal infection.

infections in both men and women requires that physicians be knowledgeable of the symptomatology and clinical findings of pelvic infections in women.

Patients with pelvic peritonitis present with a complaint of lower abdominal pelvic pain that is associated with a fever ranging from 100°F to 104°F. They frequently date the onset of symptoms to immediately following the last menstrual period. Usually patients are without gastrointestinal complaints, and their appetites are usually not impaired.

Positive physical findings are limited to the lower abdomen and pelvis. On abdominal examination the lower abdomen and suprapubic areas are tender, with the suggestion or presence of rebound. Intestinal sounds are commonly active. On pelvic examination there may or may not be a vaginal discharge. There is a history of a malodorous discharge before the last menstrual flow. Bimanual examination will demonstrate bilateral adnexal and uterine tenderness. This tenderness will be accompanied by guarding, and one frequently will be unable to delineate the adnexal structures clearly. Moderately sized ovarian or tubal masses may be missed. Rectal examination is mandatory because it allows demonstration of the presence of posterior pelvic masses characteristic of tubo-ovarian or pelvic abscesses.

Unfortunately the outlined physical findings may be the result of a variety of clinical entities. Such findings are observed in appendicitis associated with perforation, or an inflamed appendix that is adherent to pelvic viscera. Other gastrointestinal inflammatory states may also result in pelvic peritonitis. These include the uncommon Meckel's diverticulum and diverticulitis. Leaking ovarian cysts or twisting either of ovarian tumor or adnexa may result in similar complaints. Benign uterine tumors such as degenerating myomata can also cause similar physical findings.

The patient's history may be of assistance in suggesting an exposure to gonorrheal infection (Fig. 16–17). In such cases the collection of cervical cultures may demonstrate the gonococcus, and the patient respond rapidly to antibiotics such as penicillin or tetracycline.

RECURRENT PELVIC INFECTION

The continued destruction of ovarian and tubal architecture as a result of recurrent and inadequately treated infections may result in the evolution of tubo-ovarian abscesses or ovarian abscesses. The major problem with such abscesses is rupture with intraperitoneal leakage of their contents. This syndrome is associated with inordinate mortality if operative intervention is not prompt. Those patients who have intraperitoneal leakage develop progressive peritonitis with ileus associated with nausea and vomiting. Their heightened temperature and tachycardia do not respond to antibiotic therapy. On pelvic examination, pelvic masses will be found in at least 50 percent of the cases. These patients often require immediate exploration and cannot be treated nonsurgically.

PREGNANCY

At the moment of child-birth, every woman has the same aura in isolation, as though she were abandoned, alone.

BORIS PASTERNAK
(1890–1960)

DIAGNOSIS OF PREGNANCY

The most prominent changes in the pelvis during early pregnancy revolve around the vascular congestion that takes place. The cervix softens and the uterus grows slightly larger and softer. Subsequently cyanosis of the upper vaginal tissues and of the cervix becomes prominent (Chadwick's sign).

The initial enlargement of the uterus is not usually symmetrical but is more pronounced on one horn, apparently the side of conception. Subsequently globularity of the uterus becomes evident, in contrast to the anteroposterior flattening normally present. A softened area 2 or 3 cm in diameter appears on the anterior wall (Ladin's sign).

There is also fullness and congestion of the breasts and increased prominence of the superficial veins.

DIAGNOSIS OF PREVIOUS PREGNANCY

The nipples and areolae retain the brown color acquired during pregnancy and do not resume the former pink color. The linea alba remains brown. The cervical os never resumes the round and symmetrical configuration but will be irregular and slightly enlarged. The perineum may show a loss of tone, or there may be scarring of the posterior fourchette (episiotomy).

EXAMINATION OF THE ABDOMEN DURING PREGNANCY

It is contrary to nature for children to come into the world with feet first.

PLINY THE ELDER
(23–79)

The initial prenatal visit calls for a complete examination and an estimation of the capacity of the pelvis. Subsequent examinations in the average case call only for a brief interval history and a limited examination. The patient's weight and blood pressure should be obtained, and the urine should be examined for albumin and sugar.

Abdominal examination should be performed on every visit. The height of the fundus of the uterus above the pubic bone should be measured to estimate continued and appropriate uterine growth. The uterus first rises above the symphysis pubis at about the third month. Thereafter, the number of centimeters divided by four equals the months of pregnancy. This rule is only approximate, but marked deviations from it suggest the possibility of twins or hydramnios if the measurement is great, or of fetal abnormality or death if the fundal height fails to increase.

Palpation of the fetus within the uterus usually begins about the fifth month with an attempt to locate the fetal head by grasping it above the pubic bone with the thumb and middle finger. If the pole of the fetus in this area gives the impression of being pointed rather than firm and rounded, the head should be sought in the fundus, with both hands placed flat on the abdomen and parallel to the uterine axis. The back of the fetus can also be located with the hands flat on either side and the fingers parallel to the uterus. The fetal small parts feel knobby and irregular in comparison with the back, on which the hand can be fitted flat.

SECTION VI

NEUROMUSCULAR SYSTEM

17. MUSCULOSKELETAL SYSTEM
  Lee H. Riley, Jr.
18. NERVOUS SYSTEM
  Sid Gilman
  Faith T. Fitzgerald

*As to diseases, make a
habit of two things, to help
or at least to do no harm.*
HIPPOCRATES
(460?–377? B.C.)

1. Patient sitting
   a. General inspection
   b. Cranial nerve testing (may be done as part of head examination
      —see Section III)

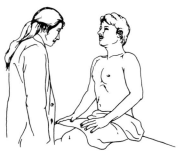 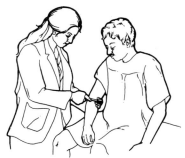

   c. Motor function upper extremities including reflexes
   d. Joint examination—neck and upper extremities
   e. Cerebellar testing (begin)

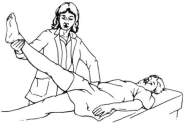 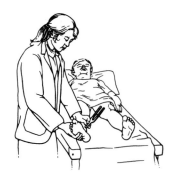

2. Patient recumbent
   a. Motor function lower extremities
   b. Joint examination—lower extremities
   c. Reflexes
   d. Sensory examination
   e. Cerebellar testing (finish)

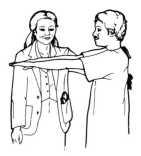 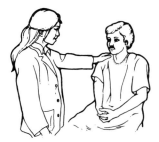

3. Patient standing—posture, station, gait, deformities, Romberg test
4. Patient sitting again—mental status, reflexes

CHAPTER 17

MUSCULOSKELETAL SYSTEM

No muscle uses its power in pushing but always in drawing to itself the parts that are joined to it.

LEONARDO DA VINCI
(1452–1519)

Trauma, arthritis, degenerative change, congenital and acquired deformities, and general aches and pains are prevalent complaints in the American population. The increasing emphasis on sports and fitness has led to a burgeoning number of orthopedic injuries.

The musculoskeletal examination of an individual who has not been acutely injured differs greatly from the examination of an acutely injured patient. For example, the active and passive range of motion of the cervical spine should be determined when the patient shows symptoms of a nontraumatic disorder of the neck and upper extremity. However, this determination is not performed in an individual who has been acutely injured until the mechanical stability of the cervical spine has been demonstrated by roentgenogram. The importance of this distinction cannot be overemphasized.

The physical examination of an adult differs in some respects from the physical examination of a child and especially from that of an infant. The method detailed here is that used for the examination of an adult.

ANATOMY

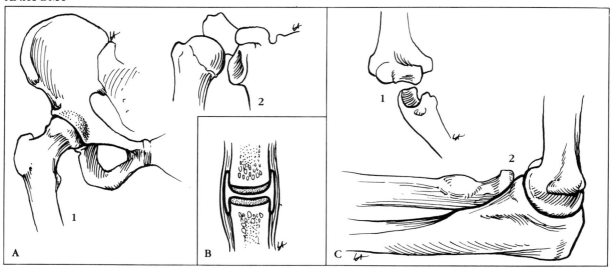

FIGURE 17–1
Types of joints. A. Ball-and-socket: hip (1), shoulder (2). B. Synovial. C. Hinge: elbow disarticulated (1), elbow articulated (2).

415

HISTORY

Some men ('gainst Raine) doe carry in their backs
Prognosticating Aching Almanacks;
Some by a painefull elbow, hip or knee
Will shrewdly guesse, what weather's like to be.

JOHN TAYLOR ("The Water Poet")
(1580–1653)

Pain, deformity, and **limitation of function** are the major symptoms of musculo-skeletal abnormality. Limitation of function in itself may be due to pain associated with movement, to bone or joint instability, or to the restriction of joint motion. The joint restriction in turn may be due to muscle weakness from neurologic disease or trauma, muscle contractures from previous injury or disease, bony fusion, or a mechanical block by bone fragments or torn cartilage within the joint.

Pain is a significant symptom. Its characteristic location and relation to the patient's activity should be noted. The pain of bone erosion caused by tumor or aneurysm is usually described as deep, constant, and boring. It is apt to be more noticeable and more intense at night, and it may not be relieved by rest or position. The pain of degenerative arthritis and muscle disorders is an aching type that is often accentuated by activity and lessened by rest. The discomfort may be increased by certain positions or motions. For instance, the pain resulting from degenerative changes in the cervical spine is often accentuated by maintaining the neck in extension. Subjective paresthesias that do not follow a dermatome distribution are often noted by the patient with degenerative changes involving the cervical or lumbar spine. These paresthesias are often described as a "sandy" feeling or as if the foot (or arm) were "going to sleep." The pain of fracture and infection of bone is severe and throbbing and is increased by any motion of the part. Acute nerve compression causes a sharp, severe pain radiating along the distribution of the nerve. It is often associated with weakness of muscles supplied by the nerve and sensory changes over the area supplied by it.

Referred pain is that perceived by the patient in an anatomic location removed from the site of the lesion. Pain resulting from a disorder of the hip is often first noted by the patient in the anterior and lateral aspect of the thigh, or in the knee. Pain from a shoulder lesion may be felt at the insertion of the deltoid muscle on the lateral aspect of the proximal portion of the humerus. Pain from the lower cervical spine is often referred to the interscapular region of the back, along the vertebral aspect of the scapula, or to the tips of the shoulders and lateral aspects of the arms.

PHYSICAL EXAMINATION

1. Inspect posture and gait. Look for obvious deformities and inflammation of joints, muscles, and bones.

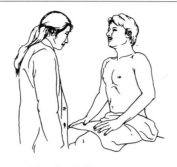
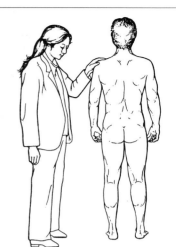

2. Inspect, palpate, and examine range of motion* for the following:

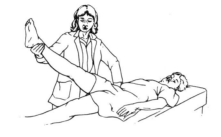

   Cervical spine
   Thoracic spine
   Lumbar spine
   Shoulder
   Elbow
   Wrist
   Hand
   Hip
   Knee
   Ankle
   Foot

3. Inspect, palpate, and test the strength of muscle groups as you follow the sequence of joint examination in (2).

   *Emphasis, of course, is on those joints to which history or gross inspection casts suspicion of disease.

Science is the father of knowledge, but opinion breeds ignorance.

> HIPPOCRATES
> (460?–377?
> B.C.)

GENERAL

POSTURE AND GAIT

Begin the examination by observing posture and gait as the patient enters the examining area. Gait is divided into two broad phases—stance and swing. The stance phase includes heel-strike (as the heel strikes the ground), midstance (as the body weight is transferred from the heel to the ball of the foot), and push-off (as the heel leaves the ground). The swing phase includes acceleration, swing-through (as the foot travels ahead of the opposite foot), and deceleration (as the foot slows in preparation for heel-strike). Observe each phase and note any awkwardness or change in rhythm. For example, a patient with a painful callus on the ball of the foot will not bear weight normally on that part of the foot during midstance and push-off.

TABLE 17–1. Some Causes of Antalgic Gait

Bone disease
    Fracture
    Infection (osteomyelitis)
    Tumor
    Avascular necrosis (if in childhood, often called by eponym)
        Femoral head (Perthes' disease, Legg-Calvé disease)
        Tibial tubercle (Osgood-Schlatter disease)
        Tarsal navicular (Köhler's bone disease)
Muscle disease
    Traumatic rupture, contusion
    Cramp secondary to fatigue, strain, malposition
    Inflammatory myositis
Vascular disease
    Claudication of arterial insufficiency
    Thrombophlebitis
Joint disease
    Traumatic arthritis
    Infectious arthritis
    Immune arthritis (rheumatoid, lupus, vasculitis of other sorts)
    Crystalline arthritis (gout, pseudogout)
    Hermarthrosis (hemophilia, scurvy)
Neurologic disease
    Lumbar spine disease with nerve root irritation or compression
    Pelvic masses involving sacral roots
Other
    Foot trauma (including blisters, ingrown toenails)
    Foreign bodies of the foot
    Corns, bunions

Abnormalities in gait may be caused by

1. Mechanical or structural abnormalities
2. Pain (antalgic gaits—Table 17–1)
3. Muscle disease
4. Neurologic disease
5. Psychiatric disease

Look for gross deformities, areas of swelling, and areas of discoloration. The presence of ecchymoses suggests previous trauma. A red swollen area that is warm and tender to palpation suggests inflammation. If such an area is about a joint and is associated with fluid within the joint, acute synovitides such as rheumatoid arthritis, gouty arthritis, or infectious arthritis are suspected. If such an area is over the diaphyseal region of an extremity, infectious lesion of the underlying bone or soft tissues or noninfectious inflammatory lesion (e.g., thrombophlebitis) is suspected.

TABLE 17–2. Testing for Muscle Strength

100%	5	N	(normal)	Complete range of motion against gravity with full resistance
75	4	G	(good)	Complete range of motion against gravity with some resistance
50	3	F	(fair)	Complete range of motion against gravity
25	2	P	(poor)	Complete range of motion with gravity eliminated
10	1	T	(trace)	Evidence of slight contractility No joint motion
0	0	0	(zero)	No evidence of contractility

EXAMINATION OF A JOINT

Observe the joint and note any gross deformity and swelling. Swelling within a joint may represent either fluid or thickened synovial tissue. In the former, a fluid wave can be demonstrated; in the latter, the firm and somewhat boggy tissue can be palpated and no fluid wave is noted unless, of course, excessive fluid is also present. Palpate about the joint for masses and for points of tenderness that may indicate a torn ligament, an area of osteoarthritis or synovitis, or the torn attachment of a meniscus. Determine the active and passive range of motion of the joints, comparing those on opposite sides. Palpate the joint during active and passive motion to detect crepitation. Test the ligaments that help stabilize the joint and the muscles.

EXAMINATION OF A MUSCLE

. . . and at the same time as the sparks were obtained, there were produced wonderfully strong contractions in each muscle of the joints just as if an animal in tetanus had been used.

LUIGI GALVANI
(1737–1798)

In the examination of a muscle or a muscle group, ascertain the status of the muscle fibers as well as the nerves that supply them. Inspect the muscle for gross hypertrophy or atrophy and for fasciculations, which are isolated contractions of a portion of the fibers. Look for areas of muscle spasm that can be easily palpated and often are accentuated as the joint they span is moved passively. Areas of muscle spasm are tender to palpation. Measure the circumference of an extremity at a given point above and below the patella or above and below the olecranon and compare this measurement with that of the opposite side. Test the strength of the muscle according to the criteria given in Table 17–2. Note the consistency of the muscle to palpation and the presence of tenderness over the muscle or its tendon. The spinal segments and the peripheral nerves that generally innervate major muscle groups of the extremities are listed in Table 17–3. Common causes of atrophy and weakness are listed in Tables 17–4 and 17–5.

TABLE 17–3. Innervation of the Muscles of the Extremities

Upper Limb Muscles	Nerve	C2	C3	C4	C5	C6	C7	C8	T1
Sternocleidomastoid; trapezius	Spinal accessory	X	X	X					
Diaphragm	Phrenic		X	X					
Deltoid	Axillary				X	X			
Supraspinatus	Suprascapular				X	X			
Infraspinatus	Suprascapular				X	X			
Teres minor	Axillary				X	X			
Subscapularis; teres major	Subscapular				X	X			
Serratus anterior	Long thoracic				X	X	X		
Rhomboideus	Dorsal scapular			X	X				
Clavicular pectoralis major	Lateral and medial pectoral				X	X	X		
Biceps; brachialis	Musculocutaneous				X	X			
Brachioradialis	Radial				X	X			
Latissimus dorsi	Thoracodorsal					X	X	X	
Sternal pectoralis major	Lateral and medial pectoral					X	X	X	X
Flexor carpi radialis; pronator teres	Median					X	X		
Extensor carpi radialis, longus & brevis; extensor digitorum communis; extensor indicis proprius; extensor carpi ulnaris; extensor pollicis, longus & brevis; abductor pollicus longus; triceps	Radial					X	X	X	
Flexor digitorum sublimis	Median						X	X	X
Flexor digitorum profundus	Volar interosseous; ulnar						X	X	X
Flexor carpi ulnaris	Ulnar						X	X	X
Pronator quadratus	Volar interosseous						X	X	X
Interossei	Ulnar							X	X
Lumbricals; flexor pollicis brevis	Median; ulnar							X	X
Adductor pollicis; opponens digiti minimi	Ulnar							X	X
Biceps tendon reflex	Musculocutaneous				X	X			
Brachioradialis reflex	Radial				X	X			
Triceps tendon reflex	Radial						X	X	

Lower Limb Muscles	Nerve	L1	L2	L3	L4	L5	S1	S2	S4	S5
Hip flexion	Lumbar plexus; femoral; superior gluteal; obturator		X	X	X	X	X			
Hip adduction	Obturator		X	X	X					
Knee extension	Femoral		X	X	X					
Hip abduction	Superior gluteal				X	X	X			
Foot inversion & dorsiflexion	Peroneal				X	X	X			
Toe extension	Peroneal				X	X	X			
Great toe extension	Peroneal				X	X	X			
Foot eversion	Peroneal				X	X	X			
Foot inversion & plantar flexion	Tibial					X	X			
Toe flexion	Tibial					X	X			
Great toe flexion	Tibial					X	X			
Hip extension	Inferior gluteal					X	X	X		
Knee flexion	Peroneal; tibial					X	X	X		
Foot plantar flexion	Tibial					X	X	X		
Cremasteric reflex	Genital-femoral	X	X							
Patellar tendon reflex	Femoral			X	X					
Achilles tendon reflex	Tibial						X	X		
Anal reflex	Pudendal							X	X	X

Muscle rows detail:

- Hip flexion: Iliopsoas; sartorius; rectus femoris; tensor fasciae latae
- Hip adduction: Adductor magnus; adductor brevis; adductor longus
- Knee extension: Quadriceps femoris
- Hip abduction: Gluteus medias; gluteus minimus; tensor fascia femoris
- Foot inversion & dorsiflexion: Tibialis anterior
- Toe extension: Extensor digitorum, longus & brevis
- Great toe extension: Extensor hallucis, longus & brevis
- Foot eversion: Peroneus, longus & brevis
- Foot inversion & plantar flexion: Tibialis posterior
- Toe flexion: Flexor digitorum, longus & brevis
- Great toe flexion: Flexor hallucis longus
- Hip extension: Gluteus maximus
- Knee flexion: Biceps femoris; semimembranosus; semitendinosus
- Foot plantar flexion: Gastrocnemius; soleus

TABLE 17–4. Some Causes of Muscle Atrophy

Old age
Generalized wasting diseases
  Malignancy
  Tuberculosis or other chronic infections
  Starvation
  Thyrotoxicosis
  Diabetes mellitus
  Cushing's disease
  Addison's disease
Disuse atrophy (affects unused muscle mass locally)
  Fractured bone
  Casting or immobilization
  Painful or ankylosing joint disease
  Hysterical paralysis
Lower motor neuron lesions with flaccid paralysis
  Spine
    Disc disease
    Syringomyelia
    Cord tumor
    Poliomyelitis
    Amyotrophic lateral sclerosis
  Spinal root
    Disc disease
    Tumor entrapment
    Radiculitis due to meningitis
  Peripheral nerves
    Infective mononeuropathy or polyneuropathy
    Vasculitic mononeuropathy or polyneuropathy
    Trauma

EXAMINATION OF A BONE

Observe the soft tissues covering a bone for obvious deformity, such as bowing, angulation, and tumor. Palpate the bone for areas of tenderness and for masses (Table 17–6). Tenderness of a bone suggests underlying tumor, inflammation, or the sequelae of trauma. This impression is strengthened when percussion of the bone at a site distant from the site of tenderness produces pain, not at the site of percussion but at the point of tenderness to palpation. Test the gross structural integrity of a bone by noting its ability to resist a deforming force. Lack of resistance suggests a fracture or the result of a fracture (pseudoarthrosis).

SPECIFIC EXAMINATIONS

CERVICAL SPINE

In the cervical part of the spine evaluate the vertebrae, the articulations between them (the facet joints posteriorly and the intervertebral discs anteriorly), and the structures that are totally or partially contained within these bone structures (the spinal cord, the cervical nerve roots, and the vertebral artery).

Inspect the spine for gross deformities and visible muscle spasm. Among the possible deformities are absence of the normal cervical lordosis, or abnormal

TABLE 17–5. Some Causes of Muscle Weakness

Congenital
  Muscular dystrophies: limb-girdle,
    facioscapulohumeral, Duchenne,
    myotonic
  Glycogen storage diseases: Pompe's,
    McArdle's
  Inherited spinal muscular atrophies,
    myositis ossificans

Infectious
  Virus: influenza
  Bacteria: tuberculosis, pyogens, syphilis
  Parasites: trichinosis, toxoplasmosis,
    trypanosomiasis

Toxic
  Alcohol
  Heavy metals: mercury, lead, arsenic
  Corticosteroids
  Organophosphates
  Drugs: vincristine, Adriamycin, heroin,
    chloroquine, etc.
  Botulism

Metabolic
  Hyperthyroidism
  Hypothyroidism
  Hypokalemia
  Hypophosphatemia
  Hypocalcemia
  Hypomagnesemia

Hypoglycemia
Diabetes mellitus
Cushing's disease
Addison's disease
Hyperparathyroidism
Hyperaldosteronism
Acromegaly
Malnutrition

Vascular insufficiency

Immune/idiopathic
  Myasthenia gravis
  Scleroderma
  Systemic lupus erythematosus
  Polyarteritis nodosa
  Rheumatoid arthritis
  Polymyalgia rheumatica
  Sarcoidosis
  Polymyositis/dermatomyositis

Traumatic
  Exercise
  Injury
  Seizure

Neoplastic
  Carcinomatous myopathy
  Eaton-Lambert syndrome
  Carcinoid myopathy

TABLE 17–6. Some Causes of Bony Masses or Swelling

Trauma
  Heterotopic bone; myositis ossificans
  Fracture callus
  Fracture

Infection
  Osteomyelitis
  Tuberculosis
  Syphilis
  Typhoid periositis

Metabolic disease
  Rickets
  Scurvy
  Acromegaly
  Paget's disease

Tumor
  Osteoma
  Chondroma
  Fibrocystic disease
  Giant cell tumor
  Angioma/angiosarcoma
  Osteogenic sarcoma
  Periosteal fibrosarcoma
  Ewing's sarcoma
  Metastatic tumor to bone
  Myeloma
  Neurofibroma

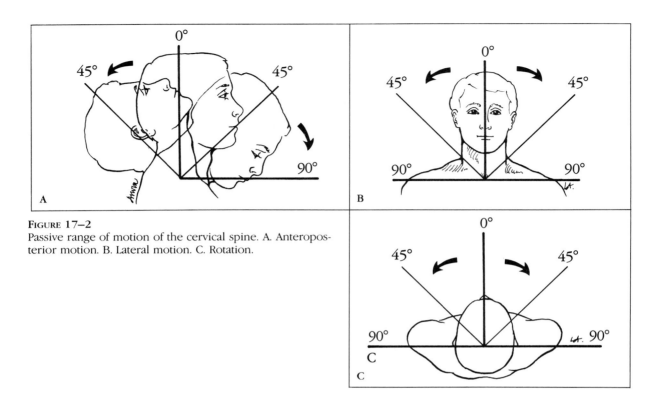

FIGURE 17–2
Passive range of motion of the cervical spine. A. Anteroposterior motion. B. Lateral motion. C. Rotation.

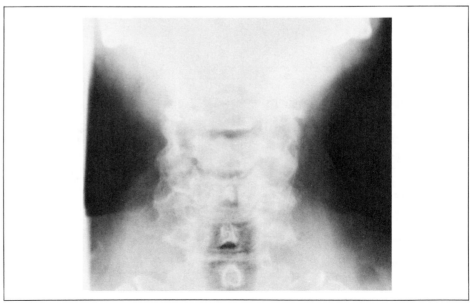

FIGURE 17–3
Roentgenogram showing osteoarthritis of the cervical spine.

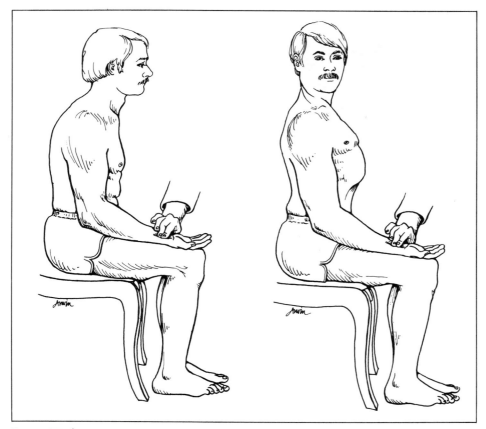

FIGURE 17–4
Adson maneuver.

shortness of the neck, which may be associated with congenital malformation of the cervical vertebrae. Determine the active and passive range of motion of the cervical spine in flexion, extension, lateral bending, and rotation (Fig. 17–2). *Do not* perform this maneuver on patients with severe rheumatoid arthritis or those who have sustained recent neck injury, as serious damage to the spinal cord may result. Transient giddiness or even unconsciousness that is induced by a particular head or neck position suggests temporary occlusion of a vertebral artery within the neck. This diagnosis may be suspected on physical examination but must be confirmed by arteriography.

Palpate the tips of the spinous processes for general alignment and for points of tenderness. Palpate the cervical muscles—which include the posterior paraspinal muscle group, the trapezius muscle, the sternocleidomastoid muscle, and the scalene muscles—for tenderness and muscle spasm. Decreased motion of the cervical spine associated with points of tenderness to palpation over the spinous processes is commonly seen in tumors and infections of the cervical vertebrae, as well as in degenerative, prolapsed, and herniated cervical intervertebral discs (Fig. 17–3).

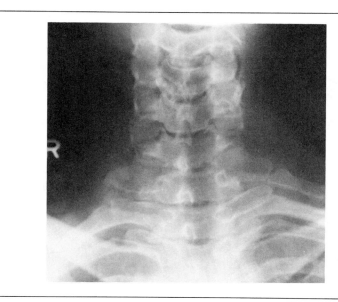

FIGURE 17–5
Roentgenogram showing cervical rib.

Palpate the cervical spine anteriorly, with the palpating finger passing medial to the carotid vessels and lateral to the trachea and esophagus. Tenderness is noted in the presence of disc lesions, infections, and certain tumors.

Maintain the neck in extension by having the patient look at the ceiling for 60 seconds. This test will produce discomfort in the base of the neck, the interscapular region of the back, or the lateral aspect of the shoulders or arms when there are degenerative changes involving either the cervical intervertebral discs (anteriorly) or the facet joints (posteriorly). Vertically compress the extended cervical spine by pressing on the head. This will intensify discomfort in the same areas in the presence of degenerative, prolapsed, or herniated intervertebral discs.

Increase in the symptoms on vertical compression of the extended cervical spine with the head tilted to the side indicates degenerative changes in the facet joints or the uncovertebral articulations (so-called joints of Luschka).

Examine the *thoracic outlet* routinely as part of the examination of the cervical spine. Palpate the supraclavicular fossae for muscle spasm, vascular thrills, masses, and points of tenderness. Perform the *Adson maneuver* with the patient sitting with the forearms in supination and resting on the thighs (Fig. 17–4). Palpate the radial pulse on the side to be tested. Instruct the patient to extend the neck and turn the chin to the side to be tested. The transient disappearance of the radial pulse during inspiration signifies temporary occlusion of the subclavian artery as the anterior scalene muscle is tensed (by extension of the neck and rotation of the skull) while the "floor" of the thoracic outlet rises during inspiration. This may be due to the presence of a cervical rib, for example (Fig. 17–5). Compression of the

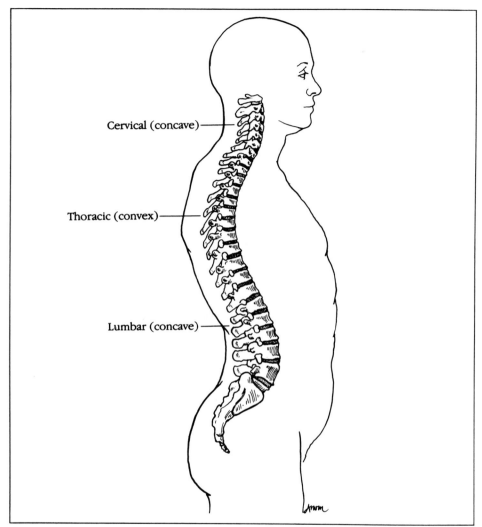

FIGURE 17–6
Normal spinal contours.

brachial plexus in the supraclavicular fossa is suggested by intensification of pain and paresthesia in the arm as the Adson maneuver is performed, by tenderness to palpation over the brachial plexus, and by neurologic changes in arm and hand (particularly a decrease in the ability to appreciate light touch over the fourth and fifth fingers of the hand). These signs may be intensified as the shoulder is abducted and externally rotated. Measure the circumference of the upper arm and forearm and compare the measurements with those of the opposite arm. Test muscle strength, sensory modalities, and deep tendon reflexes in the upper extremity.

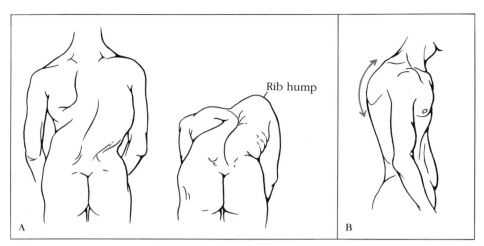

FIGURE 17–7
Deformities of the thoracic spine. A. Scoliosis. B. Kyphosis.

THORACIC SPINE
Palpate the tips of the spinous processes for general alignment and points of tenderness. Test the motion of the thoracic spine during flexion, extension, and lateral bending and observe the symmetry of the ribs. Small rotational deformities of the thoracic spine that produce asymmetry of the rib cage are best appreciated by inspecting the flexed thoracic spine and rib cage from the rear (Fig. 17–7).

LUMBAR SPINE
Note the contour of the lumbar spine with the patient standing. A lumbar lordosis is normally present; its absence suggests a spinal abnormality. Palpate the paraspinal muscles for tenderness and spasm; palpate the tips of the spinous processes, noting their general alignment and any points of tenderness that may be present. Carefully differentiate spinal tenderness from flank tenderness, which would indicate an abnormality in the retroperitoneal space. When a spondylolisthesis is present, anterior displacement of the superior spinal segment produces a "step" deformity in which the spinous processes of the superior (cephalad) segment can be palpated anterior to those of the inferior (caudal) segment. Test the range of lumbar motion in flexion, extension, lateral bending, and rotation (Fig. 17–8). Limitation of flexion exerted by tightness of the hamstring muscles in the posterior aspect of the thigh is associated with spondylolisthesis and less commonly with tumors, arachnoiditis, and herniated intervertebral discs in the lumbar and lower thoracic regions (Fig. 17–9).

Perform the straight-leg-raising test with the patient lying supine on the examining table. Flex the hip with the knee in full extension by raising the foot (Fig. 17–10). A sharp pain traveling from the lower back or buttock down the posterior aspect of the leg indicates irritation of the sciatic nerve or its roots of origin within the spine (Table 17–9). In the absence of such irritation, this maneuver may be limited by muscle tightness at the back of the thigh but not by sharp pain.

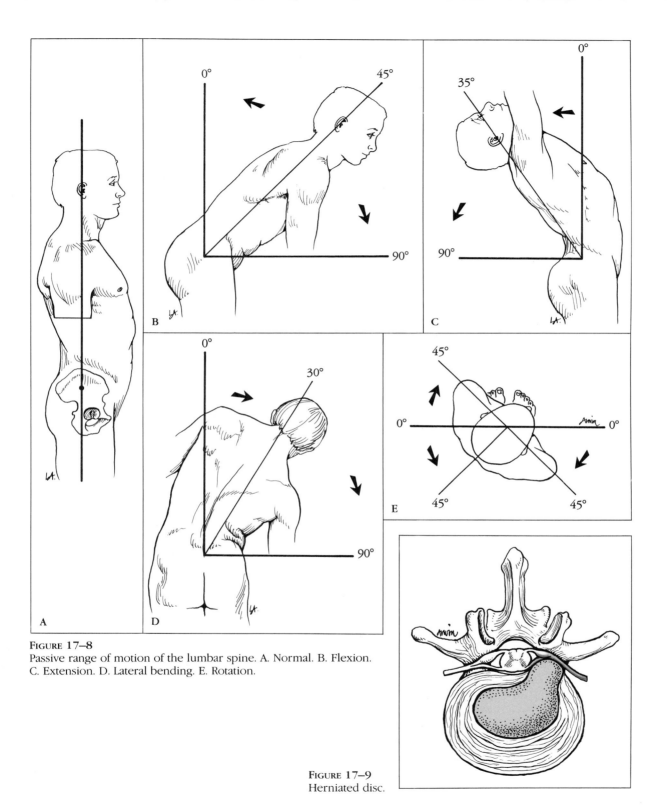

FIGURE 17–8
Passive range of motion of the lumbar spine. A. Normal. B. Flexion.
C. Extension. D. Lateral bending. E. Rotation.

FIGURE 17–9
Herniated disc.

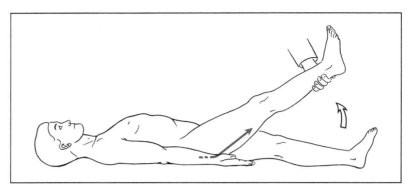

FIGURE 17–10
Straight-leg-raising test.

TABLE 17–7. Signs of Disc Disease of the Lumbar Spine

Diminished or obliterated lumbar lordosis
Decreased flexion of spine
Painful extension of spine
Asymmetrical limitation in straight-leg raising
Percussion tenderness over affected disc
Atrophic change in muscle mass of affected leg (occasionally seen)
Focal muscle weakness in affected leg
Sensory loss in a dermatomal distribution
Absent deep tendon reflex (patellar or achilles)

As part of the complete physical evaluation you will, of course, perform a rectal examination, a brief evaluation of the urinary tract, an examination of the abdomen, and an evaluation of the femoral pulses. Prostatic disease in men, pelvic abnormalities in women, and diseases of the kidneys and ureters may produce discomfort in the lower back. Occlusion of the distal aorta or of the hypogastric arteries, as well as an abdominal aortic aneurysm, may produce pain in the lower back or in the buttocks.

Tenderness to palpation over the lumbar spinous processes associated with limited motion of the spine may indicate disc lesions, osteoarthritis, spondylolisthesis, tumor, or infection. Laxity of the sacroiliac joints may be detected by palpation while the patient, standing erect, lifts first one knee and then the other ("marching in place"). A click can be felt if subluxation of the sacroiliac joint occurs. With the patient supine, stress the articulation between the fifth lumbar vertebra and sacrum by acutely flexing the patient's hips and knees. Resultant pain in the lower back suggests a mechanical abnormality at the lumbosacral articulation. Tilting the pelvis in this position by rocking the knees to the left and right causes pain when abnormalities of the sacroiliac joint are present.

Measure the leg length from the anterosuperior spine to the medial malleolus.

TABLE 17–8. Localization of Ruptured Disc of the Lumbar Spine

Disc	Pain	Paresthesias	Weakness	Atrophy	Reflexes
L_3–L_4 (3–5%)	Anterior thigh	Anteromedian thigh	Quadriceps	Thigh	Decreased or absent knee jerk
L_4–L_5 (45%)	Posterior thigh, calf, top of foot	Medial dorsal foot, great toe	Anterior tibialis, dorsiflexors, toes	Lower leg	Normal knee jerk, normal or slightly decreased ankle jerk
L_5–S_1 (50%)	Posterior thigh, calf, ankle	Lateral dorsal foot, small toe	Calf, plantar flexors, toes	Calf	Decreased or absent ankle jerk

TABLE 17–9. Some Causes of Sciatica

Nerve root compression
In the spinal cord
  Protruded disc
  Tumor
  Abscess
In the intervertebral foramen
  Arthritis of the spine
  Vertebral collapse
  Tumor of the nerve in the foramen
  Extruded disc
  Inflammatory synovitis of the facet
    joint (Marie-Strümpell disease)
In the pelvis or buttocks
  Intrapelvic tumor
  Intrapelvic or gluteal abscess

Inflammatory, metabolic, or vascular disease of the nerve
Toxins
  Alcohol
  Heavy metals
Diabetes mellitus
Syphilis
Direct trauma to the nerve

Measure the circumference of the thigh and calf and compare the measurements with those of the opposite leg. Test muscle power of the dorsiflexors and plantar flexors of the foot and ankle by having the patient support the body weight on the toes and on the heels. Test deep tendon reflexes at the knee and ankle and the sensory modalities of light touch, pain, and position sense.

SHOULDER
Inspect the shoulder anteriorly and posteriorly and look for loss of normal contour and muscle atrophy. Three major muscles are easily visible about the shoulder: (1) deltoid (which covers the shoulder anteriorly, laterally, and posteriorly), (2) supraspinatus, and (3) infraspinatus, the last two of which originate on the posterior border of the scapula above and below the scapular spine. Visible atrophy of the deltoid muscle follows disuse, injury to the axillary nerve, diseases of muscle, and diseases of the nervous system, such as amyotrophic lateral sclerosis. Visible atrophy of the supraspinatus and infraspinatus muscles is seen following nerve injury, diseases of the nervous system, tears of the insertion of these muscles into the rotator cuff of the shoulder, and calcific tendinitis involving that portion of the

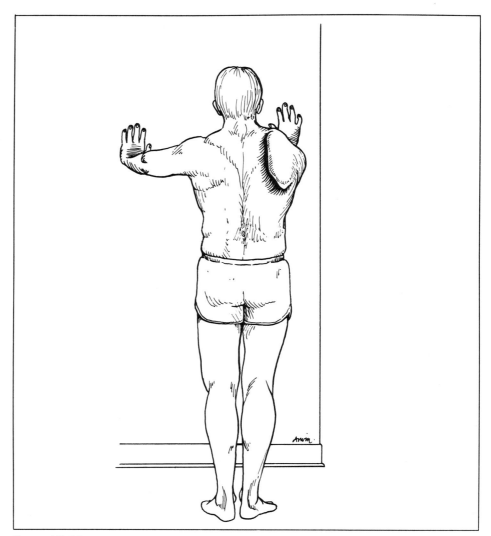

FIGURE 17–11
Winging of the scapula in injury of the nerve to the anterior serratus muscle.

rotator cuff that represents their insertion. Determine the function of the anterior serratus muscle by having the patient push with both hands against a wall. The medial border of the scapula is not held firmly against the chest wall but is displaced posteriorly ("wings") when weakness of the anterior serratus muscle is present (Fig. 17–11). Weakness of this muscle frequently follows injury to the long thoracic nerve of Bell either in the neck or in the axilla.

Note the bony contour of the shoulder and the position of the humeral head. Flattening of the lateral portion of the shoulder is seen when the humeral head is not in its proper position but is displaced, as in a subcoracoid dislocation of the shoulder. Prominence of the distal end of the clavicle indicates a dislocation of the acromioclavicular joint or a tumor of the distal end of the clavicle.

Carefully palpate the structures about the shoulder, particularly the rotator cuff, for points of tenderness. The rotator cuff of the shoulder represents the insertion of the subscapularis, supraspinatus, infraspinatus, and teres minor muscles into the proximal humerus. Tenderness to palpation of a segment of the rotator cuff indicates a rotator cuff tear or calcific tendinitis. Diffuse tenderness over the entire cuff suggests pericapsulitis (frozen shoulder) or synovitis of the joint. Tenderness over the long head of the biceps tendon as it lies in the bicipital groove between the greater and lesser tuberosities of the humerus suggests tendinitis of the biceps tendon. This diagnosis is further suggested if shoulder pain is accentuated when the forearm is flexed and supinated against resistance.

Determine the effects of active and passive motion of the shoulder and compare with the opposite side (Fig. 17–12). If passive motion of the shoulder is normal but active motion is limited, a tear of the rotator cuff or muscle weakness about the shoulder should be suspected. If active and passive motion are both limited to an equal degree, contractures, arthritis, or a mechanical block (such as calcific tendinitis) should be suspected. Test sensation over the lateral portion of the shoulder, which is supplied by the axillary nerve.

Before putting the patient who gives shoulder pain as a major complaint through vigorous maneuvers, ascertain by careful history and physical examination of other systems that the shoulder pain is not referred from the heart or abdomen (Table 17–10).

ELBOW

Note the contour and the carrying angle of the elbow. The latter is the angle formed by the upper and lower arm when the elbow is observed from the front with the forearm in full extension and supination (Fig. 17–13). Change in this angle may be seen following damage to the elbow from trauma, rheumatoid arthritis, or osteoarthritis. Determine the relationship between the olecranon and the medial and lateral epicondyles, which form a triangle. Note points of tenderness and the presence of palpable effusion of synovitis within the joint. Palpate the head of the radius and the tissue just anterior to it for points of tenderness as the forearm is supinated and pronated.

Tenderness lateral or anterior to the radial head may indicate lateral epicondylitis ("tennis elbow") and may be accentuated as the patient pronates the forearm and extends the wrist against resistance (Fig. 17–14). Palpate the ulnar nerve in the groove in the posterior aspect of the medial condyle of the humerus. Localized tenderness over the ulnar nerve at this spot suggests irritation of the nerve, which frequently follows fractures about the elbow. It may be associated with pain and paresthesia in the fourth and fifth fingers and weakness of those muscles in the hand supplied by the ulnar nerve (adductor pollicis, third and fourth lumbricales, interossei, flexor carpi ulnaris, flexor digitorum profundus III and IV, and abductor digiti minimi) (Fig. 17–15). Test the active and passive ranges of motion of the elbow in flexion, extension, supination, and pronation and compare with the opposite side (Fig. 17–16). Palpate the subcutaneous surfaces of the proximal ulna

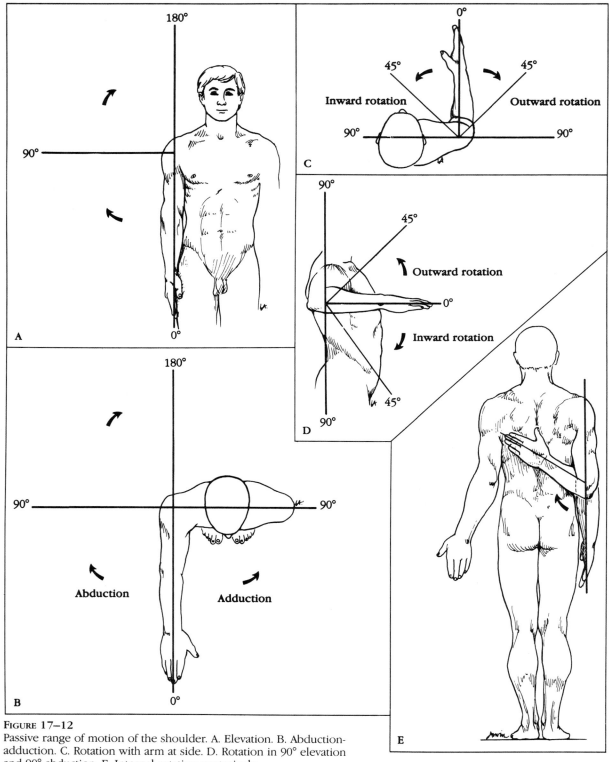

FIGURE 17–12

Passive range of motion of the shoulder. A. Elevation. B. Abduction-adduction. C. Rotation with arm at side. D. Rotation in 90° elevation and 90° abduction. E. Internal rotation posteriorly.

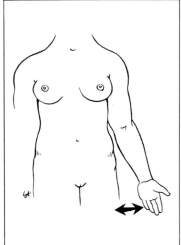

FIGURE 17–13
Normal carrying angle of the elbow.

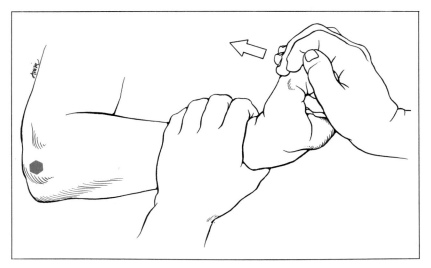

FIGURE 17–14
Cozen's test. Dorsiflexion of the wrist against resistance causes pain in the area of the lateral epicondyle in epicondylitis (tennis elbow).

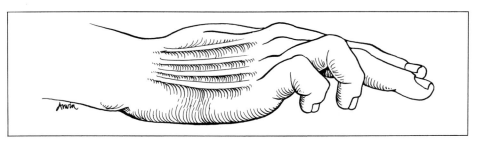

FIGURE 17–15
Position of fourth and fifth fingers and atrophy of hand muscles in ulnar nerve palsy.

TABLE 17–10. Some Causes of Shoulder Pain

Originating in the shoulder
Trauma
Arthritis
Bursitis
Myositis
Neuritis (brachial plexus)
Tendinitis (calcific tendinitis)

Originating outside the shoulder (referred pain)
Cardiac ischemia or infarction
Pleuritis
Lung tumor
Pneumothorax
Gastric or duodenal disease
Gallbladder or liver disease
Pancreatic disease
Subdiaphragmatic irritation (fluid, pus)
Neurologic disease of cervical spine

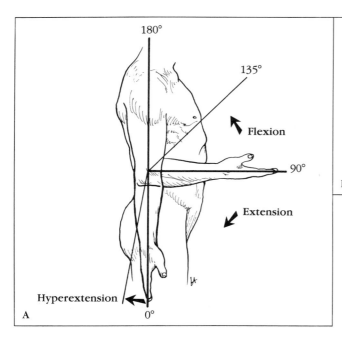

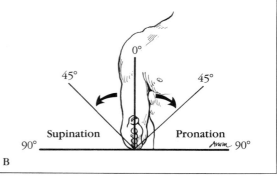

Figure 17–16
Passive range of motion of the elbow. A. Flexion and extension. B. Forearm (elbow and wrist).

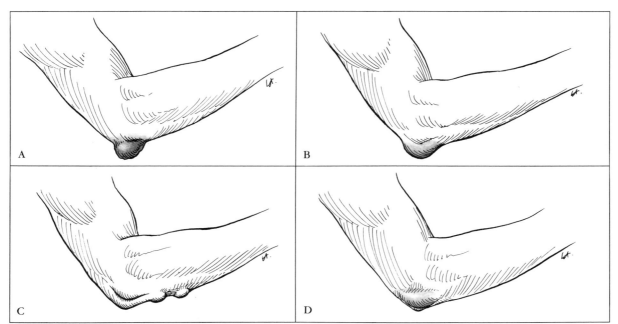

Figure 17–17
Some lesions of the elbow. A. Gouty tophus is deposited over the olecranon. Elbow may be inflamed, tender, and firm to palpation and may drain chalky material. B. Bursa may be inflamed or swollen or both. Bursitis may be caused by trauma, infection (staphylococcus), or rheumatoid arthritis. Elbow is tender and boggy. C. Rheumatoid nodules are firm, non-tender nodules at pressure points on the ulna. D. The arthritic elbow has fluid or boggy synovium in the groove between the epicondyle and olecranon. Elbow is inflamed, tender, and swollen.

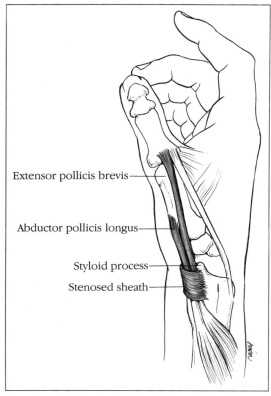

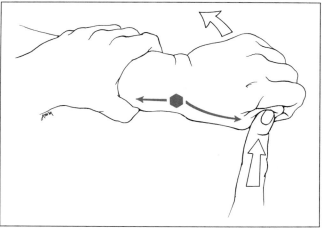

FIGURE 17–19
Finkelstein's test. The patient makes a fist enclosing the thumb. Pressure on the fist into ulnar deviation induces pain in the radial styloid process that may radiate to the thumb or toward the elbow.

FIGURE 17–18
De Quervain's disease. This condition occurs only in adults, generally women. In chronic circumstances a small swelling may be felt just proximal to the styloid process. Fine crepitus may also be present.

for nodules that are often found with rheumatoid arthritis, even when rheumatoid involvement of the elbow is not present (Fig. 17–17).

WRIST
Observe the contour of the wrist and note any fullness about the joint. Palpate the bony and tendinous structures about the wrist for tenderness and nodularity. Tenderness over the anatomic snuffbox in the lateral aspect of the wrist may be associated with abnormality of the navicular or greater multangular bones. Tenderness over the lateral aspect of the distal radius suggests inflammation of the tendon sheaths of the extensor pollicis brevis and the abductor pollicis longus, *de Quervain's disease* (Fig. 17–18). The diagnosis is confirmed when a tender nodule can be felt within one or both of the tendons over the lateral aspect of the distal radius and when a positive Finkelstein's test is noted. Perform *Finkelstein's test* (Fig. 17–19) by moving the wrist rapidly into ulnar deviation as the patient holds the thumb

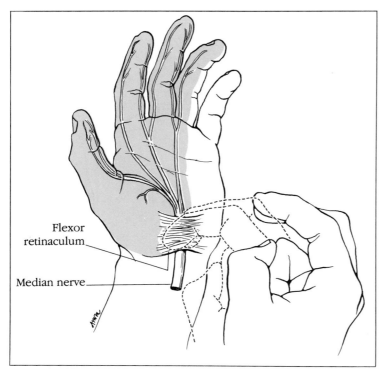

FIGURE 17–20
Tinel's sign. Strike the median nerve in the wrist as it passes through the carpal tunnel. A tingling sensation radiating from the wrist to the hand is a positive test.

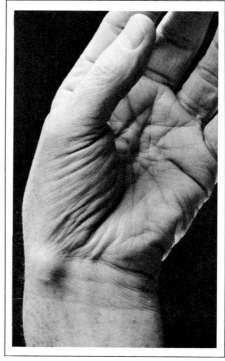

FIGURE 17–21
Ganglion of the wrist.

TABLE 17–11. Some Causes of the Carpal Tunnel Syndrome

Idiopathic
Local trauma
Synovitis of the wrist or flexor tendons
Ganglion of the wrist
Acromegaly
Hypothyroidism
Pregnancy
Fracture about the wrist

flexed in the palm. The test result is positive if it induces sudden pain that extends to the thumb or toward the elbow.

Compression of the median nerve at the wrist causes tenderness over the nerve, loss of normal sensation in the portion of the hand supplied by this nerve—the flexor surfaces of the thumb, the index and middle fingers, and the lateral half of the ring finger—and weakness of those muscles of the thumb supplied by the

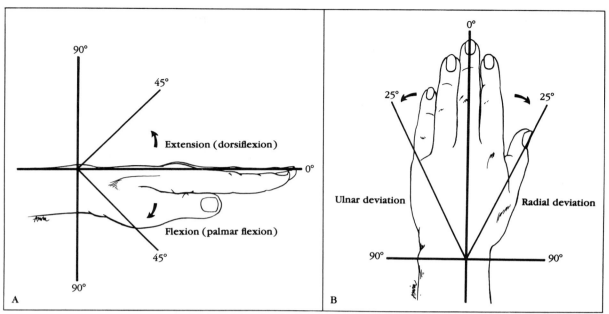

FIGURE 17–22
Passive range of motion of the wrist. A. Flexion and extension. B. Lateral deviation.

median nerve, i.e., carpal tunnel syndrome (some causes of which are presented in Table 17–11). In addition, percussion over the median nerve at the wrist will produce pain or tingling radiating distally into the hand—a positive *Tinel's sign* (Fig. 17–20).

A *ganglion* is the result of myxomatous degeneration of a portion of connective tissue in a joint capsule. The cystlike swelling may occur on ankle, foot, or finger, but is more common on the wrist (Fig. 17–21). The swelling is not inflamed but may be slightly tender.

The wrist may also be the site of arthritis (rheumatoid, infective, gouty) and trauma.

HAND

Inspect the hand for deformities. Test active and passive ranges of motion of the fingers for evidence of nerve injury, tendon rupture, muscle fibrosis, joint contracture, or arthritis. Test the function of each muscle to the fingers and wrist. The normal range of motion of the wrist is illustrated in Fig. 17–22. The presence of nodules within the palm, associated with firm fibrous bands that limit extension of the fingers suggests *Dupuytren's contracture*. A palpable nodule within a flexor tendon overlying a metacarpophalangeal joint, associated with a palpable click as the finger is flexed or extended, suggests a *trigger finger* in which a nodular enlargement of a flexor tendon snaps into or out of the fibrous tunnel through which it passes.

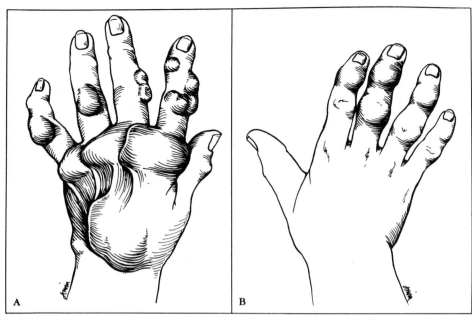

FIGURE 17–23
A. Rheumatoid arthritis. B. Osteoarthritis.

TABLE 17–12. Some Differential Diagnostic Aids to Distinguish Rheumatoid from Degenerative Arthritis

Features	Rheumatoid Arthritis	Osteoarthritis
Age at onset	Younger, but may occur at any age	Older (40+ years)
Onset	May be explosive or gradual	Generally insidious
Systemic symptoms (fever, malaise)	Present	Absent
Joint involvement	Often symmetrical, progressive	Localized, affects the most active joints
Inflammation	Common	Less common
Effusion	Common	Uncommon
Subcutaneous nodules	May be present	Absent
Activity	Increases pain in active joint	Ameliorates pain in active joint
Extra-articular involvement	May be present	Absent
Sedimentation rate	Increased	Often normal
X-ray changes	Erosion	Hypertrophy

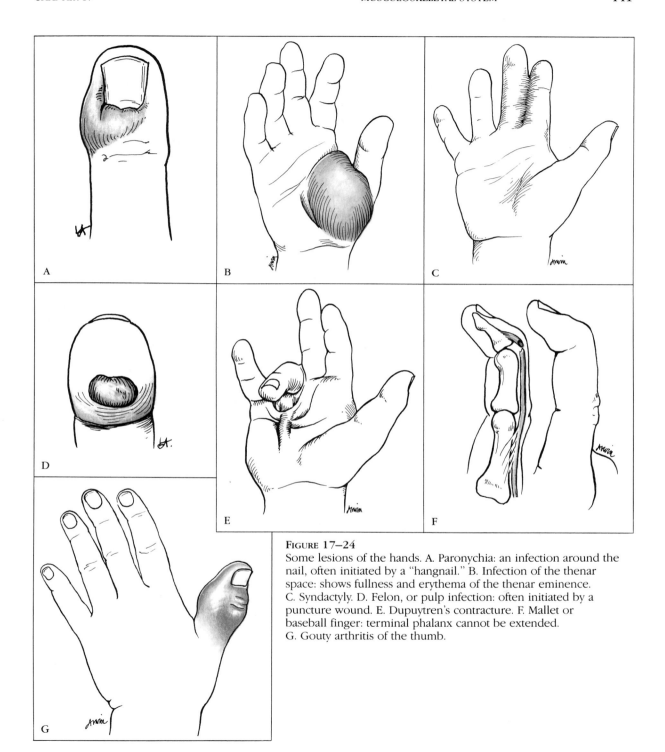

FIGURE 17–24
Some lesions of the hands. A. Paronychia: an infection around the nail, often initiated by a "hangnail." B. Infection of the thenar space: shows fullness and erythema of the thenar eminence. C. Syndactyly. D. Felon, or pulp infection: often initiated by a puncture wound. E. Dupuytren's contracture. F. Mallet or baseball finger: terminal phalanx cannot be extended. G. Gouty arthritis of the thumb.

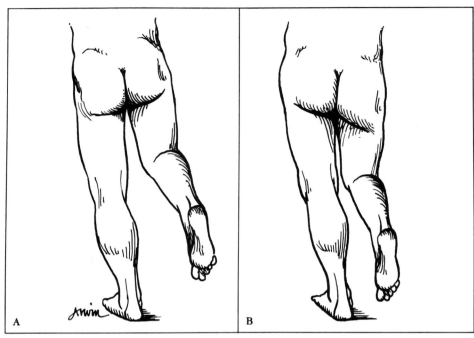

FIGURE 17–25
Trendelenburg's sign. A. Normal. The right side of the pelvis rises when weight is borne on the left leg. B. Positive Trendelenburg's sign of the left hip. The right side of the pelvis falls when weight is borne on the left leg.

Nodules along the distal interphalangeal joints *(Heberden's nodes)* occur in degenerative osteoarthritis. These nodules must be distinguished from the *tophi* of chronic gout. Carpal, proximal, and middle interphalangeal joint deformity, swelling, and erythema—all of which symmetrically involve both hands—are characteristic of rheumatoid arthritis (Table 17–12 and Fig. 17–23). Figure 17–24 illustrates some common lesions of the hand.

HIP
Examination of the hip begins with the initial evaluation of the patient's gait. Leg-length inequality, muscle weakness, habit patterns, fusion, contractures, and pain-producing lesions of the hip, knee, ankle, and foot all may produce abnormalities of gait. Fairly specific for abnormality of the hip, however, is the *Trendelenburg gait,* which is marked by a fall of the pelvis, rather than the normal rise, on the side opposite the involved hip when it is weight bearing (Fig. 17–25). This indicates weakness of the abductor muscles due to intrinsic muscle disease, lack of normal innervation of the muscle, or an unstable hip joint. In the antalgic ("antipain") gait of hip disease, the patient attempts to minimize the force borne through the hip by leaning over the involved hip as weight is borne through it. This moves the body's center of gravity toward the hip joint, decreasing the force exerted on the hip and thus decreasing the discomfort.

Palpate the hip anteriorly for points of tenderness and fullness within the joint. The location of the femoral head is approximately 1 inch distal and 1 inch lateral to the point at which the femoral artery crosses the inguinal ligament. In addition, palpate the greater trochanter laterally and the ischial tuberosity posteriorly. Inflamed bursae in either of these locations may account for pain in the hip region. Although more than 18 bursae have been described about the hip, only four of these are commonly affected clinically. When the iliopectineal bursa is inflamed, tenderness may be present over the anterior hip at about the midpoint of the inguinal ligament. Pain will occur on extension, internal rotation, or adduction of the hip and may radiate down the front of the leg.

Patients with ischiogluteal bursitis have great tenderness over the ischial tuberosity. It develops in those whose jobs require long periods of sitting on hard surfaces *(weaver's bottom)*.

Deep trochanteric bursitis may present as pain on any movement of the hip, radiating down the back of the thigh. There is tenderness over the greater trochanter.

Superficial trochanteric bursitis presents as pain and swelling over the bursa, without pain on motion of the hip. Test the range of motion of the hip in flexion, extension, abduction, adduction, and rotation (Fig. 17–26). Test for flexion contracture of the hip by maximally flexing the opposite hip with the patient supine on the examining table. In this maneuver the pelvis is flexed on the lumbar spine, and any lumbar lordosis present is eliminated (Fig. 17–27). If a flexion contracture is present, the involved thigh will flex. The angle that the involved thigh forms with the surface of the examining table indicates the degree of contracture (Thomas test). Determine the strength of the flexor, extensor, abductor, and adductor muscle groups by having the patient move the thigh against the resistance of the examiner's hand.

KNEE

Inspect the knee for joint swelling and gross deformity, and the thigh for atrophy of the quadriceps muscle group, which may indicate a significant knee abnormality.

Test for excessive fluid within the knee joint by pressing the patella against the femur with the knee in full extension and gently tapping one side of the joint while feeling for a fluid wave on the other side of the joint. In addition, note whether ballottement of the patella is possible (Fig. 17–28). Palpate about the joint line, about the circumference of the patella, over the attachments of the medial and lateral collateral ligaments, over the anserine bursa (on the medial posterior aspect of the proximal tibia about 1 inch distal to the joint line), and in the popliteal fossa. When tenderness is noted over the medial or lateral joint line, a torn meniscus is suspected (Fig. 17–29). Tenderness about the patella suggests osteoarthritis or chondromalacia. The diagnosis is confirmed if crepitation and pain are elicited when the patella is moved medially, laterally, proximally, and distally while it is firmly pressed against the underlying femur. Tenderness over the medial or lateral collateral ligament suggests a tear of the ligament or an inflamed bursa between the ligament and the bone. Tenderness over the prepatellar bursa or in the popliteal fossa suggests symptomatic bursitis in these regions (Fig. 17–30).

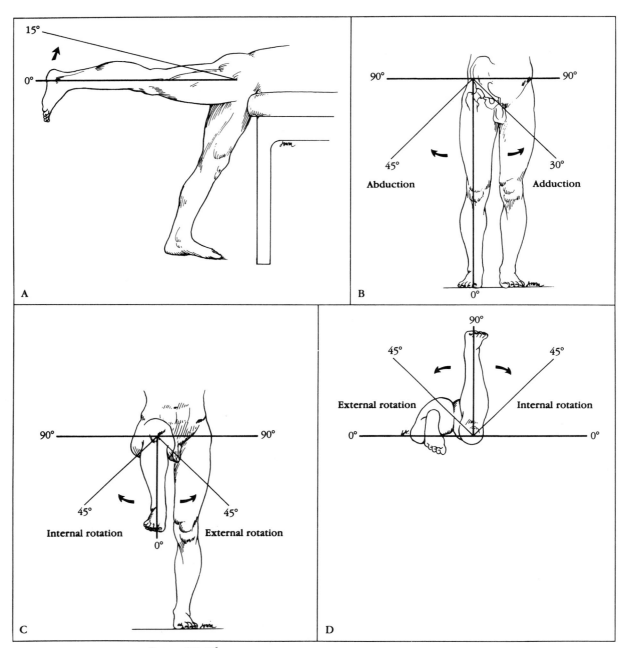

FIGURE 17–26
Passive range of motion of the hip. A. Extension. B. Lateral motion. C. Rotation in flexion. D. Rotation in extension (prone).

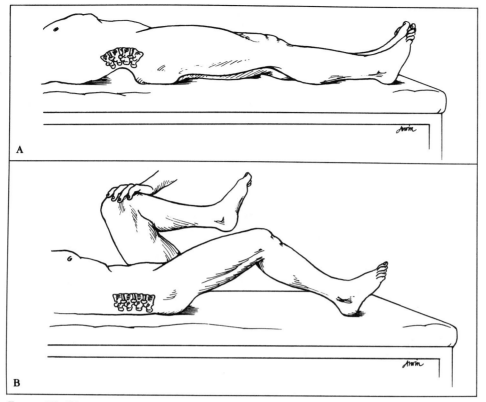

FIGURE 17–27
Thomas test. A. With the patient supine, a flexion contracture of the hip may be masked by lordosis of the lumbar spine. B. When the lumbar lordosis is eliminated by maximally flexing the left hip, the angle that the right thigh makes with the examining table designates the degree of flexion contracture in the right hip.

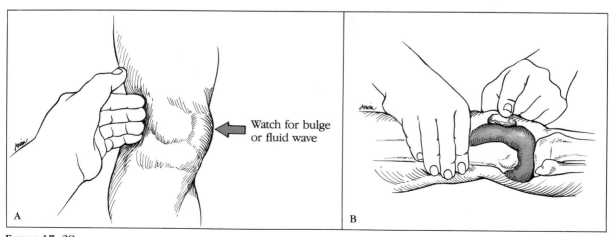

FIGURE 17–28
Testing for fluid in the knee joint. A. The bulge sign. B. The patellar tap will suggest fluid in the knee as the patella clicks against the femur. With greater amounts of knee fluid, the patella will be ballotable.

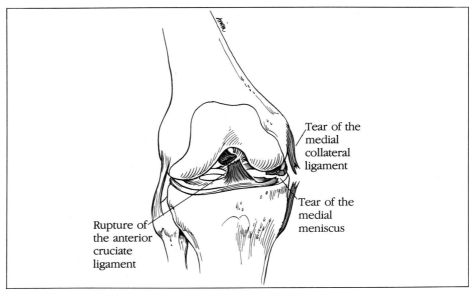

FIGURE 17–29
Three common severe injuries of the knee.

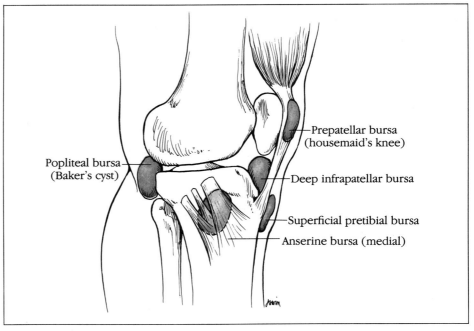

FIGURE 17–30
Common sites of bursitis in the knee.

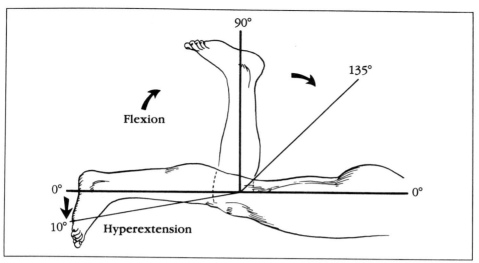

FIGURE 17–31
Passive range of motion of the knee.

Determine the range of motion and compare with the opposite side. Full extension and at least 120 degrees of flexion from full extension are normally present (Fig. 17–31). Palpable crepitation within the knee joint during flexion and extension suggests a mechanical incongruity of the joint that may be the result of arthritic changes, a tear of the medial or lateral meniscus, or a loose fragment of cartilage or bone within the joint. Locking of the joint during flexion or extension signifies a mechanical block within the joint, most commonly a torn meniscus or a bone fragment. A mechanical block preventing full extension, or a contracture of the posterior capsule, is suggested when the knee cannot be fully extended passively. Test for a positive spring sign, which indicates a mechanical block with the consistency of cartilage, by maximally extending the knee passively and then forcibly extending the knee further. The joint will extend and then quickly snap back into flexion when the sign is positive. A torn meniscus is further suggested by a positive McMurray sign. To evoke this sign (Fig. 17–32), flex the knee fully with the patient recumbent, steadying the knee with one hand, and slowly extend the knee while holding the tibia in internal rotation. A palpable or audible snap associated with momentary discomfort as the knee is extended suggests a tear in that portion of the lateral meniscus that was between the femoral condyle and the tibial plateau when the snap occurred. This test is repeated with the tibia held in external rotation, which tests the posterior aspect of the medial meniscus. This test is generally not positive when the tear involves the anterior one-third of either meniscus.

Test the integrity of the medial collateral ligament by attempting to force the knee into valgus (knock-knee) deformity with the knee in full extension. If more than 5 to 10 degrees of deformity can be produced, instability of the medial collateral ligament is suspected. Test the lateral collateral ligament by attempting to force the knee into varus (bowleg) deformity with the knee in full extension (Fig. 17–

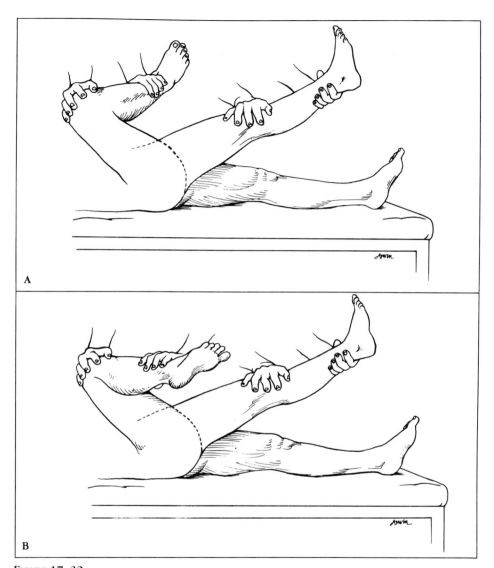

FIGURE 17–32
McMurray maneuver. A. Extension in internal rotation. A palpable or audible snap suggests a lesion in the lateral meniscus. B. Extension in external rotation. A palpable or audible snap suggests a lesion in the medial meniscus.

33). Again, if more than 5 to 10 degrees of deformity can be produced, instability of the ligament is suspected. Test the cruciate ligaments with the patient sitting with the knees flexed to 90 degrees. If the tibia can be pulled anteriorly from under the femur (a positive drawer sign), laxity of the anterior cruciate ligament is present (Fig. 17–34). If the tibia can be pushed posteriorly under the femur, laxity of the posterior cruciate ligament is present.

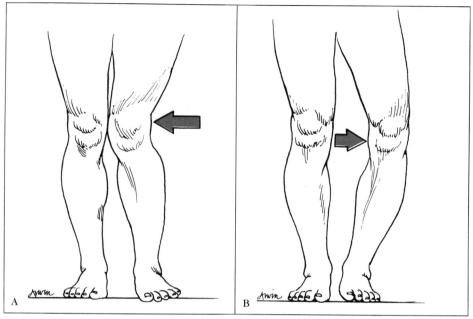

FIGURE 17–33
Forced valgus and varus. A. Forced valgus suggests instability of the medial collateral ligament. B. Forced varus suggests instability of the lateral collateral ligament.

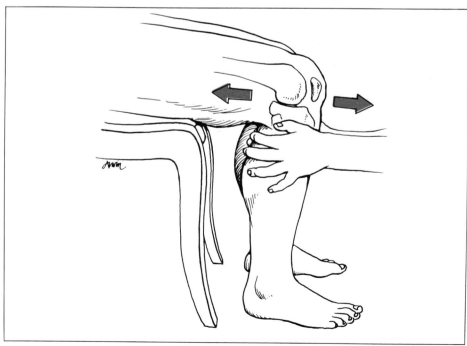

FIGURE 17–34
Drawer sign.

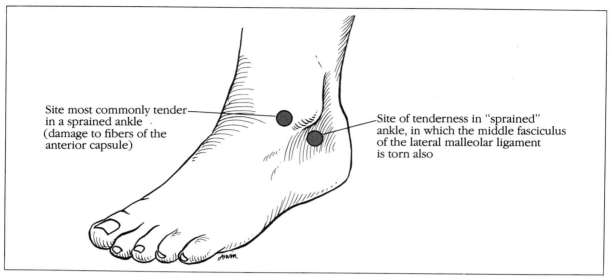

Site most commonly tender in a sprained ankle (damage to fibers of the anterior capsule)

Site of tenderness in "sprained" ankle, in which the middle fasciculus of the lateral malleolar ligament is torn also

FIGURE 17–35
Sprained ankle. A *sprain* implies that no fracture has occurred but the ligaments of the ankle have been stretched, with but a few fibers torn. In more severe injury the term *ligament rupture* should be used.

ANKLE

Inspect the ankle for gross deformity or swelling and palpate for points of tenderness or fullness within the joint. Tenderness over the medial or lateral malleolus suggests previous injury to these bony structures. Tenderness distal to the tip of the medial or lateral malleoli but over the medial or lateral ligaments of the ankle suggests previous injury to these ligaments. Common sites of tenderness with acute trauma (sprain) are shown in Figure 17–35. Tenderness just anterior to the Achilles tendon at its insertion into the calcaneus suggests an inflamed bursa, often noted in patients with rheumatoid arthritis. Tenderness over the posterior tibial tendon as it lies just posterior to the medial malleolus or tenderness over the peroneal tendons just behind the lateral malleolus suggests inflammation of these structures. Occasionally tenosynovitis of the posterior tibial tendon or the peroneal tendons, similar to de Quervain's disease of the wrist, is seen. In such cases tenderness is present over the tendon at the point of the constriction posterior to the malleolus. Passive motion of the foot will intensify the discomfort, and a palpable nodule may be present within the tendon itself.

Test the active and passive motions of the ankle joint (Fig. 17–36). At least 10 degrees of plantar flexion and 15 degrees of dorsiflexion should be present. Test the stability of the joint, particularly in inversion and eversion. Normal ankle motion is dorsiflexion and plantar flexion. If tilting of the talus can be demonstrated as the ankle is forced into eversion, instability of the medial collateral ligament is present.

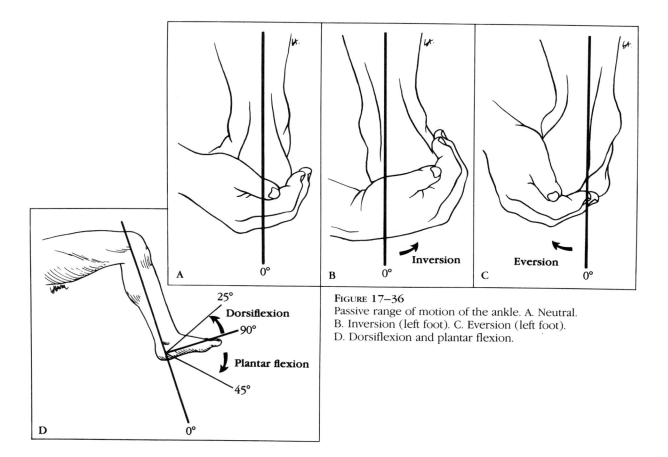

FIGURE 17–36
Passive range of motion of the ankle. A. Neutral.
B. Inversion (left foot). C. Eversion (left foot).
D. Dorsiflexion and plantar flexion.

Determine the strength of the muscles crossing the ankle joint by having the patient support body weight first on the heel and then on the ball of the foot.

FOOT
Inspect the foot for obvious deformities and swelling. Observe the heel from the rear. The axis of the heel is normally a continuation of the long axis of the lower leg. If the heel is tilted toward the midline of the body, the heel is in varus—a deformity frequently associated with clubfoot and cavus foot (Fig. 17–37). If the axis is tilted away from the midline, the heel is in valgus—a deformity associated with flatfeet. A bony prominence just anterior to and below the medial malleolus suggests the presence of an accessory navicular bone, which may be associated with flatfeet and which makes proper shoefitting difficult. A swelling over the medial aspect of the metatarsophalangeal joint of the great toe is termed a bunion and may be associated with a medial deviation of more than 15 degrees when compared with the lateral four metatarsals (metatarsus primus varus), or with lateral deviation of the great toe (hallux valgus). Inspect the toes for abnormalities such as claw-toe, in which the proximal interphalangeal joint is acutely flexed while the

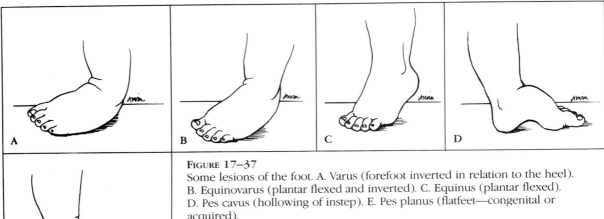

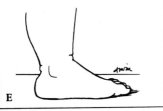

FIGURE 17–37
Some lesions of the foot. A. Varus (forefoot inverted in relation to the heel).
B. Equinovarus (plantar flexed and inverted). C. Equinus (plantar flexed).
D. Pes cavus (hollowing of instep). E. Pes planus (flatfeet—congenital or
acquired).

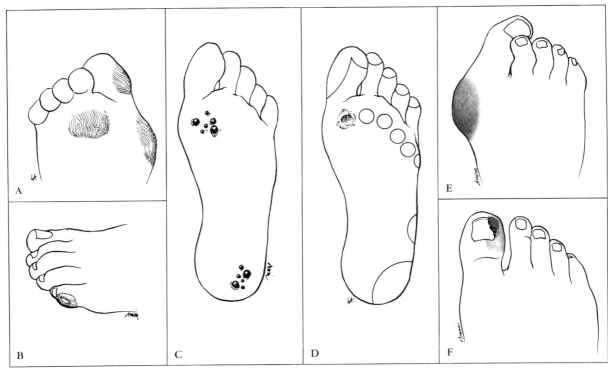

FIGURE 17–38
Some other lesions of the foot. A. Callosity: hard protective layer of skin over stress site. B.
Hard corn: highly compressed keratotic cells with central white core. C. Plantar warts: a viral
infection giving a dark pearl on the skin of the sole; very painful. D. Neurotrophic ulcers:
painless perforations seen in peripheral neuropathies. Most common sites are outlined. E.
Hallux valgus with bunion: proximal phalanx in valgus, often congenital. A bunion is an
inflamed bursa over a hallux valgus. F. Ingrown toenail.

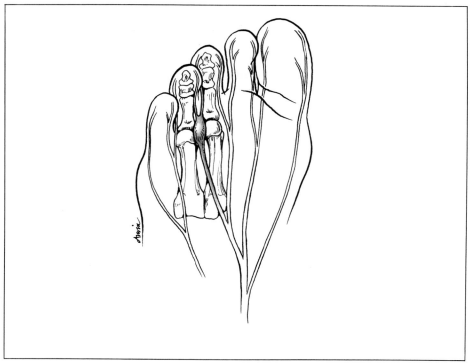

FIGURE 17–39
Plantar neuroma just above the division of the plantar nerve into its terminal branches.

metacarpophalangeal joint remains in neutral position. Inspect the sole of the foot for the presence of calluses over the metatarsal heads (Fig. 17–38). Observe the state of nutrition of the tissues of the foot by palpating the skin, noting the presence or absence of hair on the dorsum of the toes, and palpating the dorsalis pedis and posterior tibial pulses.

Test inversion and eversion of the foot by rocking the heel medially and laterally while stabilizing the lower leg, rotating the foot by supinating and pronating the metatarsals as a unit while stabilizing the heel, and flexing and extending the toes. Test the individual muscles by having the patient perform the appropriate movements against the resistance of the examiner's hand.

Palpate for points of tenderness indicating inflammation of bursae or joints. Diffuse tenderness over the calcaneus itself is often associated with early rheumatoid arthritis or with Reiter's syndrome. Inflammation detected in any of the joints of the foot may be caused by septic arthritis, rheumatoid arthritis, osteoarthritis, or gout. Tenderness to palpation over the metatarsal heads on the ball of the foot indicates metatarsalgia; tenderness between the metatarsal heads on the dorsum of the foot suggests interdigital neuroma. The latter possibility is strengthened if a sensory abnormality can be demonstrated on the opposing surfaces of the contiguous toes supplied by the involved interdigital nerve, and if medial to lateral compression of the forefoot induces metatarsal pain that radiates into the involved toes.

A lancinating pain in the toes and metatarsal tenderness, especially in women, suggests a neuroma just above the division of the plantar nerve into its terminal branches (Fig. 17–39).

CHAPTER 18

NERVOUS SYSTEM

*From the brain, and from the brain only, arise our pleasures, joys,
laughter and jests, as well as our sorrows, pains, griefs, and tears.*

HIPPOCRATES
(460?–377? B.C.)

With practice, the medical student will quickly learn to make a screening neurologic examination part of every physical examination and will find that many parts of the neurologic assessment are already incorporated into the general history and physical examination (e.g., eyes, skeletal-muscular examination).

Evaluation of patients with complaints relevant to the nervous system requires an approach similar to that used in most other branches of medicine. A clear statement of the chief complaint and a coherent chronological history of the principal symptoms and the past history must be obtained. Then a general physical and neurologic examination should be performed. Following this workup, most experienced physicians can localize the patient's neurologic problem and construct a short list of possible differential diagnoses. Often only a few laboratory tests will be needed to complete the evaluation and then treatment can be instituted. Many patients with neurologic disorders can be treated effectively with medications.

ANATOMY

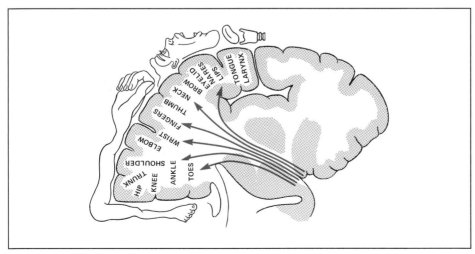

FIGURE 18–1
The cortical topography of neurologic function: Sensory homunculus (sensory cortex); motor homunculus (area 4, anterior central gyrus).

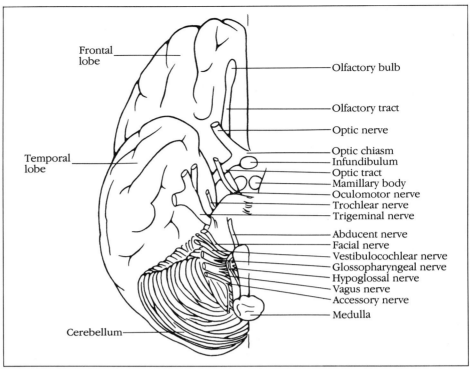

FIGURE 18–2
Brain stem with cranial nerves.

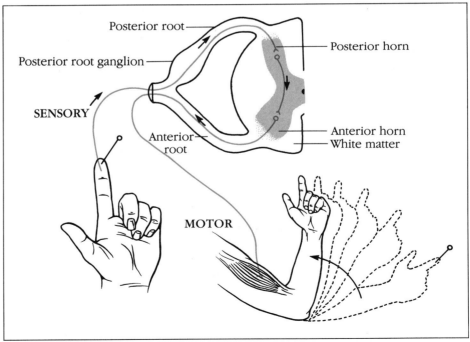

FIGURE 18–3
Spinal cord with sensory and motor reflex arcs.

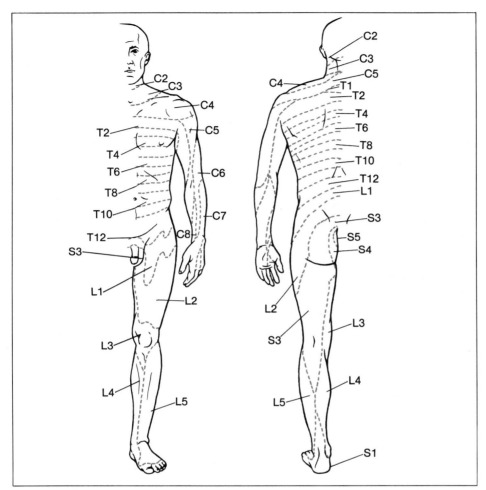

Figure 18–4
Dermatomes.

HISTORY

The Brain—is wider than the Sky—
For—put them side by side—
The one the other will contain
With ease—and You—beside—

EMILY DICKINSON
(1830–1886)

The history of a patient with neurologic symptoms should be obtained from the patient and, if necessary, from a close relative or friend as well. Some patients with neurologic problems have disease of the central nervous system, and this can affect memory, perception, or speech, making the history difficult to obtain. Patience and care must be used to obtain the best history from the patient or other persons. The history of progression of signs and symptoms in patients with neurologic diseases is often of crucial importance, because this gives clues to the type of pathology that may be present. In gradually progressive diseases such as brain tumors, symptoms usually increase gradually. With lesions that occur intermittently, such as those seen in multiple sclerosis, symptoms often are exacerbated, and then in remission. Rapidly occurring symptoms, such as sudden loss of neurologic function, frequently result from vascular disease. The following symptoms are particularly important in patients with neurologic complaints and should be explored fully in the history:

Changes in consciousness. The state of awareness of the patient may vary from mild drowsiness to unresponsive coma. Coma may be transient or permanent; there are many causes of coma, some of which are presented in Table 18–1.

Disturbances of vision may be due to drugs or eye disease, but organic lesions of the central nervous system may present with a history of visual field loss (stroke, brain tumor), double vision (multiple sclerosis, trauma, basilar artery insufficiency, chronic basilar meningitis, tumor), flashing lights (migraine, seizure disorder), visual hallucinosis (seizure disorder, drugs), and transient blindness (vascular lesions, migraine).

Disturbances of smell and taste suggest a focal lesion of the olfactory nerves.

Seizures (fits, convulsions) are important symptoms. Ascertain the situation in which they occurred, the prodromal symptoms, the focal components of the seizures, and obtain a minute description of the seizure itself from the patient and a witness, if possible.

Vomiting may result from disease of the cerebral hemispheres, especially if it is unaccompanied by nausea and is projectile in its force. Vomiting may also occur with migraine, cerebellar and brain stem disease, and psychiatric disorders.

Difficulty with bladder and bowel control, as well as **sexual dysfunction,** may signal spinal cord or autonomic dysfunction. Other autonomic symptoms include palpitations and abnormal patterns of sweating and flushing.

Disturbance of gait should be categorized as due to motor weakness or incoordination or due to sensory dysfunction.

Disturbance of speech may be noted by the physician as the history is given or may be the patient's major complaint. Try to discern if the difficulty is one of articulation *(dysarthria)* or of word command *(aphasia).*

Abnormal involuntary movements often indicate disease of the basal ganglia. Tremor often results from disease of the cerebellum or brain stem.

Numbness usually indicates peripheral nerve or spinal cord (posterior column) involvement but may also be due to sensory pathway interruption in the brain stem, thalamus, or parietal cortex.

Weakness may result from abnormalities of muscle, myoneural junction, or nerve, or of the corticospinal tract in the spinal cord, brainstem, internal capsule, or motor cortex. Involvement of other central pathways also may produce weakness.

TABLE 18–1. Some Causes of Coma*

Cerebral vascular accidents	**Brain tumors**
Cerebral infarction	**Postepileptic coma**
Cerebral hemorrhage	**Cerebral hypoperfusion**
Cerebral embolism with infarction	Arrhythmias
Subarachnoid hemorrhage	Stokes-Adams disease
Cerebral trauma	Severe congestive heart failure
Concussion	**Psychiatric "coma"**
Cerebral contusion	Hysteria
Subdural hematoma	Schizophrenia
Epidural hematoma	**Other**
Drugs and toxins	Akinetic mutism
Alcohol	Locked-in syndrome
Narcotics	
Barbiturates	
Insulin	
Aspirin	
Carbon monoxide	
Heavy metals (lead, arsenic)	
Other sedatives and drugs	
Endogenous toxins or states	
Diabetic coma	
Uremia	
Hepatic failure	
Hypoxemia	
Hypoglycemia	
Myxedema	
Hypothermia	
Hypercalcemia	
Hyponatremia	
Adrenal insufficiency	
Avitaminosis	
(B_{12}, thiamine)	
Profound anemia	
Heat stroke	
Infections	
Severe systemic sepsis	
Central nervous system infections	

*Not listed in order of frequency.

TABLE 18–2. Some Causes[a] of Chronic Dementia[b]

Dementias associated with systemic disorders	Dementias associated with other neurologic signs
Avitaminosis (B_{12}, thiamine)	Huntington's chorea
Hypothyroidism	Slow virus disease (e.g., Creutzfeldt-Jakob)
Hypercorticosteroidism	
Dementias associated with some cancers	Demyelinating disorders (e.g., Schilder's disease)
Hepatolenticular degeneration (Wilson's disease)	Lipid storage disease (e.g., Tay-Sachs)
Syphilis	Myoclonic epilepsy
Chronic alcoholism and/or drug use	Parkinson's disease
Porphyria	Hereditary ataxias
Dementias in which dementia may occur as the sole evidence of disease	Cerebral atherosclerosis (multiple stroke syndrome)
Senile and presenile dementias (Alzheimer's disease)	Brain tumor
Some brain tumors of the frontal lobes or central structures.	Brain trauma (multiple, old)
	Normal pressure hydrocephalus

[a]Not listed in order of frequency.
[b]*Dementia:* A clinical state characterized by failing memory and loss of other intellectual functions due to chronic, progressive, degenerative disease of the brain.

Dizziness usually means one of three things: vertigo, imbalance, or faintness. *Vertigo* indicates the subjective sensation of spinning, either of the patient or of the environment. It usually is caused by dysfunction of the inner ear balance mechanisms or the vestibular portion of the eighth cranial nerve or its central connections. *Imbalance* implies difficulty in walking in a straight line and may result from disease of peripheral nerves, posterior columns, cerebellum, or other central pathways. *Faintness* indicates a feeling that the patient is about to lose consciousness and may be associated with generalized weakness. It results from a variety of disorders, including postural hypotension, hypotension from other causes, cardiac arrhythmias, and seizure disorders.

Fainting or loss of consciousness results from loss of function of the brain due to decrease or loss of blood supply, inadequate nutrition (oxygen, glucose), imbalance of nutrients, abnormal cerebral electrical discharge (epilepsy), or cerebral injury due to any cause.

Pain is due to activation of pain endings and pain fibers of peripheral nerves or of the central pain pathways (spinothalamic tracts) in the spinal cord, brain stem, or thalamus.

Headache is caused by distortion of or traction on blood vessels or the meninges or other covering structures of the brain, or by pressure, distortion, traction, or displacement of almost any extracerebral structure in the head, including the skull, paranasal sinuses, scalp, and posterior suboccipital muscles of the neck.

Defective memory or thinking. Difficulty with these two cerebral functions may result from a lesion in almost any area of the brain, although a specific memory defect may result from small lesions in the hypothalamic-thalamic-temporal lobe structures (Table 18–2).

PHYSICAL EXAMINATION

1. Assay mental status (history, recent and remote memory, judgment, affect).
2. Auscultate and palpate the head and the carotids in the neck.

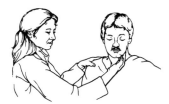
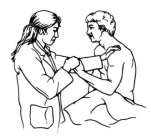

3. Test cranial nerves II–XII (cranial nerve I not generally tested in routine examinations).
4. Test motor function (abnormal movements, muscle mass and tone, strength, deep tendon reflexes, and plantar responses).
5. Test cerebellar function (finger to nose, heel to shin, rapid fine and alternating movements).

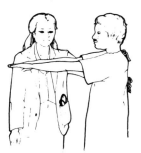
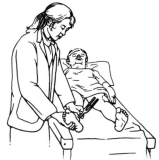

6. Test station and gait (Romberg test included).
7. Test sensation (temperature, superficial pain, vibration, light touch, deep pain).

The auditory nerves were atrophied. . . . The convolutions of the brain, which was rather soft and edematous, seemed to be twice as deep and twice as numerous as normal.

> Report of autopsy on Ludwig van Beethoven
> JOHANN WAGNER
> (1800?–1833)

GENERAL

Some observers prefer to examine the nervous system by regions rather than by systems; that is, the arms are examined as to motor, sensory, reflex, and cerebellar responses, and then the legs are examined, and so forth. This approach has advantages but probably should be left to those with considerable experience. It is not necessary to do the examination in the order listed here, however. It is often better to examine first the part or function involved in the presenting complaint and then return to the established routine.

The examiner should have available a reflex hammer, tuning forks (128 and 256 cps), an ophthalmoscope, a small flashlight, tongue blades, sharp pins, and cotton or a camel's-hair brush. A stethoscope and otoscope are also usually required.

MENTAL AND PSYCHIATRIC STATUS

You will have obtained considerable information about your patient's recent and remote memory, affect (mood), judgment, basic intelligence, and alertness during the history and physical examination already done. Take care not to confuse cultural difference or deafness with poor cognition, language difficulty with limited intelligence, or aphasia with dementia. In the history, assess the patient's socioeconomic and educational level so that you will be able to analyze any deficit found in cognitive function.

GENERAL BEHAVIOR

Describe the patient's appearance, including facial expression, general attitude, and manner of dress. Describe any special postures or gestures, the stream of speech, and any distractability, flight of ideas, or inappropriate comments.

ORIENTATION

Ask the patient to identify the day, date, and year, the name of the hospital and city, and his own name.

AWARENESS

Ask the patient to identify the president of the United States, and the vice president, secretary of state, mayor, and governor. Ask about recent events that have made headlines in the local newspapers.

MEMORY

Remote past: Ask for facts of the patient's life that can be verified with the patient's relatives or friends. Ask for the dates of birth, marriage, school attendance, and military service. Ask for the dates of major events in the history of the United States such as World War II, the Korean War, the Vietnam War. *Recent past:* Ask about the events of the last few days or weeks. *Immediate recall:* Give the patient the names of three objects (e.g., doll, book, dog) with instructions to remember them, and then ask the patient to repeat them in 5 minutes. Don't forget to ask for them when the 5 minutes are up.

CALCULATIONS

Give the patient simple arithmetic problems to solve, including serial subtraction, addition, multiplication, and division. A convenient standard test is the 100 minus 7 test. Ask the patient to subtract 7 from 100 (93), then 7 from that (86), then 7 from that (79), and so on as far as the patient can go. Record both the accuracy of the computations and the final number.

ABSTRACT THINKING

Ask the patient for the meaning of the old saying, "People who live in glass houses shouldn't throw stones." The patient should give an abstract interpretation such as, "nobody is perfect, so people shouldn't criticize others." A concrete interpretation suggests organic cognitive dysfunction or psychosis. Thus, the answer "They'll break the glass" is an abnormal response. Other proverbs that could be used include, "Every cloud has a silver lining" and "Make hay while the sun is shining." Ask for the similarity between a lemon and an apple, bicycle and automobile, and bird and airplane.

JUDGMENT AND INSIGHT

Ask the patient what he would do if he found a stamped, addressed, sealed envelope lying on the ground. The correct answer is to put it in a mailbox, give it to a mail carrier, or give it to a police officer. Also ask the patient what he would do if he were in a theater and saw a fire. The correct answer is to notify the responsible authorities and walk out, since running or shouting "fire" may provoke a panic.

PSYCHIATRIC DISORDERS

Symptoms and signs of emotional, mental, and psychosomatic illness are common in patients seen by all physicians. Some of these are easily recognized and understood even by the inexperienced clinician (e.g., the anxiety of the student who experiences palpitations just before every university examination); others are more subtle (e.g., the gradual decline in memory that may occur in a variety of dementias).

Certainly no patient with organic disease is free of emotional responses to it. Organic disease may also, as you know, induce mental and emotional changes directly (e.g., the psychosis that can accompany certain vitamin deficiencies), or emotional-mental disease can present with major or minor physical symptoms.

In psychiatry, as in the rest of medicine, accurate diagnosis depends on a comprehensive history, taken in a nonjudgmental way. Pain originating "all in my head" is no less painful than that which comes from distal sensory nerve stimulation. Because most medical education emphasizes the diagnosis of organic diseases rather than psychiatric or nonorganic disorders, inexperienced clinicians often denigrate diagnoses in which there are few or no physical, roentgenologic, or laboratory "abnormalities." Although some psychiatric disorders are associated with such "objective" findings, it remains true that the history (from the patient and his or her family, friends, or attendants) is the principal diagnostic tool of psychiatric diagnosis.

As the clinician takes the "routine" history from the patient in search of organic disease, clues to psychiatric dysfunction may present themselves, especially in the "mental status" portion of the neurologic exam. These may be present either *in addition* to those of concurrent organic dysfunction or as the paramount and sole causes of the patient's distress.

Psychiatric symptoms tend to fall into three major categories: (1) perception disorders; (2) cognitive disorders; and (3) affective disorders.

PERCEPTION DISORDERS

In these disorders, the patient "misinterprets" reality and presents with such symptoms as *depersonalization* (the sensation that one is not fully "in" one's body, i.e., is detached somehow from self or the world), *derealization* (the feeling that the world is unreal), and *illusions* (misrepresentation or misinterpretation of a genuine external experience). In all of these symptoms, the patient is aware that his or her experience is strange and that the altered perception is abnormal. These may occur secondarily from stress, drugs, and organic diseases, or as a primary psychosis.

More serious disorders of perception include *hallucinations* (false sensory perceptions in the absence of real external stimuli) and *delusions* (fixed false beliefs that are illogical and unaccounted for by the patient's cultural background). These suggest more severe brain disease, drug intoxication, or psychosis.

Drugs involved in perceptual difficulties include "street" hallucinogens, sedative-hypnotics (especially in the older patient), and others, including digoxin, propranolol, anticholinergics, antihistamines, and antiparkinsonian drugs, as well as steroids. Alcohol is one of the most common drugs that may lead to such symptoms and must always be suspected, even if the patient is "too nice to be a drinker." Direct inquiry is called for concerning *all* drugs and medications used, including over-the-counter medications.

Brain tumors and migraine may also present with perceptual difficulties as may, of course, psychiatric disease such as schizophrenia.

COGNITIVE DISORDERS

These include dementia, delerium, and amnestic syndromes, which are all characterized by loss of intellectual function and/or major memory deficits, with consequent behavioral dysfunction.

Dementia is a state in which there is loss of intellectual capacity, including memory; learning new tasks; orientation to time, place, and person; logic; abstract thought; judgment; language; and problem solving. Depending on the cause, some areas of intellectual function may be severely compromised while others remain relatively intact. Clinical clues to subtle dementias include family reports of irritability, forgetfulness, trouble at work, and loss of interest or ability in formerly well-loved activities. Mental status testing will often show defects in short-term memory, backward spelling, and occasionally errors in judgment. Emotional lability may be present.

Some causes of dementia include Alzheimer's disease, multiinfarct dementia, chronic alcoholism and use of other drugs, degenerative and slow viral central nervous system diseases, and as a residual effect of head trauma and cerebral hypoxia. Hydrocephalus, metabolic dementias (B_{12}, thiamine, or niacin deficiency; hypothyroidism) are potentially reversible dementias (see Table 18–2).

Specific psychometric testing occasionally must be used to define the exact extent and nature of dementia.

Delirium is a more acute state of dementia and is a clouding of consciousness often associated with perceptual difficulties, illusions, and hallucinations, often generating fear and physical hyperresponsivity. Causes of delirium include drug (alcohol and other) intoxication or withdrawal; systemic and cerebral infections; hypoxemia; hypoglycemia; renal and hepatic failure; cerebral vasculitis; thiamine, vitamin B_{12}, and niacin deficiencies; hypothyroidism; and electrolyte imbalance.

Delirium is a medical emergency and requires full evaluation with history, physical examination, and laboratory and x-ray studies directed at the most likely cause.

Amnesia (mild memory defects, simple forgetting) is common (as every medical student knows). More serious memory defects, such as those associated with vascular injury to the brain, thiamine deficiency, head trauma, brain tumors, and degenerative or infectious central nervous system disease, require detailed documentation through mental status examination, memory testing, and diagnostic workup to determine etiological factors.

AFFECTIVE DISORDERS

These are among the most common of psychiatric disorders in human medicine and refer to those states in which mood is exaggerated to the point of compromising the patient's function.

Depression, for example, may be minor, transient, and appropriate (as in the patient who has just heard of a poor prognosis for his cancer) or major and debilitating. It can occur unassociated with any external event evident to the examiner. Because depressed patients often have a feeling of futility and low self-regard, suicide is a risk and should be asked about ("Have you considered suicide?" "Do you have any plans as to how or when you might kill yourself?"). Studies have shown that mentioning suicide to the depressed patient—far from "giving them the idea"—allows them to express their deepest fears and plans and may save their lives.

Physical correlates to severe depressions may include early morning awakening and other disturbance of sleep pattern, fatigue, loss of appetite and loss of weight, constipation, loss of sexual interest, abnormal sweating, and even hallucinations and delusions. You may discern a "flattening" of affect and a monotonality of speech during the interview. Some patients, those with the most severe depressions, may even make you feel depressed ("infectious depression"), a clue to their diagnosis. Abnormal elation, inappropriate elevation of mood, may signal drug use (e.g., amphetamines), neurologic illness (e.g., multiple sclerosis), or psychiatric disorder (schizophrenia, bipolar disorder with mania).

Anxiety is a common feeling shared by all human beings. In the absence of an appropriate external stimulus, however, or disproportionate to a stimulus, anxiety may be debilitating. Specific questioning about anxiety, including whether the patient believes it is interfering with his or her function, is appropriate. Drug use and hyperthyroidism, along with organic brain disease and major psychiatric disorders, should be considered as possible contributors to anxiety.

As you question the patient, exercise tact and gentleness. Many patients with impaired mentation are frightened by their perceived loss of ability and will have erected defenses to its discovery. In breaking through those defenses the physician may become threatening to them. Patients who lack formal education may interpret your probing as an attempt to belittle their intelligence. If you meet with a hostile or disturbed response during mental status testing, back off for a while and come back to it later.

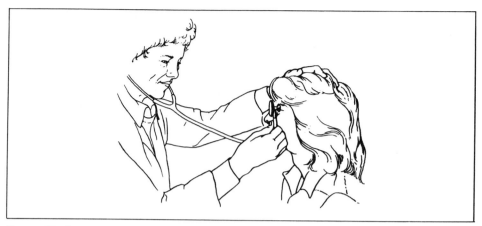

FIGURE 18–5
Auscultation of the orbit.

EXAMINATION OF THE HEAD AND NECK

Palpate the common carotid arteries in the neck and the temporal arteries just in front of the ears. Palpate both radial arteries at the wrist, noting both strength and simultaneousness of impulse.

With the bell of the stethoscope listen for a bruit over each eyeball after asking the patient to close both eyes. Place the bell over one eyeball firmly and ask the patient to open the other eye and look steadily at an object (Fig. 18–5). Listen also for a bruit over both carotid arteries high in the neck at the angle of the jaw and in each supraclavicular space. If a bruit is heard in either of the latter two spaces, compare blood pressure in the arms.

The carotid pulses are usually equal, and when absent or markedly decreased, may be occluded. However, complete or partial occlusion can take place in the presence of what is apparently a normally palpable carotid artery. If the common carotid artery in the neck gives a full pulse, but the pulse in the temporal artery on the same side is decreased or absent, there is presumptive evidence of occlusion of the external carotid. The subclavian, brachial, and radial pulses and also the dorsalis pedis, posterior tibial, and femoral pulses, if absent or definitely decreased, may give hints of occlusion of the main branches of the aorta, and this may be helpful in neurologic diagnosis.

Auscultation of the skull and orbits may reveal a bruit. Such a bruit may be heard on the side of increased or decreased blood flow through the carotid or vertebral arterial territories. Increased flow may be due to occlusion on the opposite side or to an arteriovenous anomaly or tumor on the same side. A bruit due to decreased flow occurs with partial or complete occlusion on the same or opposite side, or even in the absence of vascular disease.

A bruit in the supraclavicular space may indicate partial or complete occlusion of the subclavian artery with possible production of the "subclavian steal" syndrome. With this syndrome there may be also a decrease in the blood pressure in the affected arm and a delay in the radial pulse on the same side. Proximal obstruc-

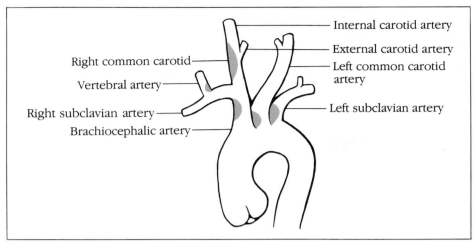

FIGURE 18–6

Frequent sites of atherosclerosis in the aortic arch. Eighty percent of lesions are at the bifurcation of the common carotids. Obstruction may also occur at the take-off of the great vessels from the aorta, at the origin of the vertebral artery, or at the origin of the subclavian arteries. Subclavian occlusion may (rarely) produce the "subclavian steal."

tion in the subclavian artery decreases the pressure in that artery at the point of origin of the vertebral artery (Fig. 18–6); this condition may result in an actual reversal of flow in the vertebral artery, with blood draining from the basilar artery into the arm as it is exercised.

SUPPLENESS OF THE NECK

The most easily tested of the meningeal signs is that for *nuchal rigidity* (stiff neck). Ask the patient to relax, and then with both hands flex his neck on his chest. If nuchal rigidity is present, there will be resistance and pain. *Brudzinski's sign* is flexion of the hips when the head is flexed in this manner. Test for *Kernig's sign* by flexing the hip on the trunk, allowing the knee to flex at the same time. When the hip is flexed to 90 degrees, extend the knee. In the presence of meningeal irritation there will be resistance, pain, and sometimes a tendency toward flexion of the neck.

APHASIA

When a patient has difficulty expressing himself, the examiner must determine whether the patient is suffering from aphasia or a general confusional state. Aphasia consists of the defective comprehension and formulation of verbal symbols in the absence of general confusion. You will have gathered a good idea of the patient's ability to express himself and to understand what is said to him in the course of the initial history. If aphasia is suspected, carry out the following tests.

ABILITY TO UNDERSTAND SPOKEN WORDS. Give the patient a series of verbal commands, such as "close your eyes," "raise your left arm," and "take hold of my hand."

Follow these with more complicated two- or three-step commands, such as "put out your tongue, then close your eyes, and then raise your left hand." Do not indicate by gesture the desired response.

ABILITY TO UNDERSTAND WRITTEN WORDS. Present the patient with a series of written commands in order of increasing complexity. Provide these in legible handwriting or in block capitals. Use commands such as, "open your mouth," "put out your tongue," "put your hand on top of your head," and "point to your left eye."

ABILITY TO EXPRESS IDEAS IN SPEECH. There is no formal test for this, but you should take note of the patient's spontaneous speech, including any defect of grammar and syntax, the occurrence of jargon, the capacity to finish sentences, and failures in the production of words.

ABILITY TO EXPRESS IDEAS IN WRITING. Give the patient a pencil and sheet of paper and ask him to write his own name, the name of his home town, some account of the weather, a statement about his own complaint, or recent news in the newspapers.

NAMING OBJECTS. Ask the patient to name a series of common objects that are shown to him. These can include a coin, button, handkerchief, pencil, wrist watch, fountain pen, collar, necktie.

READING ALOUD. Ask the patient to read aloud a paragraph from a book or newspaper. Choose a passage whose meaning the patient should be able to understand. Note any mistakes, including mispronunciation and repetition.

It is important to know the handedness of the patient, although if this cannot be ascertained it is usually safe to assume that the left cerebral hemisphere is dominant (Fig. 18–7). (About 98 percent of all people, including at least half of those who are left-handed, have left-hemisphere dominance.) Involvement of the dominant hemispheres by any type of disease often produces aphasia or dysphasia (partial aphasia).

Aphasia must be distinguished from dysarthria, which consists of difficulty with articulation. This may progress to the point of anarthria in which the patient is completely unable to speak in spite of having fully intact comprehension. The ataxia of speech that occurs with cerebellar and brain stem disturbances must be differentiated from the dysarthria that results from lesions of the cerebral cortex or subcortex.

Aphasia can be classified into three broad groups: expressive, receptive, and conductive. In expressive (Broca's) aphasia, comprehension is intact, but the patient cannot express himself effectively in speech. In receptive (Wernicke's) aphasia, the patient is unable to understand spoken language and often written language as well. In conductive aphasia, receptive and expressive aphasia are combined. If the patient's aphasia is mainly expressive, the lesion is likely to be in the front half of the dominant hemisphere. If the aphasia is receptive, the lesion is in the back half

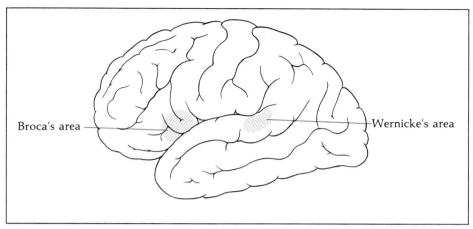

FIGURE 18–7
Cerebral cortical areas important for language. Injury to Broca's area results in nonfluent aphasia with good comprehension of language. Injury to Wernicke's area leads to fluent aphasia with poor comprehension of language.

of the dominant hemisphere. If the aphasia is conductive, the lesion may be between the front and back halves of the dominant hemisphere.

EXAMINATION OF THE CRANIAL NERVES
A large part of the cranial nerve examination is commonly done at the time of examination of the head, eyes, ears, nose, throat, and neck (see Chaps. 8–10, Sec. III).

I: OLFACTORY
Ask the patient to identify, with his eyes closed, any common nonirritating odor, such as coffee, tobacco, vanilla, turpentine, or cloves. Do not use noxious substances such as ammonia. Test each nostril separately. If these scents are not readily available, items at the bedside, such as oranges, flowers, and cigarettes, may be used. Normally the patient should be able to approximately identify familiar odors. Care must be taken here to differentiate between inability to smell the substance and inability to identify it properly. Many patients smell the substance correctly but are unable to name it. For this reason very familiar odors are probably best. Loss of the ability to smell (anosmia) is abnormal but does not usually indicate disease of the nervous system and is therefore of little localizing value. Local nasal disorders are far more common as a cause of loss of smell.

The most common neurologic causes of anosmia are head injuries and tumors, especially meningiomas of the olfactory groove. The ability to smell commonly decreases with advancing age.

II: OPTIC

Examination of the optic nerve is divided into three major subdivisions: (1) vision, (2) visual fields, and (3) funduscopic.

Visual acuity is best tested with standardized charts or with small pocket-size testing cards. If these are not available, the examiner can use any printed material and compare his own visual ability (assuming he knows his own acuity) with the patient's. Because we are interested in lesions of the retina and optic pathways and not in errors of refraction, the patient should be tested with his glasses on. Test each eye separately. If the acuity is so diminished that the patient cannot read even large print, ask him to count extended fingers at various distances. If even this is impossible, test his ability to see moving objects or to distinguish light from dark. Visual acuity, with correction, should be 20/20. In youth, the visual acuity is usually better than this, and in fact an acuity of 20/20 in the young can represent some loss of vision.

Check the *visual fields* by the confrontation method. Ask the patient to cover one eye and with his other eye look straight into your eyes. Slowly bring from behind the patient one constantly moving finger held 12 to 18 inches from his head. A small test object such as a cotton applicator may be used. As the test object is moved forward, the patient will let you know when he first sees it. All four quadrants should be tested at 45-degree angles from the horizontal and the vertical. Each eye must be tested separately, but most field defects of central nervous system origin can be found with both of the patient's eyes open. Finer testing can be done with small test objects and screens made for the purpose. Many scotomas cannot be found without such special equipment. Extinction consists of the perception of a stimulus when it is presented alone but lack of perception of the same stimulus when it is given simultaneously with another stimulus. Test for extinction by moving a finger in one visual field and determining whether the patient perceives the movement; then repeat the stimulus while simultaneously moving a finger in the opposite visual field. Normally, both movements will be seen. With extinction, only one of the moving objects will be observed.

The *optic fundi* should be examined with an ophthalmoscope. The presence of a sharp disc outline and of spontaneous pulsations of the veins on the discs is of particular interest from a neurologic standpoint, because these findings indicate a normal intracranial pressure. The two most common funduscopic abnormalities of concern during neurologic testing are swelling or edema of the optic disc and optic atrophy. Papilledema first appears as a loss of distinctness of the disc margins that progresses until all evidence of margin disappears. It then may become raised above the surrounding retina, and the edema may spread into the retina. Do not attach great significance to minimal indistinctness of the disc margins along the nasal or medial aspect of the disc, since this is often normal. Optic atrophy is usually manifested by a combination of pallor of the lateral aspect of the disc and a lack of normal vascularity in that area.

The most common gross visual field defect of neurologic importance is that of a homonymous hemianopia, in which, for instance, the right visual field is lost in both the right and left eyes. This would indicate that the left optic tract or visual radiation is injured somewhere between the optic chiasm and the left visual cortex.

A homonymous quadrantanopic defect usually indicates disease involving the visual radiations as they pass through the parietal or temporal lobes. An upper quadrantanopic defect usually indicates involvement of the visual radiations in the opposite temporal lobe, and a lower quarter field defect indicates involvement of the opposite parietal lobe. Bitemporal field defects (involvement of the lateral half of the visual field in each eye) indicates a lesion in the center of the optic chiasm interrupting the fibers as they cross from one optic nerve to the opposite tract. The most common lesion causing this defect is a tumor of the pituitary gland.

A fuller discussion and illustration of the optic examination and its relationship to neurologic evaluation are provided in Chapter 8.

III, IV, AND VI: OCULOMOTOR, TROCHLEAR, AND ABDUCENS

These nerves supply the muscles of eye movement and are tested as a unit. Each eye is tested separately and then both together. Ask the patient to follow an object such as a fingertip, keeping his head motionless. Move the object laterally from side to side, and then vertically up and down when lateral gaze is reached. Test elevation and depression with the eyes in the midposition also. Pause for a moment at each end point and inspect for nystagmus and weakness of eye muscle. The test object is then brought from a distance of 3 or 4 feet to within an inch of the patient's nose. In this way both convergence and the normal pupillary constriction to convergence are tested.

Loss of function of cranial nerve III results in a dilated pupil, external deviation of the eyeball, and ptosis of the upper lid. Cranial nerves IV and VI carry no parasympathetic fibers, and their paralysis results only in weakness of the appropriate muscles. The eye is deviated inward with *paralysis of cranial nerve VI* (lateral rectus muscle weakness). Sixth-nerve weakness has only moderate localizing value because it may result from increased intracranial pressure regardless of cause, especially in children. *Loss of function of cranial nerve IV* is not quite so easy to detect and is rare. There is weakness of internal rotation of the eyeball and of gaze downward and inward. The patient may tilt his head so that the eye with the paralyzed superior oblique muscle is elevated somewhat above the plane of the normal eye. This is done to bring the horizontal axes parallel and thus prevent diplopia (see Chap. 8).

The eyes are inspected for *ptosis,* and any difference in the width of the palpebral fissures is noted. Check the *pupillary response to light.* The light is directed into one eye, watching for pupillary constriction in the eye being tested (direct light reflex) and in the other eye (consensual light reflex). At rest, depending on the amount of light in the examining room, the pupils are normally equal and about 2 to 3 mm in diameter. They react quickly to light both directly and consensually and also to convergence.

Anisocoria (unequal pupils) may be a normal phenomenon or it may be caused by a variety of abnormalities. Smallness of one pupil may indicate a sympathetic lesion (Horner syndrome). In this situation, the small pupil will be accompanied by ipsilateral ptosis, decreased sweating on the same side of the face, and the impression that the eye is somewhat retracted into the socket (enophthalmos). A small pupil can also result from the use of drugs such as eye drops for ocular disease.

A unilaterally dilated pupil often occurs with increased intracranial pressure, and in this case it is an early sign of injury to cranial nerve III. The dilated pupil is usually on the side of the lesion causing the increased pressure. The Argyll Robertson pupil is usually equal on the two sides. The pupil is very small (< 1 mm), irregular, and reacts to accommodation but not to light. The pupil does not respond to mydriatic agents. Adie's pupil usually is a unilaterally dilated pupil that reacts only slowly to light and darkness. Adie's pupil is found in young women with decreased or absent deep tendon reflexes and no other neurologic abnormalities. (Table 8–8 describes abnormal pupils.)

When the eyes are moved to the limit of lateral gaze in any direction, there normally may be minimal *nystagmus* (repetitive beating movements of the eye). Normally there should be *no* nystagmus on elevation and depression of the eyes, even at the extremes.

Nystagmus often gives a definite clue as to location and even type of neurologic disease present. Of special importance is the *dissociated nystagmus* with lesions of the medial longitudinal fasciculus. In this type of nystagmus the eye on the side to which the gaze is directed participates strongly with a horizontal nystagmus, whereas the opposite eye will show less nystagmus but will show some weakness of internal rotation. Multiple sclerosis is the most common cause of this type of nystagmus when the nystagmus is bilateral. Unilateral dissociated nystagmus occurs somewhat more commonly with stroke than with multiple sclerosis.

Nystagmus is common in diseases of the cerebellum and brain stem, in which case it is usually more pronounced on looking toward the side of the lesion. There also may be a minimal to moderate nystagmus with strictly cerebral lesions, in which case it is usually more evident in looking away from the side of the lesion.

V: TRIGEMINAL

Test the areas supplied by the three divisions of the trigeminal nerve (Fig. 18–8) for their sensitivity to light touch (cotton), pinprick, and temperature. If a medullary or upper cervical cord lesion is suspected, it is important to test pain, temperature, and touch on the face; with a lesion involving the descending tract of the trigeminal nerve, touch may be intact with absence of pain and temperature. In such lesions, the loss of pain and temperature sensation extends exactly to the midline. It may, however, involve only the first, second, or third divisions of the trigeminal nerve because of the arrangement of these divisions in the descending tract. For this reason it is important to test all three divisions.

The corneal reflex is important and can be tested by carefully placing a fine, elongated wisp of the cotton on the cornea while the patient is looking away from the approaching cotton (Fig. 18–9). *Both eyes should blink quickly with this stimulation.* Test each eye separately.

The corneal reflex may be diminished unilaterally from either a peripheral or a central lesion. With a peripheral lesion, the decreased corneal reflex may result from injury to the fifth or the seventh cranial nerve. With a lesion of the fifth cranial nerve, the patient will not feel the cotton touching the cornea, and there may be

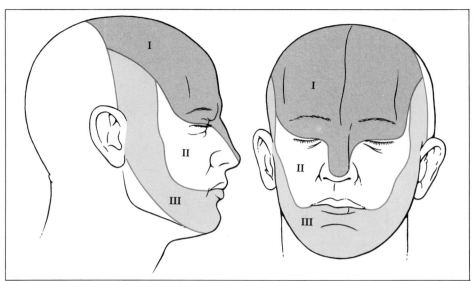

FIGURE 18–8
Three sensory divisions of the trigeminal nerve: ophthalmic (I), maxillary (II), and mandibular (III).

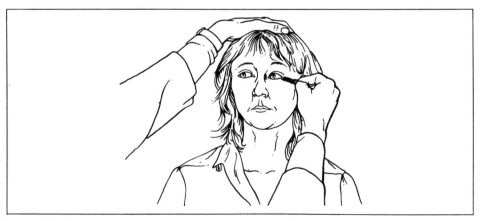

FIGURE 18–9
Testing the corneal reflex.

no blink on both the side of the stimulated cornea and the opposite side. In the
presence of a seventh nerve lesion preventing the corneal reflex from occurring,
there should be an obvious severe weakness of the face. The patient will feel the
cotton touching the cornea, and there will be blinking of the contralateral eyelid.
When the corneal reflex is diminished by a central lesion, there usually are other
signs of disease of the brain stem or cerebral hemisphere, including hemiplegia
and hemisensory loss.

TABLE 18–3. Right Facial Weakness

Central (Upper Motor Neuron)	Maneuver	Peripheral (Lower Motor Neuron)
	I. Face at rest	
Loss of nasolabial fold on right Corner of mouth droops on right To a limited degree, widening palpebral fissure on right		Loss of nasolabial fold on right Corner of mouth droops on right Widening palpebral fissure on right

	II. Elevation of eyebrows	
Patient can elevate both eyebrows		Unable to elevate eyebrow on right

The masseter and temporalis muscles should be palpated with the patient clenching his jaws. Deviation of the jaw on opening the mouth should be assessed. Test also the strength of the jaw on lateral movement. Check the strength of jaw closure by asking the patient to grip a tongue blade with his teeth on each side while you try to extract the blade.

With cerebral lesions there may be some decrease in sensation on the opposite side of the face, but this usually does not extend exactly to the midline. There is usually no appreciable weakness of the masseter and pterygoid muscles on the side opposite a "central" (cerebral) lesion.

TABLE 18–3. (Continued)

Central (Upper Motor Neuron)	Maneuver	Peripheral (Lower Motor Neuron)
	III. Closing eyes	
Patient can close both eyes		Right eye does not close and eyeball turns up (Bell's phenomenon)

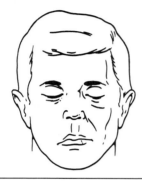 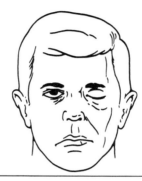

IV. Emotion

Smile symmetrical   Smile asymmetrical

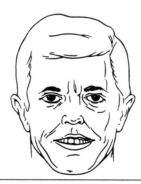 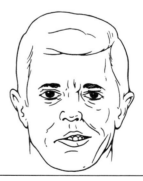

VII: FACIAL

Test the facial nerve by asking the patient to show his teeth and smile, close the eyes against resistance, elevate the eyebrows, and contract the platysma (Table 18–3). Each of these maneuvers may be first shown to the patient by movements of your own.

All facial movements should be equal bilaterally. Some individuals, however, habitually talk and smile more out of one side of their mouth than the other. These habit patterns must be kept in mind while looking for possible evidence of weakness.

In a "central" *(upper motor neuron)* weakness of the face, as commonly seen with cerebral lesions, there is moderate to marked weakness of the opposite lower facial muscles, including the platysma, the orbicularis oris, and sometimes the lower part of the orbicularis oculi. With a small lesion there may be only minimal drooping of the opposite corner of the mouth at rest and some weakness of that corner of the mouth on voluntary movement. The patient, however, will be able to close his eye and wrinkle his forehead fairly strongly on the side opposite the cerebral lesion. With weakness of the face due to a lesion of the seventh-nerve nucleus or of the nerve itself (peripheral facial paralysis, *lower motor neuron disease,* Bell's palsy) there is weakness of all parts of the face on the side of the lesion. The patient will be unable to wrinkle his forehead, close his eyes, or show his teeth.

Weakness of one side of the mouth, even though minimal, may be an important clue in determining whether the lesion responsible for the accompanying weakness of an arm (or an arm and a leg) on the same side is in the spinal cord, the brain stem, or the cerebrum. If the lesion is in the spinal cord, there should be no weakness of the face. If it is in the pons, the facial weakness will be on the side opposite that of the affected arm and the leg. If the lesion is above the brain stem, weakness of the face, arm, and leg will be all on the same side.

Test *taste* with a solution of sugar or salt. Dab a very small amount of the solution with an applicator onto the coarse folds at the lateral edge of the anterior two-thirds of the tongue about halfway back from the tip. Have the patient put the tongue out to the opposite side and nod if he tastes anything. Then ask him to describe the taste. Test each side of the tongue separately.

VIII: AUDITORY

The two divisions of the auditory nerve—the cochlear and the vestibular—are tested separately. The patient's ability to hear a watch tick or a whispered voice at a definite distance from each ear may be all that is necessary to test. Hearing may also be tested with a tuning fork of 256 or more cycles per second. Normally the patient's hearing should be equal in both ears, and air conduction should exceed bone conduction.

Decreased air conduction with preserved bone conduction indicates that there is *conductive* (middle ear or external ear) deafness. If both air conduction and bone conduction are reduced, the deafness is *perceptive* (nerve) or mixed. With unilateral nerve deafness the patient will hear the tuning fork when it is placed on the midline of the skull (Weber's test) in his good ear, whereas if the defect is in the middle ear or external ear the patient will hear it in his deaf ear. Lesions central to the cochlear nuclei do not cause unilateral deafness; therefore, unilateral perceptive deafness indicates a lesion of the cochlear nuclei (rare), cranial nerve VIII, or the end-organ (cochlea). To differentiate between these it is sometimes helpful to test the vestibular portion of cranial nerve VIII. There is no need to test vestibular function in the routine neurologic examination. In more directed inquiries, it may be tested by syringing each ear with cold water, provided the ear drum is intact. This process will produce nystagmus if vestibular function is intact. The ves-

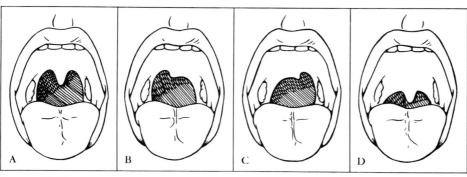

FIGURE 18–10
Tests of uvular deviation (cranial nerves IX and X). A. Normal. B. Left IX and X palsy. C. Right IX and X palsy. D. Bulbar palsy.

tibular function will be preserved if deafness is caused by a lesion of the cochlear nuclei but may be lost in lesions of the nerve or end-organ.

Tests of hearing are described in detail and illustrated in Chapter 9.

IX AND X: GLOSSOPHARYNGEAL AND VAGUS

These two complex cranial nerves are tested together and, in fact, are rather simple to evaluate. Note the quality of the patient's voice and his ability to swallow. Ask him to open his mouth and say "ah." Observe the position of the soft palate and uvula at rest and with phonation (Fig. 18–10). Check the gag reflex with a tongue blade by touching each side of the posterior pharyngeal wall separately. Taste on the posterior one-third of the tongue can be examined when an abnormality is suspected.

Normally the uvula and palate rise in the midline with phonation. It is important to test this function with the patient's head in the midline and not turned to either side.

If there is unilateral paralysis of cranial nerves IX and X, the palate and uvula will deviate to the unparalyzed side during phonation. The distance between the soft palate and the posterior pharyngeal wall will be decreased on the paralyzed side. The arch of the palate at rest on the paralyzed side will droop lower than on the normal side. The sensory component of the gag reflex is mediated by cranial nerve IX and the motor by X. However, paralysis of cranial nerve IX alone is difficult to detect, since sometimes there may be no apparent sensory loss in the pharynx. If there is any doubt about the presence of a vagus paralysis, the vocal cords should be visualized to see whether there is unilateral or bilateral weakness.

Marked palatal and vocal cord paralysis on the same side indicates a lower motor neuron lesion. However, some patients will show moderate and temporary palatal weakness of the side opposite a large upper motor neuron lesion such as that caused by a large cerebral infarct. Marked unilateral paralysis of the palate, pharynx, and vocal cords without evidence of long sensory or motor pathway involvement nearly always indicates that the lesion is outside the brain stem and involves the

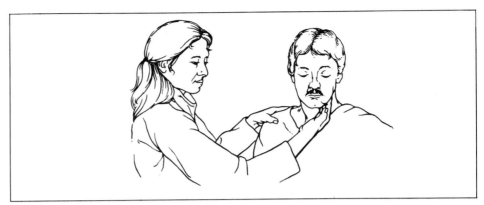

FIGURE 18–11
Testing the strength of the sternocleidomastoid muscle (cranial nerve XI).

cranial nerves IX and X after they have left the medulla. Bilateral weakness can result from lesions of the upper motor neurons bilaterally, giving a pseudobulbar palsy, or from involvement of the nuclei in the medulla, the nerves, or the muscles, giving a bulbar palsy.

XI: SPINAL ACCESSORY

Examine the sternocleidomastoid and trapezius muscles for fasciculations and atrophy before testing for muscle strength. Ask the patient to turn his head to one side forcefully against your hand. Meanwhile palpate the opposite sternocleidomastoid muscle (Fig. 18–11). Palpate the trapezius muscle and test the strength of the patient's "shrug" while you press down on the shoulders with both hands. Normally the strength of the sternocleidomastoid and trapezius muscles is equal bilaterally.

If unilateral weakness and atrophy of the trapezius and sternocleidomastoid muscles are found, the responsible lesion is outside the brain stem, because the nerve has its origin in the upper cervical cord. Marked bilateral weakness and atrophy of these muscles often occur in primary muscle disease, such as muscular dystrophy.

XII: HYPOGLOSSAL

Ask the patient to protrude his tongue in the midline, and observe any deviation or atrophy. Another test for weakness or deviation of the tongue is to ask the patient to stick his tongue into his cheek while the examiner presses against the bulging cheek. Unilateral tongue weakness is manifested by a deviation of the protruded tongue toward the weak side and often by atrophy and fasciculations on the affected side. When the tongue is lying in the mouth, however, it will be pulled toward the strong side (Fig. 18–12). The reason for this pull is that the sets of tongue muscles in action when the tongue is protruded are different from those sets in action when the tongue is resting in the mouth.

It is important to check the tongue carefully for fasciculations; they may be the earliest sign of lower motor neuron disease affecting the hypoglossal nerve nuclei. Normally a few small tremulous movements are seen in the tongue. These move-

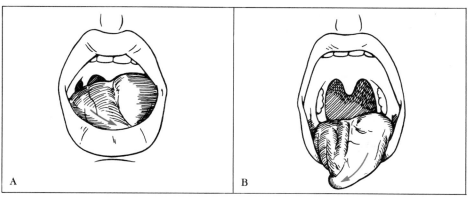

FIGURE 18–12
Hypoglossal nerve (cranial nerve XII). A. Right XII paralysis, tongue at rest. B. Right XII paralysis tongue protruding.

ments should not be confused with the continuous "wormy" movements (fasciculations) over the entire tongue seen in amyotrophic lateral sclerosis. Occasionally, as with the palate and pharynx, there may be temporary unilateral weakness of the tongue on the side opposite a large acute upper motor neuron lesion. Associated with this weakness may be a transient dysarthria; both usually clear within a few days. With a bilateral upper motor neuron lesion there may be anarthria and inability to protrude the tongue beyond the lips.

EXAMINATION OF THE MOTOR SYSTEM

INSPECTION

Observe the patient's musculature for abnormal movements, either large (capable of moving a joint) or small (within the belly of the muscle itself). Fasciculations consist of small, flickering, involuntary contractions of groups of muscle fibers. True fasciculations result from abnormal impulses from diseased anterior horn cells in amyotrophic lateral sclerosis and usually are accompanied by atrophy and weakness. Benign fasciculations can occur and are not associated with weakness or atrophy. Fasciculations induced by muscular contraction or percussion of the muscle are generally without pathologic significance.

Atrophy (Fig. 18–13) and *hypertrophy* may give important clues in the diagnosis of muscle disease. If atrophy is present or if a progressive disease that might cause atrophy is suspected, the circumference of the muscle should be measured bilaterally; record the point at which the measurement is taken. The limbs of the normal individual at rest do not demonstrate any movement either of the joints or in the body of the muscles themselves except for an occasional rare and random fasciculation. A concept of normal muscle bulk is gained only by experience. Great variation is normally present among persons of different ages, sexes, and occupations. Chronic illness in itself may produce generalized wasting of the muscles.

Abnormal movements should be carefully observed and described (Table 18–4). The abnormal movement of parkinsonism is a *resting tremor* (4 to 5 per sec-

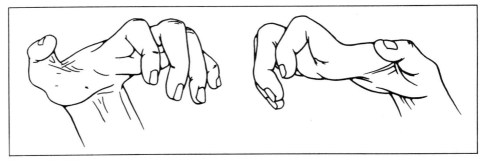

Figure 18–13
Hand muscle atrophy.

Table 18–4. Some Causes of Abnormal Movements

Tremor Type	Characteristics	Seen In
Simple tremor		
Essential, familial, or senile tremor	Not present at rest, except in head	Persons with a family history: Fatigue Advanced age Stimulants Fever Hyperthyroidism
Parkinsonism (resting tremor)	Present in hands at complete rest Associated with rigidity; decreased associative movements, small steppage gait, masked face	Parkinsonism of all types
Cerebellar tremor	Worse with motion and associated with cerebral signs	Multiple sclerosis Wilson's disease Hereditary ataxia
Chorea	Jerky, irregular, sudden movements; intermittent fidgeting	Acute rheumatic fever (Sydenham's chorea) Huntington's chorea
Athetosis	Upper limbs predominate Slow, sinuous, writhing movements	Cerebral palsy Torsion dystonia
Myoclonus	Sudden jerks of single muscles or muscle groups	Epilepsy Encephalitis Hyponatremia Hyperosmolar state Some degenerative CNS diseases
Tetanic spasms	Sustained contractions of single muscles or muscle groups	Tetanus Strychnine poisoning Tetany Spasticity
Hemiballismus	Flinging movements of arm and leg on one side	Infarction of the subthalamic nucleus

TABLE 18–5. Grading of Muscle Strength

Grade	Percentage	Criteria
0		No movement of the muscle
1 (trace)	0–5	Trace movement
		Cannot move the joint
2 (poor)	6–20	Minimal movement
3 (fair)	21–50	Can move the joint against gravity
4 (good)	51–90	Good power but not normal
5 (normal)	91–100	Normal strength

ond) that is usually more evident in the hands but is also found in the arms, head, face, tongue, and legs. It may be associated with rigidity (increased resistance to passive manipulation) of the muscles and thus may produce the typical *cogwheel effect,* which is a rhythmic increase and decrease in resistance superimposed on passive movements produced by the examiner. *Essential* (familial or senile) *tremor* is not present at rest but is pronounced with sustained posture or with movement. It is not associated with any alteration in resistance to passive manipulation and is more likely to involve the head than is the tremor of parkinsonism. The *kinetic (intention) tremor* characteristic of lesions of the cerebellum is usually combined with some degree of ataxia and is brought out with purposeful movement such as the finger-to-nose test.

Choreic movements are irregular, involuntary, spontaneous movements usually involving more than one joint. They are purposeless but may not appear so at first glance. They are most easily characterized as being similar to the "fidgets" or normal restlessness seen in children. They involve the extremities, the face, the mouth, and the tongue. They are not associated with an increase in tone. *Athetoid movements* are characteristically slow, writhing movements involving mainly the proximal parts of the extremities and also the trunk and face. They are often associated with other neurologic abnormalities found in cerebral palsy. *Myoclonus* is a sudden brief contraction of a group of muscles that usually causes movement across joints. Myoclonic movements usually are more rapid than choreic movements.

STRENGTH

In testing the strength of all appropriate muscle groups, pay particular attention to the relative strength of the two sides and the differences between proximal and distal groups. Special attention should be paid to any area that the patient considers weak. It is not necessary to do a complete detailed muscle examination on every patient, especially if he does not complain of weakness. A screening examination would logically include testing the strength of dorsiflexion and plantar flexion of the feet, extension of the wrist, and flexion and extension of the forearm and shoulders. Strength can be graded from 0 to 5. A system of grading by percentage of the normal may also be used (Table 18–5).

The strength of different individuals varies greatly. The handgrip normal for a society matron would certainly not be considered normal for a farmer. The difference in strength between the nondominant and dominant sides of the body is usually minimal and should not be used as an explanation for unilateral weakness.

It is important to test both distal and proximal muscle groups in both the upper and lower extremities. In some muscle diseases, such as muscular dystrophy, there may be marked weakness of the shoulder and hip girdle musculature and surprising strength of the hands and feet. If weakness is present, detailed tests of all muscle groups are indicated to determine the extent, distribution, and degree of weakness. Much diagnostic information can be obtained in this way.

The muscular weakness of myasthenia gravis will characteristically be accentuated by repetitive or continuous use of the muscles (arms held over the head, eyes fixed upward in a steady gaze, or hands clenched in a continuous grip). Strength testing before and after a trial dose of edrophonium chloride is the most certain method of identifying this disease.

A tendency to slowed relaxation of the muscles is characteristic of such diseases as hypothyroidism, myotonia, and myotonic dystrophy. It is most evident in patients with myotonia. It may be demonstrated by percussion of affected muscles, such as the quadriceps, the forearm groups, or the thenar muscles, with the reflex hammer. The percussed muscle will contract and then relax at a rate several times slower than normal.

Feigned muscle weakness may fool the most sophisticated observer. A tendency to "give way" in a jerky fashion is characteristic of nonorganic muscular weakness, but some tendency toward giving way may be found in certain definitely organic diseases.

MUSCLE RESISTANCE TO PASSIVE MANIPULATION ("TONE")

Check muscle resistance to passive manipulation by both fast and slow flexion and extension at the elbows, wrists, shoulders, knees, and ankles. Ask the patient to relax as much as possible during this examination. In healthy cooperative adults the muscles are normally somewhat hypotonic. The normal patient should be able to relax his extremities sufficiently so that the examiner can easily test for tone. In some patients, particularly those who are tense or anxious, there is marked difficulty in producing the necessary relaxation of the extremities. The patient tries to cooperate and voluntarily moves the arm in the same manner as the examiner, thus defeating the examiner's purpose. In a few people it may be impossible to assess resistance to passive manipulation adequately for this reason.

Muscle resistance to passive manipulation is normally decreased in diseases of the anterior horn cells and peripheral nerves and in uncomplicated diseases of the cerebellum. An increase in resistance to passive manipulation is found in upper motor neuron diseases (pyramidal tract), in which case it is characterized as *spasticity*. Spasticity is the most common abnormality of resistance to passive manipulation and is classically of the clasp-knife type. The resistance varies from normal as one rapidly extends or flexes the joint to a marked increase when full flexion or extension is approached. With continued pressure the muscle then gradually gives way.

On the other hand, *rigidity*, which characterizes the extrapyramidal group of diseases such as parkinsonism, is characterized by an increase of resistance that is present throughout the full range of motion of the joint, producing steady resis-

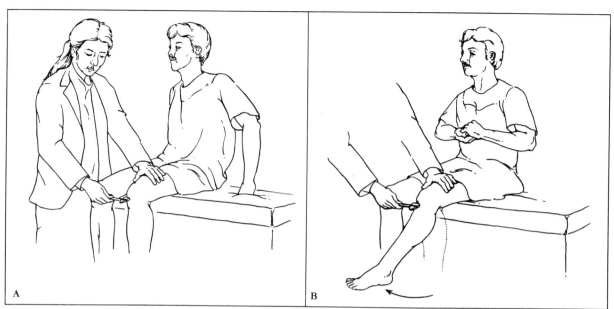

FIGURE 18–14
Reinforcement of the patellar reflex. A. Patient at rest. B. Patient pulls against his own fingers just as tendon is struck.

tance to the examiner's superimposed movement. In addition there may be a "cog-wheeling," as mentioned above.

REFLEXES

Examine the biceps, triceps, radial periosteal, patellar, and Achilles reflexes in all patients. Strike the tendon directly and smartly with the reflex hammer. The limb to be tested should be relaxed and in a flexed or semiflexed position. The biceps reflex is best tested by tapping the examiner's finger or thumb, which has been placed over the patient's tendon.

In normal young adults, reflexes may be minimal or apparently absent and may be elicited only by asking the patient to "reinforce" by pulling with one hand against the other at the time the tendon is tapped (Fig. 18–14). A reflex is not considered truly absent until there is proof that it cannot be elicited by this maneuver. In certain patients the reflexes may be extremely active, but sustained *clonus* (persistent involuntary flexion and extension of the joint under extension or flexion pressure) is never present in the absence of central nervous system disease.

It is good to develop the habit of charting all the reflexes completely. This is easily done by drawing the figure of a man, labeling the sides right and left, and placing the state of the reflex represented by 0 through 4 + at the appropriate joint. An abbreviated chart may also be used for this purpose. Reflexes should be represented as follows: 0, absent; 1 +, decreased; 2 +, normal; 3 +, hyperactive; 4 +, hyperactive with clonus. These methods are illustrated in Figure 18–15.

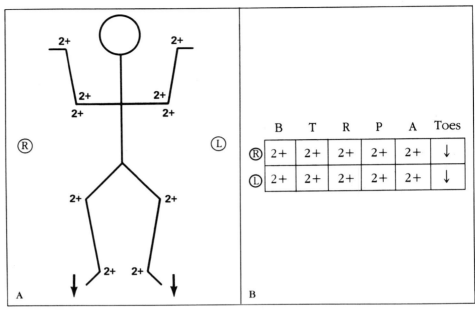

	B	T	R	P	A	Toes
Ⓡ	2+	2+	2+	2+	2+	↓
Ⓛ	2+	2+	2+	2+	2+	↓

FIGURE 18–15
Recording the reflexes. One may record the deep tendon reflexes by drawing them on a stick figure (A) or in a table. (B) in the written physical.

Reflex asymmetry has more pathologic significance than the absolute activity of the reflex. That is, 3+ hyperreflexia bilaterally in the knee jerks may occur as a result of anxiety, for example, and is less diagnostic of neurologic abnormality than a 3+ reflex in the right knee with 2+ in the left. The reflex examination is one of the most important parts of the neurologic examination because abnormalities in this sphere are difficult to feign and thus represent an objective assessment of the patient's neurologic status. Anything that interferes with the anterior horn cell, the sensory or the motor part of the reflex arc, the motor end-plate, or the muscle may eliminate or decrease the reflex. On the other hand, a pathologic increase in reflexes almost invariably represents chronic disease of the upper motor neuron. The lesion, of course, can be anywhere from the cerebral cortex to just above the appropriate anterior horn cell. Any isolated reflex change, either increase or decrease, requires special consideration by the examiner.

It is important to memorize a few reflex arc levels that are helpful in determining the level of spinal cord lesions (Table 18–6).

PATHOLOGIC REFLEXES. The pathologic reflexes are extremely important and should be carefully looked for. There are two basic pathologic reflexes—the *Babinski* and its variants, and the *Hoffmann* and its variants.

Test for the plantar response by stroking the sole of the foot with the blunt end of a reflex hammer or with a key, moving the test object from the heel along the lateral edge and then across the ball of the foot medially. A flexor plantar response

TABLE 18–6. Reflex Examination

Name	Technique	Reflex Arc Level
Biceps		C 5–6

| Triceps | | C 6–7–8 |

| Radial periosteal | | C 5–6 |

TABLE 18–6. (Continued)

Name	Technique	Reflex Arc Level
Patellar		

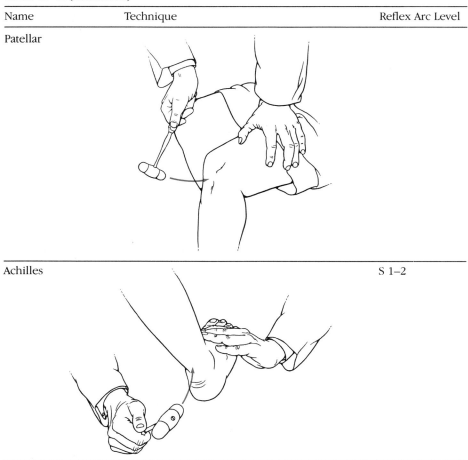

Name	Technique	Reflex Arc Level
Achilles		S 1–2

consists of a downward flexion motion of the great toe. An extensor plantar response consists of an upward extension of the great toe. Often there is corresponding dorsiflexion of the ankle, flexion of the knee, and flexion of the hip. This is called the triple flexion response. An extensor plantar reflex indicates the presence of Babinski's sign or the Babinski reflex. The Babinski reflex is either present or absent; there is no positive or negative Babinski's sign. Many patients withdraw their limbs with even gentle plantar stimulation, making the plantar response difficult to evaluate. A series of variants of the Babinski reflex have been described that avoid direct plantar stimulation. In all of these, a pathologic response consists of dorsiflexion of the great toe. At times, dorsiflexion of the toe will be accompanied by fanning of the other toes, but this is not a required response. Elicit the *Chaddock reflex* by stroking the lateral edge of the foot from the heel to the toes just above the sole. Evoke the *Oppenheim reflex* by firmly pressing down on the shin with the knuckles from the knee to the ankle. The *Gordon reflex* can be tested by squeezing the calf firmly. Normally, after infancy, there is no extensor response of the foot and toes to any of these maneuvers. The presence of these reflexes is an unequivocal sign of disease of the pyramidal tract (Table 18–7).

There are several sources of difficulty in interpreting the plantar response. At times the response may be equivocal with perhaps only fleeting dorsiflexion of the large toe and no fanning of the other toes. There may be no response to plantar stimulation at all; when this occurs, it is usually significant if there is a difference in the responses of the two feet. Another source of difficulty is the tendency of some patients voluntarily to withdraw their lower extremity when the sole of the foot is stimulated. Often this can be overcome by simply asking them not to withdraw. Some plantar responses are strongly abnormal, with withdrawal of the entire lower extremity, and yet they are stated to be equivocal because the examiner incorrectly thinks that the withdrawal is voluntary and not part of the reflex. It is only with experience that the examiner learns to differentiate between these two types of withdrawals.

Babinski's sign is one of the most reliable signs in neurology and should be tested for in all patients.

Test the *Hoffmann reflex* by quickly extending or flexing the last joint of the middle finger. While suspending the limp hand by its middle finger, quickly flip the tip of the finger upward or downward (Fig. 18–16). Normally there is very little if any response to this maneuver. A positive Hoffmann reflex consists of a flexion movement of the thumb and fingers. This may be present under normal circumstances and is significant only when it is markedly exaggerated or unilaterally present. In this case, it may indicate pyramidal tract disease.

Clonus is tested by quickly flexing or extending a joint and maintaining the joint in flexion or extension (Fig. 18–17).

Test for the *jaw jerk* by placing your finger on the patient's jaw, asking the patient to open his mouth slightly, and then tapping your finger with a reflex hammer. The jaw jerk consists of rapid closure of the jaw. The jaw jerk is graded the same as other deep tendon reflexes. It is an important reflex because it tests the integrity of a myotatic reflex arc within the pons. It is the only deep tendon reflex that can be easily tested above the level of the neck, and it can be important in differentiating spinal disease from disease located at a higher level of the nervous system.

SUPERFICIAL SKIN REFLEXES. The main superficial reflexes are the abdominal and cremasteric reflexes. The *abdominal reflex* is elicited by stroking with a firm or slightly irritating object (such as a somewhat sharp stick) over all four quadrants of the abdomen. The stroke can be directed toward, away from, or at right angles to the umbilicus. Normally the umbilicus moves toward the stimulus. The *cremasteric reflex* in men is elicited by stroking along the internal aspect of the upper thigh. A normal response results in an upward movement of the testicle of the side stimulated due to involuntary contraction of the cremaster muscle (Fig. 18–18).

Both of these reflexes are normally present in the young, relaxed patient, but their absence is common and may be due to a variety of causes. Diseases of either the upper or the lower motor neurons will eliminate the superficial reflexes. In addition the superficial reflexes may be difficult to elicit in the tense, obese, preg-

TABLE 18–7. Reflex Examination in Pyramidal Tract Disease

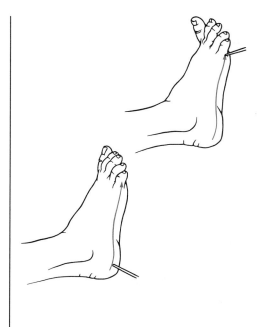

Babinski's	Firmly hold the knee or ankle to prevent withdrawal
	Stroke the lateral sole of the foot with a blunt point (a key is good for this); the stroke must not be painful
	A Babinski sign (extensor plantar response) is dorsiflexion of the great toe, often with fanning of the other toes
Chaddock's	Stroke with a blunt point around the side of the foot, from lateral malleolus to the small toe
	In a positive test, there is dorsiflexion of the great toe

Oppenheim's

Firmly press down on the shin and run the thumb and the knuckles along the anterior medial tibia toward the foot
In a positive test, there is dorsiflexion of the great toe

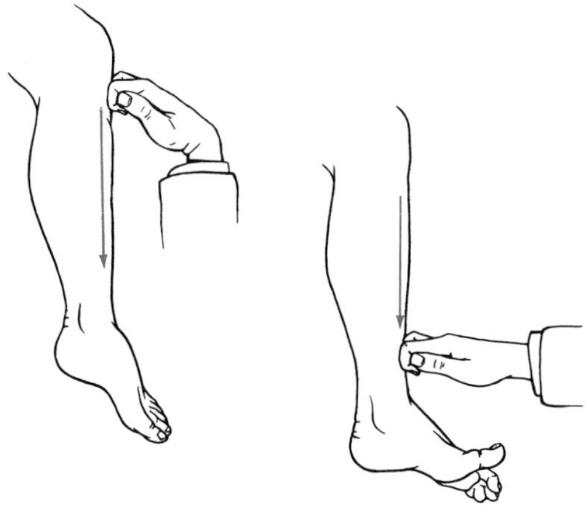

Gordon's

Firmly squeeze the calf
In a positive test, there is dorsiflexion of the great toe

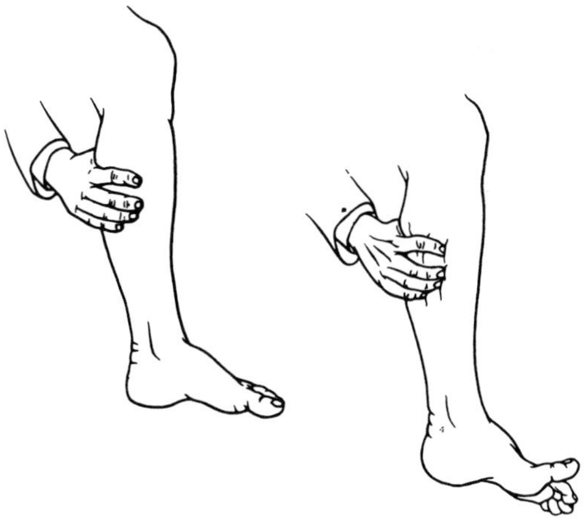

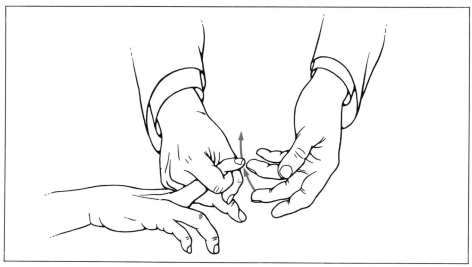

FIGURE 18–16
Hoffmann reflex.

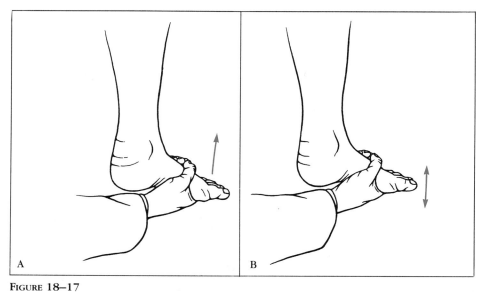

FIGURE 18–17
Testing for clonus at the ankle. A. Grasp and quickly dorsiflex the foot. B. Holding the foot in dorsiflexion, you will feel the rhythmic contractions ("beats") in your hand.

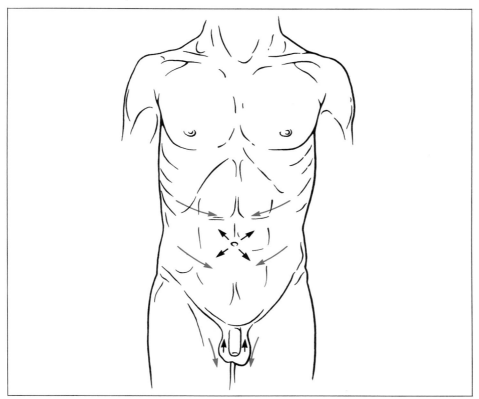

FIGURE 18–18
Abdominal and cremasteric reflexes. Sites of testing for these superficial reflexes are indicated by red arrows. Reflex response is indicated by black arrows.

nant, or uncooperative patient. Although their absence can be significant, they are not usually of diagnostic importance. Unilateral absence or absence of either the upper or lower abdominals may be helpful in ascertaining the "sidedness" of a lesion or the level of a lesion in the spinal cord. In this regard it is important to remember that the upper abdominals are innervated by segments T7 through T9 and the lower by T9 through T11.

CEREBELLAR FUNCTION
Coordination and the ability to perform skilled and rapid alternating movements in the upper and lower extremities are tests of cerebellar function.

UPPER EXTREMITIES. Ask the patient to supinate and pronate his hand alternately as rapidly as possible on each side. He should be able to perform rapid alternating movements nearly as well with his nondominant as with his dominant hand. Direct the patient to touch the index finger of one hand from the tip of his nose to the tip of your finger, which you hold at full arm's length from the patient (the finger-

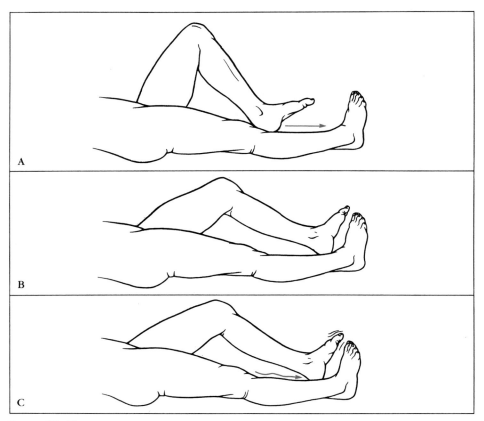

FIGURE 18–19
Heel-knee-shin test. A. Beginning the test. B. Normal result: The heel runs smoothly and straight down the shin. C. Abnormal result: The heel is ataxic and jerky and may even fall off the shin.

nose-finger test). This should be performed accurately without tremor and without missing either target. Patients with cerebellar disease develop a proximal side-to-side tremor on approaching the target. Ask the patient to perform rapid opening and closing movements of each hand.

LOWER EXTREMITIES. Ask the patient to tap his foot against the floor as rapidly as possible, then direct him to touch one heel to the opposite knee and run it slowly down his shin to the big toe (heel-knee-shin test) (Fig. 18–19). These maneuvers should be performed rapidly without any wavering or tremor. Patients with cerebellar disease perform these movements slowly and, during the heel-knee-shin test, there is side-to-side movement of the heel, with the heel often falling off the shin. The abnormal coordination seen with cerebellar disease is termed *ataxia*. This consists of *dysmetria,* which is difficulty in reaching the target precisely for each movement, and abnormalities in the rate and regularity of each movement.

TABLE 18–8. Some Causes of Ataxia

Generalized weakness or fatigue of any cause

Drugs and toxins
  Alcohol
  Sedative-hypnotics
  Phenytoin (Dilantin)
  Narcotics

Sensory defects
  Posterior column disease
    Vitamin B_{12} deficiency
    Tabes dorsalis (syphilis)
    Diabetes
  Peripheral neuropathy (if severe)
    Diabetes
    Alcoholism
    Guillain-Barré syndrome
    Vasculitis (rare)
    Porphyria
    Carcinomatous neuropathy
    Nutritional disorders
  Multiple sclerosis of the spinal cord
  Lesions of the thalamus, internal capsule, sensory cortex

Cerebral lesions
  Multiple sclerosis
  Alcoholism
  Vascular events
    Thrombosis
    Bleeding
  Hereditary ataxia
  Tumor

Hysteria

Many things may interfere with cerebellar testing or give false cerebellar signs. Among these are sensory loss, especially loss of proprioception. In addition, pyramidal tract disease may lead to slowness in movement; marked weakness of lower motor neuron or peripheral nerve origin may also result in slowness. A combination of these defects may produce cerebellarlike signs that make it difficult to determine whether the ataxia is really of cerebellar origin. Certainly one should be careful to do adequate sensory testing on any patient with apparent cerebellar disease to determine whether proprioception is intact.

Disease of one cerebellar hemisphere produces signs on the same side of the body. That fact is important to remember when attempting to localize a lesion because the thalamic, pontine, and occasionally frontal lobe lesions of the opposite side may produce ataxia similar to that from involvement of the cerebellum itself. Since ataxia may be drug-induced and therefore transitory, it may be necessary to test the patient more than once. Some causes of ataxia are presented in Table 18–8.

STATION AND GAIT

Ask the patient to walk as normally as possible for some distance. Notice his general posture, the size of his steps, the lateral distance between his feet as he places them on the ground, the amount of associated arm swinging present, and his balance while walking. Test his ability to start and stop on command. Sometimes walking will be normal but running impossible. Ask the patient to walk in a straight line, putting one heel directly in front of the toes of the other foot. This is called *tandem walking.*

Abnormalities in gait should be described as accurately as possible. A difference in length of stride between the feet should be mentioned. Any tendency toward dragging of the toes and high lifting of the knees due to weakness of the dorsiflexors of the feet (*footdrop gait* of peroneal palsy or multiple neuritis) (Fig. 18–20) also should be described. The *hemiplegic gait* (Fig. 18–21) with circumduction of the affected leg, weakness of dorsiflexion of the foot, and some tendency toward flexion at the knee on the affected side is a classic characteristic of corticospinal tract damage. Similarly, the wide-based *ataxic gait* (drunken gait) (Fig. 18–22) is the classic gait of cerebellar dysfunction. Also diagnostic is the typical *gait of parkinsonism* (Fig. 18–23), with small shuffling steps, lack of normal arm swing, flexion of the trunk, and a tendency to increase the speed and fall forward. The dancing gait of advanced *Huntington's chorea* is distinctive, as are the wormlike, athetoid movements of the limbs and trunk in athetosis. The spastic form of cerebral palsy (Little's disease) produces a *scissors gait* (Fig. 18–24), with a tendency toward internal rotation of both legs and scraping together of the semiflexed knees as the patient drags them forward. The typical gait of *tabes dorsalis* is characterized by ataxia, foot slapping, and a tendency for the patient to watch his feet (since he does not know where they are) when he walks.

Test the patient's balance by asking him to stand on one foot and then to hop on that foot. Test for Romberg's sign by asking him to stand with his feet together, first with his eyes open and then with his eyes closed. Be ready to catch the patient as he may fall when the eyes are closed. Romberg's sign can be tested only when the patient does not fall with his eyes open. A positive Romberg's sign occurs when the patient falls after closing his eyes (Fig. 18–25). A positive Romberg's sign is diagnostic of position sense loss in the lower extremities. This occurs in the presence of severe peripheral neuropathy, dorsal root disease, or dorsal column disease. Cerebellar disease should not produce a positive Romberg's sign; people with cerebellar disease often cannot stand with the eyes open and may be somewhat worse with the eyes closed.

SENSORY EXAMINATION

GENERAL

The sensory examination is difficult to perform well and interpret correctly. It is subject to great variation, depending on the experience and skill of the examiner and the cooperation and emotional balance of the patient. It is of primary importance, however, and can give clues to a diagnosis that can be obtained in no other way. Sensory testing is usually done with the patient's eyes closed.

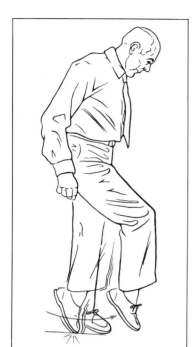

FIGURE 18–20
Steppage or footdrop gait. To avoid dragging his toes against the ground (since he cannot dorsiflex the foot), the patient lifts his knee high and slaps the foot to the ground on advancing.

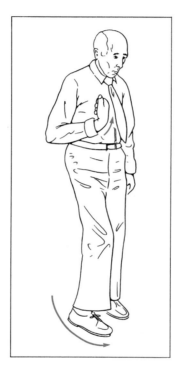

FIGURE 18–21
Hemiplegic (hemiparetic) gait. The arm is carried across the trunk, adducted at the shoulder. The forearm is rotated; the arm is flexed at elbow and wrist and the hand at the metacarpophalangeal joints. The leg is extended at the hip and knee. The patient swings his affected leg outward in a circle (circumduction).

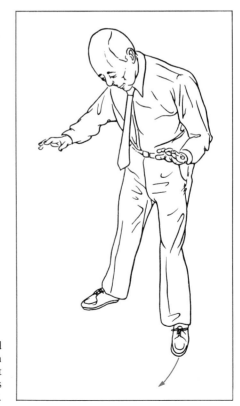

FIGURE 18–22
Ataxic gait. In *cerebellar ataxia* the patient has poor balance and a broad base; therefore he lurches, staggers, and exaggerates all movements. In *sensory ataxia* the patient has a broadbased gait and, because he cannot feel his feet, slaps them against the ground and looks down at them as he walks. In both types of ataxias the gait is irregular, jerky, and weaving.

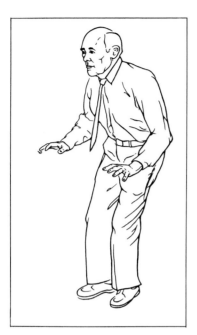

FIGURE 18–23
Parkinsonism. The head, trunk, and knees are flexed; the arms are held rather stiffly with poor associative movement. The gait is shuffling or characterized at times by short, rapid steps (marche à petits pas). The patient may lean forward and walk progressively faster, seemingly unable to stop himself (festination).

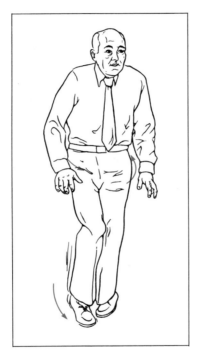

FIGURE 18–24
Scissors gait. Spasticity of thigh adduction, seen in spastic paraplegics, draws the knees together. The legs are advanced (with great effort) by swinging the hips.

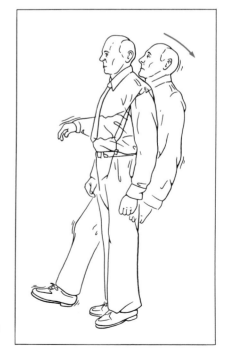

FIGURE 18–25
Positive indication of Romberg's sign. The patient falls backward only when his eyes are closed.

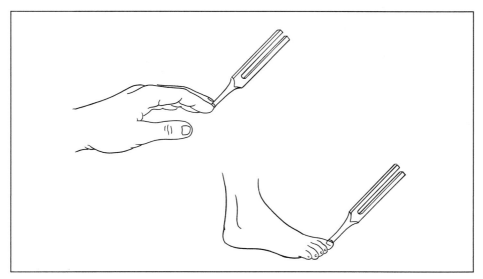

FIGURE 18–26
Testing for vibration sense. A. Upper extremity. B. Lower extremity.

VIBRATION, MOTION, AND POSITION (POSTERIOR COLUMN SENSES)
Apply a vibrating tuning fork (128 cycles per second) in succession to the tip of a finger on each hand and to the great toe of each foot, and determine whether the patient can feel the vibration. Normally, this should be perceived by individuals up to the age of about 65. In people older than 65, vibration sense may be lost at the great toe, but it remains intact on other parts of the foot and on the lateral malleolus of the ankle. A quantitative estimate of vibratory sense can be obtained by striking the tuning fork with the same strength and holding it with the same degree of firmness against each prominence (Fig. 18–26), testing in succession the first knuckle of each hand and the lateral malleolus of each ankle. Vibration sense can be used also to determine the level of a spinal cord lesion. If vibration sense is lost in the lower extremities, "walk" up the body with a tuning fork, moving from bony prominence to bony prominence until the patient feels vibration. The level of sensory perception in the bones corresponds very well to that of the skin over them. Vibration sense is mediated by both the posterior columns and the lateral columns.

With the patient's eyes closed, test position sense by grasping one toe or finger of each of the four extremities and move it briskly upward or downward (Fig. 18–27). Ask the patient to tell you whether the digit moved up or down. Grasp the digit by the sides rather than by the top and bottom if possible. Patients normally can perceive movements of 1 mm accurately. Loss of vibration and position sense can occur with dorsal column lesions, but also with disease of the peripheral nerves and posterior roots.

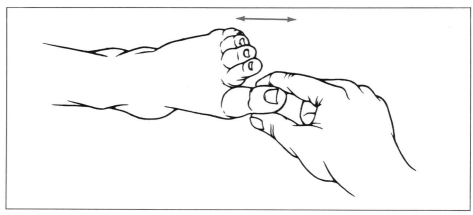

FIGURE 18–27
Testing for position sense in the lower extremity.

PAIN AND TEMPERATURE

Test pinprick sensation by touching all four limbs lightly with a sharp pin, and ask the patient to say whether the pinprick feels equally sharp in all limbs. Test more systematically any area in which the patient complains of sensory loss. It may be helpful to ask the patient to quantitate the degree of sharpness. Determine whether the patient perceives a 10 percent decrease, which is often not significant, or a 50 percent decrease in sharpness. Outline the areas that show definitely reduced pinprick sensation (Figs. 18-28 and 18-29). Use a new pin for each patient.

Pinprick sensation is tricky to test, and one may easily obtain abnormal responses in a normal person. Such difficulties are partly due to the natural variations in the pressure put on the pin and the sensitivity of different areas of the skin. Some patients may report pinprick decrease that is not significant. In this case the examiner is wise to go to some other part of the examination and then return later so as not to emphasize the "abnormality" that he has found. Another problem in examining with a pin occurs when testing one side of the body against the other. The second or last side tested will often apparently be more sensitive to the pinprick. In this case the examiner should reverse the order of the sides tested.

Pinprick testing is the most common way of determining the sensory "level" caused by a spinal cord lesion. There is usually an area of increased response to the pin at the level of the lesion, normal response above the level, and decreased response below.

Deep pain sensation may be assessed by firmly pinching the Achilles tendon or the thenar eminence.

Temperature sensation can be tested with any cool or warm object. The tines of the examiner's tuning fork or the metal handle of the reflex hammer often will serve well enough. If necessary, fill one test tube with warm water and another with ice water for more refined testing. The sensations of pain and temperature are thought to be mediated by the same central pathways, but it is often useful to test both modalities. This is particularly helpful in patients with conversion reac-

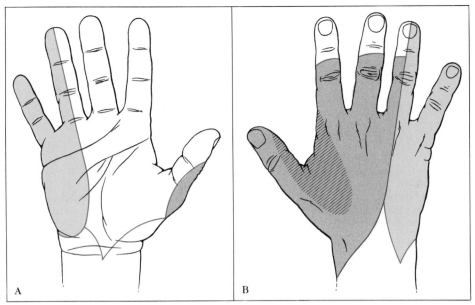

FIGURE 18–28
Sensory change on the hand with peripheral nerve injury. A. Palm. B. Dorsum. Pink indicates the area of sensory loss with ulnar nerve lesions; white, loss with median nerve lesions; and shaded area, loss with radial nerve lesions. In some patients with radial nerve lesions, only the area shown with cross-hatching will be affected.

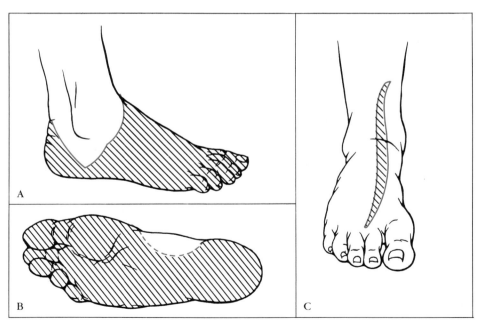

FIGURE 18–29
Sensory change on the foot with peripheral neuropathy. A. Sciatic nerve. B. Tibial nerve. C. Common peroneal nerve.

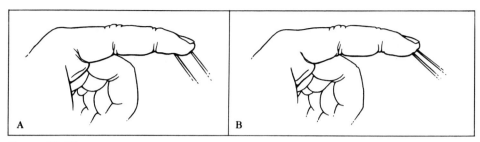

FIGURE 18–30
Two-point discrimination. A. The patient perceives the touch of two wooden sticks at 33 mm apart as two distinct stimuli. B. When the sticks are less than 3 mm apart, the touch is felt as though one stick were being used.

tions. They are unaware that the distributions should be the same for these two modalities.

FINE SENSORY MODALITIES

Fine sensory modalities include touch, two-point tactile sensation, stereognosis, and graphesthesia. Test for *light touch* with a wisp of cotton on the surfaces of the body. Include the trunk and all four extremities, and test one side against the other.

Two-point tactile discrimination is tested with two dull points. Ask the patient to close his eyes; then simultaneously touch two places on the same extremity. Compare one side of the body to the other. The threshold at which the patient feels two distinct points, or conversely at which he feels them as one, is recorded. Two-point discrimination is usually tested on the tips of the fingers. The threshold on the tip of the index finger on a normal person is about 3 mm, that is, the points are 3 mm apart or less when they are perceived as one (Fig. 18–30).

Stereognosis is tested in the hands. Ask the patient to close his eyes and identify objects placed in his hands by moving them around and feeling them with his fingers. Any convenient objects, such as coins and keys, can be used. A normal person can differentiate between a penny, nickel, quarter, and half dollar.

Before stating that a patient has astereognosis, one should be careful to determine that there is no more obvious sensory loss in the extremity. If there is a definite sensory loss in the extremity and stereognosis is also decreased, the loss would better be called stereoanesthesia and does not necessarily indicate parietal cortex dysfunction.

Test *graphesthesia* by drawing numerals on various parts of the patient's skin and asking him to identify them. The size of the identifiable numeral will naturally vary with the area.

Extinction can be detected by the method of double simultaneous stimulation. Have the patient close his eyes, and touch him, for example, on the back of the hand. Ask him where he was touched. Touch him then on the identical spot on the other side of his body and repeat the question. The third time, touch him in both places simultaneously and with equal pressure. Extinction is present when the patient can perceive touch on each side of the body separately, but perceives touch only on one side of the body when the stimulus is applied to both sides simultaneously. This is commonly seen in the presence of parietal lobe disease, but it may occur with lesions in other parts of the nervous system, including the peripheral nervous system.

Since motion, position, and vibratory senses have already been checked to test the function of the posterior columns, most of the finer modalities do not need to be tested in the usual patient. However, they are useful in evaluating parietal cortex function and should be tested when disease is suspected in that region.

Because these finer sensory modalities are mediated by in the posterior columns of the spinal cord, they also may be useful in the analysis of hysterical (conversion reaction) sensory loss. Some patients with hysterical sensory loss have loss of vibration but good stereognosis. The reverse of this may also occasionally be true.

CONVERSION REACTION

Many patients with psychological disorders present with complaints of disturbed neurologic function. In evaluating such patients, it is important to look for objective signs of neurologic dysfunction. These include abnormalities of the deep tendon reflexes, downward drift with pronation of an extended arm when the patient's eyes are closed, and abnormalities of gait, some of which are difficult to feign. Patients with conversion reaction often show a sensory disturbance that does not match anatomical distributions of peripheral nerves or nerve roots. In addition, the patient often will show inconsistent responses, with absence of sensation over a patch of skin at one moment and presence of sensation at another moment. The presence of "give-way" weakness is often a sign of conversion reaction. In give-way weakness, the patient puts out good effort in the initial phase of strength testing, but then the effort rapidly decreases. Patients with conversion reactions at times will claim to have complete loss of all sensation on one half of the body. The sensory defect will include loss of vibration sense. Such patients will claim to feel a vibrating tuning fork only on one half of the skull and on one half of the sternum. This is physically impossible because vibration is transmitted across bone very rapidly, and even people with severe sensory loss on one side of the body will perceive a vibrating tuning fork when applied to the skull or sternum on the half of the body with a decrease of sensation.

The diagnosis of conversion reaction should be made only with great caution. Many patients with organic disease of the nervous system will show motor and sensory defects that appear to be hysterical in origin, including give-way weakness and a variable sensory defect. Some patients with organic pathology also will embellish their responses to testing. Thus, one must be wary of making an easy diagnosis of hysteria. Often repeated neurologic examinations and extensive laboratory and imaging tests are needed to establish a correct diagnosis.

SECTION VII

SPECIAL EXAMINATIONS

19. PEDIATRIC EXAMINATION
   Patricia O'Connor
   George H. Lowry
20. GERIATRIC EXAMINATION
   James K. Cooper
21. INJURED PATIENT
   Gerhard Schmeisser
   George D. Zuidema

*. . . one man in his time
plays many parts,
His acts being seven ages.
At first the infant,
Mewling and puking in
the nurse's arms.
Then the whining
schoolboy with his satchel
And shining morning
face, creeping like snail
Unwillingly to school. And
then the lover. . . .
Then a soldier. . . .
And then the justice. . . .
The sixt age shifts
Into the lean and slipper'd
pantaloon,
With spectacles on nose
and pouch on side;
His youthful hose well
sav'd, a world too wide
For his shrunk shank, and
his big manly voice,
Turning again toward
childish treble, pipes
And whistles in his sound.
Last scene of all,
That ends this strange
eventful history,
Is second childishness and
mere oblivion —
Sans teeth, sans eyes, sans
taste, sans everything.*

WILLIAM SHAKESPEARE
(1564–1616)

CHAPTER 19

PEDIATRIC EXAMINATION

*Science is essentially a matter of observation, inference, verification,
generalization. The mind of Sydenham, interested in a sick child and
humanely preoccupied with its cure, did not, insofar as it functioned
scientifically, operate differently from that of Galileo, interested in cosmic
physics. Both alike observed, reflected, verified, generalized.*

ABRAHAM FLEXNER
(1866–1959)

Physical examinations of children present challenges and rewards not found when
dealing with adults. The child is not a miniature adult. Although children follow
general predictable patterns of growth and development, many individual variations are found in healthy children.

Growth and development consist of continuous, expansive, progressive changes
occurring at a generally rapid pace, especially in infancy (the first year of life) and
in adolescence. The normal child is continuously becoming bigger, more able,
more adept, and more mature in various organ functions. Children of the same age
will vary considerably in size, personality, coordination ability, and in maturity, for
example, but will also be comparable in many of these same characteristics. Understanding these likenesses and differences in the growing child makes monitor-
ing and fostering growth and development a fascinating and rewarding activity.

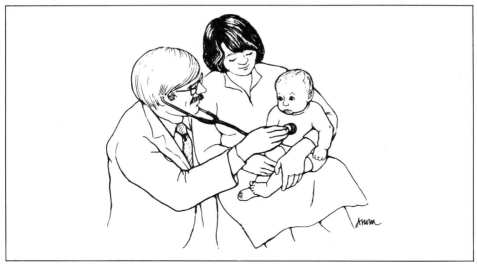

FIGURE 19–1
Examining the child in the mother's lap.

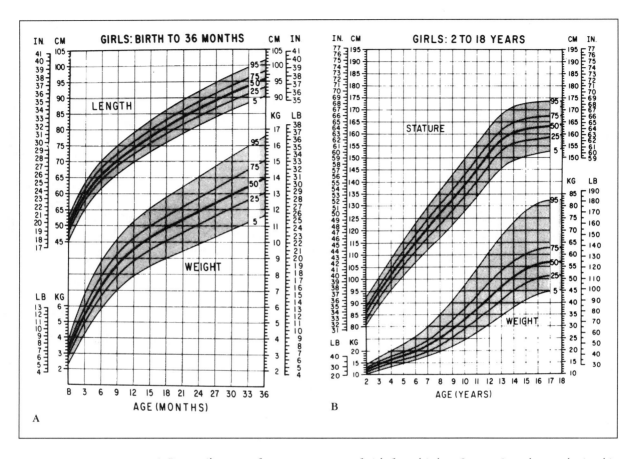

A. Percentile curves for measurements of girls from birth to 3 years. Length was obtained in a recumbent position during the first 3 years, thereafter as standing height. Where the length and height measurements overlap, the results have been modified to result in a smooth uninterrupted curve. B. Percentile curves for measurements of girls from 2 to 18 years. (Reproduced by permission of the National Center for Health Statistics.)

GROWTH AND DEVELOPMENT

I'll just have to save him. Because, after all,
A person's a person, no matter how small.

            "Dr. Seuss" (Theodor S. Geisel)
                 (1904–)

See Figs. 19-2 and 19-3 and Tables 19-1, 19-2, 19-3, and 19-4.

HISTORY

Infants do not cry without some legitimate cause.

                 Ferrarius
                 (16th century)

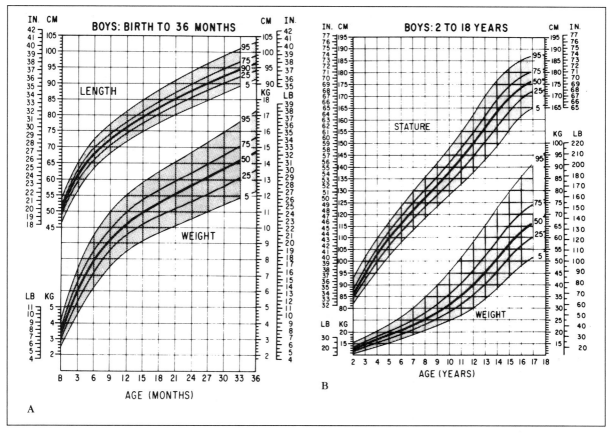

FIGURE 19–3
A. Percentile curves for measurements of boys from birth to 3 years. See legend for Figure 19-2A. B. Percentile curves for measurements of boys from 2 to 18 years. (Reproduced by permission of the National Center for Health Statistics.)

GENERAL

Histories and physical examinations of children will vary in relation to the age of the child. Different approaches will be appropriate for the infant and toddler, the young child, and the older child and adolescent.

For all ages, a calm, reassuring, nonjudgmental approach, which allows parents and the older child to express their concerns in their own words is a good way to initiate history taking. The child is often fearful of the visit to the doctor and needs to be handled gently and supportively. Open-ended questions addressed to parents and to the older child are often most useful. If tangential or unrelated information is obtained in this way, more specific questions aimed at eliciting factual data can be used to guide the history-taking process.

TABLE 19–1. Average Head Circumference of American Children

Age	Mean		Standard Deviation	
	Inches	Centimeters	Inches	Centimeters
Birth	13.8	35.0	0.5	1.2
3 mo	15.9	40.4	0.5	1.2
6 mo	17.0	43.4	0.4	1.1
12 mo	18.3	46.5	0.5	1.2
18 mo	19.0	48.4	0.5	1.2
2 yr	19.2	49.0	0.5	1.2
3 yr	19.6	50.0	0.5	1.2
4 yr	19.8	50.5	0.5	1.2
5 yr	20.0	50.8	0.6	1.4
6 yr	20.2	51.2	0.6	1.4
7 yr	20.4	51.6	0.6	1.4
8 yr	20.6	52.0	0.8	1.8
10 yr	20.9	53.0	0.6	1.4
12 yr	21.0	53.2	0.8	1.8
14 yr	21.3	54.0	0.8	1.8
16 yr	21.9	55.0	0.8	1.8
18 yr	22.1	55.4	0.8	1.8
20 yr	22.2	55.6	0.8	1.8

Source: From G. H. Lowrey, *Growth and Development of Children* (7th ed.). Chicago: Year Book Medical Publishers, 1978.

TABLE 19–2. Some Developmental Milestones*

Age	Activity
1 mo	Head sags when in sitting position
	Smiles
	Regards faces
3 mo	Holds head erect when in sitting position
	Follows large objects with head and eye
6 mo	Rolls over
	Reaches and grasps objects
8 mo	Sits erect
	"Talks" jargon and imitates vowel sounds
10 mo	Effects finger-thumb grasp
	Pulls self to standing position
	Says and means ma-ma and da-da
12 mo	Walks with one hand held or alone
	Releases cube in cup after demonstration
	Helps in dressing
18 mo	Walks up stairs with support
	Builds tower of three or more cubes
	Follows simple verbal directions

*These are examples of developmental stages that will be accomplished by more than half the children in an average population. What is important is that the individual makes steady progress with advancing age.

TABLE 19–3. Secondary Sexual Characteristics in American Children

Characteristic	Age (yr)
Female fat deposition about pelvis	8–10
Initial breast hypertrophy	9–11
Mature breast development	14–18
Female pubic hair	9–12
Female axillary hair	10–13
Menarche	11–15
Enlargement of penis and testes	10–13
Male pubic hair	10–13
Male axillary hair	11–15
Male facial hair	12–15

TABLE 19–4. Pediatric Vital Signs

Variations in Respiratory Rates (quiet breathing)		Average Heart Rate at Rest	
Age	Rate per minute	Age	Rate per minute
Premature	40–90	Birth	130–150
Newborn	30–80	1–6 mo	120–140
1 yr	20–40	6–12 mo	110–130
2 yr	20–35	1–2 yr	110–120
4 yr	20–35	2–4 yr	90–110
10 yr	18–20	6–10 yr	90–100
Adults	15–18	10–14 yr	80–90

Normal Blood Pressure for Various Ages (mm Hg)

Age	Systolic	2 S.D.	Diastolic	2 S.D.
1 mo	86	20	54	18
6 mo	90	26	60	20
1 yr	96	30	65	25
2 yr	99	25	65	25
4 yr	99	20	65	20
6 yr	100	15	60	10
8 yr	105	15	60	10
10 yr	110	17	60	10
12 yr	115	19	60	10
14 yr	118	20	60	10
16 yr	120	16	65	10

Source: From G. H. Lowrey, *Growth and Development of Children* (7th ed.). Chicago: Year Book Medical Publishers, 1978.

In addition to the history obtained from the parents and the older child, hospital records and reports from physicians, teachers, psychologists, and others who have cared for the child should be consulted when these are available and pertinent.

With the infant and toddler, the parent or caretaker is the major source of the history. Physician observation during the history and examination and hospital or clinic records are also very useful when evaluating very young children. Previous weights documented in hospital records, for example, are important in the evaluation of an infant with a feeding problem or a problem with diarrhea. In taking the history, objective data should be sought. Parents should be asked or records should be checked for Apgar scores, maximum bilirubin level in the neonatal period, frequency of breast feedings, specific brand and method of preparation of the infant's formula, total amount of formula taken per day, use of fluoridated water, use and kind of vitamin supplements, frequency and kind of bowel movements, for example. If an infant has a chronic medical problem, further specific information is required such as kind and dose of medications, settings for respiration and heart rate limits on monitors, and the like.

As language develops, the child becomes more able to provide some of the history. "My tummy hurts" or "Johnny hit me" are generally honest and accurate statements from a preschool child. With the increased concern about possible child abuse, dolls with anatomically correct external genitalia are being used to help elicit histories from preschoolers who may have been abused. Generally, however, the physician must rely on parents or caretakers for specific points in the history.

The older child and adolescent become increasingly competent in providing history about acute illnesses. Their knowledge of past medical history such as birth history is generally scant. They also may tend to downplay their symptoms for fear of shots or of being restricted from desired activities. In cases of eating disorders, sexual promiscuity, and substance abuse, denial is very common. Teenagers may be more open and frank when parents are absent and they can speak confidentially with the physician. It is desirable for the physician to provide an opportunity for interaction with the teenager alone, in most instances. Parents or caretakers often provide additional insight when the physician speaks privately with them.

The outline of the history given below will vary in order and in detail depending on the reason the child is being seen. The history of a 2-year-old who appears to be developmentally delayed would require considerable detail relating to such points as the course of pregnancy, method of delivery, birth weight, early feeding problems, times of accomplishing the developmental milestones, and similar developmental patterns in other family members. Conversely, the history of a 12-year-old who has been well but now has a fever and sore throat would not include such details.

The history of a sick child should indicate the background of the child and his family and should answer to some degree the question "In what sort of a child did this sickness develop?" As with the adult, the informant should be guided by the examiner, but he or she should be given the freedom to report in his or her own words. Detailed psychosocial histories may be indicated in certain cases, but often these are most appropriately done at another time because of the need to focus on

History Form

Name _____   Informant _____
Birth date _____   Reliability _____

Chief complaint:

Usually a single symptom in the informant's own words, duration.

Present illness:

Initial symptoms, date of onset, subsequent symptoms chronologically, pertinent negative data by direct questions.

Past history:

1. Birth and neonatal: prenatal care, mother's illnesses during pregnancy; gestation time; labor, delivery (position, instruments, etc.); birth weight; Apgar score; immediate cry, cyanosis (duration, therapy); jaundice (duration, maximum bilirubin, therapy); days hospitalized; early feeding (breast, bottle, difficulties); early weight gain.
2. Developmental milestones (examples are given in Table 19–4): toilet training, grade in school, school difficulties and progress. Do parents consider the child either unusually easy or difficult to manage?
3. Feeding history (mainly for young children): breast feeding (duration, etc.); formula (ingredients, changes in formula and why); schedule, duration and quantity per feeding (apparent cause of prolonged feeding time); weight at various ages; solids (when started and how received); vomiting (relation to feeding, character of material, projectile, etc.); stools (frequency, quantity, color, consistency); adolescent diets, fads and cults.
4. Immunizations (reactions): pertussis, tetanus, diphtheria, poliomyelitis, measles, rubella, mumps, *Hemophilus influenzae* type B vaccine, others (include boosters).
5. Illnesses (frequency, severity, complications, operations, fractures, accidents, allergies, etc.)
6. Habits (sleep, naps, bowel and bladder, nail biting, tics, behavior with other children, etc.)

Family history:

Many complaints about a child may result from problems within the family. Examples are parental conflicts, chronic or recurrent absence of one or both parents, intense sibling rivalry, rigidity of discipline or disagreement of parents in the methods or use, unrealistic expectations of the child's performance. Since many of these factors may not be recognized or may be suppressed by either parent or child, a direct question concerning them is often unrewarding. Clues may be obtained from remarks about changes in behavior, withdrawal from friends, poor schoolwork, etc. In addition to these aspects the usual family history as previously outlined should be recorded.

Social history:

Because of its influence on the child this may be very important—type of home, own room for child or shared, number of people in home, income, interfamily relations, etc.

Systems review:

Similar to that for the adult.

specific medical data in a limited amount of time. Often it is clear after a brief interview that there are significant problems requiring referral to a social worker, psychologist, or psychiatrist. The physician who is being asked to check for an organic cause for the child's stomach pain, for example, should first concentrate on evaluating organic pathology as a cause of this complaint.

COMMON SYMPTOMS IN PEDIATRIC PATIENTS

FEVER

This is a very common symptom in children. Throughout the early part of a child's life, the febrile response is usually higher than that of an adult to a similar cause. The premature and newborn infant, however, may have little or no fever even with very severe infections, and such reactions as an irregular temperature course, poor appetite, vomiting, and irritability may be the only symptoms that should prompt careful and thorough evaluation of the infant.

Most fevers in children are due to infections in the respiratory tract or to generalized viral illnesses. Infections in other organ systems, particularly in the renal system and genitourinary tract, should always be considered in severe or unexplained febrile illnesses. Central nervous system infections such as meningitis also must be considered in severe or unexplained febrile illnesses, particularly in infants who may not show the usual signs of meningitis such as a stiff neck, headache, and sensorium changes. Chills, delirium, and convulsions often accompany high fever in children and require prompt diagnosis and treatment.

Prolonged or recurrent fever with no apparent cause may be a symptom of a number of diseases. In addition to chronic or recurrent infections of the respiratory and genitourinary tracts, conditions that must be considered are neoplasms, leukemia, rheumatoid arthritis and immune diseases, hypersensitivity reactions, inflammatory bowel disease, and diseases of the central nervous system. Chronic infections such as tuberculosis and localized abscesses such as dental abscesses should also be considered.

ABDOMINAL PAIN

Abdominal pain is a common complaint in children and one that is often difficult to evaluate. It is often associated with illnesses such as streptococcal tonsillitis and pneumonia that do not directly involve abdominal organs.

In infants, abdominal pain or abdominal disease should be considered when there is persistent screaming and crying often associated with flexion of the thighs on the abdomen, vomiting, grunting respiration, and changes in pattern of bowel movements. Abdominal distention, bilious (yellow to yellow-green) vomiting, and passage of blood in the stools are signs of serious abdominal distress in infants and require emergency evaluation. Volvulus with twisting of the intestine around the mesentery and compromise of blood supply to the intestine, intussusception (a telescoping of one segment of the bowel on an adjacent segment), and incarcerated inguinal hernia are of particular importance in infants and young children and require prompt attention by a surgeon skilled in pediatric care.

Colic, a condition seen in the first few months of life, is characterized by periodic crying and some degree of gaseous abdominal distention. The crying is often relieved by burping, rocking, walking with the infant, or by feeding. Colic symptoms tend to recur at the same time of day or night. Parents find this very disturbing. Physicians have to be sure that something serious is not causing the crying. Consolability, lack of progression of symptoms, and lack of other findings, such as hernias, vomiting, or blood in the stool, tend to support a diagnosis of infantile colic.

Older children are able to identify complaints localized to the abdomen. As in infants, infections outside the abdomen may result in abdominal pain. In addition, appendicitis, genitourinary tract infection, gastroenteritis, peptic ulcer disease, gall bladder disease, pancreatitis, intestinal obstruction due to volvulus or intussusception, hematomas or bleeding secondary to trauma, and inflammatory bowel disease may cause abdominal pain in children. One of the most common causes of abdominal pain in children is constipation due to poor dietary and toileting patterns.

VOMITING

Like abdominal pain, vomiting often accompanies disturbances unrelated to the intestinal tract or central nervous system, two areas frequently involved in serious disease. In young children, vomiting is frequently associated with acute infections, indiscretion in diet, fear or severe anxiety, and pain. Regurgitation is the nonforceful vomiting of small quantities, often seen in early infancy. Occasionally this kind of vomiting may persist, as in the ruminating child. Esophageal atresia is manifested by vomiting shortly after birth and by the presence of large amounts of mucus in the baby's mouth. Choking and cyanosis indicate aspiration. In the newborn period, vomiting of bile-containing material always indicates bowel obstruction until proved otherwise. Vomiting caused by pyloric stenosis in infants is associated with visible peristaltic waves in the upper abdomen and becomes increasingly projectile, but since there is no nausea, refeeding is easily accomplished. In pyloric stenosis, when the stomach is empty the "olive" shape of the hypertrophied muscle at the pylorus may be palpated. In vomiting secondary to lesions of the central nervous system, nausea is often present. In the very young subject, this may be possible to detect only by the facial expression. Excessive dosage of drugs, such as theophylline or salicylates, will produce nausea and vomiting. Many metabolic disturbances may cause vomiting, including diabetes mellitus with acidosis, galactosemia, adrenogenital syndrome with salt loss, excessive hydration resulting in cerebral edema, and dehydration and ketosis.

FAILURE TO GAIN WEIGHT AND LOSS OF WEIGHT

These symptoms are important, since infants and young children normally show a progressive though somewhat variable weight gain (see Figs. 19–2, 19–3; Table 19–5). Even the older child and adolescent, except when purposely dieting, will show only brief periods when weight is not gained. Obviously, any of the causes discussed under vomiting will result in failure to gain weight if the condition persists. Malnutrition, with or without psychosocial deprivation, will produce this symptom. Defects in assimilation of food, as in cystic fibrosis of the pancreas and

TABLE 19–5. Some Causes of Short Stature*

Constitutional slow growth (delayed adolescence)

Psychosocial (emotional deprivation)

Intrauterine dwarfism
    Extreme prematurity
    Multiple births
    Maternal infection
    Maternal drug ingestion (e.g., drug abuse, therapeutic drugs, alcohol, smoking)
    Placental dysfunction

Malnutrition (primary or secondary)

Genetic
    Racial (pygmies)
    Familial short stature
    Chromosomal abnormalities (e.g., Down syndrome, Turner syndrome)

Chronic disease
    Infection (e.g., parasites, malaria, cystic fibrosis)
    Renal failure
    Heart disease (especially congenital)
    Metabolic (e.g., glycogen storage disease, mucopolysaccharidosis, galactosemia, diabetes
        mellitus)

Endocrine
    Hypopituitarism (isolated growth hormone or multiple deficiencies; may involve
        hypothalamic releasing factors or end-organ response)
    Hypothyroidism
    Sexual precocity (rapid early growth, but early puberty reduces potential)
    Hypothalamic dysfunction

Skeletal diseases
    Bone dysplasias (many types including achondroplasia, osteochondrodystrophy,
        osteopetrosis congenita)
    Rickets

Iatrogenic
    Corticosteroid therapy
    Others

*Difficulty arises in any such listing, since there is considerable overlap of categories; for example, cystic fibrosis may cause growth retardation from both malnutrition (malabsorption) and lung infection.

the various malabsorption syndromes, lead to a failure to gain. Most chronic disease will eventually result in failure to gain, because of loss of appetite as well as other less obvious factors, including fever, pain, infection, and impairment of organ function, such as heart failure. Failure to progress in normal statural growth will frequently accompany poor weight gain, as in hypothyroidism, hypopituitarism, achondroplasia, and hereditary dwarfism. The abused ("battered child") or emotionally neglected infant or child may show profound weight loss or failure to grow. Observation of the mother's handling and feeding of her child may be most helpful in determining the proper cause for a failure to thrive. Obviously, a careful investigation of the kind and quantities of food ingested is important and, where appropriate, a detailed analysis of formula preparation.

STRIDOR

This is a harsh, high-pitched, crowing noise that is most distinct during inspiration. In contrast to wheezing, it originates high in the respiratory tract, usually in the trachea or larynx. It indicates obstruction of the airway and may be combined with cough, dyspnea, hoarseness, retractions of the chest wall with respiration, and tachypnea. The small size of the infant airway is conducive to increased frequency and severity of obstruction. Slight stridor with crying is normal in some babies. In the newborn period, congenital structural abnormalities are the most common cause. These include flaccidity of the epiglottis, laryngeal web, cysts, and defects in the tracheal cartilaginous rings. In the older child, acute spasmodic laryngitis (croup) is the most common cause and typically has its onset suddenly and at night with little or no fever. Stridor may also be caused by laryngeal edema due to serum sickness, irritation due to smoke or chemicals, and obstruction by a foreign body. Extrinsic factors, such as a neoplasm or abscess in surrounding tissue, can result in obstruction and stridor.

SLOW DEVELOPMENT (MENTAL RETARDATION)

This may be suspected by parents at any age (the most severe forms at an early age), by comparing their children to siblings or other children. The presence of some physical stigmata (as seen in Down syndrome, microcephaly, hydrocephaly, and some of the chromosomal defects) may be important clues. One cannot outline the developmental diagnosis for each age in a brief space, but it can be emphasized that delay in appearance of normal achievements in several areas of behavior is almost always significant (see Table 19–2). The areas of behavior are divided into motor, language, adaptive (reaction to environment and manipulation of it), and personal-social. These areas overlap to a considerable extent. Mental retardation is a symptom with many causes. Any physician who deals with children should become adept at recognizing the child with mental retardation; the degree of impairment may then be determined by a trained psychologist.

DYSPNEA

Labored respiration, or dyspnea, is a symptom that must be discussed in relation to the age of the subject. We have noted the changes in respiratory rate with age (see Table 19–4). In the premature infant a periodic pattern of breathing is normally encountered with short periods of apnea. Gradually this pattern disappears. In the newborn period, dyspnea may be associated with atelectasis or the respiratory distress syndrome (most common in premature babies and those born to diabetic mothers). Aspiration of amniotic fluid, and congenital anomalies such as lung cysts and diaphragmatic hernia, are often associated with dyspnea. Labored breathing may also be seen with congenital heart disease, with or without failure. Later in life, dyspnea is more apt to be caused by pulmonary infection and asthma. Hyperventilation, which is seen in diabetic acidosis, fever, aspirin poisoning, and occasionally with intracranial lesions, must be distinguished from dyspnea.

CONVULSIONS

Convulsions form another symptom complex that varies in causation with age. In the newborn infant, intracranial bleeding, congenital defects of the brain, metabolic abnormalities, and anoxia may cause seizures. Hypocalcemic tetany most commonly is seen in the first 2 months of life and is often accompanied by carpopedal spasms and laryngeal stridor. The convulsive seizures of this metabolic abnormality are not easily distinguished from seizures due to other causes. Convulsive disorders are characterized by seizures of great variety, from grand mal to petit mal, to partial seizures, and may or may not be associated with other neurologic symptoms or signs between attacks. Throughout childhood the most common cause of convulsive seizures is high fever, regardless of whether the cause of fever is an infection of the respiratory tract, meninges, urinary tract, or gastrointestinal tract. The threshold for "febrile convulsions" appears to rise with age. Convulsions in children are occasionally associated with metabolic abnormalities, such as severe electrolyte imbalance or hypoglycemia, and with anoxia, intracranial bleeding, trauma, tumors, and drug intoxication or poisoning.

PHYSICAL EXAMINATION

The childhood shews the man,
As morning shews the day.
    JOHN MILTON
    (1608–1674)

BEGINNING THE EXAMINATION

Sitting by the bed or examining table is often less threatening than standing and leaning over the older infant and young child. The examiner must proceed nonchalantly and in a confident manner. Especially in children from about 1 to 6 years of age, some resistance is to be expected. A friendly attitude with conversation and casual play at the child's level is helpful. The physician must never convey feelings of either frustration or anger.

An explanation of what is to be done and showing the child the instruments to be used beforehand may contribute to his cooperation. Often part or all of the examination may best be accomplished with the patient in the mother's lap (see Fig. 19–1). In some patients several attempts with utmost patience may be necessary to perform abdominal palpation or some other portion of the examination. Skill in this respect comes with experience, and the student should not be discouraged by initial failures.

Respect the child's sense of modesty and level of understanding. In the young child undressing may be interpreted as a loss of personal identity and is best done in stages. A gown and sheet should be provided for the older child and adolescent and undressing should be accomplished in the physician's absence.

Order of procedure should delay the most objectional parts until last. It is sometimes desirable to examine first that part of the body from which the chief complaint arises. This is because cooperation is often best early in the examination before fatigue or discomfort is experienced. Listening to the chest or palpating the abdomen before the child frets or cries may be important. Examination of the throat and ears is frequently disagreeable to the infant and young child and may be delayed to the end. The fact that restraint is often necessary in this portion of the examination accounts in part for the patient's objection.

Warm and clean hands and instruments are appreciated by both patient and parent.

These preliminary considerations cannot be emphasized too much. They may mean the difference between a satisfactory and unsatisfactory physical evaluation. Both physician and patient can enjoy the examination, and this attitude should prevail. It might also be emphasized that the short time the examiner spends with the child should not be used as an opportunity to try to correct faults in disciplinary training.

With the very ill child or the smaller premature infant, the physical examination may be carried out in brief stages to permit periods of rest. In the premature infant this may be necessary to conserve body temperature and to maintain adequate humidity or oxygen administration in an incubator.

GENERAL APPEARANCE

Observation of the patient during the interview often reveals evidence of mental retardation, parent-child conflicts, parental attitudes concerning discipline, posture related to pain or weakness, and facial expression related to specific questions in the older child. The mother's handling of the infant while dressing or undressing him and while feeding often reveals her level of understanding and emotional reaction to the infant; it may also indicate errors in feeding techniques. Ambulation, relative to the age of the child, is an important observation that is too often neglected in the usual examination. Giving the child objects with which he can play will also help in the examination of general dexterity and his developmental level.

Height and weight measurements are always a routine part of the examination. Together they have great value in estimating the state of nutrition, general health, and some aspects of endocrine balance and maturation. Often the first recognized sign of disease is either failure to gain normal increments in weight or stature or an actual loss of weight (see Figs. 19–2, 19–3, and Table 19-3). Growth charts are extremely useful for sequential evaluations of a child. A single set of measurements should be interpreted with caution. Some 15 percent of children could be considered obese when their heights and weights are plotted. In the final analysis of the growth of a child, the expected rate of gain is of greater value than any single measurement.

Speech and cry are very important. Hoarseness is often present with laryngitis, hypothyroidism, and tetany. A high-pitched, piercing cry in the infant may indicate increased intracranial pressure. Pharyngeal paralysis due to poliomyelitis or diphtheria will influence speech, producing a nasal quality. A monotone type of verbalization may indicate hearing loss.

Posture, muscle tone, and coordination may be observed during the history taking. Pain in the abdomen can result in flexion of the thighs on the abdomen in infants and younger children. Opisthotonos indicates meningeal irritation (Fig. 19–4). A "position of protection" is often assumed in the presence of pain or tenderness. Lack or limitation of motion may indicate paralysis, fracture or dislocation, joint inflammation, or an intracranial lesion. Spasticity, scissors gait, and poor coordination are found as a result of cerebral injury, often present since birth. Many of the muscular dystrophies are first manifested in an abnormal gait and either

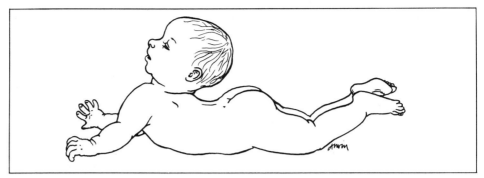

FIGURE 19–4
Opisthotonos. Some causes of opisthotonos are meningitis, tetanus, and strychnine.

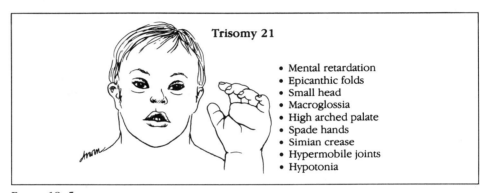

FIGURE 19–5
Down syndrome.

hypotonicity or hypertonicity. The general lack of tone of all muscle groups characterizes Down syndrome (Fig. 19–5).

VITAL SIGNS
Temperature is usually obtained rectally until the age of 3 years or over. A normal temperature in infancy and early childhood may be a degree or more above the adult average (98.6°F or 37°C).

Pulse and respiratory rates are more rapid in younger children and change with age. These rates should be obtained when the child is quiet. Both of these are fairly sensitive measures of fever, increasing about 15 to 20 percent with each degree rise in temperature. The respiratory rate and depth of breathing may increase with either respiratory or metabolic acidosis, and such changes are often the initial physical findings of the underlying abnormality. Cardiac and pulmonary diseases are also reflected by deviations from the normal.

Blood pressure also changes with age. A cuff of proper width is necessary for accurate readings. It should cover approximately one-third to one-half of the upper arm. Most children need to be reassured that the procedure will not be very uncomfortable, and the readings should be considered true values only when the subject is quiet and emotionally undisturbed. Doppler devices provide more accurate readings.

Changes with age in normal heart rate, respiratory rate, and blood pressure are presented in Table 19–4.

SKIN

The skin and subcutaneous tissues reflect the general state of hydration and nutrition. The status of tissue turgor in the infant and child is of particular importance, and it is best demonstrated by picking up a fold of abdominal skin between the thumb and index finger. Normally on release the skin rapidly returns to its former position. In some states of dehydration or undernutrition the skin remains creased and raised for a varying period of time.

In the premature and newborn infant the skin appears thin and almost transparent. It is red and wrinkled under normal conditions. Small red patches (nevus vasculosus), which are not raised and which blanch with pressure, may be present over the occiput, forehead, and upper eyelids. These patches are commonly seen in the newborn. The soft, moist, white or clay-colored material covering all newborn infants is the vernix caseosa. Some flaky desquamation occurs shortly after birth and varies in degree with individuals. For the first few weeks of life, very small, white to yellow, raised lesions that are discrete are present normally in groups, especially over the face. They are caused by plugging of the as yet poorly functioning sebaceous glands, and collectively they are known as milia. Miliaria is the red "prickly heat" rash noted during the summer or in overly dressed infants.

A blotchy blue appearance of the hands and feet (acrocyanosis) is normal in early infancy but is not a constant finding. Bluish, irregularly shaped areas that are not raised and vary greatly in size are sometimes present over the sacral and buttock areas are called mongolian spots. These spots occur most frequently in dark-skinned individuals such as Africans and Orientals. They gradually decrease in intensity and disappear with increasing age. They have no pathologic significance and should not be confused with bruises.

Physiologic jaundice is present to a mild degree in many infants, starting after the first day of life and usually disappearing by the eighth or tenth day. Jaundice that appears during the first 24 hours of life often indicates excessive hemolysis, that is, hemolytic disease of the newborn, due to the presence of maternal antibodies against the infant's red cells. If jaundice persists and gradually becomes more intense over the first few weeks of life, congenital anomalies of the biliary tract with obstruction should be suspected.

Cradle cap, or seborrheic dermatitis, in the newborn is characterized by a greasy yellowish scale over the scalp that sometimes involves other areas of the head, especially behind the ears. Another common dermatitis of childhood is tinea capitis, or ringworm of the scalp. Hair on the involved area is broken off close to the scalp and edema, reddening, and crusting are usually present.

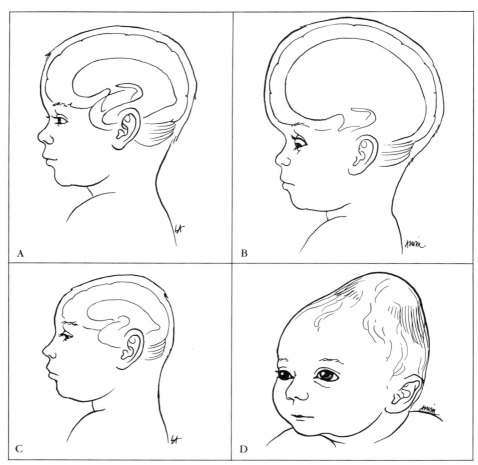

Figure 19–6
Some cephalic shapes. A. Normal. B. Hydrocephalus. C. Microcephalus. D. Caput succedaneum.

Lymph Nodes

The lymph nodes have a distribution in children similar to that in adults but are
more prominent up to the time of puberty. They are easily palpable as shotty, small,
bean-sized nodules, and usually undergo considerable hypertrophy in response to
infections throughout childhood. Anterior cervical nodes that are shotty, moveable,
and nontender are common in children.

Head

size and shape

Head size is relatively larger in children than in adults; the younger the child, the
more this is evident. Head circumference measurements have a relatively narrow
range for any age and are directly related to intracranial volume; they therefore

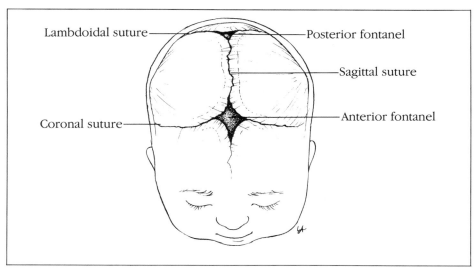

FIGURE 19–7
Skull of a child.

permit an estimation of brain growth. Rate of growth is of vital importance in patients with suspected hydrocephalus or microcephalus. The measurement is obtained by passing a tape measure over the occipital protuberance and just above the supraorbital ridges (Fig. 19–6; see Table 19–1). Children with a head circumference of more than 2 standard deviations below or above the mean should be carefully evaluated for mental retardation or other neurologic abnormality.

The head of the newborn often undergoes some distortion in shape as it passes through the birth canal. There may be overlapping of the large flat bones, which are easily palpable. Depending on the degree of molding, as this process is called, a few days to a few weeks may pass before normal anatomic relationships are reestablished. Soft tissue molding of the scalp at the time of birth results in caput succedaneum, a soft, poorly outlined swelling that pits on pressure from the edema present. It may overlie the suture lines (Fig. 19–7).

Asymmetry of the head may result from premature closure of some of the sutures. It may also be seen in the normal infant who always lies in the same position, since the bones at this time are very soft. Flattening of a portion of the cranium may occur in normal infants but is frequently associated with certain pediatric diseases, such as torticollis or mental retardation, due to the tendency for such children to maintain a constant position. Cephalhematoma is a swelling resulting from bleeding beneath the periosteum of the cranium and is therefore limited to a single cranial bone. Palpation usually reveals a small, firm, elevated margin of the lesion, which is becoming organized into a clot and later may be calcified. This and the superficially similar-appearing caput succedaneum are limited to the newborn period. Cephalhematoma may continue to increase in size following birth; caput succedaneum does not.

Careful and frequent measurements of head circumference constitute an important method of appraisal when compared with tables for normal growth rates (see Table 19–1). The posterior fontanel is closed to palpation in a few months. The anterior fontanel varies greatly in size throughout early infancy but is usually palpable only as a slight depression by 12 to 18 months of age. Normally, until the fontanels close, some arterial pulsation is transmitted through them.

Head control and movement of the head are important in evaluation of neuromuscular development. By 2 months, the head is held relatively steady when the baby is supported in an erect position, and he can raise it from a prone position. By 4 months, head control is good, with no unsteadiness.

Separation of the sutures, which have previously been approximated, and the bulging with tenseness of the anterior fontanel are indicative of increased intracranial pressure, regardless of cause. The veins over the head may also be prominent in such cases. Microcephaly, a head circumference more than two standard deviations below the normal for a given age, may indicate premature synostosis but is more commonly an associated finding in mental retardation with an underlying brain defect. Transillumination of the head is a valuable method of examination in infants. It is done in a dark room with a bright flashlight fitted with a soft rubber collar to ensure a lightproof fit against the scalp. In severe hydrocephalus and anencephaly, nearly the whole skull will transmit light. In hygroma, a localized subdural collection of fluid, a sharply delineated area of transillumination is obtained on the side of the lesion. Ultrasound of the infant skull through the anterior fontanel is an extremely useful technique for evaluating such cranial variations noninvasively.

FACE

Examine the face for shape and symmetry. Paralysis may be elicited only by making the child smile or cry. Thickening and puffiness of the features may be present with edema or hypothyroidism. Chorea is associated with uncontrolled grimacing and must be differentiated from tics and habit spasms. Epileptic seizures may be localized to the face or begin in this area in children. A lack of expression is characteristic of severe mental retardation.

EYES

The eyes of the newborn may be difficult to examine since they are tightly closed most of the time. Holding the baby upright usually results in at least a brief opening of the eyes; if he is then slowly rotated, the eyes follow in that direction. A bright light shined in the eyes will cause blinking and some dorsiflexion of the head. These two procedures permit examination of the sclerae, pupils, irides, extraocular movements, and light perception. The corneal reflex is present in all normal infants. The red reflex is elicited by setting the ophthalmoscope to "0" and viewing through the pupil at a distance of 10 to 12 inches. The normal red-orange color may be distorted if there are lesions of the cornea, anterior chamber, lens, or retina. The pupillary reflex is present at birth.

Conjugate eye movements are present shortly after birth, but true tracking movements may not be present for several days to a few weeks. Conjugate fixation on a large object (e.g., the human face) is often present at birth. Searching nystagmus normally appears for brief periods in the first few days and then normally disappears. Intermittent alternation of convergent strabismus may be observed in normal infants for the first 4 to 6 months of life. Divergent strabismus should always be considered a sign of pathologic significance. By 2 to 3 months, accurate, coordinated following of moving objects is present. Sensitivity to light and large or asymmetric corneas should alert one to consider glaucoma as a possible cause.

In early childhood, before age 6 years, the most important part of the eye examination is to determine the condition of amblyopia ex anopsia. If it is detected after that age, therapy may be unable to prevent serious loss of visual acuity. The usual causes are weakness of extraocular muscles or a refractive error in one eye resulting in visual disparity. If muscle weakness causes medial deviation it is termed *esotropia;* if lateral, *exotropia.* Two useful and simple tests to detect muscle weakness of strabismus are outlined. Both require some cooperation but are not difficult to accomplish.

1. The *cover test* has the subject look at a light source held in the middle of the examiner's forehead. Then, alternately, each eye is "covered" by placing the thumb or fingers in front of one and then removed. Each eye is observed for movement both before and after covering. If either eye moves, strabismus is present. Analysis of the results permits a differential diagnosis of the strabismus, if present (see details in Chap. 8).

2. The *Hirschberg test* also has the child look at the light in the same position as noted for the cover test. The position of the light reflection in the cornea is noted, and then the child's head is slowly turned to the right and then left. The reflection in each cornea normally will be symmetrical in all positions. If strabismus is present the reflections will be asymmetrical, and analysis of the resulting pattern will indicate whether esotropia or exotropia is present.

Visual testing with a Snellen E or other appropriate chart can be accomplished by age 2½ to 3 years. Prior to that time, parental observation of the child's awareness of surroundings, exploration, and developmental milestones may indicate normal or abnormal visual response.

Dilation of the pupils may be necessary for adequate funduscopic examination. Many neurologic diseases in infancy and childhood have retinal manifestations (e.g., toxoplasmosis, subdural hematoma, Tay-Sachs and Niemann-Pick diseases, generalized systemic candidiasis).

EAR, NOSE, AND THROAT

The ear, nose, and throat examination is best delayed to the last in the infant and young child, as restraint is often required (Figs. 19–8 and 19–9). Small, simple, deformed and low-set external ears (auricles) may indicate other congenital anomalies, such as renal agenesis or chromosomal abnormalities involving multiple systems. For a few days after birth the ear canal is filled with vernix caseosa, obscuring the tympanic membrane. In early infancy the light reflex on the membrane is less sharply delineated than later. Because middle ear infections are so common in

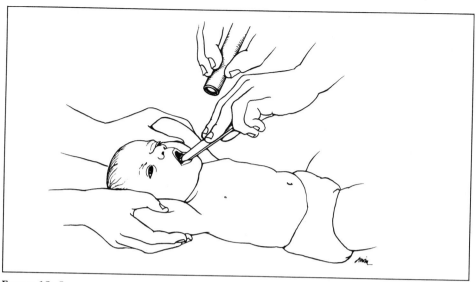

FIGURE 19–8
Examination of the throat. Note how the child's head is immobilized by using its own arms as a "vise."

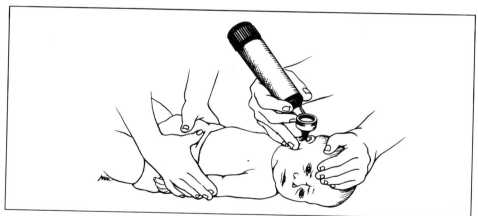

FIGURE 19–9
Examination of the ear. Note that the examiner's hand, holding the otoscope, rests on the child's head so that any sudden movement will be transmitted to both the hand and the instrument, minimizing trauma to the external canal.

early childhood, the physician who will be caring for this age group should use every opportunity during training to observe normal and pathologic conditions and to become familiar with the use of the pneumatic otoscope. When examining the ears of infants and young children it is important to minimize discomfort. The external auditory canal is relatively shallow in the infant and the bony part of the canal is very tender. The speculum should remain in the outer or cartilaginous part of the canal and the tympanic membrane visualized by angling the speculum to see all parts of the membrane.

Hearing in infancy can be tested by the child's response to sounds ranging in loudness from a small bell to a sharp clap of the hands. Responses may vary and may include cessation of activity, turning the head toward the sound, blinking, or even a verbal response. Defective or absent hearing may not be apparent for several months and should be suspected if there is a delay in vocalization or diminished smiling and laughing; what vocalization is present may be monotonal and unmodulated. Extreme visual and tactile attentiveness may be suggestive symptoms. Parents should be alerted to check their infant's response to sounds of varying tone and loudness. Tympanometry and audiometry provide quantitative measurements for evaluating and following auditory status.

The tonsils and adenoids are relatively large and cryptic in many children. The presence of enlarged tonsils does not necessarily indicate chronic infection. With acute pharyngitis in children, the tonsils are nearly always red and enlarged and may have small areas of whitish exudate.

NECK

Small bean-sized lymph nodes are easily palpable in the necks of older infants and young children. They are often enlarged in association with infections of the tonsils and pharynx. Torticollis, a condition in which the head is tilted with the chin rotated toward the opposite shoulder, is usually associated with a palpable hematoma in a sternocleidomastoid muscle in the newborn. Torticollis in older children is usually traumatic in origin or due to a respiratory infection. An unusually short neck may indicate spinal anomalies such as Klippel-Feil syndrome. A webbed neck is part of Turner syndrome. Palpable and visualized masses in early infancy may include cystic hygroma, brachial cleft cysts, and thyroglossal duct cysts as well as abscesses following infections. Generalized cervical (anterior and posterior) lymph node enlargement is present in several types of viral infections especially rubella, measles, and infectious mononucleosis.

CHEST

Asymmetry of the chest with bulging over the heart may be present in children with prolonged cardiac enlargement.

The chest in the infant and young child has a relatively greater anteroposterior diameter than in the adult. The chest wall is so thin that diseased underlying structures may be more easily discovered by auscultation and percussion than in the adult. Small nodular breast hypertrophy is found in most newborn infants and may be associated with small amounts of milklike secretion for a few days. Some breast hypertrophy, not always symmetrical, is usually present transiently in adolescent boys. Obese children often have apparent breast hypertrophy; however, this is due to adipose tissue and not to glandular hypertrophy.

Auscultation reveals breath sounds that normally are loud, harsh, and somewhat bronchial in character as compared with those of the adult. Pathology is actually more readily apparent than in older subjects, once the physician has gained experience by listening to the normal chest. Percussion note over the lung fields is more resonant in the child and even approaches being tympanitic in quality. In the infant, respiration is largely under control of the diaphragm, with little or no intercostal movement. This leads to the so-called abdominal type of respiration that lasts for about the first 6 years of life. Examination of the chest in a crying infant or child has considerable value and should not be considered as meaningless. Deep respiratory sounds are actually enhanced. Even slight changes in the position of the infant, such as turning the head, may influence the relative positions of the intrathoracic structures and therefore the intensity of breath sounds or the degree of resonance.

Rhonchi transmitted from the trachea or large bronchi often confuse the student who is listening to the chest of an infant. Their character, position, and differentiation may be facilitated by holding the stethoscope an inch or 2 from the infant's mouth or nose and comparing these sounds to those heard over the chest.

The heart in early life fills relatively more of the thoracic cavity than it does in later life, and the apex is one or two intercostal spaces above that which would be considered normal in the adult. Sinus arrhythmia, with acceleration of the heart rate on inspiration, is a physiologic phenomenon prominent throughout infancy and childhood. This finding is so constant that its absence suggests cardiac abnormality.

The heart sounds during childhood are of a higher pitch and shorter duration with greater intensity than during later years. Until adolescence the pulmonary second sound is regularly louder than the aortic. Functional murmurs are the rule during childhood. They are less common in the newborn than later. Between the ages of 6 and 9, over one-half of the children have murmurs that are obvious to the examiner. The most common areas of maximum intensity in the order of frequency are the third to fourth intercostal area at the left border of the sternum, the pulmonic area, and the apex. Parasternal murmurs become less frequent as adolescence approaches, while pulmonic ones become more prevalent. These murmurs usually are of grade II intensity or less, well localized, and are either blowing or vibratory in character. Change in intensity or complete disappearance may follow a change in position. With increased use of noninvasive study of the heart by echocardiography and Doppler studies, some murmurs previously identified as functional are now being related to some variations in cardiac structure. Mild pulmonary artery stenosis, mitral valve prolapse, and bicuspid aortic valve are examples of these conditions. A venous hum is also common in childhood. It is a continuous purring sound that is best heard either above or below the clavicles. It is accentuated in the upright position. It should not be confused with the murmur of patent ductus arteriosus. With the exception of the venous hum, all the functional or innocent heart murmurs are systolic in time, are rarely transmitted to areas beyond the point of maximum intensity, and do not obscure other normal heart sounds.

ABDOMEN

The abdominal examination, because a child may cry, may be somewhat more difficult to perform here than in the adult. If the child is frightened, repeated attempts may be necessary. Distraction from the examining hand can often be accom-

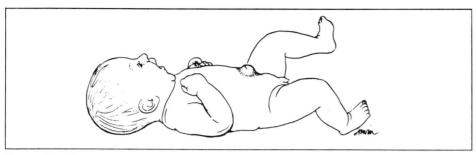

FIGURE 19–10
Umbilical hernia.

plished by conversation of interest to the child or by attracting his attention with a toy.

The liver edge is often palpable in infancy and childhood, and the spleen is normally palpable on deep inspiration in some children.

Inspection of the abdomen of the crying child may best demonstrate hernia, diastasis recti abdominis, or localized bulging due to regional paralysis. Palpation is sometimes done with the child in a prone position, because he relaxes best if he is not looking directly at the examiner. In the infant, relaxation may be obtained during bottle feeding. This procedure may also be used to demonstrate peristaltic waves and for the palpation of a tumor such as that found in hypertrophic pyloric stenosis. Umbilical hernia (Fig. 19–10) is particularly common in infants, sometimes in association with hypothyroidism and Down syndrome.

GENITALIA

The size of the genitalia must be evaluated in relationship to age and not necessarily to body size. The penis and scrotum often appear disproportionately small in obese boys. It must be remembered that throughout most of childhood or until the increased release of pituitary gonadotropins with the onset of puberty, there is virtually no increase in size of the penis or testes.

The precocious appearance of sexual hair may be caused by adrenal lesions (in early infancy by congenital adrenal hyperplasia), brain lesions, gonadal tumors, and a few other rare conditions. Delayed appearance or absence of sexual hair may be found in pituitary, thyroid, or gonadal insufficiency and in certain chronic illnesses. Some degree of retarded growth is usually an accompaniment. Tufts of hair over the spine may indicate an underlying spinal dysraphism.

Actual enlargement of the penis or clitoris, often accompanied by the appearance of pubic hair, is seen as a result of virilizing adrenal lesions or other causes of precocious development. Partial fusion of the labia minora is common in prepubertal girls. Because of the patency of the inguinal canal and the sensitive cremasteric reflex, several examinations should be carried out before diagnosis of undescended testicle is made.

Secondary sexual development shows great individual variation as to the time of

TABLE 19–6. Abnormal Sexual Development

Conditions associated with delayed onset of puberty
  Hypopituitarism, usually with short stature (i.e., multiple deficiencies)
  Hypothyroidism
  Hypogonadism (agenesis, e.g., Turner syndrome; atrophy, surgical or traumatic
      castration; may be incomplete as in testicular feminization syndrome)
  Hypothalamic syndromes
  Any severe chronic illness

Conditions associated with precocious sexual development
  Hyperadrenalism
    Congenital adrenal cortical hyperplasia
    Adrenal cortical tumors
  Hypothalamic lesions
  Pineal gland tumors (predominately in boys)
  Gonadal tumors
  McCune-Albright syndrome (polyostotic fibrous dysplasia)
  Exogenous source of sex hormones

onset. Table 19–3 gives averages of the range for normal American children. Conditions associated with abnormal sexual development are outlined in Table 19–6.

RECTAL EXAMINATION

The rectal examination is an extremely important part of a child's checkup. Digital examination must be done with adequate lubrication, slow and steady pressure with the finger until it passes the sphincter, and the use of the little (fifth) finger in infants and young children. A nasal speculum may be used for examining the anal region in infants.

MUSCULOSKELETAL SYSTEM

The extremities are comparatively short during the first few years of life (the span of the outstretched arms is less than the standing height until approximately age 10 years in boys and 14 years in girls). These proportions, plus the abundant subcutaneous fat, give the infant a rotund appearance. Going into the second and third years the child normally becomes more linear and lean. Recognition of these changes is important in counseling worried parents and avoiding feeding problems precipitated by parents who desire to maintain the plumpness, mistaking it for an indication of good health.

The muscular and skeletal systems are examined as in the adult, taking into account the fact that ambulation is not present in the early months of life. Lack of motion, weakness, and distortion of normal relationships must be looked for in the child even more carefully than in older subjects.

Congenital dislocation of the hip may be demonstrable at birth or not until later. Checks must be done in the newborn period and at every routine examination during infancy. In congenital dislocation of the hip, the head of the femur is located posterior and superior to the acetabulum. There will therefore be limited abduction of the flexed hip and, if only one hip is dislocated, apparent shortening of the affected leg with asymmetry of popliteal folds and gluteal creases. If there is acetabular dysplasia with a potential for dislocation, a click can be heard and felt as the femoral head slips back into the acetabulum as the femur is maneuvered.

Brachial plexus injuries, osteochondrosis, rickets, scurvy, amyotonia congenita, and muscular dystrophies are particularly important in the child. The spine is more flexible in the infant and child than in the adult. Some degree of lordosis and "pot belly" is natural until midchildhood.

NEUROLOGIC EXAMINATION

The neurologic examination will often evaluate the expected behavior and responses to certain stimuli as well as the more formal elicitation of reflexes, muscle tone, and sensation. For example, what the 9-month-old infant does with three cubes or blocks may be as important as his Achilles reflex. Does he grasp firmly, reach accurately, transfer from hand to hand, use fingers as well as palm in grasping?

The changing pattern of reflex behavior in early infancy is important in estimating neurologic integrity. At birth, tonicity and activity are equal bilaterally. The premature newborn has decreased tonicity and activity compared to the normal infant. The premature infant lies in a flaccid position with hands open. The full-term infant assumes a flexed position with hands fisted, and efforts to straighten out the extremities meet considerable resistance. When the baby is supported by one hand under the abdomen in a horizontal position, he raises his head and legs toward the plane of his body. This Landau reflex, which is normally easily elicited in the newborn, may be absent in the premature infant. The full-term infant firmly grasps an object (e.g., a finger) placed in its palm and can be lifted up so that most or all of its weight is supported. The greater the degree of prematurity, the less strong this grasp reflex becomes; under 36 weeks of gestation the response may be absent or very weak. The full-term infant sucks vigorously on a finger placed in the mouth. When the cheek is lightly stroked, the infant turns his head toward the stimulated side and the lips may protrude in preparation for sucking. This reaction is termed the rooting reflex. The newborn responds to sudden change in position, jarring, or loud noises by the Moro reflex. This is characterized by a tensing of muscles, a wide embracing motion of the upper extremities, and some extension of the legs. Normally this reflex disappears by 5 months of age.

Blinking, sneezing, gagging, and coughing to appropriate stimuli are easily elicited in the full-term infant and in all but the smallest of those born prematurely. Although a typical Babinski reflex is seldom demonstrable in the newborn, dorsiflexion of the great toe to the usual stimulus is present in most infants and may persist throughout much of the first year. Due to the often relaxed Achilles tendon from fetal positioning, the ankle jerk may not be demonstrable, but all other deep tendon reflexes are present at birth. All the superficial reflexes—abdominal, anal, and cremasteric—are present at birth, although they may be somewhat difficult to elicit.

In early infancy there may be insufficient development of the nervous system to

TABLE 19–7. Apgar Score for the Newborn*

Signs	Score		
	0	1	2
Heart rate	Absent	<100	>100
Respiratory effort	Absent	Weak	Good
Muscle tone	Limp	Some flexion	Well-flexed extremities
Response to stimulus to feet	None	Some motion	Motion and crying
Color	Pale or blue	Acrocyanosis	Completely pink

*The score is computed at 1 and 5 minutes following delivery by assigning 0, 1, or 2 to each item. A total score of 10 indicates optimum. A total score of 0 indicates a moribund infant.
Source: From V. Apgar, D. A. Holaday, L. S. James, I. M. Weisbrot, and C. Berrien. Evaluation of the newborn infant: Second report. *J.A.M.A.* 168:1985, 1958. Copyright 1958, American Medical Association.

give reliable neurologic signs. Meningitis in this age group may not be associated with obvious nuchal rigidity, or Brudzinski's or Kernig's signs. Lethargy, anorexia, vomiting, and other symptoms and signs of seemingly less specific significance may be the only findings to indicate meningeal irritation.

EXAMINATION OF THE NEWBORN

If she find it warm, not black, she should blow into its mouth; but if, as sometimes happens, the anus is closed by a little skin, she should cut it with a sharp knife . . .

PAULUS BAGELLARDUS
(1472–?)

Because no other period of life carries as great a risk of morbidity and mortality as the first weeks of life, it is appropriate to devote special emphasis to the examination of the newborn infant. The 1-minute and 5-minute Apgar scores are a general indication of the viability of the infant and the effects of labor (Table 19–7). Scores of 6 or less indicate actual or potential problems.

A limited examination that includes a search for major defects should be done immediately. If no problems are apparent, a more complete evaluation can be delayed for several hours. Auscultation of heart and lungs and palpation of the abdomen can best be accomplished while the infant is quiet or asleep. At birth or soon thereafter the umbilicus should be examined for the presence of a single artery. Normally there are two arteries and one vein. A single artery is often associated with anomalies of the heart, central nervous system, and gut.

Not all infants of low birth weight (under 2,500 gm) are premature. A significant number have had full-term gestation but suffered intrauterine malnutrition from maternal disease or poor placental function. An attempt should be made to correlate the baby's gestational age and birth weight. The premature infant is vulnerable to sepsis and hyaline membrane disease (respiratory distress syndrome). He will also show organ immaturity, as in liver function with jaundice. The malnourished baby is particularly susceptible to hypoglycemia. Unusually large babies (over 3,800 gm) are often born to mothers with diabetes mellitus or to prediabetics.

Because menstrual histories are often inaccurate, more objective means of estimating gestational age are required. These include the following: Before 36 weeks, only one or two transverse creases are present on the sole of the foot, the breast nodule is less than 3 mm in diameter, no cartilage is present in the earlobe, and the testes are seldom in the scrotum, which has few or no rugae. By 40 weeks, many creases are present on the sole, the breast nodule exceeds 4 mm, cartilage is present in the earlobe, and the testes have descended into the scrotum, which is covered with rugae. Increasing muscle tone with the assumption of a posture of predominantly flexed extremities is another sign of increased maturity.

The premature infant often has brief periods of apnea lasting up to 15 seconds. Apnea in excess of 15 seconds may be a harbinger of cardiopulmonary or central nervous system pathology. Respiratory distress is indicated by an increased respiratory rate, grunting, retraction of intercostal and subcostal spaces and suprasternal notch, seesaw sinking of the chest with rising abdomen in contrast to the normal synchronous motions, and flaring of the nostrils.

Nasal and esophageal patency can be assured if a soft catheter will pass through the nose, pharynx, and esophagus into the stomach. The resting newborn is an obligatory nose breather, so obstruction, such as atresia of choanae or syphilitic rhinitis, may result in serious respiratory difficulty. Excessive collection of mucus in the nose and mouth characterizes atresia of the esophagus. Passing a tube into the stomach rules out esophageal obstruction.

Visual inspection of the oral cavity as well as palpation with a gloved finger will rule out such defects as a cleft palate. Thrush (candidiasis) is an infection of the mucous membranes with slightly raised dull white patches and can be easily distinguished from Epstein's pearls, which are pearly white nodules limited to the palate and are transient. It is important to remember that respiratory distress, with or without cyanosis, is not limited to intrinsic lesions of the lungs at this period. Intracranial lesions, including anomalies, hemorrhage, or damage due to anoxia, may be responsible. Congenital heart disease and diaphragmatic hernia are further possibilities to be ruled out and often require a chest x-ray for definitive diagnosis.

Some breast hypertrophy at birth, occasionally with small secretions of "milk," is not uncommon and is transient.

The genitalia should be carefully examined for anomalies such as hypospadias, hydrocele, hernia, and ambiguous development indicating possible abnormal sexual development due to endocrine influences. Failure to pass meconium or urine within 24 to 48 hours requires investigation.

Evaluation of the central nervous system depends on observations of spontaneous alertness and activity, strength and character of the cry, response to stimuli, vigor of sucking and feeding, and postural tone. Head measurements and examination have been described earlier in this chapter, and some of the reflexes also have been mentioned.

CONCLUSION

Lucy: Don't tell me you took that blanket to school today?
Linus: Sure, why not? It calms me down and helps me get better grades.
Lucy: But don't the other kids laugh at you?
Linus: Nobody laughs at a straight "A" average!

CHARLES M. SCHULZ
(1922–   )

In this chapter an attempt has been made to emphasize some of the important differences between the child and the adult. The fact that the child is a changing organism is important to remember and is extremely helpful in evaluation of the history and the physical findings. Failure to grow in stature or weight is always significant. Delay in both physical and mental maturation as well as in growth may indicate endocrine or deficiency disorders or chronic infectious disease. Fortunately fever, emotional response, fatigue, general behavior, intestinal upsets, and the like are more labile in the child than in the adult and therefore are important indicators of disease. Special attention to behavior and facial expression before and during the actual examination is of the utmost importance. If these facts are kept in mind, the examination of the infant or child can be an exciting and rewarding experience for the physician.

CHAPTER 20

GERIATRIC EXAMINATION

The proportion of older people in the United States is increasing each year. By the year 2000, about 20 percent of the population will be over age 65. With the exception of pediatricians, other physicians—family practitioners, internists, gynecologists, cardiologists, and virtually all subspecialists—will be seeing more and more older patients.

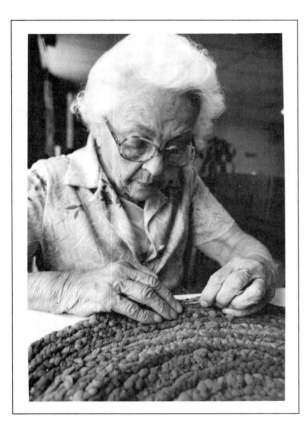

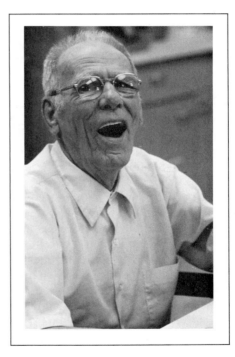

The experienced physician uses several special techniques for examining older patients: (1) efficiently obtaining the medical history; (2) using information sources other than the patient (such as the family or caretaker); and (3) separating normal aging changes from changes of disease.

HISTORY

An efficient process of obtaining a medical history may be difficult to achieve for a number of reasons. Older people have a longer life history; their greater life span has exposed them to a greater risk of disease, and they probably have accumulated a number of maladies and problems along the way. Further, they are not likely to be sophisticated in differentiating their critical symptoms from trivial but annoying symptoms, so that many symptoms, important and trivial, may be recounted. Finally, the patient's combination of some memory loss and some hearing loss can make history taking uncomfortable and frustrating for the examiner.

Recognition of the problems in history taking leads to rational approaches to solving them. All older people have some hearing deficit. The examiner should situate himself or herself to have direct eye contact with the patient. This improves communication by allowing lip reading and also allows paralanguage communication with facial expressions.

The most common type of hearing deficit in the elderly is sensorineural hearing loss. In sensorineural hearing loss, comprehension is worse when there are competing sounds or noises. It is useful to obtain the medical history in an environment as free of competing sounds as possible. Because most hearing loss in the elderly is high-frequency loss, speaking in a low pitch is also useful. With high-frequency loss, high-frequency speech sounds (such as "s" and "f") cannot be heard; low-frequency sounds are heard normally. The person's understanding of speech is hindered, even though the patient believes he or she is hearing sounds adequately. Shouting, which is the natural response in dealing with a patient with a hearing loss, is usually counterproductive. It will irritate the patient, especially one who does not feel there is a hearing problem, and it probably will not improve understanding anyway.

Besides eye contact and dealing with hearing problems, there are some other useful techniques. In the long run, it is preferable to avoid addressing the patient by his or her first name. It shows a lack of respect. If we call the patient by his first name, and we allow nurses and others to do so, we are probably being paternalistic, and we may contribute to the patient's dependency and infantilism. A major goal in geriatrics is to reduce dependency. It is also preferable to avoid speaking to a family member or caretaker in the room with the patient, referring to the patient in the third person; this creates a self-defeating triangle in which the patient feels excluded and ignored. Discussion with the family member can occur later, privately.

The "present illness" of an older patient often will have no volunteered "chief complaint." As problems accumulate in the older person, there is a tendency for them to merge and become seen as one entity. It is important to determine why the patient is being seen at this time. What is different? What is new? Most disease is not dormant and reveals itself in new symptoms.

Sometimes the patient's loneliness and memory loss team up to make history taking a long, drawn-out activity. Closed questions or multiple choice questions, frowned-on for younger patients because they can be leading or "can put words in the patient's mouth," may be necessary when interviewing the older person. Forcing a limited response may be required. For example, "Is the pain worse in the

TABLE 20–1. Normal Aging Effects on Physical Examination

Decreased skin turgor
Slower pupil reflex
Weaker upward gaze
Increased residual lung volume
Decreased intestinal peristalsis
Enlarged prostate
Vaginal or testicular atrophy
Shorter-paced gait

shoulder or in the stomach? (You have to tell me which one)," is a useful questioning style.

All historical information does not have to be obtained at one time. When the patient becomes fatigued, it is time to postpone further questions. Otherwise, the responses are likely to be invalid.

Direct communication with the patient should be augmented by communication with family members or caretakers. Memory loss, denial, depression, or embarrassment may cause the patient to omit important historical details. One phone call to the family sometimes reveals more information than an hour of questioning the patient. No geriatric history is complete without talking to the patient's family, caretaker, or companion.

AGING VS. DISEASE

The ability to separate normal aging from disease is necessary for the interpretation of the history and the physical examination. Normal aging changes often are not clinically important (Table 20–1). A rule of thumb is that differences due to aging are generally less than differences simply due to biologic variability among individuals. There is wide variation found in examining older people. Put another way, "If you've seen one older person . . . you've seen one older person." (J.W. Rowe, Geriatric medicine conference, March 31, 1986, Boston.)

Normal aging affects the neurologic system by reducing hearing, near vision, smell, and taste. Some recent memory loss is considered normal. The pupillary response is slower, motor reaction time is slower, and vibratory sense is diminished. Yet, in spite of these neurologic changes, elderly patients can be expected to be alert and have a normal level of consciousness and agility. Age does not affect language use or comprehension. Although there may be some decline in coordination, physical examinations will normally reveal no particular muscle weakness.

Likewise, the cardiovascular system does not normally show any significant decline. Early studies that showed a decrease in cardiac output with age did not exclude all individuals with coronary artery disease. When they are excluded, cardiac output is not found to decline with age, either at rest or with exercise. Systolic hypertension was also thought to be a normal aging process, but current thinking considers it a treatable disease.

Age causes changes in the lungs similar to those of emphysema. Both closing volume and residual volume increase with age, resulting in a decrease in vital capacity. There is an increase in chest wall stiffness and a counteracting increase in lung compliance. However, the similarity of aging and emphysema is in direction only, not in extent. Age changes are much less than changes due to smoking, for example.

In the gastrointestinal tract, normal changes include decreased peristalsis, decreased absorption, and decreased hepatic blood flow. These changes usually have no demonstrable effect except to increase complaints of constipation and to decrease the hepatic metabolism of drugs and other substances. When nutritional intake is marginal, decreased absorption can be important.

Due to a variety of changes within the kidneys, the creatinine clearance typically decreases with age, requiring a downward dosage adjustment of renally excreted drugs. It is important to remember that these changes are not universal; in one-third of older people creatinine clearance does not decrease. The only way to be sure what the patient's creatinine clearance is is to measure it.

Skin changes include loss of elasticity and turgor. Increased dryness is common. The stratum corneum is not thinner and its barrier function remains intact.

Musculoskeletal changes include decreased calcium content of bones and joint changes that are difficult to distinguish from osteoarthritis. However, to consider osteoarthritis as simply "normal wear and tear" of joints rather than a treatable disease would allow widespread unnecessary suffering.

Endocrine changes include the menopause in women and some tapering of testosterone levels in men. Changes in the ratio of estrogen to testosterone in men is related to prostatic hypertrophy, especially within the prostate's surgical capsule, causing some urethral obstruction. Thyroid hormone level stays essentially constant. When corrected for body protein content, the basal metabolic rate also stays essentially constant.

SYMPTOMS IN THE ELDERLY

PAIN

Pain complaints are paradoxical. Older people often have accumulated a number of problems causing aches and pains, so they have many pain complaints. Yet visceral pain seems to be blunted in older people. This can mask disease, making painless or "silent" myocardial infarction more common, for example. Hip fracture causes less pain, as does appendicitis. So, while chronic pain may be more prevalent, new pain, even minor, may be quite significant. The key is to separate the two.

Headache, a common cause of pain in young people, is relatively rare in older people. Certainly headache in individuals not previously bothered with chronic headaches, or headaches of a different nature, are much more likely to be due to organic disease in the elderly than such headaches are in the young. One cause of headache, temporal arteritis, can lead to blindness if not treated. Brain tumor, encephalitis, and subdural hematoma are also potentially fatal causes of headache and cause a higher proportion of headaches in the elderly than in younger people.

Chest pain may be myocardial, but the clinician must also consider the higher incidence of arthritis, which can cause pain at the costosternal joints and in the shoulder. As noted, myocardial infarction can be painless. Coronary insufficiency, or "angina," may also be painless, and sometimes shows up only as shortness of breath due to pulmonary edema. The pulmonary edema results from myocardial dysfunction due to ischemia, with decreased pump efficiency and a backup of venous pressure in the lungs.

Abdominal pain has great significance in the older patient. If coupled with early increased peristalsis (emptying reflex) and then ileus, it may signal an abdominal catastrophe such as mesenteric artery thrombosis, a disease found almost exclusively in the elderly.

FEVER

Fever also may not be as straightforward a symptom or sign in the older person as it is in the younger. The absence of fever does not rule out the presence of infection as readily in the older patient; one-third of older patients with pneumonia may be afebrile. Urinary tract infections (UTIs) may also have no febrile response; sometimes the only manifestation of a UTI is mental confusion. Further, a "normal temperature" may actually represent a low-grade fever, as many older people have a baseline temperature 0.5 to 1° below the nominal 98.6°F that is considered normal. This emphasizes the value of having baseline observations, so the significance of subsequent observations can be assessed appropriately.

Although the absence of fever is less likely to preclude or rule out infection, the presence of fever is also less likely to mean infection, because other causes of fever are more prevalent in older people, including drug-fever, collagen-vascular diseases, and cancers.

WEIGHT LOSS

Loss of appetite is common in the elderly. Anorexia has the same differential diagnoses as in the young, but anorexia due to cancer, depression, or drugs is highly characteristic of the older population.

SHORTNESS OF BREATH

Changes in the pulmonary system are expected with age, but shortness of breath is a symptom that always must be taken seriously and investigated thoroughly. Older people generally are less physically active than younger people, but they should be able to do what they are accustomed to doing without shortness of breath. Shortness of breath may be due to pulmonary or heart disease, anemia, or metabolic disorders.

URINARY INCONTINENCE

A major source of embarrassment, social withdrawal, and expense, urinary incontinence may not be volunteered as a complaint. The examiner must specifically ask about incontinence. About one-half of the cases of incontinence can be significantly improved by simple interventions such as stopping or starting different medications and frequent toileting. Many other causes of incontinence can be approached surgically.

FALLS

Older people live with a justified fear of falling. Falls may easily lead to hip fracture, with attendant loss of mobility and unexpectedly high 2- or 3-year mortality. Falling must be separated from syncope, which includes loss of consciousness. Risk factors for falling include poor vision, poor coordination, weakness, and environmental hazards such as loose rugs and dim lighting. Orthostatic hypotension may cause transient dizziness and decreased consciousness, leading to falling down. Orthostatic hypotension is more prevalent in older people because of the increased use of prescription medications, a greater prevalence of dehydration, and decreased baroreceptor reflexes. True syncope has a more ominous prognosis in the elderly because it is more often due to cardiac disease.

MEMORY LOSS

The clinician must answer two critical questions about the patient's memory loss. First, is the memory loss within the limits of normal age-associated changes? A formal mental status examination, e.g., the Folstein mini–mental exam, helps answer this question. The second critical question is whether the memory loss is due to some treatable condition. The differential diagnosis includes depression, thyroid disease, central nervous system lesions such as brain tumors and subdural hematoma, and metabolic disorders. The history and physical examination should give clues to the possibility of any of these disorders.

PHYSICAL EXAMINATION

The format for the physical examination of the older patient follows the same pattern as that in any adult. Special attention should be paid to "vital signs," and blood pressure determinations should be made on both arms with the patient sitting, then on either arm with the patient supine, then immediately on standing, and then after the patient has been standing 2 minutes. Any symptoms that occur while the patient is standing should be noted.

The skin should be carefully examined because of the increased incidence of skin cancer.

The pupils are generally smaller, and pupillary reflexes are slower in the elderly. Arcus senilis is not associated with disease. Conjugate upward gaze may be weak, but downward gaze should be normal. Inability to understand a forced whisper in one ear from 5 feet represents severe hearing loss. Deep tendon reflexes and muscle strength should be normal and symmetrical, although a symmetrical decreased ankle jerk reflex is common and may be unassociated with any disease. Plantar reflexes should be flexor.

A formal mental status examination is not necessary unless the patient exhibits memory loss or unusual behavior. However, the three "A's" should be observed and recorded: appearance (is the patient properly dressed and well groomed?); affect (is the patient sad-appearing, or slow moving?); and appropriateness (are the flow of conversation and other behavior appropriate?). A quick check of the patient's orientation to time, place, person, and purpose (why they are there) should be made.

TABLE 20–2. Diseases with Atypical Presentations in the Older Patient

Dementia
Depression
Hyperthyroidism
Hypothyroidism
Myocardial infarction and angina
Pneumonia, pulmonary embolism
Tuberculosis
Urinary tract infection

In young people, an S_3 cardiac gallop may be normal, but in the elderly any gallop rhythm suggests disease.

Because of the increased closing volume and other changes of aging, crackles may be heard in the lungs with no associated disease. Nevertheless, finding crackles requires correlation with any symptoms and usually requires some follow-up. The anteroposterior diameter of the chest wall may be increased due to kyphosis and some vertebral collapse.

Abdominal examination may reveal some decrease in peristaltic sounds. Because of increased vascular disease, bruits should be listened for, and some estimation should be made of whether the abdominal aorta is dilated with an aneurysm.

Periodic genital examination should be performed, even though positioning the patient with arthritis may cause discomfort. Genital examination always requires the examiner's sensitivity and courtesy. With older people, this requirement is heightened still further. For many older women, their last genital examination was at the time of their last childbirth, which may have been even before the examining physician was born. Besides being unaccustomed to such examinations, having grown up in a different cultural era, may make an otherwise simple procedure painfully difficult for the patient. The examining physician must be aware of the older person's possible or probable cultural difference in attitudes towards sexuality and sexual organs, just as the physician would be aware of and sensitive to any other cultural differences.

The female genital examination will normally reveal vulvar atrophy, disappearance of labial furrows, and thin, dry, vaginal mucosa. The bimanual examination is not different from that of younger women. The male genital examination will show atrophic (smaller) testes and a larger prostate.

A functional assessment should be completed. Data from the history and physical examination are combined to assess if the patient can do the practical functions of daily living—putting on clothes, walking, eating, and toileting.

LABORATORY EXAMINATION

Initial laboratory examinations will, as in the young, be directed by the history and physical examination, but an awareness of atypical presentations of diseases (Table 20–2) and the higher prevalence of certain diseases generally will lead to more testing in the old than in the young. Routine "preventive medicine" tests could justifiably include an electrocardiogram and urinalysis and screening for thyroid disease, glaucoma, occult fecal blood, and anemia. Periodic Papanicolaou (Pap) tests and mammograms should be obtained in women. Periodic sigmoidoscopy should be done in both sexes.

APPROACH TO THE GERIATRIC PATIENT

There are many differences between older people and younger people. Still, most disease in older people produces the same symptoms and signs as the same disease would in the young. However, because of the increased likelihood of multiple diseases (resulting in multiple complaints), and use of multiple drugs (resulting in multiple drug side-effects), sorting the historical and physical findings into typical disease patterns becomes an important skill. And, often enough, disease in older people has an atypical presentation. For example, anorexia, weight loss, and constipation suggest the presence of colon cancer. This is true in the elderly as well as younger persons. But in the elderly, these symptoms, surprisingly enough, may also result from hyperthyroidism, which more classically produces increased appetite, weight loss, and diarrhea.

In general, physicians will be caring for more and more older patients. An understanding of the changes due to aging compared to the changes due to disease is essential. So is the ability to sort out specific disease symptoms from multiple complaints. Finally, awareness of the possible surprising diagnosis is not only essential, it also keeps the geriatric examination an interesting challenge.

CHAPTER 21

INJURED PATIENT

Though the experienced practitioner may, by a process of apparently instinctive "short circuiting" achieve a diagnosis so swiftly that he seems to be guided by something called "clinical instinct," we may be quite sure that, as a matter of fact, the processes actually involved are observation, elimination of the irrelevant, inference—in other words induction—even though the pace has been so rapid that the several steps are indistinguishable.

ABRAHAM FLEXNER
(1866–1959)

GENERAL PRINCIPLES

The aim of this textbook is to present the principles of examination and diagnosis. The first aim of the examining physician is the preservation of life. When dealing with acute trauma it is often impossible to separate diagnostic and therapeutic measures; indeed, it would be improper to dissociate these features completely. The care of the acutely injured patient imposes certain important restrictions on the examiner. It may be impossible to obtain a detailed or even cursory history from the patient. The examiner is often forced to rely heavily on physical findings for diagnosis. The initial examination is as likely to be performed in the field or beside a highway as in a well-equipped hospital emergency room. Some attempt at determining the mechanism of injury, severity of force or speed involved, and direction of impact should be made and is valuable in predicting patterns of injury.

When confronted with an acutely injured patient you should ask yourself the following questions, in rapid order:

1. Is the airway patent?
2. Is breathing impaired? by chest injury?
3. Is there significant hemorrhage?
4. Is there serious or potential brain or spinal cord injury?
5. Is there a fracture? are the extremities deformed, suggesting fracture or dislocation?
6. Is there peripheral nerve injury?

The most urgent requirement is the evaluation of the patient's **airway and breathing**. Death may ensue in minutes if adequate ventilation is not possible. The problem may be compounded by unconsciousness, by aspiration of blood or vomitus, or by serious injuries to the chest wall or lung parenchyma. When evaluating the status of the patient's airway, the head should be maintained in neutral position to avoid potential injury to the cervical spine. It may be necessary to lift the chin or to exert traction on the tongue to maintain an oral airway. If tracheal obstruction exists, endotracheal intubation should be undertaken. If this is not possible, an emergency cricothyroidostomy or tracheostomy may be indicated. If ventilation is inadequate, mouth-to-mouth resuscitation should be initiated without hesitation.

Prompt recognition of this need may be life-saving. It should be noted that cardio-pulmonary resuscitation (CPR) is not useful in traumatic cardiac arrest.

The second important threat to life is **massive hemorrhage.** In the patient with an injured extremity, control of visible sources of bleeding is best achieved by direct manual pressure. Elevation of the limb may help to control blood loss. Only in exceptional instances will arterial blood loss be a major problem. In these rare circumstances a tourniquet should be applied proximal to the wound. The time should be carefully noted and surgical control of bleeding obtained as soon as possible in an operating room. Compression by MAST suit or air splint is an alternative to a tourniquet. Bleeding from pelvic and large bone fractures is easy to underestimate unless you are alert to this possibility.

When adequate airway and ventilation are ensured and hemorrhage is controlled, it is time to perform a rapid physical examination to assess the extent of coexisting injuries. This should be initiated as soon as possible and, though brief, should be thorough and systematic. Failure to carry out this kind of survey will lead to errors in diagnosis and management that may have serious consequences or may result in disability or loss of life. The information obtained by this preliminary examination provides valuable baseline data by which to follow the patient's progress and also aids subsequent management. Examination for life-threatening neurologic injury is next.

The examination should rule out the possibility of **spinal injury**, since if such a patient is moved roughly or improperly, sudden paralysis may occur. Pain medication should be withheld until a clear indication for it exists and brain injury is ruled out. If narcotics are given before the examination is completed, diagnostic evaluation becomes clouded and neurologic signs are difficult to interpret. When given, the analgesic should be administered intravenously because of the uncertainties of absorption associated with hypotension, which often accompanies massive trauma.

There is a great tendency, based on our natural curiosity, to probe, explore, and investigate open wounds, but in most instances this should be avoided. In general, even in the face of hemorrhage, open wounds should be explored only in the operating room. Anesthesia should be adequate to permit thorough study, cleansing should be performed with copious amounts of sterile saline, and sterile technique should be strictly observed. Anything short of this fosters an incomplete and inadequate examination, is likely to lead to infection, and may result in failure to find foreign bodies or may cause inadvertent nerve or vessel injury. The ideal method of early management calls for application of a dry, sterile (or at least clean) dressing to prevent additional soilage. Definitive care should be given as soon as conditions permit.

RADIOLOGIC EXAMINATION

X-ray examination is a valuable adjunct to the physical examination in evaluating the extent of injuries. Selected studies often provide information that may be obtained in no other way. In addition, a standard-size chest film is worth obtaining. In many ways physical examination of the heart and lungs is limited, and every physician realizes that the x-ray is sometimes more accurate and effective in detecting subtle pulmonary, mediastinal, and cardiac changes.

Cervical spine films should be obtained in obtunded or unresponsive patients or those with cervical tenderness or pain. A flat film of the abdomen and pelvis may be useful if abdominal trauma has occurred. Major long bones and joints that are painful or deformed should be x-rayed.

X-ray examination of the skull plays no part in the evaluation of patients with head injury. Computed tomographic (CT) scan is the preferred method of evaluating intracranial injury. The principal value of skull films lies in the recognition of skull fracture, which requires specific treatment only if the fracture is depressed. As a general rule, radiologic studies should be completed as soon after head injury as the general condition of the patient permits.

Common sense should dictate when radiologic studies will contribute to successful management.

HEAD INJURIES

CEREBRAL TRAUMA

Obtundation, agitated behavior, or other abnormal neurologic signs may be the result of airway obstruction or ventilatory problems. This requires primary attention. The neurologic examination may then be performed. The three aims of emergency neurologic evaluation are (1) to determine whether the patient is in need of emergency surgical intervention to relieve subdural or epidural hematoma; (2) to establish the nature and severity of any existing head injury; and (3) to obtain baseline neurologic information for comparison purposes later.

A time-consuming, detailed, elaborate neurologic examination is not appropriate for the early care of patients with head injury. On the contrary, a few carefully selected studies may be obtained using simple equipment. The state of consciousness should be evaluated. Does the patient open his eyes or speak spontaneously? Does he move both sides of the body? Record the patient's response to verbal or painful stimulation, for example, response to loud voice, to supraorbital pressure, pinprick, or pressure on the sternum with the knuckles. Observe and record the condition of the pupils, their relative size, equality, and response to light. A dilated, nonreactive pupil in an obtunded patient may signify intracranial hemorrhage. Dilated, fixed pupils have a poor prognosis. Inequality of the pupils may reflect local brain damage or may result from drugs or alcohol or ocular injury.

CHARACTER OF RESPIRATION

Irregular or depressed respirations may accompany severe intracranial injury. If this situation exists in the presence of an adequate airway, the prognosis is grave.

DEGREE OF MOTOR ACTIVITY

If the patient is conscious, motor activity may be appraised by having him squeeze the examiner's hands or by testing his ability to resist passive motion of the extremities. In the comatose patient the degree of flaccidity may be evaluated by lifting the extremity and letting it drop. It is important to examine both sides of the patient. This permits comparison and provides baseline information should his condition deteriorate under observation. Extensor rigidity of all extremities implies a bad prognosis. Although alcoholism or drug intoxication may confuse this observation, complete flaccidity and areflexia usually indicate severe central nervous system damage or spinal cord injury. Rectal sphincter tone should be determined by digital examination.

EVALUATION OF DEEP TENDON REFLEXES

A detailed examination may be inappropriate at first. Study of the triceps, biceps, radioperiosteal, plantar, knee, and ankle reflexes, together with the test for the presence of ankle clonus, should be adequate for initial evaluation.

TYPES OF HEAD INJURIES

The seriousness of a head injury in most cases relates to the nature and extent of the cerebral injury, rather than to that of the overlying scalp or skull structures. Therefore, consider first whether the injured patient has loss of consciousness or the presence of a deficit in neurologic function. Look for injury to the skull second and the scalp third. Head injuries may be classified as minor or major depending on whether there is loss of consciousness and as open or closed depending on whether the protective coverings of the brain are breached (by a gunshot wound, for example).

Minor closed-head injury, the kind most frequently seen, occurs after a blow to the head and is associated with momentary or very brief loss of consciousness and amnesia for the precipitating event. The person is alert and has no concommitant symptoms such as nausea or vomiting. There is usually no permanent brain damage associated with minor closed-head injury, and the episode usually is called a "concussion" by lay persons. Delayed sequelae of true minor closed-head injury, such as chronic subdural hemorrhage, are rare.

Major closed-head injury is diagnosed when loss of consciousness lasts more than a minute, is associated with retrograde amnesia (i.e., loss of memory for the injury and events preceding), or with neurologic abnormalities, such as an altered level of consciousness, muscular weakness, or slurred speech. It is difficult to briefly define altered levels of consciousness, but persons who appear drowsy, do not respond to questions promptly and appropriately, speak in a garbled or incoherent fashion, or fail to respond appropriately to simple instructions should be suspected of having serious underlying brain injury.

It is particularly important to identify progressive deterioration in the level of consciousness, because this is evidence of an expanding intracranial mass, such as **extradural** or **subdural hematoma.** Characteristically, a brief period of unconsciousness may be followed by a "lucid interval," then progress to confusion, drowsiness, and coma. With extradural hemorrhage, the sequence of events tends to be fairly rapid, developing over a matter of hours. With subdural hemorrhage the course of the condition may be extended over several weeks or months. In either event the presence of lateralizing neurologic signs, anisocoria, and alteration in the deep tendon reflexes and motor responses should be sufficient reason to prompt emergency neurosurgical consultation and examination of the head by CT scan.

Skull fracture may or may not occur in association with brain injury, and is usually of secondary importance unless focal trauma has caused a **depressed skull**

fracture. Depressed fragments of bone can cause brain injury by direct contact and should be treated by exploration and elevation. Clinical signs of temporal or parietal skull fracture include palpable bogginess of the overlying scalp or palpable depression of the skull. When skull fracture occurs in the petrous bone or along the base of the skull where it will not be palpable, clinical signs include leakage of cerebrospinal fluid from the nose or ears, blood behind the tympanic membranes, and extravasation of blood into the soft tissues behind the ears (Battle's sign) and around the eyes ("raccoon eyes").

Scalp laceration and contusion are common injuries and may lead to profuse blood loss because of the highly vascular nature of the scalp. Bleeding from a scalp laceration can usually be controlled by direct pressure along the edge of the wound, at least initially, and all such wounds should be explored for possible underlying skull injury before closure.

Penetrating wounds of the head can cause devastating or trivial injury depending upon the momentum of the projectile and the path it takes. One should not be misled by a small entrance wound. Early surgical exploration and debridement are often indicated, usually after CT is done to define the location and extent of injury.

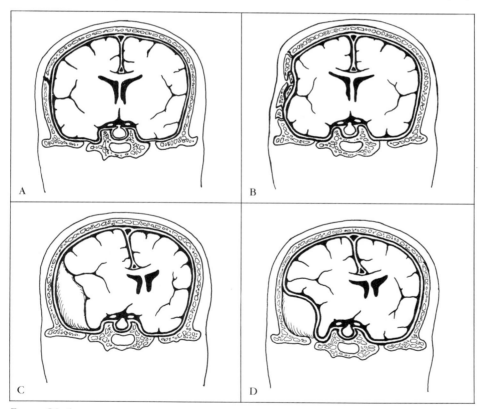

FIGURE 21–1
Some types of head injury. A. Linear skull fracture. B. Depressed skull fracture. C. Subdural hematoma. D. Epidural hematoma. E. Intracerebral hematoma.

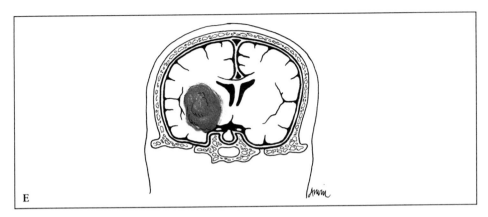

E

Figure 21–1 *(Continued)*

EXAMINATION FOR FACIAL INJURIES

In accidents in which head injury occurs, fractures of the facial bones are common. In many instances, facial fractures can be diagnosed by observation of the deformities they cause or by careful palpation of the facial bones. Fracture of the nose is often obvious because of epistaxis and deviation from the normal contour. Edema and discoloration of the skin, however, may render the diagnosis difficult. Examine the patient from above as well as from the front to detect minor degrees of asymmetry. Bimanual palpation and intranasal speculum examination may also help.

Fractures of the mandible and maxilla are identified by finding malocclusion of the teeth or pain on opening the mouth. Inspection and palpation of the gingival surface will often reveal discontinuity and tenderness, along with loosening of the teeth. A fracture on one side of the mandible is frequently accompanied by a companion fracture on the other side.

A blow on the cheek may produce a fracture of the zygoma. This fracture is frequently associated with considerable edema and subcutaneous hemorrhage, diplopia, subconjunctival hemorrhage, and anesthesia below the eye due to injury of the second division of the trigeminal nerve.

Fractures of the facial bones do not constitute surgical emergencies, although they may be associated with some degree of airway obstruction. Operative treatment may be delayed for several days, if necessary, to permit adequate treatment of the patient's other injuries.

INJURIES OF THE SPINE

Fractures or fracture dislocations of the spine result from violent trauma. These may result from automobile accidents, football injuries, diving accidents, etc. It is essential to suspect the diagnosis and transport the patient without producing further injury to the spinal cord. The cervical spine, because of its mobility, is particularly susceptible to injury. For this reason, gentle traction should be exerted on the head in the long axis of the spine when moving a patient. The patient should not be allowed to flex his neck. A general rule is to allow the patient as little motion as possible and to transport him in the prone or supine position, depending on the circumstances, using a long spine board, without permitting rotation, flexion, or extension of the spine.

Evaluate injury of the spinal cord by asking the patient to move his legs and toes. If he is able to do this, he has escaped major cord damage. If, however, the legs are paralyzed but the patient can move his hands, the cord lesion is located below the cervical region. Paradoxical motion of the chest and abdomen with respiration results from paralysis of chest wall muscles. If arm function is interfered with, cervical spine involvement is suggested. It is possible to confirm the location of cord injury by testing for loss of sensation to pinprick.

INJURIES OF THE CHEST WALL

FRACTURES

Rib fractures are common injuries. They may or may not be associated with intra-thoracic damage. To permit proper examination the patient should be stripped to the waist and asked to take a deep breath. In the presence of rib fracture there is usually limitation of motion associated with pain on the affected side. The palpation of each rib in order should be carried out to identify subcutaneous emphysema which is associated with pneumothorax. Compression of the chest cage in an anteroposterior direction and laterally may elicit pain when rib fractures are present.

Percussion and auscultation of the chest should be performed in every instance to detect the presence of pneumothorax or hemothorax which interferes with ventilation. It is well to omit compression of the chest cage if physical signs of pleural effusion, pneumothorax, or mediastinal shift are present.

Fractures of the sternum are usually secondary to considerable violence and may occur in steering-wheel injuries. This fracture is usually associated with considerable pain and rapid, shallow respiration. The sternum may show a visible depression and subcutaneous hemorrhage may be prominent. Characteristically, the patient holds his head forward in a rigid manner. This lesion is often associated with a contusion of the heart, hemopericardium, or injury to the intrathoracic aorta, which lies directly beneath the sternum. Cardiac arrhythmias or murmurs may be present.

With severe crush injuries of the ribs, resulting in multiple fractures, a portion of the chest wall may become freely movable. This condition is known as *flail chest*. With inspiration the mobile portion of the chest wall is sucked inward, resulting in decreased ventilation. In effect, the involved side ceases to function in ventilatory exchange. The result is shunting of blood through the affected lung. Diagnosis is not difficult, since the chest wall is unstable to palpation and is seen to move paradoxically. It is imperative to achieve adequate ventilation. If this condition is severe or bilateral, ventilation is usually achieved by endotracheal intubation and positive pressure ventilation. Intrapulmonary hemorrhage or contusion may also be present.

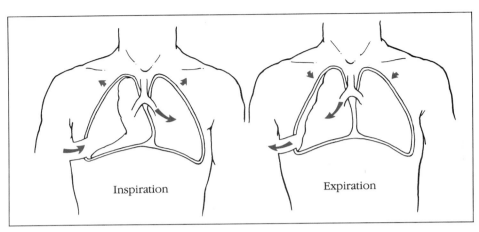

FIGURE 21–2
Intrathoracic dynamics in patient with sucking wound of the chest. Note shifts in lung and mediastinum with inspiration and expiration.

PENETRATING WOUNDS

Penetrating wounds of the chest wall should be distinguished from blunt injuries. Penetrating closed wounds of the chest are usually associated with some degree of intrathoracic visceral damage. The possibilities include hemothorax, tension pneumothorax, subcutaneous or mediastinal emphysema and cardiac tamponade.

With **an open wound** of the chest there is free communication between the pleural space and the outside. This is usually associated with great distress and signs of asphyxiation. Cyanosis and hypotension with a rapid and thready pulse are usually present. Inspiration is labored and accompanied by an audible sucking sound. Expiration is forced and often accompanied by frothy serum or blood issuing from the wound (Fig. 21–2). Subcutaneous emphysema is common. A large sucking wound of the chest is a surgical emergency that demands immediate treatment. It can usually be closed by applying a clean dressing. This should be carried out immediately, using materials at hand without regard to sterility. Ventilation may then be improved by having the patient lie on his injured side, until more definitive care can be provided.

HEMOTHORAX

The physical signs of hemothorax are those of pleural effusion—diminished breath sounds at the base posteriorly on the involved side and dullness to percussion when hemothorax is massive. The mediastinum may be shifted, and this may be detected by percussion and palpation of the trachea for shift. All degrees of hemothorax may occur, depending on the origin of the hemorrhage of the chest which can arise from the lung or from intercostal vessels adjacent the pleura. Hemothorax may also be associated with pneumothorax if the parenchyma of the lung is involved. In this situation, increased resonance and absent breath sounds will be present above the area of dullness. The physical signs of pneumothorax tend to obscure the signs of pleural effusion.

PNEUMOTHORAX

Physical signs of pneumothorax depend on the amount of air present between the lung and the chest wall. Small amounts of pneumothorax are difficult to identify, but one of any significant size should be readily recognizable. Respiratory rate is increased and dyspnea is present. Patients complain of shoulder pain with breathing. The chest wall on the affected side shows decreased movement, and cyanosis may be present. Percussion may indicate a shift of the heart and mediastinum. This may be confirmed by palpation of the trachea. The percussion note over the involved side is characteristically increased in resonance and is tympanitic.

TENSION PNEUMOTHORAX

Tension pneumothorax occurs when injury involves pulmonary parenchyma or bronchi, creating a ball-valve type phenomenon that lets air escape into the pleural space but not exit. It may develop when an open sucking wound of the chest is closed by packing or strapping, or it may be spontaneous due to rupture of a pulmonary bleb. This injury is serious and demands prompt surgical treatment. With each inspiration, air enters the pleural space on the involved side, increasing the collapse of the lung and pushing the mediastinum toward the uninvolved side. This further reduces the function of the good lung and may reduce blood return to the heart. Clinically the situation is characterized by pronounced dyspnea and cyanosis. Vascular collapse with hypotension and a rapid thready pulse are due to decreased venous return to the heart. It is important to differentiate between circulatory collapse secondary to hemorrhage or shock elsewhere in the body and that which is secondary to tension pneumothorax. The trachea and heart will be shifted toward the uninvolved side, and the percussion note is usually hyperresonant and tympanitic. It is possible, however, for tension pneumothorax to exist with minimal signs of hyperresonance and tympany. The mediastinal shift toward the uninvolved side may also be detected by percussion. Breath sounds on the involved side are generally absent or muffled. Emergency treatment, consisting of evacuation of the trapped air with a large needle or chest tube, should be instituted promptly and may be life-saving. Sufficient air should be aspirated to produce relief of symptoms.

SUBCUTANEOUS EMPHYSEMA

Subcutaneous emphysema occurs when air gains access to tissue planes around the wound or injury. Considerable subcutaneous spread may occur, characterized by local swelling, edema, and crepitation on compression. This is a common accompaniment of compression injuries to the chest involving rib fractures. It may also be seen in rupture of the parenchyma of the lung and with injuries to the trachea or larynx, with dissection of air beneath the visceropleura into the mediastinum. It may then spread rapidly to produce swelling of the neck, face, and chest wall and may even extend to the abdominal wall and scrotum. It may be associated with minimal respiratory distress. If, however, dyspnea and cyanosis are present, one should suspect a coexisting tension pneumothorax. On auscultation over the base of the heart the characteristic crackling "mediastinal crunch" may be detectable in the pneumomediastinum, but this is generally not physiologically significant.

PERICARDIAL EFFUSION

Both blunt and penetrating chest wounds may produce an accumulation of blood within the pericardium that results in progressive compression of the heart with obstruction of the great veins. Cardiac filling is impaired and cardiac output decreases. This may progress to death unless aspiration of the pericardium is carried out. **Cardiac tamponade** is associated with a high venous pressure. The neck veins are distended and the patient is dyspneic and cyanotic. On auscultation the heart sounds are distant and rapid. Systemic blood pressure is low, with a narrow pulse pressure as systolic pressure falls and diastolic pressure rises. A paradoxical pulse is present and may be demonstrated by maintaining the blood pressure cuff pressure at the level at which systolic sounds are first heard. With each inspiration the systolic sounds disappear. Echocardiography will confirm effusion. Treatment consists of aspiration of blood from the pericardium, which can be life saving.

PULMONARY CONTUSION

With blunt injury of the chest it is sometimes possible to encounter extensive pulmonary damage in the presence of an intact chest wall. An **intrapulmonary hematoma** may be associated with hemoptysis or frothy sputum and dyspnea. On percussion, dullness may be noted, whereas on auscultation breath sounds will be diminished and may be associated with coarse, bubbling rales. A high temperature may be present.

Pulmonary edema may occur as a result of severe pulmonary injury and shock or in association with severe head injury. The physical findings consist of cyanosis, dyspnea, and production of frothy white or blood-stained sputum. Coarse rhonchi may be palpable, and moist rales may be heard on auscultation. When this occurs early after severe chest injury, it carries a grave prognosis.

INJURY TO OTHER STRUCTURES

Contusions of the heart may be associated with irregular pulse or hypotension. The heart may have associated valvular damage or rupture.

Injuries of the aorta may accompany steering-wheel trauma. Rupture or dissection of the aorta may occur early in the postinjury period. The site of rupture is usually located in the descending aortic arch in the region of the left subclavian artery. Frequent x-ray examination of the chest should be employed to detect early signs of mediastinal widening or hemorrhage. These injuries are difficult to manage and many have a fatal outcome.

ABDOMINAL INJURIES

As a general rule, penetrating wounds of the abdomen require surgical exploration. If treatment is to be successful, early operation is an absolute necessity. If more than 8 hours elapse from time of injury to time of exploration, even simple wounds of the bowel are associated with a high mortality rate. Hypotension occurring early after injury is likely to be associated with blood loss, whereas hypotension developing after several hours' delay may indicate widespread infection or peritonitis.

A complete examination is extremely important. It must take into account the type of agent inflicting the wound and the position of the patient at the time of injury. When the physician is faced with multiple wounds, it is easy to be misled and to overlook small entry wounds. The buttocks, perineum, and anal canal should be carefully inspected. The appearance of the wound may provide information regarding the nature of the injury. For example, the presence of intestinal contents or bile may denote specific visceral injury. Under these circumstances prompt exploration is indicated, and little will be gained from prolonged detailed physical examination. Where entry wounds are small, however, detailed examination is important. This is particularly true when the wounds so located that intra-abdominal damage is not definitely established. The identification of blood in the gastric aspirate, urine, or rectal vault mandates surgical exploration. Careful physical examination must be directed toward eliciting evidence of even minor degrees of peritoneal irritation. This should certainly include rectal examination and may include sigmoidoscopy without the use of air insufflation. Injection of stab wounds with water-soluble contrast medium (Hypaque) is often helpful in determining peritoneal or visceral penetration. X-ray films are taken in lateral and oblique projections. Peritoneal lavage may detect early signs of peritonitis or hemorrhage. A favored policy is to do an exploratory operation on patients with peritoneal penetration. The contrast injection technique should not be used on patients with stab wounds of the chest.

Intra-Abdominal Hemorrhage

Intra-abdominal hemorrhage may be produced by laceration of the liver, spleen, mesenteric vessels, or retroperitoneum. The development of pallor, sweating, restlessness, and thirst within a few hours of the time of injury is significant. Hypotension ensues, and the pulse becomes rapid in rate and thready in quality. Tachypnea or "air hunger," poorly localized abdominal pain or pressure, and rebound tenderness may be present. With massive hemorrhage the abdomen becomes progressively swollen and full. When intra-abdominal hemorrhage is not massive, normal blood pressure may be maintained for several hours. Under these circumstances it is necessary to follow the pulse pressure and pulse rate with care, as their course is more important than their initial value. With slow, continued bleeding, progressive abdominal tenderness and spasm may become evident but are frequently absent. With sustained slow blood loss, decompensation and hypotension may occur rather suddenly when compensatory mechanisms fail. A rising pulse and respiratory rate may indicate impending decompensation.

With perforation of a hollow viscus, abdominal pain may occur and will rapidly become associated with a rigid, tender, silent abdomen and low urine output. These features are most prominent if some time has elapsed following injury. The early signs may be overlooked in the presence of multiple injuries or if analgesics or sedatives have been administered. If shock develops 8 to 12 hours or more after injury, it may be caused by generalized peritonitis. Shock may be accompanied by tachypnea and characteristic anxious facies.

Several abdominal wounds are commonly associated with hypotension. Pain and syncope may contribute, but blood loss and massive peritonitis rapidly contribute to "irreversible shock." Although the time period necessary for this to develop may vary, it is worth noting that therapy should not be withheld on the premise that the observed hypotension is irreversible. It is also true, however, that if blood pressure fails to rise after adequate volume replacement, a poor prognosis is indicated. It is equally important to be certain that some remediable lesion is not contributing to the patient's poor clinical condition. For example, tension pneumothorax or cardiac tamponade may occur in association with intra-abdominal injury. The physician should be prepared to reevaluate the patient completely at frequent intervals to be certain that his working diagnosis is accurate.

BLUNT ABDOMINAL INJURY

The liver, stomach, intestines, spleen, and pancreas are all subject to severe injury of a blunt or nonpenetrating nature. The injury may occur as the result of direct compression, translational motion with shearing, or when the viscus is crushed against the vertebral column. Frequent examination of the abdomen is of considerable importance. Peritoneal lavage, CT scan, or both, may detect injury before clinical signs are obvious and are important to consider in anyone with potentially severe abdominal injury. If there is reasonable doubt about the possibility of intraperitoneal injury, exploratory celiotomy should be done. This is a matter of judgment; the severity of other associated injuries must be weighed against the possibilities of a negative exploration.

Laceration of the liver results in intraperitoneal hemorrhage, which may vary in extent. With a disruption of large hepatic veins, exsanguination and death may result. With minor degrees of laceration, bleeding usually stops spontaneously. Injury to bile ducts is rare but bile accumulation can occur. Physical signs can include peritoneal irritation, possibly with shifting dullness, rebound tenderness, and generalized peritonitis, or they may be absent.

Splenic rupture is a common injury and should be suspected following blows on the left flank or the lower left chest. The clinical picture is characterized by abdominal pain, pain in the left shoulder, and shock. On physical examination, peritoneal irritation will usually be present and will be more marked in the left upper quadrant. Pain in the left shoulder and dyspnea may result from diaphragmatic irritation. Diagnosis may be exceedingly difficult with minor lacerations of the spleen. The diagnosis can be made by CT scan or ultrasound or suspected by peritoneal lavage. Minor splenic laceration may be managed by observation to preserve splenic function.

Mild trauma may produce a **subcapsular hematoma of the spleen** that may rupture several days or weeks later with shock, intraperitoneal hemorrhage, and rebound tenderness. The diagnosis is made in the same way as acute splenic injury. A water-soluble contrast study of the stomach and duodenum should be done on anyone in whom duodenal rupture is suspected because of a history of focal upper abdominal blunt injury (e.g., with a steering wheel, handlebar, or nightstick).

In some diseases, such as malaria, leukemia, or infectious mononucleosis, splenomegaly is a prominent feature. In these patients the spleen may rupture spontaneously or following minor trauma.

Forcible compression of the small intestine may lead to laceration. The most common location is just distal to the ligament of Treitz or in the terminal ileum, close to points of fixation. The duodenum in its position anterior to the spine is susceptible to rupture. When this occurs, bowel contents leak out and peritonitis develops posteriorly. Physical signs may appear late. Spasm and abdominal rigidity will be delayed. Peritoneal lavage may detect this injury before clinical signs occur. The white blood cell count in peritoneal lavage fluid is markedly elevated within 4 to 6 hours after bowel perforation. Free air is seen on plain films only about 10 percent of the time.

Rupture of the large intestine is not common. However, lacerations of the large bowel mesentery may occur, and necrosis and gangrene may result. The patient will present with considerable abdominal pain but usually without signs of peritonitis. The diagnosis may be extraordinarily difficult to make.

INJURY OF THE URINARY TRACT

Injuries of the kidney are usually seen in association with injury of the abdominal viscera, either the blunt or the penetrating type. Flank pain is variable but hematuria is a fairly constant finding. Blood loss may be considerable but is rarely exsanguinating. Extravasation of urine may occur into the renal fossa and flank, but is usually contained within Gerota's fascia. The combination of hemorrhage and urinary extravasation may produce muscle spasm, tenderness, and flank fullness. A mass may be palpable and may even be noted on inspection. Other physical signs include ecchymoses in the flank, nonshifting dullness in the flank, and a positive psoas sign due to extravasation of blood and urine overlying the psoas muscle.

It may be difficult to distinguish between injury of the spleen or liver and a damaged kidney. If the patient's condition warrants and he is not in shock, an echogram or intravenous pyelogram may be helpful. If other abdominal injuries are suspected, CT of the abdomen is preferred. It is important to have information regarding the involved kidney as well as on the functional state of the uninvolved side.

Bladder and urethral injuries are usually associated with fractures of the pelvis. In evaluating the possibility of this type of injury it is important to establish when the bladder was emptied prior to the accident. If the patient had not voided for some time and the bladder was known to be full at the time of the accident, rupture of the bladder is much more likely than if the bladder had been empty. The passage of bloody urine following injury helps establish the diagnosis of bladder or urethral injury. If the patient successfully voids clear urine after the accident, it is safe to assume that no serious injury to the lower urinary tract has resulted. If there is evidence of injury of the bladder neck or membranous urethra, such as blood in the urethra or perineal ecchymosis, a retrograde urethrogram should be done to detect urethral injury before any attempt is made to pass a urinary catheter. Damage may be compounded by unskilled attempts to pass the catheter in the presence of urethral damage.

Intraperitoneal rupture of the bladder occurs only if the bladder was full at the time of injury. Physical findings on examination consist of deep tenderness, muscle spasm, and peritoneal irritation. Rectal examination demonstrates tenderness and a normal prostate and membranous urethra. On completion of these initial diagnostic steps, catheterization may be performed. If bloody urine is obtained, urinary tract damage should be suspected. A cystogram may be diagnostic.

Injury of the bladder neck or membranous urethra results in extravasation of urine into the tissues surrounding the bladder and lower abdominal wall and may present as scrotal swelling. The extravasation extends laterally, and the area is markedly tender to gentle pressure. Rectal examination is important in localizing the area of injury. Damage to the prostatic urethra results in the presence of a boggy, tender mass that obscures the prostate gland. With laceration of the urogenital diaphragm, urine and blood extravasate into the perineum and perivesical space. These physical findings are indications for early surgical intervention.

Injuries to the lower urinary tract usually occur in conjunction with pelvic fractures. Lateral compression of the pelvis helps to make this diagnosis, although an x-ray study will be helpful in determining the extent of the injury.

PERIPHERAL NERVE INJURIES

Wounds in the extremities that include peripheral nerve injuries are encountered in military experience where extensive wounds of soft tissues and long bones occur. Peripheral nerve damage involves lower motor neuron axons, resulting in a flaccid type of paralysis. As a late result, muscles distal to the lesion undergo atrophy, sensory loss, and autonomic changes. The distal skin eventually becomes thin, smooth, and pale or mottled. Sweating is absent. Fingernails and toenails become brittle. These latter signs are, however, late in appearance, and early diagnosis will depend on loss of voluntary muscle power or absence of perception of pinprick.

Some peripheral nerve injuries are commonly encountered in civilian medical practice. For example, the radial nerve may be injured with fractures of the distal shaft of the humerus; the ulnar nerve may be damaged in association with fractures about the elbow; common peroneal nerve involvement may be found in connection with fractures, soft tissue wounds, or the use of tight casts that produce pressure about the knee. The lumbar plexus may be injured with widely displaced pelvic fractures involving sacroiliac joints. The sciatic nerve may be injured when dislocations of the hip occur. Lacerations about the wrists may produce damage to the median or ulnar nerves, and traction on the upper extremity may produce brachial plexus damage.

Partial damage to a peripheral nerve may be followed by a characteristic type of pain termed *causalgia,* which may develop rapidly after injury or may require several days to make its appearance. Causalgia is characterized by constant, intense, burning pain. It is made worse by moving, touching, minor trauma, excitement, and often by temperature change. The sciatic and median nerves are those most commonly involved. On neurologic examination the peripheral nerve injury is usually not complete. The skin of the involved member tends to be shiny and glossy, although not invariably so. Anesthetic block of the related sympathetic pathways characteristically produces prompt relief of the pain. This observation is of value in diagnosis.

EXAMINATION OF THE MUSCULOSKELETAL SYSTEM FOLLOWING ACUTE TRAUMA

GENERAL

The circumstances under which the injuries sustained by an accident victim are first determined usually require a different examination sequence and technique from that used in diagnosing less urgent musculoskeletal problems in the outpatient clinic or private office. In a modern community, patients who may have severe injuries are usually not seen by a physician until after they have been immobilized at the scene by emergency medical technicians and taken by ambulance to an emergency department. By the time the doctor sees them they have already been placed in a recumbent position on a backboard. Following the initial evaluation, only a limited degree of repositioning should be performed while x-ray or other special diagnostic studies are completed. Examination of the extremities does not begin until airway, breathing, and circulatory and other major organ systems have been assessed.

Fortunately the symptoms and signs of acute bone or joint injury are few and are easy to detect. The anatomy of each region is conducive to common patterns of injury that are easily identified by the experienced examiner. For example, the shoulder may sustain either a fracture through the humeral neck, with associated soft-tissue injuries, or a scapulohumeral dislocation; similarly, the elbow may sustain either a supracondylar fracture or an ulnohumeral dislocation. It is important to pay attention to pulses and motor function distal to injured areas.

For quick determination of precisely which injury has occurred, routine x-ray studies are more reliable than physical examination. Even the most experienced clinician cannot be certain of all findings without x-ray studies. Therefore, attempts to distinguish injuries within a given region by lengthy clinical examination should be avoided, especially when the examination requires diagnostic manipulations that might further injure the soft tissues. In the initial survey, on the other hand, a good screening physical examination is more reliable than x-ray films in disclosing regions of injury. X-ray studies should not be performed, therefore, until all suspicious regions have been identified.

Frequently the treatment of the injuries should be started during the course of the examination. As soon as a presumptive diagnosis of a fracture or dislocation is established, the involved region should be immobilized by splinting in order to minimize further damage to the soft tissues during subsequent examination and x-ray procedures. These splints should not be disturbed either during or following the x-ray examination until definitive treatment has been started.

POSITIONING THE PATIENT

For the initial examination, the accident victim should, if possible, be lying supine on a stretcher or backboard. Because moving an injured patient is hazardous, the stretcher frame should be detachable, so that the patient can be lifted to a table and x-rayed or operated on while he is still on the stretcher. Although no single position allows complete inspection of the patient, the full supine position offers the greatest latitude for both examination and treatment. If the victim is not initially in the supine position but is prone or on the side, turning an accident victim onto his back without regard for a possible broken spine or other serious fracture, is, of course, fraught with grave risks. On the other hand, if his condition requires immediate airway clearance, there is no choice but to turn him, using the log-rolling technique with traction on the head and the neck in neutral position.

In less critical cases the patient should be questioned for location of pain and his limbs quickly inspected for evidence of deformities that might indicate fractures or dislocations. He should be asked to move his fingers and toes; the presence or absence of paraplegia or quadriplegia is thereby established. If the patient has pain in his neck or back, a vertebral injury should be presumed until confirmed or refuted by x-rays.

If the findings suggest a vertebral injury, it is possible to turn the patient, if necessary, by straightening his back or neck and carefully avoiding any bending or twisting. The patient should be rolled with someone holding his head and turning it in harmony with the rest of his body, with care to see that his arms are extended along the sides of his body. It is remotely possible that straightening an injured vertebral column may aggravate an injury, but this possibility must be accepted since completion of the examination and treatment ultimately require a supine position.

If a limb bone injury is suspected, the patient should be turned with an attendant supporting the injured limb and turning it in gentle harmony with the rest of the body. Although splinting a limb prior to turning has been advocated, splints are most easily applied with the patient supine and are of relatively little value in maintaining fracture alignment during turning. After turning has been accomplished, splinting will afford protection during further maneuvers.

GENERAL TYPES OF FRACTURES

Fracture and *break* are synonymous terms, classically defined as "a dissolution of continuity of a solid structure," for example, a bone. If there are more than two fragments, the fracture is said to be *comminuted.* Self-explanatory terms, such as *transverse, oblique, spiral, T, Y,* are frequently used to describe the orientation of a fracture line. A fracture line may enter one side of the bone and then divide and extend across the remainder of the bone in two diverging branches, creating an extra piece of bone imaginatively denoted as a *butterfly* fragment (Figure 21–3 shows various types of fractures.)

When a long bone is subjected to bending force, the portion that is under the greatest tension usually breaks apart first. This type of break is similar to that of a broken piece of chalk. The fragments can move apart easily. In the body, the surrounding soft tissues restrain the fragments from displacement. Displacement and deformity are relative to the degree of soft tissue disruption, particularly of the periosteum. In adults the periosteum is thin; therefore, widespread displacement and severe deformity are likely. In children the periosteum is thick and is frequently torn on only one side of the bone, thereby allowing only angular deformity

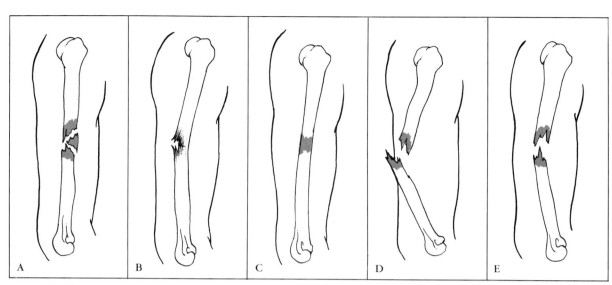

FIGURE 21–3
Some types of fractures. A. Comminuted. B. Greenstick. C. Torus. D. Compound (open). E. Simple (closed).

with little or no displacement. In either age group, if the periosteal disruption is sufficiently severe, the ends of the fragments may displace. If the fracture line is oblique or spiral, or if sufficient lateral displacement occurs in a transverse fracture, some overriding of the fragments and consequent shortening of the limb are likely. One fragment may twist with respect to the other (malrotation). Any degree of angulation may occur. The ultimate position of the fragments and the external appearance of the limb are determined by the effects of neighboring muscles as well as by the effects of gravity and the direction and magnitude of the fracture force. Although shortening of a limb because of muscle spasm is commonly observed immediately after a fracture, lengthening almost never occurs.

Since children's bones are less brittle than adults', only one side of the bone may pull apart; the other side bends. This *incomplete fracture* is referred to as a *greenstick* fracture. It exhibits only an angular deformity. Occasionally, when a child's long bone is subjected to a bending or an axial compression force, it may buckle on the compressed side of the bone. This usually occurs in the flared (metaphyseal) area. The opposite cortex of the bone appears normal on an x-ray and the limb exhibits no deformity, merely localized pain and tenderness to palpation. This type of *incomplete* fracture is referred to as a *torus* fracture.

Fractures near the ends of children's long bones have special significance. If a fracture either crushes or splits an epiphysis and its underlying epiphyseal (growth) plate, a growth disturbance may occur. More frequently, fractures in this area pass transversely along the metaphyseal side of the epiphyseal plate and then deviate into the metaphysis. The terminal fragment then consists of the epiphysis with the epiphyseal plate and a small piece of metaphysis. Although displacement of this composite fragment may be wide, little or no damage has been done to the epiphyseal plate, and an ultimate growth disturbance is unlikely.

If a wound extends from the skin surface to the fracture site, there is grave risk of infection of the injured bone regardless of whether this skin is pierced by a bone fragment from within or by a foreign body from without. Such fractures are termed *open* or *compound*. It is essential that any skin wound, however small, that might communicate with the fracture site be recognized and promptly treated. The blood in a fracture hematoma quickly darkens and contains visible globules of fat from the marrow. A skin wound in the neighborhood of a fracture that oozes fluid of this type is therefore one that communicates directly with the fracture. Any fracture, no matter how comminuted, that does not communicate with a skin wound is referred to as a *closed* or *simple* fracture. Because of frequent confusion in the designations *compound* and *simple,* the terms *open* and *closed* are now preferred in standard use.

Small bones, such as those of the spine, ankle, and wrist, may be split or crushed by the forces of trauma. Displacement of the fragments is usually minor compared with that of fragments of long bones. Deformity is seldom evident if the bones are deep beneath the skin, as in the case of vertebral fractures; however, because of their proximity to the spinal cord and nerve roots, even minor displacements of vertebral fractures may produce signs of nerve damage. Fractures of small bones in the ankle and wrist seldom exhibit deformity unless displacement is severe, but they may alter the range of motion of associated joints, as indicated by pain on local palpation or attempted motion. Fractures extending into joints cause bleeding into the joints. Motion is painful and if the joint is a superficial one, such as the knee or elbow, swelling eventually occurs.

The cardinal symptoms of a fracture are pain, tenderness, and deformity. Pain, is usually most severe at the fracture site. Tenderness may be evoked by palpation directly over the fracture or by moving the bone fragments. The former technique is safe and reliable; the latter is hazardous. Deformity results from soft-tissue swelling or displacement of fracture bone. Motion of the fragments is also likely to cause audible or palpable crepitus. The patient may be able to report that he felt or heard his bone snap at the time of injury and has felt the grating of fragments when he has been moved. The examiner should not attempt to elicit crepitus. Instablity is usually obvious, but occasionally a fracture may be quite stable, and the fact that a patient can use his injured limb does not rule out fracture, although it makes it less likely. Visible or palpable deformity may or may not be present. Swelling, ecchymosis, and increased local heat occur to a variable extent with all fractures but are late signs.

GENERAL TYPES OF DISLOCATIONS

If the articular surface of one bone is totally displaced from the articular surface of its partner, the joint is *dislocated*. A joint may be dislocated and spontaneously reduce itself, or the bones may be trapped by the surrounding structures and special maneuvers required for reduction. A *subluxation* is a partial dislocation; contact between the articular surfaces is less than normal. This term is best applied to certain malformed joints and is seldom applicable to traumatized joints with the exception of the vertebrae. In trauma the joint either is or is not dislocated; there are no intermediate possibilities.

As with a fracture, the cardinal symptom is pain, and there is local tenderness to palpation or motion. The range of motion is altered and usually reduced; in fact, the joint seems locked in an abnormal position. The examiner should not attempt to elicit motion but should take the word of the patient on this point. Deformity of adjacent structures is evident in a superficial joint. The posture of the limb distal to the joint is usually abnormal. Dislocation of some joints, such as the shoulder, increases the overall length of the limb. Swelling, ecchymosis, and heat are late signs. Ideally diagnosis should be established and the dislocation reduced before these have been allowed to develop.

X-ray studies should not be delayed in an effort to establish the details of a joint injury by physical examination, since films are far more reliable. Two points, however, should be quickly determined: (1) the presence of a wound into the joint, because an *open* or *compound* dislocation is as vulnerable to infection as an open fracture; and (2) the presence of vascular or neurologic insufficiency in the limb distal to the injury, particularly in dislocations of the knee and elbow.

Ligaments, Tendons, and Muscles

The ligaments of interest in this chapter are those that span joints and thus stabilize and control the motion of the involved bones. In the joints of the arms and legs, motion is possible primarily within a single plane; strap ligaments on either side of the joint allow very limited lateral or medial motion (abduction and adduction). With excessive leverage improperly applied to the joint, a ligament may be ruptured, torn transversely, or separated from one of its points of attachment. In any case, the point of maximum pain and tenderness to digital palpation coincides with the point of injury. If the most tender spot lies over ligament rather than bone, a ligament injury is more probable than a fracture. If x-ray films at this time indicate that no fracture is present, it is safe to test the ligament for partial or total disruption by carefully abducting or adducting the joint. If a ligament is totally divided, and if the patient is able to relax his muscles, excessive motion will be found in the joint. Such an examination is sometimes too painful for a patient to endure, and either an anesthetic must be administered or the joint allowed to "cool off" for a couple of days or weeks in some form of protective immobilization, such as a cast. *Strain* and *sprain* are words frequently used imprecisely. *Strain* is correctly used to refer to a stretch or partial tear; *sprain* is correctly used to refer to a total tear or avulsion. A dislocation cannot occur without serious tearing or avulsion of ligaments.

A tendon forms the connection between muscle and bone, converting the contraction of the muscle into motion of the bone. Tendons, musculotendinous junctions, and occasionally even muscles can be torn apart if the bone is prevented from moving or is forced to move in opposition to a strong muscle contraction. In children, avulsion of a piece of bone at the point of tendon attachment is more common than a tear in the tendon or musculotendinous junction. The opposite is true in adults. Common examples of tendon tears in adults occur in the tendons of the long head of the biceps, the tendon of the supraspinatus, and the tendo Achillis of the calf. These injuries are identified by correlating the site of pain with weakness or absence of function in a specific muscle. There may be a palpable soft-tissue defect at the point of pain and enlargement of the muscle indicating its uncontrolled recoil. X-rays that are taken for soft-tissue detail can sometimes confirm a clinical impression of tendon tear.

ARTERIAL INJURY

Fractures or dislocations may impair distal arterial blood supply by compressing or lacerating the artery at the site of injury. This occurs most frequently at the knee and elbow but can occur with bone or joint injuries in many other regions. Therefore the quality of the peripheral circulation in all four limbs should always be clearly determined and recorded during the initial examination, before any splint is applied or x-rays taken. Early signs of arterial insufficiency are lowered skin temperature, absence of wrist or foot pulses, and pallor. Later signs include hyperesthesia and paralysis. At the site of arterial injury there may be a large and pulsatile swelling, indicating massive extravasation of arterial blood; however, this is a relatively infrequent complication.

NERVES

Wherever nerves lie close to bone, fractures can injure them. The region of greatest concern, of course, is the vertebral column. Elements of the lumbosacral plexus are occasionally damaged by fractures of the pelvis. A significant percentage of posterior dislocations of the hip damage the sciatic nerve and paralyze the dorsiflexors of the foot (footdrop). Severe knee injuries and fractures of the upper end of the fibula may damage the peroneal nerve, producing a footdrop. Fractures and dislocation of the shoulder joint are occasionally associated with injury to the axillary nerve, resulting in a weak abduction. Fractures of the shaft of the humerus, especially at the junction of the middle and distal thirds, may injure the radial, median, or ulnar nerves; radial palsy signified by inability to dorsiflex the wrist (wristdrop) is most common. Elbow injuries may be complicated by the same types of nerve injuries. At the wrist, compression of the median nerve in the carpal tunnel, with resulting numbness over the first two fingers, is common. To determine whether nerves have been injured, the motor and sensory function distal to any fracture must be evaluated and recorded on initial examination. Neurologic injury can also result from ischemia associated with arterial injury or muscle compartment swelling.

SPECIFIC FRACTURES AND DISLOCATIONS

VERTEBRAL FRACTURES AND DISLOCATIONS

Paralysis and sensory loss signify spinal cord or nerve root damage with a vertebral injury. Analysis of the level of motor or sensory loss will reveal the level of vertebral injury. Charts of sensory dermatomes and muscle innervations are helpful but are not necessary if the examiner has memorized the nerve supply to a few key regions and muscles. If the patient is comatose or stuporous, the determination is difficult but not impossible. Usually such a patient will move those regions that are not paralyzed in response to painful stimuli. If coma is profound, normal muscle tone

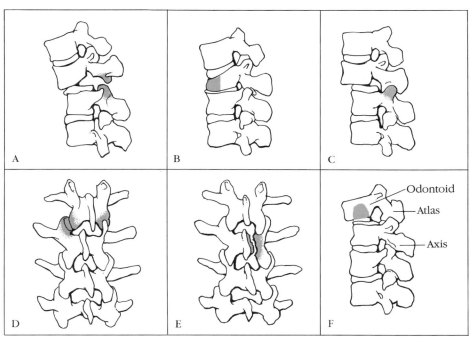

FIGURE 21—4
Common types of vertebral injury. A. Subluxation. B. Compression fracture. C. Bilateral facet joint dislocation. D. Unilateral facet joint dislocation. E. Posterior arch fracture. F. Odontoid fracture.

as well as response to painful stimuli may be absent. Usually, however, if one foot is raised and dropped directly over the other, the descending heel will not strike the other foot unless the falling limb is paralyzed. The upper limb of an unconscious patient can similarly be tested by dropping the patient's hand toward his face. When innervation is intact, the falling hand will usually either deviate to the side or decelerate just before impact.

Pain in the back or neck of an accident victim should be considered an indication for spinal x-ray. The film should include several vertebrae above and below the painful area, since pain is frequently referred below the level of injury and occasionally above. Palpation of the spinous processes for an area of maximum tenderness may facilitate precise location of injury but should not be performed if it requires turning the patient.

Because of the deep position of the vertebral column in the body, external or palpable deformity is rare. Either pain or neurologic deficit is adequate evidence for diagnostic x-rays, and the examiner should not look for deformity or abnormal vertebral motion.

X-ray studies may show any of the following types of vertebral injuries occurring individually or in combination: subluxation, body fracture, unilateral or bilateral facet joint dislocation, or fracture of the arch, odontoid, spinous process, or transverse process (Fig. 21—4).

Subluxation of an upper vertebra on a lower one is best seen in a lateral projection of the cervical spine in a neutral or forward flexed position. The interspinous ligament and sometimes the capsular ligaments of the posterior facet joints have been torn by the upper vertebra traveling too far forward on the lower, and sometimes the intervertebral disc space is narrowed. This condition represents a sprain and is an example of the so-called whiplash injury.

A vertebral body fracture is usually caused by compression forces, and the consequent reduction in height of the involved vertebral body is most conspicuous on lateral x-rays. Frequently pieces of the centrum are displaced and may impinge on the spinal cord. Compression of a thoracic vertebra into a wedge, with the narrower portion anterior and no resulting neurologic deficit, is a common finding in middle-aged and elderly persons with osteoporosis.

Dislocated posterior facet joints are rare except in the cervical spine. When unilateral dislocations occur, the vertebrae are locked in slight malrotation. For this reason the anteroposterior x-rays show a shift in the alignment of the spinous processes, with those above the dislocation shifted about ¼ inch toward the side of the dislocated facet joint. No such rotation occurs with bilateral facet joint dislocations, but the extreme forward shift of the upper on the lower vertebra is likely to cause severe spinal cord injury, in contrast to the minor neurologic deficit following a unilateral dislocation. The articular processes of dislocated facet joints can best be seen in lateral or oblique projections.

A posterior vertebral arch may sustain a fracture through the lamina, which is best visualized on an anteroposterior or oblique x-ray as a faint line near an articular facet. Usually when a ring of bone such as a vertebra is broken in one place, there is a second fracture through another part of the ring, which may be difficult to demonstrate on the x-ray. These fractures should be strongly suspected when there is a slight lateral shift of one spinous process. They may be associated with any degree of neurologic deficit. They may result from a hyperextension injury or a direct blow and are likely to be associated with significant instability of the vertebral column. Hyperextension of the spine should be carefully avoided in handling these cases.

An odontoid fracture represents a perilous injury in view of potential instability of C1 on C2 and the limited space available to the spinal cord if displacement occurs. When cord injury does occur at this level, there may be immediate paralysis of all respiratory muscles and quick death. This fracture is usually best seen on lateral films or an open-mouth anteroposterior view as a line across the waist or base of the odontoid. The overlying shadow of an upper incisor tooth frequently obscures the true outline of the odontoid in a manner that simulates a fracture. Congenital malformation of the odontoid with incomplete ossification may also confuse the findings. For a reliable diagnosis the x-ray findings must be correlated with the nature of the injury and physical symptoms.

The distal tip of a spinous process, frequently at C7 or T1, may be the site of fracture. These processes are easily palpated and are very tender if fractured. If there are no other vertebral fractures, the stability of the column is not compromised. These fractures are usually best seen on lateral x-ray projection.

Transverse processes on the lumbar vertebrae serve as points of attachment for

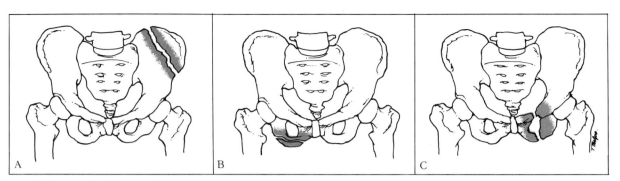

Figure 21–5
Benign fractures of the pelvis. A. Shear. B. Avulsion. C. Stable crack.

the psoas muscles and may be fractured by avulsion. This is usually accompanied by severe back pain. Retroperitoneal hemorrhage may occur, producing abdominal tenderness. The lateral edge of the psoas muscle may be obscured on the x-ray. The fractured transverse processes are best seen on an anteroposterior x-ray of the lumbar spine. Congenital malformation with incomplete ossification is common and may lead to a false diagnosis of fracture. Structural stability of the vertebral column is not impaired.

PELVIC FRACTURE

When evaluating the possibility of fracture, the examiner should think of the normal pelvis as a symmetric ring of bone with various projections serving as points of attachment for muscles. The projections may be sheared off by a direct blow or avulsed by strong muscle action. An example of a shearing injury is a fracture of the iliac crest caused by a lateral impact motor vehicle accident; local contusion and loss of normal pelvic contour are apparent. An example of avulsion is the fracture of an ischial tuberosity by a sprinter as he forcibly contracts his hamstrings while pushing away from the starting blocks at the beginning of the race. Pain and tenderness at the point of a specific muscle attachment and on contraction of the involved muscle are diagnostic signs (Fig. 21–5).

Because of the elasticity of the symphysis pubis, the pelvic ring may be broken at only one point, but simultaneous fracture in two separate areas is more likely and also more serious because of the resulting instability. Weak areas are present near the sacroiliac joints, at the ischiopubic junctions, and through the symphysis pubis. A fracture through one sacroiliac joint and the ischiopubic junctions on the same side (Malgaigne fracture) creates a large lateral fragment to which the entire lower limb is attached (Fig. 21–6). This fragment is frequently displaced proximally by the trunk muscles. It may be tilted medially or laterally. Pelvic asymmetry and shortening of the lower limb are present and easily detected. Motion on gentle compression or distraction of the iliac crests is a conclusive finding of this injury. A fracture through the ischiopubic junctions bilaterally creates an anterior fragment that may be associated with bladder rupture. If the symphysis pubis can be moved by gentle pressure, the diagnosis of this fracture is confirmed. This injury is fre-

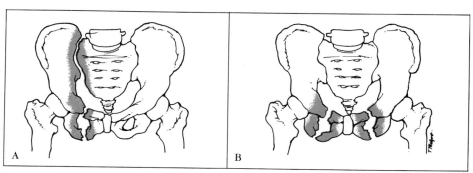

FIGURE 21–6
Unstable fractures of the pelvis. A. Malgaigne. B. Straddle.

quently caused by falling astride some large, rigid object. Contusion of the perineum may be present and the scrotum becomes distended with blood. In any of these injuries the abdomen may be tender to palpation and exhibit signs of retroperitoneal hemorrhage, which can be massive and life threatening. Various branches of the lumbosacral plexus may be injured, producing hyperesthesia or muscle weakness.

HIP JOINT AND UPPER FEMUR

Among the types of fractures sustained by the upper femur are those with stability adequate to permit ambulation initially but that ultimately separate with unpleasant consequences. These are very uncommon injuries. Significant events in the history are a fall or misstep followed by pain in the hip. Objective physical findings may be entirely negative. Good quality x-rays are necessary to establish the diagnosis, which may be that of a crack from greater to lesser trochanter, or a fracture across the neck of the femur just beneath the impacted femoral head. Although a fracture through the upper femur (broken hip) may occur at any age, it is more common among elderly persons, especially women, and more especially those with osteoporosis. Typically the limb lies in external rotation. The distance between knee and the iliac crest is reduced and any motion of the hip joint is painful. This may be hard to distinguish from a fracture of the acetabulum, except by x-ray.

Fractures of the acetabulum are frequently caused by forces that drive the femoral head into it. The femoral head may or may not be displaced medially and/or cephalad with the acetabular fragments. This is termed a *central fracture-dislocation* of the hip (Fig. 21–7). Frequently, however, this injury can be distinguished from an intracapsular femoral fracture only by x-rays.

If a person is in a sitting position with his hip in flexion and adduction at the moment of impact of a force on his knee, the femoral head may be driven over or through the posterior rim of the acetabulum and come to rest against the sciatic nerve just behind the socket. This is known as a posterior dislocation (see Fig. 21–7). Paralysis of foot dorsiflexors (footdrop) from sciatic nerve injury is common. The posture of a patient with this type of dislocation is unique. He lies with his involved limb in adduction, flexion, and internal rotation. He prefers to lie on his

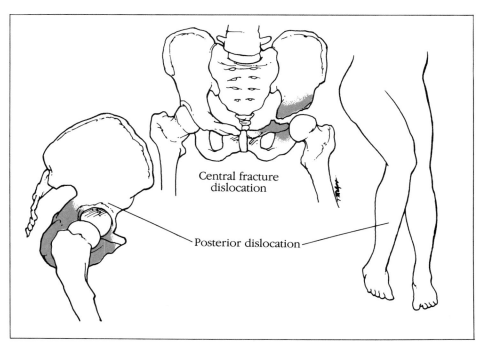

FIGURE 21–7
Central fracture-dislocation of hip and posterior dislocation of hip.

uninjured side and resists any attempt at normal positioning of his leg. Two other relatively uncommon dislocations of the femoral head occur—one into the *obturator* foramen, and the other into the region of the *inguinal* ligament. The former is an inferior dislocation and the latter, an anterior one. Both of these are caused by excessive abduction. A patient with an anterior dislocation lies in moderate abduction and external rotation, and the head is palpable beneath the inguinal ligament. A patient with an inferior dislocation lies in extreme abduction and external rotation and the head is not palpable.

SHOULDER JOINT (SCAPULOHUMERAL) AND UPPER HUMERUS
The shoulder is designed to facilitate placement of the hand in an unlimited number of positions in space. This is accomplished by a very shallow socket (glenoid) in the head of the scapula, articulating with the head of the humerus. The clavicle has a sinusoidal curve and is commonly fractured by a compression force applied longitudinally. Such a force may be applied directly by a blow on the tip of the shoulder or indirectly by a fall on the outstretched hand. This injury is one of the most common fractures in children and also in adults. The sternoclavicular joint can be disrupted by a similar force, with the result that the medial end of the clavicle dislocates medially and behind or in front of the sternum. An abrupt force downward on the tip of the shoulder can dislocate the acromioclavicular joint. Any of these injuries is easily detected by inspection and palpation, since the structures

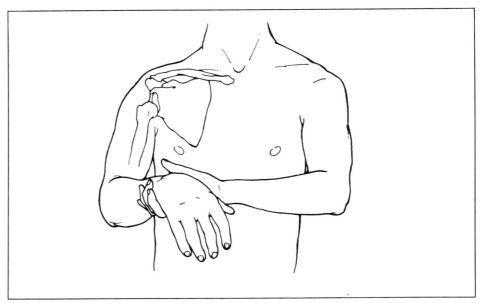

FIGURE 21–8
Anterior dislocation of scapulohumeral joint.

lie close beneath the skin. Dislocation of the medial end of the clavicle behind the sternum may create a sensation of airway obstruction due to pressure on the trachea. Clavicular fractures are frequently associated with a sizable subcutaneous hematoma and, rarely, with injury to elements of the brachial plexus and even the apex of the lung.

The common *dislocated shoulder* is an anterior or anteroinferior scapulohumeral dislocation in which the humerus ends up anterior to the glenoid (Fig. 21–8). Normally, when the humerus is abducted to the limit of its normal range of motion, it impinges against the outer edge of the acromion. If abduction is forced beyond its limit, the head of the humerus is dislocated by being levered over the anteroinferior edge of the rim of the glenoid. The patient is then unable to bring his arm in against his side or to rotate it internally. This type of dislocation frequently recurs. The first episode is extremely painful, but each recurrence is less painful, and the patient may learn to reduce the dislocation himself. The patient's appearance is unique. The deltoid bulge is flattened and the acromion is unusually prominent with an empty space just below it where the humeral head usually rests. The distance between the acromion and olecranon on the afflicted side is greater than on the opposite side. Sometimes it is possible to palpate the humeral head high in the anterior axilla.

Fractures of the head or neck of the humerus can occur from a fall on the outstretched hand. They may be found in any age group but are more common in the elderly. Any active motion of the humerus is painful. In contrast with dislocations, the deltoid bulge is accentuated by displacement, or overriding, of the fragments, and by accumulation of extravasated blood. The distance between acromion and olecranon is unchanged or decreased.

Although these injuries can be identified by physical examination, this should not be done if adequate x-ray facilities are available. The initial examination of a specific area should be limited to determining that a skeletal injury exists; x-rays of that area are then indicated as soon as all other areas have been checked.

SHAFT OF FEMUR AND HUMERUS (SINGLE-BONE SEGMENTS)

Since the thigh segment of the lower limb and the arm segment of the upper limb both contain a single long bone, fracture of the shaft of that bone creates such conspicous instability of the segment that diagnosis is usually obvious. Palpation of the bones may be difficult because of the thick muscles in these areas, but motion at the fracture site is revealed by any attempt to move the limb. The tone of the muscle tends to cause overriding of the fragments and therefore a decrease in length of the segment. If overriding is present or a hematoma has accumulated, the girth of the limb is enlarged. The ends of the sharp fragments may injure the neighboring soft tissues. In the femur, one or more of the deep veins may be torn, causing internal hemorrhage. The fractured humerus frequently damages the radial nerve, producing a wristdrop. Open fractures of these bones are especially serious injuries, and a careful circumferential check of the skin for any wound should always be made.

KNEE AND ELBOW

In the knee and elbow, bone fragments may easily be displaced; therefore no diagnostic manipulations should be performed on a deformed or painful joint until x-ray studies have been examined and found negative.

These joints link single-bone segments with double-bone segments; thus, each articulation involves three long bones. The motion of both joints is primarily within a single plane of flexion and extension. Each joint has a bony prominence that increases the mechanical advantage of the extensor muscle. For the knee this prominence is the patella; for the elbow it is the olecranon. The knee, which is subjected to high compression forces in many positions, has two semilunar wedges of cartilage called the menisci, which function as lubrication wedges, shock absorbers, and shims. Neurovascular structures lie close to the flexor aspects of distal humerus and femur (Figs. 21–9 and 21–10).

Fractures that jeopardize the arteries in these areas occur just above, between, or through the condyles and are termed *supracondylar, intracondylar,* and *condylar,* respectively. Such fractures of the humerus are especially common in children. One of the fragments, usually the distal, may be tilted by the flexor muscles toward the artery. Deformity of the elbow may range from insignificant to severe. Sometimes it may stimulate a "gunstock," with medial or lateral deviation, a fullness in the upper part of the antecubital space, and a depression posteriorly just above the olecranon. Supracondylar fractures of the femur are more common in adults. There is an increase in the circumference of the thigh just above the knee. The fracture causes hemorrhage into the knee joint with consequent swelling. The distal end of the shaft fragment may penetrate the skin near the patella. In view of the

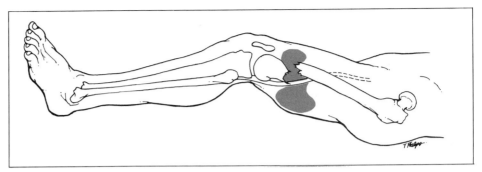

FIGURE 21–9
Injury to femoral artery by supracondylar fracture of femur.

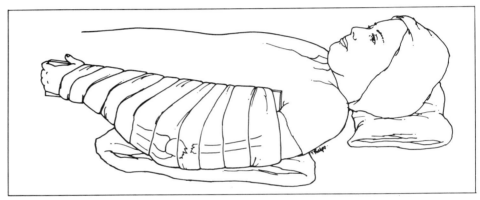

FIGURE 21–10
Supracondylar fracture of humerus.

strong possibility of arterial injury, circulation to the limb beyond the fracture must always be verified.

Both the olecranon and the patella are vulnerable to fractures from direct blows and from avulsion by muscle action. The former fractures are more often comminuted.

The patella can dislocate to the lateral side of the knee, a condition that is easily diagnosed by inspection and palpation. Dislocations of the tibia on the femur, or vice versa, cause extensive injuries that are usually accompanied by neurovascular injury. Deformity is severe and the diagnosis is self-evident.

An unfractured olecranon can dislocate only in association with the rest of the ulna, which may be displaced posteriorly and sometimes laterally. The deformity seen with posterior dislocation resembles that of a supracondylar fracture of the humerus.

If either the elbow or knee is subjected to excessive abduction or adduction stress, either the ligament fails on the side subjected to tension forces, or the bone crumbles on the side subjected to compression forces. Such fractures in the knee are called tibial plateau or tibial condyle fractures. In the elbow the counterpart of such an injury is a fracture of the radial head or neck. These fractures produce pain at the fracture site, pain on joint motion, and joint swelling. Ligament and meniscus injuries produce similar symptoms. Fractures should always be ruled out by x-rays before subjecting a joint to abduction or adduction stresses in order to ascertain ligament rupture.

If a meniscus is torn, the free part of it may become trapped between the femur and tibia and obstruct joint motion. This obstruction may be unyielding or it may be limited and variable. To detect the obstruction it may be necessary to flex and extend the joint with it twisted internally or externally and abducted or adducted. Such manipulation should never be performed if the possibility of fracture exists. A small area of acute tenderness to palpation is frequently present at the joint line close to a meniscus tear. Joint swelling is likely with this or any other knee injury and of itself may limit joint motion.

MONTEGGIA'S FRACTURE-DISLOCATION

This injury consists of a fracture of the ulna and a dislocation of the proximal end of the radius. It is usually caused by a blow on the ulnar side of the forearm near the elbow. The force breaks the ulna and then acts on the radius. If the radius does not break, the proximal radioulnar articulation is pulled apart. The annular ligament is broken, and the proximal end of the radius is displaced from its normal position of articulation against the lateral condyl (capitellum) of the humerus. The existence of this injury may be presumed if a fracture of the ulna is identified and there seems to be pain or limitation of motion of the elbow. Diagnosis is confirmed by x-rays of both the elbow and forearm.

LEG AND FOREARM (DOUBLE-BONE SEGMENTS)

The thin soft tissue covering of the bones in the leg and forearm facilitates detection of an undisplaced fracture by palpation for point tenderness directly over the bone. This technique is especially valuable in establishing the possibility of an incomplete fracture of the torus or greenstick type. Only the radius cannot be palpated throughout its length. In the proximal one-third of the radius, where this bone is covered by the extensor muscles, a fracture should be presumed if tenderness is produced by pronation or supination.

Instability may not be conspicuous if only one of the bones is broken or if both bones are broken at different levels.

Fracture of both bones in a double-bone segment is more common than fracture of only one bone. Since these fractures may occur at a considerable distance from each other, x-rays should always be taken to include the entire length of the segment.

COLLES', BARTON'S, AND SMITH'S FRACTURES

Falling on a dorsiflexed and outstretched hand may fracture the radius just proximal to the wrist joint. The distal fragment is pushed proximally and may override or impact on the proximal one. The ulnar styloid process may be avulsed, but the rest of the ulna remains intact. The hand is forced into radial deviation. The distal radial fragment is usually tilted backward and the volar edge of the end of the shaft

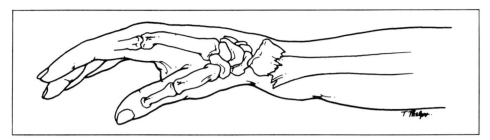

FIGURE 21–11
Colles' fracture of the wrist.

fragment crowds the flexor tendons or median nerve where they enter the carpal tunnel. The volar side of the wrist is abnormally prominent. Abraham Colles described the deformity associated with this particular fracture as resembling a dinner fork (Fig. 21–11). Sometimes the main mass of the radius remains intact, and only the prominent dorsal margin of the articular surface is broken off, permitting the carpus to dislocate posteriorly. The fracture-dislocation is called a Barton's fracture. The clinical deformity is similar to a Colles' fracture. A fracture that might be defined as a Colles' fracture, except that the distal radial fragment is tilted toward the volar rather than the dorsal side, is called a Smith's fracture.

ANKLE INJURIES (POTT'S FRACTURE)

As with the shafts of the tibia and fibula, the thin, soft tissue covering of the malleoli facilitates detection of an undisplaced fracture by palpation for point tenderness directly over the bone. When maximum tenderness to palpation is over the medial or lateral ligaments or anterior capsule, the injury is more likely due to sprain than a fracture. No other diagnostic manipulation should be performed until fractures are ruled out by x-rays. X-rays may confirm that one malleolus or both is broken. In association with these fractures, the talus may be displaced medially or laterally. Sometimes the posterior articular margin of the tibia is also broken and displaced proximally (trimalleolar fracture). If the posterior fragment includes more than one-quarter of the articular surface of the tibia, the talus also dislocates posteriorly. Pott's fracture is a generic term for ankle fractures in general (Fig. 21–12).

FOOT AND HAND

Although displaced fractures or dislocations of the bones of the feet and hands are easy to recognize on inspection, x-rays are necessary to identify certain undisplaced fractures, especially those of the carpal and tarsal bones. Fractures of the calcaneus are usually caused by a blow on the bottom of the heel, as when an accident victim strikes the ground in a standing position after falling from a ladder or scaffold. Vertebral compression fractures are commonly associated with this injury and should not be overlooked.

Fist fights result in broken knuckles and Bennett's fractures. The involved knuckle is usually depressed. The fracture is through the metacarpal neck, and the metacarpal head is tilted down into the palm. If a first metacarpal is driven proximally with excessive force, a fracture dislocation of the metacarpomultangular joint is

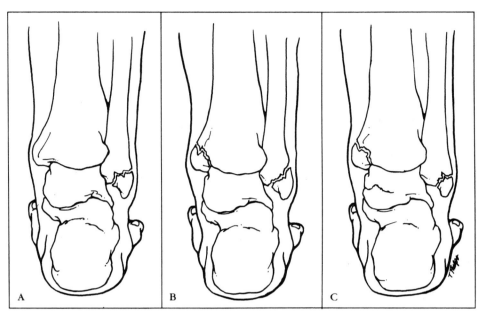

FIGURE 21–12
Some fractures of the ankle. A. Lateral malleolar fracture. B. Medial and lateral malleolar fracture. C. Trimalleolar fracture.

sustained. This is called a Bennett's fracture. The thumb is shortened, and pain is greatest at its base. Thumb abduction and extension are painful and limited.

A blow sustained on the tip of an outstretched finger may forcibly flex the tip before the extensor tendon can be relaxed. The insertion of the extensor tendon is avulsed and the patient is unable to lift the tip of his finger.

INITIAL ASSESSMENT OF THE TRAUMA VICTIM

A number of convenient approaches can ensure the complete initial assessment of the traumatized patient. Any mnemonic one uses should facilitate examination of an accident victim with injuries of unknown extent in a sequence that is easily remembered, address the priorities of resuscitation, and be sufficiently complete to detect any significant injury.

The Advanced Trauma Life Support course of the American College of Surgeons breaks the initial assessment into two phases, a brief primary survey performed initially, and a more complete secondary survey, performed after resuscitation efforts have begun.*

The *primary survey* can be remembered by the letters ABCDE (Table 21–1). The **airway** is assessed first. A patient who is alert and talking obviously has a clear airway, but one must examine obtunded persons or those with obvious facial injury carefully to be certain that blood, soft tissue, or foreign material is not compro-

*Committee on Trauma. *Advanced Trauma Life Support.* American College of Surgeons, 1984.

TABLE 21–1. Initial Assessment of the Trauma Victim

Suggested systemic approach to assessing the injured patient, following a descending
order of priorities.
A = Airway
B = Breathing
C = Circulation
D = Disability
E = Exposed

mising the upper airway. **Breathing** is assessed by inspection, palpation, and auscultation of the chest, aimed at detecting hemothorax, pneumothorax, or instability
of the chest wall. **Circulation** is assessed at first by the strength and rate of the
pulse, as well as the color and moisture of the skin, and later by vital signs and
urine output. A brief neurologic examination is done to identify obvious alterations
of consciousness, signs of expanding extradural or subdural hemorrhage, or evidence of spinal cord injury, which would be likely to cause long-term **disability**. All
surfaces of the victim should be **exposed**, to allow complete examination.

Immediate resuscitative efforts should be directed at life-threatening problems
disclosed by the primary survey, including endotracheal intubation, the starting of
large-bore intravenous lines, intubation of the stomach and bladder, electrocardiogram, chest and cervical spine films, urinalysis, and drawing of blood for analysis
as well as typing and cross-matching. When this has been completed, the secondary
survey is carried out.

This *secondary survey* begins at the head and moves systematically to the toes
and includes careful examination of soft tissues, bones, joints, and pleural and
visceral cavities. The scalp is inspected and palpated for contusion or laceration,
followed by examination of the tympanic membranes, visual acuity and ocular motion, nasal and oropharyngeal passages, teeth, and facial bones. The carotid and
other pulses, particularly those distal to fracture sites, are palpated. The larynx,
trachea, and soft tissues of the neck are examined for displacement or crepitus,
and function of the chest wall, lungs, and diaphragm is evaluated. Abdominal pain
or tenderness is elicited by gentle palpation. The spine is palpated in its entirety,
as are the pelvis, pubic symphysis, and sacroiliac joints. All long bones and major
joints are examined for stability, tenderness, and pain with active or passive motion.
Peripheral motor and sensory function is evaluated, particularly distal to sites of
potential fracture of dislocation. The rectal examination should record sphincter
tone and the presence or absence of blood.

Examination of the trauma victim should be carried out aggressively to identify
potential injuries and to confirm or exclude them. Injuries that are not thought of
and looked for will be missed. Repeat examinations should be carried out frequently, lest changes in a patient's condition be overlooked, with potentially serious consequences.

SECTION VIII

THE ART AND SCIENCE OF MEDICINE

22. CLINICAL PROBLEM SOLVING
Thomas L. Schwenk
Richard D. Judge

23. USE OF THE
CLINICAL LABORATORY
Faith T. Fitzgerald

24. PRACTICAL POINTS FOR
THE WARDS
Faith T. Fitzgerald

Day and night, thou shall endeavor for the relief of patients with all thy heart and soul. Thou shall not desert or injure thy patient, even for the sake of thy living.

HINDU OATH OF INITIATION INTO THE MEDICAL PROFESSION

CHAPTER 22

CLINICAL PROBLEM SOLVING

Medicine is a science of uncertainty and an art of probability.

Sir William Osler
(1849–1919)

A 38-year-old married male executive is sitting in your office, the first patient on your busy afternoon schedule. The patient's wife is in the waiting room. The man tells you he had an episode of "discomfort" in his chest that morning during a particularly stressful meeting with the owner of his company. The discomfort felt like heavy pressure and lasted about 10 minutes. He had no associated symptoms except that his "stomach felt a little upset." He tells you he is not particularly worried about it now, and, in fact, he would like to get back to work as quickly as possible and only came in because of his wife's worry about how hard he's been working lately. He reports that a friend "a little older than I am" died suddenly from a heart attack, but he's sure his problem is nothing like that. He wants you to tell his wife that there's no problem. What do you do?

The doctor's job is to solve the patient's problems. The main difficulty in doing so is that patients don't bring problems to the doctor. They bring symptoms ("My chest hurts."), worries ("I'm worried that I might have an illness that will keep me from working."), the worries of others ("My wife thinks I might be having a heart attack."), perceptions ("I just don't seem to be as energetic as I used to be."), socioeconomic dilemmas ("My boss doesn't think I can work today because of this pain."), and solutions of their own ("I want a prescription for nitroglycerin because I'm having angina."). The physician's real job is to understand the patient's perceptions of what is needed, collect appropriate data in the form of the history, physical examination, and laboratory testing, and organize these data in a way that explains the patient's difficulties *and* leads to some form of treatment or management.

Some studies of physician's clinical reasoning abilities suggest that they sometimes fail to accomplish this seemingly short list of tasks. They may fail to collect the data they need, to pay attention to its significance, to use their knowledge effectively in making interpretations of the data, or to make a careful consideration of alternative risks and values in the actions they take.

One of the reasons for this less-than-optimal performance is that clinical problem solving is infrequently taught in a systematic fashion. Most of you spend 2 years trying to memorize everything you see and hear and then enter your clinical rotations where you are expected to put it all together. Clinical problem solving is learned more by example and role modeling than by a systematic teaching approach. Clinical teachers have great difficulty in articulating exactly how they solved a particular problem, what specific steps they followed, why they collected the data they collected, and how those data were used in making decisions. For these reasons, the purpose of this chapter is not to teach how to teach clinical problem solving, but to teach you, the student, how to learn it.

BARRIERS TO LEARNING HOW TO SOLVE CLINICAL PROBLEMS

Given your responsibility to learn clinical problem solving, what are some of the barriers to this learning? There are at least four, including:

1. An inappropriate devotion to thoroughness in data collection, rather than thoroughness in hypothesis formation
2. An excessive reliance on the inductive method of scientific research, rather than on the deductive method of decision theory and clinical problem solving
3. The forced use of the deductive method of problem solving at times when more powerful pattern-recognition methods are better
4. A lack of accounting for sociological and psychological influences on problem solving

A hallmark of excellence in practicing medicine is thoroughness. Walsh McDermott, who was an eminent internist and medical educator, has described thoroughness as the most enduring and critical quality of the excellent physician. Unfortunately, as medical research has made an explosive amount of biomedical data available to physicians, thoroughness has been defined in terms of data collection, rather than in terms of early and aggressive development of competing sets of hypotheses or possible diagnoses. Many educators have noted that medical education emphasizes a routine and uncritical approach to data collection. Rather than being encouraged to generate early and appropriate hypotheses, you are often warned "not to jump to conclusions," because "more mistakes result from lack of thoroughness than from lack of knowledge." While these dicta are correct in their proper context, they may be misinterpreted by you as encouraging passive (and massive) data collection. Many studies on the learning of problem-solving skills have shown that thoroughness of data gathering was uncorrelated with obtaining the correct diagnosis.

For example, Howard Barrows and his colleagues* found that (a) on the average, even experienced physicians collected only about two-thirds of the available significant data, (b) they obtained most of that information within the first 10 minutes of the interview, and (c) the interview could have been stopped after 10 minutes with no adverse effect on the accuracy of the physician's diagnostic interpretations. This work, and that of other researchers, suggests that medical schools can facilitate and enhance the learning of clinical problem solving only if medical school teachers are willing to abandon their advocacy of thorough, unguided data collection. Data collection must be absolutely accurate, yet selective, while hypothesis formation must be thorough. This is the fundamental difference between the inductive and deductive methods of problem solving.

Abraham Flexner conducted a major study of the process of medical education in the early 1900s. His name is linked with a major connection between medical education and biomedical research. This connection is often an advantage, especially with regard to the development of powerful diagnostic and therapeutic tech-

---

*See Barrows, H.S., and Tamblyn, R.M. *Problem-Based Learning: An Approach to Medical Education.* New York: Springer, 1980.

nologies that have conquered many previously frightening medical problems. The linkage of research to education has, however, resulted in the transfer of inappropriate problem-solving methods from research to the practice of medicine. Clinical medicine, as are other applied sciences, is basically deductive in nature, whereas research is mostly an inductive science.

Inductive reasoning is based on the technique of fitting large masses of data, collected in an uncritical and comprehensive manner, to a variety of possible hypotheses. Inductive problem-solving requires nearly unlimited data collection—the more the better. From this mass of unorganized data spring, almost magically, certain hypotheses or generalizations that require yet more data for proof. Deduction works in just an opposite fashion. The problem solver accepts certain generalizations as true early in the thinking process and attempts to apply them to a specific patient problem from the moment of collecting even the first piece of data.

Inductive hypothesis testing is open-ended and can lead to unbounded testing. Deductive reasoning, on the other hand, is more parsimonious in its approach, because it is knowledge-driven. Each piece of data suggests a set of hypotheses, and a limited data set is relatively thorough in hypothesis formation. Early hypothesis formation guides future data collection in a less all-encompassing fashion. Physicians can seek only data that directly prove or disprove the limited set of diagnoses. Deduction is more explicit, whereas induction is more intuitive. Deduction is the skill of reasoning from general rules to specific diagnoses, which is the purpose of clinical medicine. Having said this, we must also suggest that the deductive method is still not the most powerful method of problem solving, although it is a good way to begin and a good way to learn more powerful problem-solving abilities.

Despite the enthusiasm for the "generate and test" method of solving problems, considerable research suggests it is still a weak method of solving problems. Weak methods are based on a generic set of cognitive steps that may work in almost any situation but likely trade away efficiency and power for their generic applicability. For instance, a basic deductive method applied to a gynecologic problem may also work in cardiology, but is likely not the way that physicians experienced in each field solve their respective problems. Strong methods are dependent on a highly organized, yet illogical, collection of knowledge and experience that experienced physicians apply to problems in a pattern-recognition scheme. These methods almost always yield the right answer, but are only utilized by experienced physicians with highly organized sets of huge amounts of experience.

Your goal, then, is to make every patient and teacher meeting into a problem-solving exercise, so that as much information and experience as possible becomes organized into your long-term memory in a way that is useful for future applications. We know that expert knowledge in medicine, as in any profession, is very complex. The generation of appropriate diagnoses early in the patient encounter may result from a pattern-recognition process that draws on past experiences in memory, which are in turn a product of extensive experience with patients in addition to formal education.

As if the learning of complex biomedical problem-solving skills were not difficult enough, complex interpersonal and sociological issues play an important role. Actual clinical decisions are influenced by interactions between the doctor, the patient, and the sociocultural environment. Characteristics of the patient, characteristics of the physician, and characteristics of the physician-patient interaction all play an important role in decision making. By their very nature, these characteristics make teaching the decision-making process extremely difficult. For example, social class is known to be directly related to the frequency with which certain surgical procedures, such as appendectomies and tonsillectomies are performed. There is no known alternative to explain why patients of higher social class experience higher rates of such operations.

The patient's mere physical appearance has a strong effect on decision making. We know that obese patients are judged by medical students to be more nervous, less competent, and less well educated than patients of normal weight. How can you account for these factors in your own solving of clinical problems? As many as 20 percent of all hospital admissions may be made on the basis of sociological, rather than biomedical, reasons. What is there about these patients that caused their doctors to admit them to the hospital? Several types of patients have been shown to be perceived as "undesirable" by physicians, including those that are old, dirty, uneducated, poor, of a minority race or religion, ungrateful or obnoxious, or who cause inconvenience to the physician. How can you account for these factors as you try to solve the problems of patients with these characteristics?

SPECIFIC GUIDELINES FOR DEVELOPING CLINICAL PROBLEM–SOLVING SKILLS

The solution of patient problems is, in certain regards, deceptively simple. All that is required is accurate and selective information about the patient (a data base), an understanding of the characteristics of disease and illness (an information base), and a method of comparing the first to the second that yields a diagnosis and corresponding treatment. There are perhaps dozens of "methods" of solving clinical problems, but the problem-solving procedure used by experienced physicians usually includes all or part of the following scheme*:

1. Aggregation of groups of findings into patterns
2. Selection of a key finding
3. Generation of a list of causes based on the key finding
4. Pruning of the list according to selected pieces of diagnostic data
5. Selection of a diagnosis
6. Validation of the diagnosis through further selected testing

We will now provide you with some guidance about how to apply this method of clinical problem solving and how to move as rapidly as possible to strong, sophisticated methods of problem solving that make use of an expanding information base of experiences and knowledge arranged in a useful fashion. The following six

*See Eddy, D.M., and Clanton, C.H. The art of diagnosis: Solving the clinicopathologic exercise. *N. Engl. J. Med.* 306: 1263–1268, 1982.

guidelines are helpful both for solving problems and for learning how to solve clinical problems:

1. Form hypotheses early in the diagnostic process.
2. Develop a personal epidemiology of clinical experience, focusing on problems that are common, treatable, and/or serious.
3. Use decision theory for clinical problems that are more complex and less clear.
4. Use computers as an adjunct to clinical problem solving.
5. Account for sociological and psychological influences in all problem solving.
6. Avoid making errors that are expected and predictable.

Form hypotheses early in the diagnostic process. You may be taking a big chance at times when you form hypotheses early and offer these to your instructors. You may ask, "How can I form hypotheses early, before adequate training?" Perhaps you are in a sort of Catch-22, in which you cannot solve problems until hypotheses are developed, but cannot learn to develop hypotheses until some problems have been solved successfully. Yet, many studies show that, when asked to do so, most of you could advance reasonable diagnostic hypotheses even before receiving any formal training in clinical medicine. The improvement in diagnostic accuracy as you progress in your medical training is not due to the evolution of problem-solving strategies but to increased thoroughness and generation of more appropriate initial diagnostic hypotheses.

Hypotheses that are generated early are sorted and discarded according to a variety of strategies. The degree to which hypotheses suggest diseases that are common, treatable (or curable or manageable), or serious has an important role in determining which ones will be pursued. However, thinking of the particular illness, disease, syndrome, condition, or explanation in the most critical first step. Having a "high index of suspicion" is a paramount characteristic of an excellent problem solver.

Develop a personal epidemiology of clinical experience, focusing on problems that are common, treatable, and/or serious. Ultimately, only problems having at least one of these three characteristics is worth diagnosing. A problem with all three is worthy of major diagnostic efforts. Large patient populations have only one distribution of diseases, but each subgroup of patients, cared for by one physician, has a different distribution. Your job is to learn as much about that subgroup as possible, because the epidemiologic characteristics will strongly influence your accuracy of problem solving. Common maxims of problem solving require a complete understanding of the types of diseases to be found in a particular group of patients.

1. "Common diseases occur commonly." This may seem obvious but requires constant reminder. Clichés are still true, and "when you hear hoofbeats, you should think of horses, not zebras," no matter how experienced you are.
2. "Uncommon manifestations of common diseases are more common than common manifestations of uncommon diseases." This aphorism is really a function of Bayesian logic, in which the prevalence of a disease in a patient population

has a nearly overpowering influence on its importance in clinical problem solving.

3. "No disease is rare to the patient who has it." After a physician has carefully considered the more common diagnostic possibilities, a "high index of suspicion" is still required to consider diagnoses that are less common, but only if more common diseases do not fit the clues and data base.

The critical factor in developing and using strong methods of problem solving is the accumulation of a set of useful clues: key findings, pivotal clues, diagnostic clusters, and syndromes. Those found to be useful may vary from one physician to the next, again dependent on the physician's personal epidemiology, but a collection is essential. Some diagnoses are dependent on only one look—at a skin rash, for example. If a physician looks and does not know the diagnosis, all the history taking and physical examination in the world may not help. On the other hand, some clues only narrow the field (e.g., pain in the costovertebral angle or cloudy discharge from the nipple), and further exploration of a narrowed field of possibilities is required. Some clues are better at narrowing the field than others. Learning about nonspecific symptoms such as fatigue, dizziness, or nausea helps nearly not at all, because each of these has literally hundreds of causes. Amenorrhea, on the other hand, points to a fairly selective differential diagnosis.

Sometimes a small cluster of clues is almost diagnostic of one disease. For example, the combination of fever, a heart murmur, and evidence of multiple needle punctures on the skin is highly suggestive of infective endocarditis. On the other hand, the patient could be a medical student on a plasmapheresis donor program who has always had a benign murmur and now has influenza. Which is more likely? It depends on your particular patient population. Clues quite often come in triads, tetrads, and other small clusters. They are almost always worth remembering.

When small clusters of clues build up to become large clusters of clues, you have moved into a strong method of solving complex problems: pattern recognition. This simply means that physicians can recognize the diseases of some patients, no matter how complex, because they remember past experiences, compare them to the current patient, and seek a match. A complex case has dozens, perhaps hundreds, of features and no one feature is diagnostic. The pattern, however, is diagnostic or at least strongly suggests a diagnosis that can be proved or refuted with only a few maneuvers or further pieces of data. The clinicopathologic cases in the *New England Journal of Medicine* are examples of this method of problem solving.

These patterns and syndromes cannot be memorized from a book or lecture, but only learned from working with patients. Thus, we again emphasize that clinical problem solving can be learned, but not taught. You are responsible for studying each patient as carefully as possible and for making use of the experience through aggressive questioning and active learning. Here are a number of questions that you should ask of yourself as patients are seen, or if you are lucky, they will be asked by your instructor. These questions are all open-ended and divergent. They require that you clarify, support, defend, justify, correlate, critique, evaluate, analyze, interpret, or predict. Answering questions that require only one or a few words does little to promote problem-solving skills.

Based on the history just presented, what physical examination findings will be particularly important to note?

If a historical, physical, or lab finding were present (absent) instead of being absent (present), how would it change my thinking?

Based on this history and physical examination, what further lab tests would you recommend?

What would you do if the lab test were unavailable?

Can you justify the cost of the lab test, both in dollars and in risk to the patient?

Explain the pathophysiology of the abnormal finding just presented.

What did you expect to learn from asking that specific question?

How does the information just provided change the most likely diagnosis (hypothesis)?

What are the most likely diagnoses (hypotheses)?

What are the most serious or emergent diagnoses?

What diagnoses are most treatable?

What pieces of information tend to support your best hypothesis?

What pieces of information tend to detract from your best hypothesis?

Can you build a case to support an alternative hypothesis?

Use decision theory for patient problems that are more complex and less clear. Some problems do not lend themselves to being solved by pattern recognition, either because the problem is too complex or vague, or because the physician is inexperienced with this particular problem. Decision theory can be relied upon to help out, albeit in a somewhat tedious and cumbersome fashion at times. This method requires the construction of an elaborate branching diagram, the branching points of which represent decisions to be made, based on the likelihood that a particular outcome or next step will occur, and the degree to which finding that outcome to be true would be useful (i.e., treatable, pointing to a sure diagnosis, suggesting a management plan). For example, if a patient presents with chest pain, the possibilities are many and the potential seriousness quite great. The character of the pain (location, radiation, associated symptoms) suggests myocardial ischemia as a possible diagnosis. In a 55-year-old man who smokes, this diagnosis is quite likely. In a 25-year-old woman, it is far less so—in fact, nearly impossible. This first decision point will lead to very different diagnostic strategies, depending on assigning specific probabilities to an outcome with the same potential seriousness.

Successful use of decision analysis depends heavily on accumulating a large reservoir of bayesian probabilities (the probability that a patient has a particular disease, given the presence of a set of particular symptoms and signs). It is much more important, to both you and your patient, for you to know the possible causes of an effect, rather than to know the possible effects of a cause. Beyond this, it is useful to know the relative likelihoods and consequences of each "cause of an effect," so as to move through a decision tree with efficiency and effectiveness. These decision trees can take on the appearance of flow charts and algorithms in retrospect, but only for simple problems with few decision points. Decision analysis is better applied to complex cases with many possible decision points and dozens of possible outcomes ranging in importance from trivial to castastrophic. While cumbersome, it may be the only successful method to be used in such cases.

Learn to use computers as an adjunct to problem solving and as an adjunct to learning how to solve problems. Computers are most helpful in learning how to solve clinical problems, because they provide a convenient, reproducible, cheap, and safe method for practicing problem solving. Since problem solving is a skill, like tennis, that requires constant and never-ending practice, we recommend computers as an aid to that practice. Computers are, at this time, less useful for actually solving real patient problems, probably because the complexity of solving medical problems has yet to be accurately described to the necessary degree of completeness. Considerable work is in progress in this area, however, and future developments and possibilities are exciting.

Several promising systems are in use or in development. Examples (and the types of clinical problems which they address) include: MYCIN (meningitis), PUFF and CENTAUR (interpretation of pulmonary function tests), AI/RHEUM (rheumatology), CASNET (glaucoma), ONCOCIN (chemotherapy protocols for cancer), PIP (edema), KMS.HT (dizziness), ABEL (electrolyte abnormalities), and CADUCEUS (general internal medicine).

Recognize and account for sociological influences on clinical problem solving. Despite our interest in making clinical problem solving as "objective" as possible, it never has been and never will be. The care of patients is an intensely personal and interpersonal process. Clinical problem solving becomes more accurate, more reliable, and more understandable when the physician acknowledges the intensely personal nature of solving patient problems, rather than by denying its importance or existence.

You can learn to understand the psychosociological influences on your medical decision making by asking yourself the following questions as you grapple with patient problems:

What am I feeling right now about this patient?

What is there about this patient, and what is he/she doing or saying, that causes me to feel this way?

What is there about my past experiences or attitudes that causes me to feel this way?

Can I accept these feelings as valid and real so that I can learn how to cope with them?

In what ways can I be more helpful and comforting to the patient?

Do I have to like the patient before I can be more helpful to him/her?

What can I say to this patient whose medical situation makes me feel sad, angry, helpless, or hopeless?

What further help for me and the patient might be available from other professionals?

Am I able to continue caring for this patient?

There are several predictable errors made in clinical problem solving. Try to avoid them. Research in cognitive psychology has identified a number of errors made by physicians trying to solve patient problems. These errors are inherent in any attempt to process large amounts of complex data, but awareness of their existence has considerable preventive value. Here are several types of errors that can reasonably be anticipated and, hopefully, avoided:

An inappropriate bias toward positive and confirmatory evidence

An inappropriate bias towards favoring data collected early in the contact with the patient

Anecdotal, rather than probabilistic, thinking, such that personal experiences with one patient are more influential than the experience of others with thousands

Gambler's fallacy, in which past random events have an undue influence on the prediction of future events ("the coin came up 'heads' the last five times, so it has to be 'tails' this time")

Pseudodiagnosticity, in which irrelevant data are collected

Premature closure, in which hypothesis formation is stopped before all reasonable possibilities are considered

Anchoring, in which the physician clings to a diagnosis, despite the appearance of contradictory evidence

You will be interested to learn that the last two errors, premature closure and anchoring, are at least as prevalent in experienced physicians as in novices.

Clinical problem solving is an incredibly complex activity that is the core of the physician's professional role. The mental processes by which physicians process large quantities of ill-defined and complex data are not fully understood, but most physicians do, in fact, accurately and rapidly make hundreds of medical decisions daily. This discrepancy between what we know about problem-solving skills and what we actually do suggests that clinical problem solving may be a skill that can be learned but not directly taught. The responsibility for learning clinical problem-solving lies with you, the student, who must make the most out of every patient you meet. This inquisitive, reflective approach to critical thinking is a paramount behavior throughout the lifetime of the successful practicing physician. In the process of learning, you will pass through several phases, from the early struggles of understanding large amounts of confusing data whose significance is unclear, to a more precise ability to use decision analysis to sort through consequences of varying probability and value, and finally to the point where complex problems are solved almost magically with speed, accuracy, and parsimony of data collection. The diligence with which this difficult progression is approached has considerable ability to predict your eventual success as a physician.

CHAPTER 23

USE OF THE CLINICAL LABORATORY

The advent of multichannel automated screening of blood samples, newer nuclear diagnostic techniques, the technological revolution of computed tomography, and magnetic resonance imaging, and the availability of sophisticated endoscopy have all broadened the range of vision of today's diagnostician. We can now ask questions about the status of our patients that not long ago could be answered only on the operating or autopsy table.

But the armamentarium of modern laboratory techniques is a very mixed blessing. There are dangers in every procedure. It is essential that you have an understanding of the "therapeutic ratio"—that is, the risk involved in the test compared to the potential gain to the patient—of each laboratory or other study you consider ordering. Ask the following questions of each test:

1. Why am I getting this test? The best clinicians are directed in their use of the laboratory by carefully thought-out reasoning that underlies everything they do. One may order a glucose test on a patient because he or she has polyuria and a family history of diabetes. Or one may want a thyroid function test on a woman with cold intolerance, constipation, and decreased mentation. To order tests "just to be complete" is more comforting to the doctor than it is to the patient; but it is the patient who pays for them, and that payment may be more than monetary. For example, if a man has a uric acid level drawn as part of a "routine screening," though he is without complaints suggestive of gout or kidney stones, it is entirely possible that the uric acid test will come back showing a level somewhat over the normal. Now what? Generally the doctor feels compelled to draw another one, "just to check it out." What if this one is just at the upper level of normal? The doctor can draw a third level and average them (this is a very common sequence of events, by the way). Suppose the third level also comes back from the laboratory marginally high. Is an abnormal uric acid level a disease? If so, we have just discovered a disease in a previously healthy man. Should it be treated? Drugs may have complications associated with their administration. What if the doctor in this case gives a drug for the high uric acid, and the patient has an allergic reaction to it? What good has the doctor done the patient? The patient, previously well, has paid for three uric acid tests and for the drug he was prescribed, and has suffered the complications of that drug.

But suppose the routine screening does show a significant abnormality—for example, a very low hematocrit that can be corrected. It is a well-known event on the ward that a test result comes from the laboratory and, on returning to the bedside, the patient now gives a history and has physical findings fully supportive of the abnormality "discovered" in the lab. The anemic patient mentioned above, on direct requestioning, admits to extra heavy menstrual periods. All this means is that

585

the initially taken history and physical examination were incomplete. It is axiomatic that the best clinicians are rarely surprised by any laboratory test. They take pride in knowing that the laboratory usually confirms their clinical impression rather than creates it. The laboratory test has become, in modern hospital practice, the anonymous critic of our clinical acumen.

2. Is this test necessary? Probably the best way to assay whether or not the study under consideration is important for the best care of your patient is to ask yourself "How would I approach this patient differently if the test were positive? Negative? Equivocal?" If your diagnostic or therapeutic approach would *not* be significantly altered by the test, it is probably as well not to do it. In an elderly woman with disseminated terminal cancer, there is evidence of progressive renal failure. Should you get an intravenous pyelogram to evaluate it? Since she is dying and kept comfortable by appropriate analgesics, there is little reason to do the x-ray: It would be of no added benefit to her. Ask yourself, on each occasion, if any study you may want to do is designed to help the patient feel better or if you are treating *your own insecurity* by doing it.

3. Is this test reliable? There is a considerable amount of "faddism" in medicine. A new test or procedure appears on the horizon, and the published reports are very positive about its sensitivity (ability to detect an abnormality if it is present) and specificity (ability to fail to detect an abnormality if it is not present). It is well to keep in mind that authors seldom publish negative initial results, so that most early reports on any test will tend to be enthusiastic about it. Each physician must learn the inherent fallibility of each test or procedure in his or her own hospital. Even if a certain scan, for example, is marvelous at detecting hidden abscess at one medical center, the same technique in the hands of less practiced individuals at another medical center may be far less reliable.

Although it is difficult for students and house officers to accept, their own clinical judgment is often superior in accuracy to any laboratory test. This is true if only because the individuals caring for the patient have much more information about that patient in his or her entirety than the laboratory physician or technician, who has only a serum sample or a single organ scan. For example, a 38-year-old man presented to his physician with crescendo angina. Because of a normal ECG, he was allowed to go home. Within the next 12 hours he had a massive myocardial infarction and is now crippled by a ventricular aneurysm. One wonders, in this real case, whether the doctor—whose initial impulse was to hospitalize the patient—may not have been falsely reassured by the lack of ECG abnormality. In this instance the test probably delayed proper therapy. So if a test result runs counter to your best judgment, and you have carefully scrutinized all data available to you, trust your judgment.

4. How much does this test cost? Even if you decide that a given test is necessary, reliable, and likely to be helpful, you are obliged to consider it in terms of hard cash. Health insurance covers many laboratory procedures, but it does not pay for them all. And nothing, even health insurance, is free. It costs somebody—usually your patient—in higher premiums. Ask yourself, as you consider ordering a test, whether you personally would be willing to pay for it out of your own pocket. Indeed, as a taxpayer at times you *will* be paying for it out of your own pocket! Keep abreast of the costs of a variety of common diagnostic tests done in your own hospital. It frequently proves astonishing to students to discover that the scan they ordered "for interest" or "for teaching purposes" has a fee of $500 attached to it.

But there is another cost attached to the indiscriminate use of the laboratory. It is not uncommon for students to turn to the laboratory to answer questions for them that they had not been able to answer by their own wits. Such students slavishly take their direction from the printed laboratory result sheet, rather than directing the laboratory to specific questions. The cost to these students, and thus to the physicians they will become, is enormous. If you need a chest x-ray to diagnose lobar pneumonia, an ECG to tell you that your patient has had a myocardial infarction, or a panel of liver function tests to turn your attention to the gallbladder, you have become an extension of the laboratory rather than the other way around.

CHAPTER 24

PRACTICAL POINTS
FOR THE WARDS

Experience is the mother of science.
PROVERB

HISTORY AND PHYSICAL—EXAMPLE OF THE WRITE-UP

TRADITIONAL WRITE-UP

HISTORY AND PHYSICAL EXAMINATION

Mrs. Jane Doe
Registration #12345
432 Maple Avenue
Babylon, California
Tel #(123)-456-7899

August 31, 1989
2:00 P.M.

CHIEF COMPLAINT
This 45-year-old married mother of two has had episodic right upper quadrant "knife-like" pain for the past 2 days.

HISTORY OF PRESENT ILLNESS
Mrs. Doe was in her usual good state of health until 2 days ago (August 29) when, having just finished a pork chop dinner, she had severe "knifelike" pain in the right upper quadrant of her abdomen, radiating to her epigastrium. She concurrently felt "sick to her stomach" (without vomiting), "sweaty," and faint (without loss of consciousness). She immediately lay down on her bed and felt better "after a minute." The severe pain grew rapidly less, as did the nausea, but she had a "dull ache" in her right upper quadrant for several hours. She took no medication. Position did not affect the pain. She felt well enough after an hour to clean up the dinner table, and slept well that night. She has had two subsequent almost identical "attacks," the first at lunch yesterday (August 30) following a hamburger and french fries. The most recent episode was at breakfast today after two slices of bacon.

   She's had no fever, chills, vomiting, or diarrhea. She denies past history of similar episodes. She has no current or past history of jaundice, white stools, dark urine, or change in bowel habits. She is unaware of a history of anemia (other than a mild "low blood" associated with her first pregnancy). She has not had tarry or black stools, hematemesis, burning abdominal pain or other "indigestion," kidney stones, polyuria or hematuria, hepatitis, or foreign travel. She has had no cough, shortness of breath, or pleurisy. She has no calf pain. She regularly examines her breasts and has noted no masses. There is a history of breast cancer in her mother. She has no known heart disease. She denies trauma to her chest, back, or legs. Her menses have been normal. She takes no regular medications and specifically denies the use of antacids, aspirin, clofibrate (Atromid), or alcohol.

She currently feels quite well.

PAST MEDICAL HISTORY

Childhood illness: Mumps and chickenpox as child. No measles, rheumatic fever, scarlet fever.

Adult illness: None significant. Hospitalized only for childbirth (Soma Hospital, Babylon—1968 and 1970).

Trauma: Fractured left clavicle as child. No sequelae.

Surgery: Tonsillectomy as child of 6 (Soma Hospital). Episiotomy with each childbirth.

Allergies: Penicillin—urticarial rash without wheezing, stridor, (last dose 1976, at which time reaction occurred).

Medications: None at present. Has taken occasional aspirin for headache in past.

Travel: Never outside California.

Habits: Has never smoked tobacco or cannabis. Occasional dinner wine (none in past 2 weeks). No illicit drugs. Regular diet, 3 meals a day.

Immunizations: Does not remember childhood shots other than oral polio vaccine in early 1950s. Last tetanus shot 7 years ago.

FAMILY HISTORY

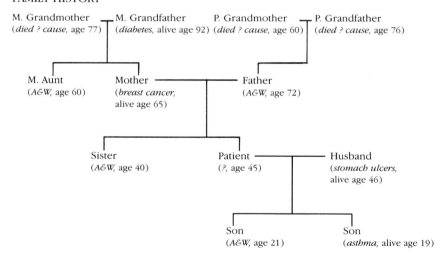

No family history of renal disease, liver disease, hypertension, anemia, tuberculosis.

SOCIAL HISTORY

Mrs. Doe was born and raised in Babylon, where she married her current husband after her graduation from high school in 1962. She worked as a secretary in his construction firm until their first child was born in 1968. She remained at home to raise her two sons, both of whom are college students (majoring in art and mathematics, respectively), and has recently returned to night school to gain college credits herself.

She describes her life as full and her marriage as happy. Activities include housekeeping, gardening, and reading "romantic novels." Her husband's medical coverage extends to her, and she is not worried about money. She does admit to some unhappiness at not having gone to college as a young woman, but "is making up for it now." She is worried that her pain may represent an illness that will interfere with her studies, and she has "a test coming up next week." She is also fearful of cancer, as her mother has metastatic cancer of the breast, which is painful and emotionally draining on Mrs. Doe, who visits her in a nursing home every day.

REVIEW OF SYSTEMS

General: See HPI. No weight change.

Head: Occasional "stress" headache. No dizziness. "Faintness" with her recent attacks as described in HPI.

Eyes: Last tested 1 year ago at 20/20. No blurring, double vision, pain, discharge.

Ears: No decreased hearing, tinnitus, pain. Otitis media once as a child (R ear).

Nose: No epistaxis, sinusitis.

Throat and mouth: Teeth in good repair. Infrequent sore throats.

Chest: See HPI. No wheezing, hemoptysis, sputum. Chest x-ray normal on screening exam 1 year ago. Negative TB skin test 1 year ago.

Heart: No pain, palpitations, orthopnea, cyanosis, edema. No history hypertension.

GI: See HPI.

GU: See HPI. No dysuria, frequency, urgency, incontinence. No history venereal disease or urinary tract infection.

Menstrual: Menarche age 13. Periods light flow for 3 days every 28 days and regular, with slight cramping on 1st day of flow. Last period normal, ended August 19, G2P2A0.

Neuromuscular: Faintness as in HPI, without syncope. No vertigo, dysesthesias, seizures. No history emotional disease.

PHYSICAL EXAMINATION

August 31, 1989
2:30 P.M.

General: Mrs. Doe is a slightly obese, pleasant, 45-year-old white woman who is somewhat anxious but in no acute distress.

Vital Signs: BP R arm Sitting: <u>140/90</u>   P85 regular R 12

           L arm sitting: <u>148/92</u>

                        T 99° F orally

           L arm standing: <u>155/95</u>

              Height: 5'6"   Weight: 152 lb

Skin: Warm and dry. No petechiae, purpura, excoriations. Anicteric. Hair and nails normal. No cutaneous lesions or rashes.

Nodes: No cervical, supraclavicular, epitrochlear lymphadenopathy: <u>1 × 1 cm, soft, nontender, mobile node R axilla. Scattered shotty inguinal nodes bilaterally.</u>

Head: Normocephalic, without trauma. No scars, tenderness, bruits.

Eyes: Conjunctivae normal. Slight scleral icterus bilaterally. Lids without lesions. Pupils equal, round, and react to light and accommodation. Vision grossly normal (reads newspaper). Visual fields full to confrontation. Extraocular motions full, without strabismus or nystagmus. Fundus shows normal discs and vasculature. No arterio-venous nicking, silver-wiring, hemorrhage, or exudate.

Ears: External ears normal. Tympanic membranes normal bilaterally. Weber midline. Air conduction greater than bone bilaterally.

Nose: Nasal mucosa normal, without inflammation, obstruction, or polyps.

Mouth: Lips, buccal muscosa without lesions. Tongue well papillated, pink, midline. Teeth in good repair. Uvula midline. Oropharynx without inflammation or lesions.

Neck: Supple. Trachea midline. Thyroid not enlarged and without nodules. Jugular veins flat. Venous pulses normal. Carotids 4+ without bruits, normal pulse contour bilaterally.

Chest and lungs: Chest wall contour normal, with symmetrical full expansion. No rib tenderness to palpation. Tactile fremitus normal. Diaphragmatic excursion 5 cm bilaterally. No percussion dullness. Lungs are clear to auscultation save for an isolated musical wheeze on forced expiration at the right base posteriorly. There is no egophony over this area. No rubs heard.

Heart: No visible lifts, PMI palpable 8 cm from the L sternal border in the 6th intercostal space, tapping in quality. No palpable thrills, lifts, heaves. Rhythm regular, rate 80. S_1 normal, S_2 physiologically split. There is no S_3, but a soft S_4 at the apex. There is a ⅔ systolic ejection murmur at the L sternal border, without radiation. No rubs, no diastolic murmurs.

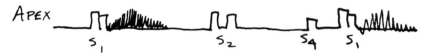

Breasts: R breast slightly larger than L. No retractions, visible dimpling or skin changes. Nipples normal, everted. 2 × 2 cm cystic, mobile, nontender mass without skin fixation in upper outer quadrant R breast. No nipple discharge.

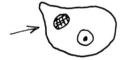

Abdomen: Slightly protuberant. No scars or visible masses. Venous pattern normal. Bowel sounds normal. No hepatic or splenic rubs. No bruits. Liver is 15 cm to percussion, and is 3 cm below the right costal margin. Liver edge is smooth and tender to palpation, with positive Murphy's sign. No epigastric tenderness. Spleen and kidneys not palpable. No shifting dullness or fluid wave. No hernia.

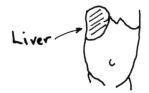

Pelvic and rectal: External genitalia normal, including Bartholin's and Skeine's glands. Vaginal vault without lesions or discharge.

Cervix parous, without lesions or discharge. Pap smear taken.

Bimanual: Fundus normal in size & position. No tenderness. Ovaries and broad ligament felt and are without masses or tenderness.

Rectovaginal: Confirms bimanual

Rectum: No anal lesions. Sphincter tube normal. No ampullary masses. Stool is <u>clay-colored</u> and negative for occult blood.

Extremities: Pulses full and symmetrical, without bruits. Skin and hair normal on extremities.

Pulses:

		Carotid	Supra-clavicular	Radial	Brachial	Aorta	Fem-oral	DP	PT
4+ = NL	R	4+	3+	4+	4+	0	4+	4+	4+
	L	4+	3+	4+	4+	0	4+	4+	4+

No clubbing, cyanosis, or edema. No swelling, redness, tenderness, limitation of movement of joints. No visible varicosities. No calf tenderness or cords. Muscle mass normal bilaterally.

Back: Slight cervical kyphosis. No spinal tenderness, CVA tenderness, or sacral edema. Full range of motion spine.

Neurologic:

Mental status: Alert, oriented. Memory, judgment, mood normal.

Cranial nerves: I—Not tested.
                       II—Pupils react to light. Reads newspaper.
                  III, IV, VI—No strabismus. EOM normal.
                       V—Corneal reflex intact.
                       VII—Face symmetrical.
                       VIII—Hearing normal.
                  IX,X—Uvula elevates symmetrically. Gag normal bilaterally.
                       XI—Trapezius, sternomastoid normal.
                       XII—Tongue protrudes midline.

Cerebellar: Gait, finger-nose, and heel-shin normal.

Station and gait: Romberg negative. Heel-toe walk normal.

Motor: Muscle mass normal. Good strength in arms, legs.
        Deep tendon reflexes: 2+ = Nl
        No pathologic reflexes.

Sensory: Normal to touch, pinprick, vibration.

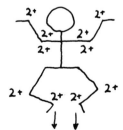

LABORATORY FINDINGS

Hemogram: Hgb 14.2, Hct 45%, WBC 8500, Polys 65, Bands 5, Monos 10, Lymphs 19, Eos 1, Baso 0.

Peripheral smear: Normocytic, normochromic RBCs. No fragments, targets, nucleated RBC. WBC morphology normal. Platelets abundant on smear.

Urine: Clear, dark yellow. SG 1015. *Dipstix* neg. heme, protein, glucose, ketones. 3 + for bilirubin. pH = 6. *Micro:* 0–1 WBC, 0 RBC, no organisms per high-power field. No crystals, casts.

Serologies:

Electrolytes: Na = 140, K = 4.2, Cl = 100, CO_2 = 28, Ca = 10, P = 3,4, Albumin = 4.0, Glob = 3.5, SGOT = 123, SGPT = 85, Alk P'tase = 210. Bili: total = 4.0, direct = 3.5. Amylase serum = 236, Gl = 123, Cr = 1.0, BUN = 10.

Chest x-ray: Bones normal, without blastic or lytic lesions. Heart shows slight straightening L heart border. Parenchyma clear except for slight linear atelectasis R base posteriorly (R lower lobe, basal seg.). No evident effusion.

KUB: Bones normal. Psoas shadows seen. Nephrograms show normal-size kidneys. Bowel gas normal. No evident ascites. Speckled calcification medial RUQ in area gallbladder.

ECG: Rate = 80, rhythm = sinus, PR = .15, QRS = .10, QT = .32, axis = +30. P waves normal. QRS normal. No T wave flattening or ST segment abnormalities. No LVH by voltage. Impression—normal ECG.

IMPRESSIONS

1. RUQ pain

   a. Probable cholecystitis with cholelithiasis. This is supported by the historical relationship of RUQ sharp pains associated with fatty foods, scleral icterus, hepatomegaly, and + Murphy's sign, clay-colored stools, and laboratory findings of bilirubinuria, abnormal liver function studies with an obstructive pattern, hyperamylasemia, and calcifications on KUB that might represent gallstones. The RLL atelectasis on chest film is not inconsistent with an intra-abdominal process.

     (1) R/O carcinomatosis of the liver. With her family history of breast cancer and the breast mass and axillary node on physical examination, this diagnosis must be considered. The episodicity of her pain, the lack of nodularity of the liver, and the absence of evident disease elsewhere makes this less likely.

     (2) R/O pulmonary embolism. Though unlikely, the RLL wheeze on P.E. and atelectasis on chest film could represent the site of lodgment of pulmonary embolism from the legs (for which there is no local evidence of phlebitis) or peripelvic (she has had 2 children) areas. The liver disease in this circumstance would represent congestive hepatopathy from transient R heart failure of pulmonary embolism.

     (3) R/O myocardial infarction or ischemia. This is very improbable with her history, but should be considered in light of her recent stress in classes and the association of her pain with eating. Her hypertension, though mild, could predispose her. In this circumstance, her liver disease would be transient congestive hepatopathy.

2. R breast mass and axillary node with FH cancer of the breast

   Although the cystic lesion of the breast probably does not represent a malignancy, her FH and deep concern are troublesome.

3. Hypertension

   Although this might be due to anxiety, the presence of the S_4 and the straightening of the L heart border on chest film suggests a fixed hypertension rather than a labile one.

4. Allergy to penicillin

   Her urticarial response could presage anaphylaxis.

5. Systolic heart murmur
   This is probably a flow murmur.

   Although other diagnoses are possible (infective pneumonia, pancreatitis, infective or toxic hepatitis), there is little to support them in the history or physical examination.

PLAN
1. RUQ pain
   Plan: I will hospitalize her today and obtain an ECHO of her gallbladder and biliary tree, as the most immediately available and least invasive of studies.
      I will ask the surgeon to see her today, should another attack require emergency surgical intervention.
      Serial physical examination, urine, bilirubin testing, and serum liver function tests will allow monitoring of her progress.
2. R breast mass and axillary node with FH cancer of the breast
   Plan: Mammography and probably biopsy of the mass are in order.
      These can be done on this hospitalization.
3. Hypertension
   Plan: I will monitor her pressures in hospital. Should they remain elevated, salt restriction, weight loss, and probably diuretic therapy will be instituted.
4. Allergy to penicillin
   Plan: I will instruct the nurses to flag her chart as allergic to penicillin. On discharge, Mrs. Doe should obtain a Medic-Alert to the effect that she is allergic to this drug.
5. Systolic heart murmur
   Plan: Observe

J.H.Galen MD

I. H. Galen, M.D.

The history and physical examination detailed above are a *full and formal,* written H and P. Other situations (emergency visits, pregnancies, readmissions to hospital, etc.) will demand less broad detail, or other emphases. How "long" a written history and physical "needs to be" (a frequent question asked by students) depends on a judicious balance of the patient's need and the clinician's time available. In all cases, the written history and physical examination *needs to be* as long as is necessary to convey pertinent data clearly and completely. Moreover, as in other fields of science, the clinician need not *say* (or write) everything he knows—but he should *know* everything he says.

STANDARD ORDERS
GENERAL
1. Follow a systematic sequence (see below) to ensure completeness.
2. Write legibly. A misinterpreted word or drug may harm your patient.
3. Be sure to review your orders frequently and to specifically cancel the old order before a new one is entered.

4. Consider prn orders as generally undesirable but occasionally necessary. Be certain to review prn orders regularly (every other day).

5. Do not order things that your patients do not need (e.g., sleeping pills should not be routine).

6. Record date, time, and legibly sign *all* orders. If an order is immediate or important, discuss it with the responsible nurse.

AN ORDER FOR ORDERS

1. Admitting diagnosis.
2. Patient's condition (critical, poor, fair, good).
3. Known allergies, if any.
4. Activity permitted (e.g., bed rest, or bathroom privileges, up ad lib.).
5. Diet (e.g., 2 gm sodium, low potassium).
6. General orders
   a. Weights (how often).
   b. Fluids (input and output).
   c. Turning (if bedridden).
   d. Precautions (e.g., seizures, confused, myocardial infarction).
7. Vital signs: frequency, and specifics for which you want to be called (e.g., "Notify MD if temp. greater than 102°F").
8. Medications and IV fluids
   a. Specific to diagnosis (1) IV solution and rate. (2) Antibiotics. (3) Cardiac drugs, etc.
   b. General: Drugs for fever, bowels, sedation, etc.
9. Specimens and tests: e.g., "Please obtain sputum for MD and for culture" or "Draw glucose in morning before breakfast."

Sign —————————————————————
Print name —————————————————————

COMMON ABBREVIATIONS

Although this glossary has potential value to the beginning student when he or she is first translating and understanding medical records, the editors present it to you with a certain reluctance.

Abbreviations are said to be useful in saving the writer's time. What you will discover is that they may waste the reader's time if he cannot understand them. Moreover, abbreviations—unstandardized and subject to misinterpretation (note below how often the same symbol represents several widely different things)—may obscure rather than clarify the chart. We fervently hope that no student using this appendix will do so for any purpose other than translating *back* into English most of the codelike abbreviations he or she encounters. To adopt the habit of using all of the abbreviations below would be to invite error deliberately. If you do abbreviate, and some abbreviations *are* useful, be certain to define your more specialized abbreviations at least once in a written workup. Since this sort of terminology is extremely variable from place to place, not all terms could be included, and the list below is both imprecise and incomplete.

A: anorexia, aorta, artery, auscultation, albumin
a: ante (before)
A$_2$: aortic second heart sound
AA: Alcoholics Anonymous, arteries
AAA: abdominal aortic aneurysm
AAL: anterior axillary line
ab: abortion
ABE: acute bacterial endocarditis
ABD: abdomen, abduction
ABG: arterial blood gas
ABO: classic blood type system
AC: air conduction
ac: ante cibum (before meals)
ACTH: adrenocorticotropic hormone
AD: to or toward
ADA: American Diabetes (or Dental or Dietetic) Association
ADH: antidiuretic hormone
ADL: activities of daily living
ad lib.: at liberty, as the patient desires
AF: atrial fibrillation, aortofemoral
AFB: acid-fast bacillus
AHF: antihemophilic factor
AI: aortic insufficiency
AIHA: autoimmune hemolytic anemia
AJ: ankle jerk
AKA: above-the-knee amputation
ALK P'tase: alkaline phosphatase
ALL: acute lymphocytic leukemia
ALS: amyotrophic lateral sclerosis
AMA: against medical advice, American Medical Association
AMI: acute (or anterior) myocardial infarction, acute mitral insufficiency
AML: acute myelogenous leukemia, acute monocytic leukemia
AMML: acute myelomonocytic leukemia
Ao: aorta
AP: anteroposterior, angina pectoris, acid phosphatase
Appy: appendix, appendectomy
ARDS: adult respiratory distress syndrome
ARF: acute rheumatic fever, acute renal failure
AS: aortic stenosis, arteriosclerosis

ASA: aspirin

ASAP: as soon as possible

ASCVD: atherosclerotic coronary (or cerebral) vascular disease

ASD: atrial septal defect

ASH: asymmetric septal hypertrophy

ASPVD: atherosclerotic peripheral vascular disease

AV: arteriovenous, atrioventricular

AVM: arteriovenous malformation

AVN: atrioventricular node

AVR: aortic valve replacement

A&W: alive and well

B: bacillus, black, bruit, basophil

B-I AND B-II: Billroth's operations (I = gastroduodenostomy, II = gastrojejunostomy)

BA: brain abscess

Baso: basophil

BB: bundle branch

BBB: bundle-branch block, blood-brain barrier

BC: blood culture, bone conduction

BCG: bacille Calmette-Guérin (tuberculosis vaccine)

BCP: birth control pills

BE: barium enema, bacterial endocarditis

bid: bis in dies (twice a day)

bili: bilirubin

BF: black female

B + J: bone and joint

BJP: Bence Jones proteins

BKA: below-the-knee amputation

BM: bowel movement, black man, black male

BO: body odor

BOA: born out of asepsis

BP: blood pressure

BPH: benign prostatic hypertrophy

BRB: bright red blood

BRBPR: bright red blood per rectum

BRRB: bright red rectal blood

BRP: bathroom privileges

BS: bowel sounds, breath sounds, blood smear, blood sugar

BSO: bilateral salpingo-oophorectomy

BSU: Bartholin's glands, Skene's glands, and urethra

BUN: blood urea nitrogen

BW: black woman

C: constipation, Celsius

c̄: cum (with)

CA: cancer, cardiac arrest

Ca: calcium

CAB: coronary artery bypass

CAD: coronary artery disease

CAH: chronic active hepatitis

CAT: computed axial tomography (an x-ray)

CBC: complete blood count

CBDE: common bile duct exploration

CBS: chronic brain syndrome

cc: chief complaint, cubic centimeter

CCCR: closed-chest cardiopulmonary resuscitation

C/C/E: clubbing/cyanosis/edema

CCJ: costochondral junction

CDB: cough and deep-breathe

CF: Caucasian female, cystic fibrosis

C&F: chills and fever

CHD: congenital heart disease

CHF: congestive heart failure

CHO: carbohydrate

Cl: chloride

CLL: chronic lymphocytic leukemia

CM: Caucasian man, Caucasian male

CML: chronic myelogenous leukemia

CMV: cytomegalovirus

c/o: complains of

Coags: tests of coagulation function of the blood

COLD: chronic obstructive lung disease

COPD: chronic obstructive pulmonary disease

Cor: heart

CP: chest pain, cerebral palsy

CPAP: continuous positive airway pressure

CPC: clinocopathologic conference

CPR: cardiopulmonary resuscitation

CR: cardiorespiratory

Cr: creatinine

CRA: cardiorespiratory arrest

CRD: chronic respiratory disease

CRF: chronic renal failure

C&S: culture and sensitivity

CSF: cerebrospinal fluid

CT: computer tomography

CV: cardiovascular

CVA: costovertebral angle, cerebrovascular accident

CVP: central venous pressure

CW: Caucasian woman

CXR: chest x-ray

Cysto: cystoscopy

D: diarrhea, diabetes, dead, developed, day, diastole

d: deciliter

D. bili: direct bilirubin

D/C: discontinued, discharged

D&C: dilation and curettage

Ddx: differential diagnosis

DH: dermatitis herpetiformis

DI: diabetes insipidus

Dig.: digitalis

DIP: distal interphalangeal

DJD: degenerative joint disease

DKA: diabetic ketoacidosis

DL&B: direct laryngoscopy and biopsy

DLCO: diffusional capacity lungs to carbon monoxide

DM: diabetes mellitus

D/NS: dextrose and normal saline

DOA: dead on arrival

DOB: date of birth

DOCA: deoxycorticosterone acetate

DOE: dyspnea on exertion

DP: dorsalis pedis (pulse)

DPH: diphenylhydantoin (phenytoin) (Dilantin)

DPT: diphtheria, pertussis, tetanus immunization

DS: disease

DSS: dioctyl sodium sulfosuccinate (stool softener)

DTRs: deep tendon reflexes

DTs: delirium tremens

DU: duodenal ulcer

DVT: deep venous thrombosis

D&W: dextrose in water

Dx: diagnosis

E: edema, exudate, eosinophils

E&A: evaluation and admission

E → A: designates egophony

EBL: estimated blood loss

ECG: electrocardiogram

ECHO: echocardiogram, or sonography of abdomen

ECT: electroconvulsive therapy

EDC: estimated date of confinement

EDTA: ethylenediaminetetraacetic acid (a chelating agent)

EEG: electroencephalogram

EKG: electrocardiogram

EM: erythema multiforme

E&M: endocrine and metabolic

EMG: electromyogram

EMT: emergency medical treatment (or triage, or technician)

EN: erythema nodosum

ENG: electronystagmogram

ENT: ear, nose, and throat

EOM: extraocular motions (EOMI = EOM intact; EOMF = EOM full)

EOS: eosinophils

ER: emergency room

ERBF: effective renal blood flow

ERCP: endoscopic retrograde cannulation pancreas

ERPF: effective renal plasma flow

ERV: expiratory reserve volume

ES: (heart)—extra sound, ejection sound

ESR: erythrocyte sedimentation rate

ETOH: alcohol (ethanol)

ETT: exercise tolerance test

EW: emergency ward

F: fever, female, Fahrenheit

FB: foreign body

FBS: fasting blood sugar

Fe: iron

FEV: forced expiratory volume

FG: fasting glucose

FH: family history

FLK: funny-looking kid (used in children with odd appearance, suggesting genetic disease, but not yet diagnosed as such)

F → N: finger to nose

FROM: full range of motion

FSH: follicle-stimulating hormone

FTA: fluorescent treponemal antibody test

FTSG: full-thickness skin graft

FTT: failure to thrive

FUO: fever of unknown origin

FX: fracture

G: growth, glucose, gravida, globulin, gallop

GA: general anesthesia

GB: gallbladder

GBD: gallbladder disease

GBS: gallbladder series

GC: gonorrhea

Gen: generally, genitalia

Gent: gentamycin

GFR: glomerular filtration rate

GH: growth hormone

GI: gastrointestinal

Gl: gland, glucose

Glob: globulin

gm: gram

GNP: glomerulonephritis

GOT: glutamic-oxaloacetic transaminase (= SGOT)

GP: general practitioner, general paresis (tertiary neurosyphilis)

GPT: glutamic-pyruvic transaminase (= SGPT)

GSW: gunshot wound

GTT: glucose tolerance test

Gtt: guttae (drops)

GU: genitourinary

GYN: gynecology, gynecologic

H: history, hypertrophy, hyperopia, hydrogen, hormone, hemorrhoids

HA: headache

HAV: hepatitis A virus

HASCVD: hypertensive arteriosclerotic cardiovascular disease

HBab: hepatitis B antibody

HBag: hepatitis B antigen

HBP: high blood pressure

HBR: His bundle recording

HBs: hepatitis B surface antigen

HCG: human chorionic gonadotropin

Hct: hematocrit

HCTZ: hydrochlorothiazide

HD: heart disease

HEENT: head, ears, eyes, nose, throat

Heme: blood, hematology

Hg: mercury

Hgb: hemoglobin
HH: hiatal hernia
HHD: hypertensive heart disease
5-HIAA: 5-hydroxyindoleacetic acid
HJR: hepatojugular reflex
HMR: histiocytic medullary reticuloendotheliosis
HNKDC: hyperosmolar nonketotic diabetic coma
HNP: herniated nucleus pulposus
HO: house officer
H&P: history and physical
HPI: history of present illness
HR: heart rate
H → S: heel to shin
HS: hour of sleep (at bedtime)
HTN: hypertension
HVD: hypertensive vascular disease
Hx: history

I: iodine, intake
IADH: inappropriate antidiuretic hormone
IASD: interatrial septal defect
IBD: inflammatory bowel disease
I. bili: indirect bilirubin
ICP: intracranial pressure
ICS: intercostal space
ID: infectious disease
I&D: incision and drainage
Ig: immunoglobulin
IgEP: immunoglobulin electrophoresis
IH: infectious hepatitis
IHSS: idiopathic hypertrophic subaortic stenosis
IM: intramuscular
IMV: intermittent mandatory ventilation
IND: investigational new drug
INH: isoniazid
I&O: intake and output
IP: intraperitoneal, interphalangeal
IPPB: intermittent positive pressure breathing
IRDM: insulin-requiring diabetes mellitus
ITP: idiopathic thrombocytopenic purpura
IU: international unit
IUD: intrauterine device
IV: intravenous

IVC: intravenous cholangiogram, inferior vena cava
IVP: intravenous pyelogram
IVPB: intravenous piggyback
IVSD: interventricular septal defect

J: jaundice
JAR: junior assistant resident
JD: joint disease
JOD: juvenile onset diabetes
JRA: juvenile rheumatoid arthritis
JVD: jugular venous distention
JVP: jugular venous pressure

K: potasssium, ketones
K-F: Kayser-Fleischer (ring)
kg: kilogram
KJ: knee jerk
KOH: potassium hydroxide
KUB: kidneys, ureter, bladder (a plain film of the abdomen [x-ray])
KW: Kimmelstiel-Wilson (diabetic) renal disease

L: left, lymphocyte, lung, lobe
LA: left atrium, left arm, left anterior
L&A: light and accommodation
LAD: left axis deviation, left anterior descending (coronary artery)
LAH: left anterior hemiblock
LAP: leucine aminopeptidase, leukocyte alkaline phosphatase, laparotomy
LBBB: left bundle-branch block
LBCD: left border cardiac dullness
LBP: low back pain
LDH: lactate dehydrogenase
Le: Lewis (blood group)
LE: lupus erythematosus, left eye, lower extremities
LES: lower esophageal sphincter
LFT: liver function test
LGV: lymphogranuloma venereum
LH: leuteinizing hormone
LHF: left heart failure
LHM: left homonymous hemianopia
Li: lithium
LIH: left inguinal herniorrhaphy
LKS: liver, kidney, spleen
LLL: left lower lobe, late latent lues

LLQ: left lower quadrant
LMCA: left main coronary artery
LMD: local medical doctor
LMP: last menstrual period
LN: lymph nodes
LOA: level of activity, leave of absence
LOC: loss of consciousness
LP: lumbar puncture
LPN: licensed practical nurse
LS: lung scan, lumbar spine
LSB: left sternal border
LUL: left upper lobe
LUQ: left upper quadrant
LV: left ventricle
LVH: left ventricular hypertrophy
LVN: licensed vocational nurse

M: mother, murmur, muscle, melena, mononuclear cell
MAL: midaxillary line
MB: myocardial band of creatine kinase
MBD: minimal brain dysfunction
MCL: midclavicular line
MD: physician, muscular dystrophy
MEA: multiple endocrine adenomatosis
MEN: multiple endocrine neoplasia
MG: myasthenia gravis
Mg: magnesium
mg: milligram
MI: mitral insufficiency, myocardial infarction
MICU: medical intensive care unit
ML: midline
MM: multiple myeloma, muscles
MMCP: measles, mumps, chickenpox
MOD: maturity onset diabetes
MOM: milk of magnesia
Mono: mononucleosis, mononuclear cell
MP: metacarpophalangeal
MR: mitral regurgitation, mental retardation
MRI: magnetic resonance imaging
MS: mitral stenosis, multiple sclerosis, morphine sulphate
MSL: midsternal line
MVA: motor vehicle accident
MVR: mitral valve replacement

N: nausea, nitrogen, nerve
NA: no answer, not applicable
Na: sodium
NAD: no acute distress, no active disease
NAS: no added salt
NC: no change
NF: Negro female
NG: nasogastric
NK: not known, nonketotic
NKA: no known allergies
Nl: normal
NM: Negro man, Negro male
NMT: nebulized mist treatments
NN: nerves
NPO: nothing by mouth
NPH: neutral protein Hagedorn insulin
NR: nonreactive, not relevant
NS: not sufficient
NSR: normal sinus rhythm
NT: nasotracheal
NTG: nitroglycerin
Nullip: nulliparous
N&V: nausea, vomiting, diarrhea
NW: Negro woman

O: oxygen
OB: obstetrics
OBS: organic brain syndrome
OCG: oral cholecystogram
OD: overdose, right eye (oculus dexter)
OM: otitis media
ONC: oncology
OOB: out of bed
OPD: outpatient department
Ophthy: ophthalmology
OR: operating room
ORIF: open reduction internal fixation
Ortho: orthopedics, orthostatic
OS: opening snap, mouth, left eye (oculus sinister)
OT: occupational therapy, oxaloacetic transaminase (SGOT)
Oto: otology

P: phosphorus, parent, pupil, pulse, para, penicillin, platelet, percussion, polymorphonuclear leukocyte

P₂: pulmonic component second heart sound

p: post (after)

PA: posteroanterior, physicians' assistant, pulmonary artery, pernicious anemia

P&A: percussion and auscultation

PAB: premature atrial beat

PABA: para-aminobenzoic acid

PAC: premature atrial contraction

PAF: paroxysmal atrial fibrillation (or flutter)

PAN: polyarteritis nodosa

PAP: pulmonary artery pressure, Papanicolaou (cervical) smear

PAR: postanesthesia recovery room

PAS: para-aminosalicylic acid, periodic acid-Schiff

PAT: paroxysmal atrial tachycardia

PAW: pulmonary artery wedge

PBC: primary biliary cirrhosis

pc: post cibum (after meals)

PCN: penicillin

PCV: packed cell volume

PDA: patent ductus arteriosus

PDR: *Physicians' Desk Reference*

P.E.: pulmonary embolism, physical examination

PEEP: positive end-expiratory pressure

PEG: pneumoencephalography

PEN: penicillin

PERRLA: pupils equal, round, react to light and accommodation

PF: pulmonary function

PFTs: pulmonary function tests

PH: past history, pulmonary hypertension

PHx: past history

PI: principal investigator, pulmonic insufficiency

PID: pelvic inflammatory disease

PIP: proximal interphalangeal (joints)

PKU: phenylketonuria

PM: post mortem

PMI: point of maximum impulse

PMN: polymorphonuclear leukocyte

PMR: polymyalgia rheumatica, physical medicine and rehabilitation

PND: paroxysmal nocturnal dyspnea

PNH: paroxysmal nocturnal hemoglobinuria

PO: per os (by mouth)

Post: autopsy (used as noun)

PPD: purified protein derivative (tuberculosis skin test), percussion and postural drainage, pack per day (smoking)

prn: as necessary (pro re nata)

PRV: polycythemia rubra vera

PS: pulmonic stenosis

PSS: progressive systemic sclerosis (scleroderma)

PSVT: paroxysmal supraventriculr tachycardia

PT: physical therapy, pyruvate transaminase (SGPT), prothrombin time

Pt: patient

PTA: prior to admission

PTH: parathyroid hormone

PTT: partial thromboplastin time

PUD: peptic ulcer disease

P&V: pyloroplasty and vagotomy

PVB: premature ventricular beat

PVC: premature ventricular contraction

PWP: pulmonary wedge pressure

PZI: protamine zinc insulin

q: quaque (every)

Q̇: perfusion

qd: every day

qh: every hour

qid: four times a day

QNS: quantity not sufficient

qod: every other day

Quad: quadriplegic

R: resistance, respirations

RA: rheumatoid arthritis, right atrium, right arm, right anterior

RAD: right axis deviation

RAI: radioactive iodine

RBBB: right bundle-branch block

RBC: red blood cell

RC: Roman Catholic, respirations ceased (died)

RDS: respiratory distress syndrome

RE: regional enteritis, right eye

RF: rheumatic fever, renal failure, respiratory failure, releasing factor

RFT: renal function test

RHD: rheumatic heart disease

RICU: respiratory intensive care unit
RLL: right lower lobe
RLQ: right lower quadrant
RML: right middle lobe
RND: radical neck dissection
ROM: range of motion
ROS: review of systems
RPGNP: rapidly progressive glomerulonephritis
RPT: registered physical therapist, repeat
RR: respiratory rate
RSB: right sternal border
RT: respiratory therapy
RUL: right upper lobe
RUQ: right upper quadrant
RV: right ventricle, residual volume
RVD: rheumatic valvular disease
RVH: right ventricular hypertrophy
Rx: therapy, treatment

S: systole, sound
S$_1$: first heart sound
S$_2$: second heart sound
S$_3$: third heart sound
S$_4$: fourth heart sound
s̄: sans (without)
SA: sinoatrial, septic arthritis
SAN: sinoatrial node
SAR: senior assistant resident
SBE: subacute bacterial endocarditis
SBO: small bowel obstruction
SBFT: small bowel follow-through
SC: subcutaneously
SCCA: squamous cell carcinoma
SCM: sternocleidomastoid
SG: specific gravity
SGOT: serum glutamic oxaloacetic transaminase
SI: sacroiliac
SIADH: syndrome of inappropriate ADH
SICU: surgical intensive care unit
SLE: systemic lupus erythematosus
SOB: shortness of breath
S/P: status post (after)

SPEP: serum protein electrophoresis
SQ: subcutaneously
SSA: sickle cell anemia
SS Hgb: sickle cell hemoglobin
SSKI: saturated solution of potassium iodide
SubQ: subcutaneously
SVC: superior vena cava
SVT: supraventricular tachycardia

T: temperature, time
T$_3$: triiodothyronine
T$_4$: tetraiodothyronine
T&A: tonsillectomy and adenoidectomy
TA: therapeutic abortion
TAb: therapeutic abortion
TAH: transabdominal hysterectomy
TB: tuberculosis
T&C: type and cross (blood)
TFT: thyroid function test
TH: thyroid hormone
TI: tricuspid insufficiency
TIA: transient ischemic attack
TIBC: total iron-binding capacity
TICU: thoracic intensive care unit
TLC: total lung capacity, tender loving care
TM: tympanic membrane
TMJ: temporomandibular joint
TP: total protein
TPR: temperature, pulse, respirations
TR: tendon reflex
TS: tricuspid stenosis
TSH: thyroid-stimulating hormone
TTP: thrombotic thrombocytopenic purpura
TURP: transurethral prostatic resection

U: upper, ulcer, unit
UA: urinalysis, uric acid
UC: ulcerative colitis
UE: upper extremities
UGI: upper gastrointestinal
UGIB: upper gastrointestinal bleeding
UH: university hospital
UQ: upper quadrant

URI: upper respiratory tract infection
UTI: urinary tract infection
UV: ultraviolet

V: ventricle, vomiting, very, vision, vagus, valve, vein, vancomycin
VA: Veterans Administration, visual acuity
VAH: Veterans Administration hospital
VB: ventricular beat
VC: vena cava, vital capacity, color vision
VD: venereal disease
VDRL: Venereal Disease Research Laboratories (test for syphilis)
VF: ventricular fibrillation
VG: very good
V-gram: venogram
VH: ventricular hypertrophy
VHD: valvular heart disease
VMA: vanillylmandelic acid
VNA: Visiting Nurse Association
VO: verbal orders
V/Q̇: ventillation/perfusion ratio
VS: vital signs
VSD: ventricular septal defect
VSS: vital signs stable
VT: ventricular tachycardia
VV: veins

W: with, well, white
WA: white adult
WAP: wandering atrial pacemaker
WB: white boy
WD: well developed
W/D: withdrawal
WF: white female
WG: white girl
WM: white man, male
WN: well nourished
WNL: within normal limits
W/O: without
WPW: Wolff-Parkinson-White

X: times, for

Y: year
y/o: year-old

COMMONLY USED LABORATORY VALUES

The values given for the variety of tests below are the average normals in current units for a variety of hospitals. Because both the average values and the units may differ from laboratory to laboratory, it is essential that the student obtain local information on these tests as soon as possible.

HEMATOLOGY

Hematocrit: men 42–52% RBC count: men $5.4 \pm 0.8 \times 10^6$/dl
             women 37–47%   women $4.8 \pm 0.6 \times 10^6$/dl

Hemoglobin: men 14–18 gm/dl
             women 12–16 gm/dl

Leukocytes 5,000–10,000 (may be lower than 5,000 in normal blacks)
  juvenile neutrophilis (bands) 3–5%
  segmented neutrophils 54–62%
  lymphocytes 25–33%
  monocytes 3–7%
  eosinophils 1–3%
  basophils 0–1%

Platelets 150,000–450,000/dl

Red blood cell indices:
  Mean corpuscular hemoglobin 27–31
  Mean corpuscular hemoglobin concentration 32–36
  Mean corpuscular volume 81–99

Bleeding studies:
  Prothrombin time 70–100% of control
  Partial thromboplastin time 24–36 seconds

BLOOD/PLASMA/SERUM

Electrolytes:
  Sodium   136–145 mEq/L   Chloride   100–106 mEq/L
  Potassium   3.5–4.5 mEq/L   Bicarbonate   24–32 mEq/L
  Calcium   9.0–11.0 mg/dl
  Phosphorus 3.0–4.5 mg/dl
  Creatinine 0.6–1.3 mg/dl

Blood urea nitrogen (BUN) 10–23 mg/dl
Glucose (plasma, fasting) 60–110 mg/dl
Total protein 6.5–8.5 gm/dl
Albumin 3.5–5.5 gm/dl
Bilirubin: total 0.3–1.3 mg/dl
            direct 0.1–0.4 mg/dl
Lactic dehydrogenase (LDH) 110–250 mU/ml
Transaminase: SGOT 10–40 mU/ml
               SGPT   5–35 mU/ml
Alkaline phosphatase 30–95 mU/ml
Uric acid 4–8 mg/dl
Cholesterol 165–240 mg/dl

COMMON DRUGS, WITH BRAND NAMES AND USES

It is much easier to write upon a disease than upon a remedy. The former is in the hands of nature and a faithful observer with an eye of tolerable judgment cannot fail to delineate a likeness. The latter will ever be subject to the whim, the inaccuracies and the blunders of mankind.

WILLIAM WITHERING
(1741–1799)

In taking the history and reviewing the medical records, the student will discover that most patients are on more than one medication and not infrequently are unaware of the purpose of any.

The student should make frequent reference to pharmacology texts, the *Physicians' Desk Reference,* and other sources (including the hospital pharmacologist or pharmacist) to learn as much as possible about these drugs, their good and their harm.

Common Brand Name	Generic Name	Family of Drug
Aldactone	spironolactone	diuretic
Aldomet	alpha methyldopa	antihypertensive
Alkeran	melphalan and L-phenylalanine mustard	cancer therapeutic
Alupent	metaproterenol	antibronchospastic
Amethopterin	methotrexate	cancer therapeutic
Amikin	amikacin sulfate	aminoglycoside antibiotic
Amoxil	amoxicillin	antibiotic
Amphojel	aluminum hydroxide	antacid
Amytal	amobarbital	barbiturate
Ancef	cefazolin	antibiotic
Anturane	sulfinpyrazone	uricosuric antiplatelet
Apresoline	hydralazine	antihypertensive
Ara-C	cytosine arabinoside	cancer therapeutic
Aramine	metaraminol	vasopressor
Arfonad	trimethaphan camsylate	hypotensive
Aristocort (Aristogel, Kenalog)	triamcinolone acetonide	corticosteroid
Augmentin	amoxicillin potassium clavulanate	antibiotic
Atarax	hydroxyzine	antihistamine
Ativan	lorazepam	sedative
Aventyl	nortriptyline hydrochloride	antidepressant
Azulfidine	sulfasalazine	sulfa and salicylate (used in inflammatory bowel disease)
Bactrim	trimethoprim-sulfamethoxazole	antibacterial, antiprotozoal
Benadryl	diphenhydramine	antihistamine

Common Brand Name	Generic Name	Family of Drug
Benemid	probenecid	uricosuric
Benisone	betamethasone benzoate	corticosteroid
Benoxyl (Benzagel)	benzoyl peroxide	topical antibacterial and drying agent (acne therapy)
Bentyl	dicyclomine hydrochloride	anticholinergic
Bicillin	benzathine penicillin G	penicillin antibiotic
Blenoxane	bleomycin sulfate	cancer therapeutic
Brethine	terbutaline sulfate	bronchodilator
Bronkosol	isoetharine mesylate	bronchodilator
Bumex	bumetanide	diuretic
Burow's solution	aluminum acetate	topical antiseptic
Butazolidin	phenylbutazone	anti-inflammatory
Cafergot	ergotamine tartrate	ergot
Calcimar	calcitonin	hypocalcemic
Capoten	capropril	ACE inhibitor
Carafate	sucralfate	ulcer therapy
Cardizem	diltiazem hydrochloride	calcium-channel blocker
Catapres	clonidine hydrochloride	antihypertensive
Ceclor	cefaclor	antibiotic
Cefulac	lactulose	antiencephalopathic
Celestone	betamethasone	corticosteroid
Claforan	cefotaxime sodium	antibiotic
Cleocin	clindamycin	antibiotic
Clinoril	sulindac	anti-inflammatory
Cogentin	benztropine mesylate	anti-cholinergic
Colace	dioctyl sodium sulfosuccinate	stool softener
Compazine	prochlorperazine	phenothiazine
Cordran	flurandrenolide	corticosteroid
Cort-Dome	hydrocortisone	corticosteroid
Co-Salt	KCl, NH_4, Cl, choline, lactose	salt substitute
Cosmegen	dactinomycin	cancer therapeutic
Coumadin	sodium warfarin	oral anticoagulant
Cuemid	cholestyramine	binding resin
Cytomel	sodium liothyronine	thyroid hormone
Cytoxan	cyclophosphamide	immunosuppressive cancer therapeutic
Dalmane	flurazepam	sedative
Darvon	propoxyphene hydrochloride	analgesic
DBI	phenformin	oral hypoglycemic
Decaderm	dexamethasone	corticosteroid
Decadron	dexamethasone sodium phosphate	corticosteroid
Delta-Cortef	prednisone	corticosteroid

Common Brand Name	Generic Name	Family of Drug
Demerol	meperidine	narcotic analgesic
DiaBeta	glyburide	oral hypoglycemic
Diabinese	chlorpropamide	oral hypoglycemic
Diamox	acetazolamide	diuretic
Dilantin	phenytoin sodium	antiepileptic
Dilaudid	dihydromorphinone hydrochloride	narcotic analgesic
Diuril	chlorothiazide	diuretic
Doriden	glutethimide	sedative
DTIC-Dome	dimethyl-triazenoimidazole-carboxamide (dacarbazine)	cancer therapeutic
Dulcolax	bisacodyl	laxative
Dymelor	acetohexamide	oral hypoglycemic
Dyrenium	triamterene	diuretic
Edecrin	ethacrynic acid	diuretic
Efudex	5-fluorouracil	cancer therapeutic (skin)
Elavil	amitriptyline hychloride	antidepressant
Epsom salts	magnesium sulfate	cathartic
Equanil	meprobamate	sedative
Eskalith	lithium carbonate	antipsychotic
Euthroid	liotrix	thyroid hormone
Feldene	piroxicam	anti-inflammatory
Flagyl	metronidazole	antibacterial/ antiprotozoal
Flexeril	cyclobenzaprine	anti-spasmodic
Flurobate	batamethasone benzoate	corticosteroid
Fortaz	cefaziclime	antibiotic
Fungizone	amphotericin B	antifungal
Furacin	nitrofurazone	topical antibacterial
Furadantin	nitrofurantoin	urinary antibacterial
Gantrisin	sulfisoxazole	antibacterial
Garamycin	gentamicin sulfate	antibiotic
Gelusil	aluminum hydroxide, magnesium hydroxide, and simethicone	antacid
Geocillin/Geopen	carbenicillin	antibiotic
Glucotrol	glipizide	oral hypoglycemic
GoLYTELY	ployethylene glycol 3350 solution	cathartic
Halcion	triazolam	sedative
Haldol	haloperidol	antipsychotic
Hydrea	hydroxyurea	cancer therapeutic
HydroDiuril	hydrochlorothiazide	diuretic
Hydromox	quinethazone	diuretic

Common Brand Name	Generic Name	Family of Drug
Hygroton	chlorthalidone	diuretic
Hytone	hydrocortisone	corticosteroid
Imferon	iron dextran	iron
Imodium	loperamide	antidiarrheal
Imuran	azathioprine	immunosuppressive
Inderal	propranolol hydrochloride	beta blocker
Indocin	indomethacin	anti-inflammatory
Intropin	dopamine hydrochloride	vasopressor, cardiotropic
Iosel	selenium sulfide	antifungal (topical)
Ismelin	guanethidine sulfate	hypotensive
Isoptin	verapamil hydrochloride	calcium-channel blocker
Isordil	isosorbide	anti-anginal
Isuprel	isoproterenol	vasopressor, cardiotropic
Kaon	potassium glutamate	potassium
Kaopectate	kaolin and pectin	antidiarrheal
Kayexalate	sodium polystyrene sulfonate	K^+-binding resin
Keflex	cephalexin	antibiotic
Keflin	cephalothin	antibiotic
Ketzol	cefazolin	antibiotic
Kenacort	triamcinolone	corticosteroid
Kenalog	triamcinolone acetonide	corticosteroid
K-Lyte	potassium bicarbonate	potassium
Kwell	gamma benzene hexachloride	antiectoparasite therapy
Lanoxin	digoxin	cardiac glycoside
Lasix	furosemide	diuretic
Leukeran	chlorambucil	immunosuppressive, cancer therapeutic
Levophed	levarterenol	vasopressor
Librium	chlordiazepoxide hydrochloride	sedative
Lidex	fluocinonide	corticosteroid
Lomotil	diphenoxylate hydrochloride	antidiarrheal
Lopressor	metaprolol	beta blocker
Lotrimin	clotrimazole	antifungal (topical)
Lozol	indapamide	diuretic
Luminal	phenobarbital	barbiturate
Maalox	magnesium hydroxide	antacid
Macrodantin	nitrofurantoin	antibacterial
Mandelamine	methenamide mandelate	antibacterial (urine)
Mandol	cefamandole	antibiotic
Marplan	isocarboxazid	MAO inhibitor
Matulane	procarbazine hydrochloride	cancer therapeutic

Common Brand Name	Generic Name	Family of Drug
Medrol	methylprednisolone	corticosteroid
Mefoxin	cefoxitin sodium	antibiotic
Mellaril	thioridazine	phenothiazine
Meltrol	phenformin	oral hypoglycemic
Mercuhydrin	meralluride	diuretic
Mestinon	pyridostigmine bromide	cholinesterase inhibitor
Metahydrin	trichlormethiazide	diuretic
Metamucil	psyllium hydrophilic mucilloid	bulk laxative
Meticortelone	prednisolone	corticosteroid
Meticorten	prednisone	corticosteroid
Mexitil	mexillitomel	antiarrhythmic
Micronase	glyburide	oral hyopglycemic
Miltown	meprobamate	sedative
Minipress	prazosin	antihypertensive
Mobidin	magnesium salicylate	anti-inflammatory
Monistat	miconazole	antifungal
Monocid	cefonicid sodium	antibiotic
Motrin	ibuprofen	anti-inflammatory
Mustargen	mechlorethamine hydrochloride	cancer therapeutic
Mutamycin	mitomycin-C	cancer therapeutic
Mycelex	clotrimazole	antifungal
Mycostatin	nystatin	antifungal
Mylanta	magnesium hydroxide	antacid
Myleran	busulfan	cancer therapeutic
Myochrysine	gold sodium thiomalate	antiarthritic
Nalfon	fenoprofen calcium	anti-inflammatory
Naprosyn	naproxen	anti-inflammatory
Naqua	trichlormethiazide	diuretic
Narcan	naloxone hydrochloride	narcotic analgesic
Nardil	phenelzine sulfate	MAO inhibitor
Nembutal	pentobarbital	barbiturate
Neo-Synephrine	phenylephrine	decongestant
Nipride	sodium nitroprusside	hypotensive
Nitro-Bid	nitroglycerin	antiangina
Nizoral	ketoconazole	antifungal
Noludar	methprylon	sedative
Normodyne	labetalol hydrochloride	beta blocker
Noroxin	norfloxacin	antibiotic (urine)
Norpace	disopyramide phosphate	antiarrhythmic
Norpramin	desipramine hydrochloride	antidepressant
Oncovin	vincristine sulfate	cancer therapeutic

Common Brand Name	Generic Name	Family of Drug
Orinase	tolbutamide	oral hypoglycemic
Os-Cal	calcium carbonate	calcium
PanOxyl	benzoyl peroxide	topical antibacterial and drying agent
Parlodel	bromocryptine	dopamine receptor antagonist
Parnate	nonhydrazine tranylcypromine sulfate	MAO inhibitor
Pentam	pentamidine isothionate	antiprotozoal
Pentothal	thiopental sodium	barbiturate
Pepcid	pamotidine	H_2 blocker
Percocet	oxycodone hydrochloride	narcotic
Permitil	fluphenazine hydrochloride	phenothiazine
Persantine	dipyridamole	antiplatelet
Pertofrane	desipramine hydrochloride	antidepressant
Phenergan	promethazine hydrochloride	antihistamine
Pipracil	piperacillin sodium	antibiotic
Placidyl	ethchlorvynol	sedative
Plaquenil	hydroxychloroquine sulfate	antimalarial, antiarthritic
Premarin	conjugated estrogens	estrogen
Primaxin	imipenem-cilastin sodium	antibiotic
Pro-Banthine	propantheline bromide	anticholinergic
Procardia	nifedipine	calcium-channel blocker
Prolixin	fluphenazine hydrochloride	phenothiazine
Proloid	thyroglobulin	thyroid hormone
Pronestyl/Procan-SR	procainamide hydrochloride	antiarrhythmic
Prostigmine	neostigmine	cholinesterase inhibitor
Proventyl	albuterol	antibronchospastic
Purinethol	6-mercaptopurine	cancer therapeutic
Questran	cholestyramine	binding resin
Quinaglute	quinidine	antiarrhythmic
Regitine	phentolamine	alpha blocker
Reglan	metoclopramide	antiemetic; GI motility
Restoril	temazepam	sedative
Riopan	magnesium hydroxide	antacid
Robinul	glycopyrrolate	anticholinergic
Rocaltrol	calcitriol	vitamin D
Seldane	terfenadine	antihistamine
Senekot	extract of senna	laxative
Serax	oxazepam	sedative
Solganal	gold thioglucose	antiarthritic
Solu-Cortef	hydrocortisone	corticosteroid
Solu-Medrol	methylprednisolone	corticosteroid
Sparine	promazine hydrochloride	phenothiazine

Common Brand Name	*Generic Name*	*Family of Drug*
Stelazine	trifluoperazine hydrochloride	phenothiazine
Stimex	paramethazone	corticosteroid
Surfak	dioctyl calcium sulfosuccinate	stool softener
Symmetrel	amantadine	antiparkinsonism
Synalar	fluocinolone acetonide	corticosteroid
Synthroid	sodium levothyroxine	thyroid hormone
Tacaryl	methdilazine hydrochloride	phenothiazine
Tagamet	cimetadine	antacid
Talwin	pentazocine	analgesic
Tambocor	flecanide	antiarrhythmic
Tandearil	phenylbutazone and oxyphenbutazone	anti-inflammatory
Tapazole	methimazole	antithyroid
Temaril	trimeprazine tartrate	phenothiazine
Tenormin	atenolol	beta blocker
Tensilon	edrophonium chloride	cholinergic
Theo-Dur	theophylline	bronchodilator
Thiomerin	mercaptomerin	diuretic
Thorazine	chlorpromazine	phenothiazine
Thyrolar	liotrix	thyroid hormone
Ticar	ticarcillin	antibiotic
Tigan	trimethobenzamide hydrochloride	antiemetic
Tindal	acetophenazine maleate	phenothiazine
Tinver	sodium thiosulfate	topical antifungal
Tofranil	imipramine	antidepressant
Tolectin	tolmetin sodium	anti-inflammatory
Tolinase	tolazamide	oral hypoglycemic
Tonocard	tocainide	antiarrhythmic
Trandate	labetolol	beta blocker
Tranxene	clorazepate dipotassium	sedative
Trilafon	perphenazine	phenothiazine
Tylenol	acetaminophen	antipyretic, analgesic
Unipen	nafcillin	antibiotic
Urecholine	bethanechol chloride	cholinergic
Valisone	betamethasone valerate	corticosteroid
Valium	diazepam	sedative
Vanceril	beclomethasone	corticosteroid
Vancocin	vancomycin	antibiotic
Vasoxyl	methoxamine hydrochloride	alpha-adrenergic
Vasotec	enapril	ACE inhibitor
Velban	vinblastine sulfate	cancer therapeutic
Ventolin	albuterol	antibronchospastic
Vivactil	protriptyline hydrochloride	antidepressant

Common Brand Name	Generic Name	Family of Drug
Vistaril	hydroxyzine	antihistamine
Xanax	alprazolam	sedative
Xylocaine	lidocaine hydrochloride	antiarrhythmic, topical anesthetic
Zantac	ranitidine	H_2 blocker
Zaroxolyn	metolazone	diuretic
Zinacef	cefuroxime	antibiotic
Zovirax	acyclovir	antiviral
Zyloprim	allopurinol	hypouricemic

INDEX

INDEX

A wave, 269–270
Abdomen
  acute, 334–337
  child and, 512–513, 526–527
  distension of, 355–356
    infant and, 513
  examination of, 31, 343–357
    auscultation and, 345–346
    bladder and, 355
    elderly patient and, 539
    inspection and, 343–345
    liver and, 351–352
    pregnancy and, 411–412
    spleen and, 352–353
    uterus and, 355
  hernia and, 382–386
  pain in
    acute, 334–337
    child and, 512–513
    elderly patient and, 537
  pelvic inflammatory disease and, 410
  renal ectopia and, 372
  spinal examination and, 430
  trauma and, 550–553
Abdominal bruit, 260
Abdominal paradox, 232
Abdominal reflex, 487, 491
Abducens nerve, 471
  paralysis and, 134
Abrasion, corneal, 127
Abscess
  lung, sputum and, 202
  ovarian, 411
  pelvic, 410
  perinephric, 372
  periodontal disease and, 168
  perirectal, 358
Abstract thinking, 462–463
Acanthosis nigricans of axilla, 88
Accessory navicular bone, 451
Accident. See Injured patient
Acetabulum fracture, 564
Acetone breath, 342
Achilles tendon, 450
  newborn and, 529
Acid breath, 342
Acquired immunodeficiency syndrome
  AIDS-related complex markers and,
    173, 175, 176
  hematopoietic system and, 104
  patient history and, 51–52
Acrocyanosis, 252, 519
Acromegaly, 68
Acuity, visual, 120–122, 470

Acute abdomen, 334–337
Addison's disease
  hyperpigmentation and, 87
  observation and, 69
Adductor pollicis, 420
Adenoid tissue, 181
  child and, 525
Adenopathy, 104
Adie's pupil, 137, 472
Adrenal insufficiency
  hyperpigmentation and, 87
  nipple and, 316
Adrenocortical hormone
  excess of, 70
  insufficiency of, 69
Adson maneuver, 425, 426, 427
Adventitial breath sounds, 222
Affective disorder, 465
Afterload, 243–244
Age
  acute abdomen and, 335
  fourth heart sound and, 287
  gestational, 531
  innocent murmur and, 294
  third heart sound and, 286
Aging versus disease, 535–536
AIDS-related complex, 173, 175, 176
Air conduction versus bone
    conduction, 159
Airway
  injured patient and, 541–542
  obstruction and, 229–231
Alopecia, 94
Alternate cover test, 130, 132
Alveolitis, fibrosing, 230, 231
Amalgam tattoo, 173
Amaurotic pupil, 117, 137
Amblyopia ex anopsia, 523
Amnesia, 465
Amphoric breathing, 222
Amyl nitrite test, 303–304
Anacrotic pulse, 258, 259
Anal fissure, 360
Anal ring, 359–360
Anemia, 102
  causes of, 110
  pallor and, 108
  tongue in, 111
  yellow pigmentation and, 88
Aneurysm
  aortic
    abdominal, 355
    mediastinal mass and, 239
    rupture of, 260

carotid artery, 190
  popliteal artery, 260
Angina pectoris, 247
Angle
  costovertebral
    abdominal palpation and, 348–349
    pain and, 371
  subcostal, 209
Angular stomatitis, 109
Anisocoria, 128, 131, 471–472
Ankle, 450–451
  clonus and, 490
  fracture and, 570
Ankle jerk, 529
Ankyloglossia, 174
Anorectal fistula, 359
Anoscopy, 361
Antalgic gait, 418, 442
Anterior chamber, 128
  redness of eye and, 119
Anterior serratus muscle, 432
Anthracotic particles, 202
Anxiety, 465
  blood pressure and, 78–79
Aorta
  abdominal examination and, 355
  aneurysm and
    abdominal, 337
    mediastinal mass and, 239
    rupture and, 260
  bifurcation occlusion and, 254
  injuries of, 550
  outflow tract obstruction and, 259
  sternum fracture and, 547
Aortic arch syndrome, 264
Aortic valve
  anatomy and, 242
  murmur and, 293–294
  prosthetic, 307
  regurgitation and
    amyl nitrite and, 303–310
    carotid pulse and, 264
    diastolic murmur and, 300, 301
    Flint-Austin murmur and, 298, 301
    head nodding and, 251
    isometric exercise and, 303
    physical findings in, 306
  stenosis and, 285
Apgar scores, 530
Aphasia, 458, 467–469
Apical impulse, 273–274
Apical pulse, 74
Apnea, 206
  premature infant and, 531

Apnea—*Continued*
  sleep, 206
Appearance, general, 57–70
  child and, 517–518
  diagnosis by observation and, 67–70
  face and, 60
  habitus and, 60–61, 67–70
  hair distribution and, 66
  hands and, 61–65
  history and, 58–59
  patient preparation and, 58
Appendiceal pain, 334, 336, 385–386
Appendicitis
  pain and, 336
  pelvic inflammatory disease and, 410
Aqueous humor, 128
Arcus, white, 128
Arcus senilis, 129
Argyll Robertson pupil, 131, 134, 136
Arm. *See also* Hand
  cardiovascular disease and, 252
  neurological examination and, 491–492
Arnold's nerve, 153
Arrest, inspiratory, 351–352
Arrhythmia
  blood pressure and, 79
  physical findings and, 261, 262
  syncope and, 248
  thyroid disease and, 194
Arterial blood gas, 228
  respiratory failure and, 232
Arteriosclerosis of retinal vessel, 143
Arteriovenous shunt, lung, 242
Artery
  coronary
    anatomy of, 245
    angina pectoris and, 247
  extremity and, 253
  trauma and, 560
Arthritis
  gouty, 411
  hand and, 440
  pain and, 416
Articulation, uncovertebral, 426
Ascites, 356–357
Aspiration, bone marrow, 111
Assessment of trauma victim, 571–572
Astereognosis, 500
Asthma, 230
  wheezes of, 223
Asymmetry
  breast and, 315
  chest and, 208, 211, 525
  infant's head and, 521
  pelvic, 563
  reflex, 484
  septal hypertrophy and, 296
Ataxia, 492, 494, 495
  causes of, 493
Athetosis, 480, 481

Atresia, esophageal, 513
Atrial fibrillation, 262
  blood pressure and, 79
Atrial gallop, 287
Atrioventricular block, 262
Atrium, 242
  hemodynamics, 268–271
  septal defect and, 308
Atrophy
  lingual mucosa and, 109
  muscle and, 422, 479, 480
  optic, 148, 149, 470
  shoulder and, 431
  spinal accessory nerve and, 478
  tongue and, 176
Auditory canal, 153, 524–525
Auditory nerve, 476
Auricle, 153, 154
  child and, 523
Auscultation
  abdomen and, 345–346
  chest and, 218–225
    child and, 525–526
  heart and, 277–304. *See also* Heart sounds; Murmur, heart
  jugular venous, 271
  newborn and, 525
  skull and, 466
  thyroid and, 193–194
Auscultatory gap, 79
Austin Flint murmur, 298, 301
Autonomous neurogenic bladder, 377
Awareness, 462
Axilla
  acanthosis nigricans of, 88
  breast examination and, 320, 322
Axillary lymph nodes, 102, 107
Axillary nerve injury, 560

Babinski reflex, 484, 486–487, 488
  newborn and, 529
Back. *See also* Spine
  abdominal examination and, 357
  physical examination and, 31
Bacterial orchlamydial vaginitis, 400
Balanoposthitis, 378
Band keratopathy, 129
Banding, white, of nail, 91
Bartholin's gland, 395
  cyst and, 396
Barton's fracture, 569–570
Baseball finger, 411
Battle's sign, 545
Beading of vas deferens, 380
Beau's lines, 62, 91
Behavior
  neurologic assessment and, 462
  retardation and, 515
Bennett's fracture, 570
Biceps tendon reflex, 485
  innervation of, 420

Bifid pulse, 258, 259
Bigeminal pulse, 259
Bile pigment, 88
Biliary colic, 336
Biliary tract calculus, 336
Bimanual pelvic examination, 399, 403, 405
Biographical data, 23
Biopsy, lymph node, 111
  cervical, 399
Biot's respiration, 74
Bitter almond breath, 342
Black hairy tongue, 175
Bladder, 375–377
  male patient and, 365
  neurologic disorder and, 458
  palpation of, 355
  percussion and, 350
  sliding hernia and, 385
  trauma and, 553–554
Bleeding. *See also* Hemorrhage
  coagulation disorders and, 104
  endometriosis and, 406
  gingival, 166
  hemoptysis and, 203
  between menstrual periods, 391
  nasal, 161
  trauma and, 542
Blepharitis, 125
Blindness, 117, 138
  cortical, 134
Blister, 95
Blood. *See also* Hematopoietic system
  anterior chamber and, 128
  occult, 337
  oxygenated, 244, 245
  sputum and, 203
  urine and, 366, 367
Blood gas, arterial, 228
  respiratory failure and, 232
Blood pressure, 76–79
  abdominal wound and, 552
  child and, 509, 518–519
  intra-abdominal hemorrhage and, 551
  pulsus paradoxus and, 259–260
  renal disease and, 368
Blood smear, peripheral, 109–110
Blood vessels of retina, 142–145
Blue-gray pigmentation, 86, 89
Bluish pigmentation of oral mucosa, 173
Blunt abdominal injury, 552–553
Blurring of vision, 117
Boggy conjunctiva, 127
Bone
  accessory navicular, 451
  examination of, 422, 423
  fractures of. *See* Fracture
  hematologic disorders and, 109
  injury and, 555, 556

Bone conduction versus air conduction, 159
Bone marrow, 110
Bounding pulse, 258–259
Bowel. *See* Gastrointestinal tract
Bowel sounds, 345–346
Brachialis muscle, 420
Brachioradialis muscle, 420
Bradycardia
    pulse and, 74
    syncope and, 248
Brain injury, 544–545
Breast, 311–327
    anatomy and, 311–312
    disorders of, 316, 318, 319, 320, 324
    hypertrophy of newborn and, 525
    inspection of, 315–317
    palpation and, 317, 320–321
    patient history and, 313
    physical examination and, 31
    pigeon, 210
    pregnancy and, 411
    self-examination and, 325–327
Breath odor, 342
Breath sounds, 219
    airway obstruction and, 229
    chest auscultation and, 222
    child and, 525–526
    fremitus and, 214
    partial bronchial obstruction and, 233
    tension pneumothorax and, 549
Breathing. *See* Respiration; Respiratory system
Breathlessness. *See* Dyspnea
Broad ligament, uterine, 403
Broca's aphasia, 468
Bronchial breathing, 220, 222
Bronchial leak squeak sign, 225
Bronchial obstruction, 233
Bronchophony, 221, 225
Bronchopneumonia, 218
Bronchopulmonary system, 197–239. *See also* Respiratory system
Bronchovesicular breath sound, 220–221, 222
Brown pigmentation, 86, 88
    nipple and, 411
    oral mucosa and, 173
Brudzinski's sign, 467
Bruit
    abdominal, 260, 346
    definition of, 289
    neurological disorder and, 466–467
    thyroid and, 194
Buccal mucous membrane, 171
Bulla, 95
    pneumothorax versus, 239
Bundle-branch block, 262
Bunion, 451

Burning pain
    abdominal, 336
    eyes and, 118
    tongue and, 166
Bursa
    hip and, 443
    knee and, 443, 446
    trochanteric, 443
Butterfly bone fragment, 556

Calculations test, 462
Calculus
    biliary tract, 336
    cystitis and, 376
    prostatic, 388
    renal, 372, 373
    ureteral, 373
Canal
    external auditory, 153
    of Nuck, 386
Cancer. *See* Malignancy
Candidiasis, 174
    infant and, 531
    vaginitis and, 400–401
        saline drop test and, 397
Cannon wave, 270
Capacitance, 242
Caput medusae, 343
Caput succedaneum, 520, 521
Carcinoma. *See* Malignancy
Cardiac cycle, 281–282
Cardiac sound, 279–302. *See also* Heart sounds; Murmur, heart
Cardiac tamponade, 550
Cardiac valve, 242
Cardiomyopathy
    hypertrophic, 296
    obstructive, 259
Cardiovascular system, 241–310
    aging and, 535
    anatomy and physiology of, 242–246
    cough and, 248
    dyspnea and, 246–247
    extremities and, 253–264
        arteries and, 153–161
        clubbing and, 253
        edema and, 264
        veins and, 261–264
    findings and, 305–308
    general observation and, 251–252
    heart and, 272–310. *See also* Heart
    hemoptysis and, 204
    neck and, 264–271
    pain and, 247–248
    palpitation and, 248
    review of systems and, 25
    special diagnostic maneuvers and, 302–304, 309
    syncope and, 248, 249
Carotid pulse
    contour of, 256

disorders and, 264
    neurological, 466–467
    illustration of, 255
    palpation of, 189
Carpal tunnel syndrome, 439
Cataract
    funduscopic examination and, 141
    senile, 117
Causalgia, 554–555
Cavernous breathing, 222
Celiotomy, 552
Central cyanosis, 251–252
Centigrade scale, 72
Central nervous system. *See* Nervous system
Central vision, loss of, 117
Cephalhematoma, 521
Cerebellar function, 491–494
    ataxia and, 493, 495
Cerebellar tremor, 480
Cerebral lesion
    ataxia and, 493
    coma and, 459
    facial nerve and, 476
    trauma and, 543
    trigeminal nerve and, 474
Cervical muscle spasm, 186, 187
Cervical spine, 422–427
    dislocation and, 562
    injury and, 546–547
    osteoarthritis of, 424
    radiologic examination and, 543
Cervicofacial lymph nodes, 101, 106
Cervix, uterine
    biopsy and, 399
    carcinoma and, 404
    lesions of, 402
    palpation of, 403
Chaddock's reflex, 486, 488
Chadwick's sign, 411
Chalazion, 125
Chancre, 379
Cheek fracture, 546
Chemosis, 194
Chest, 195–327
    acute abdomen and, 357
    breast and, 311–327. *See also* Breast
    cardiovascular system and, 241–310. *See also* Cardiovascular system
    child and, 525–526
    physical examination of, 30
    respiratory system and, 197–239. *See also* Respiratory system
    review of systems and, 25
    uremia and, 368
Chest pain
    elderly patient and, 536–537
    pulmonary disease and, 203
    sources of, 205
Chest wall
    pain and, 205

Chest wall—*Continued*
trauma and, 547–550
Cheyne-Stokes respiration, 74
Chief complaint, 23
Child, 505–532. *See also* Pediatric
examination
Chlamydial infection, 408, 410
Choana, 163
Cholecystitis, 351
Chondromalacia, 443
Chorea, 480, 481
child and, 522
Huntington's, 494
Chorioretinal scarring, 149–150
Chorioretinitis, 150
Choroidal melanoma, 150
Circulation. *See also* Cardiovascular
system
systemic and pulmonary, 242
trauma victim and, 572
Circumference of head, 522
Cirrhosis, 343
Claudication, 247–248
Clavicle, fracture of, 564
Clavicular pectoralis major muscle,
420
Cleft palate, 172
Click, systolic, 288
mitral prolapse and, 298
Clinical examination
history and, 21–26
oral presentation and, 33
physical examination and, 26–31
progress notes and, 32–33
structure and recording of, 21–33
Clinical laboratory, 585–586
Clinical problem solving, 575–583
Clitoris enlargement, 396
child and, 527
Clonus, 487
reflex and, 483
ankle and, 490
Closed fracture, 558
Closed-head injury, 544
Cloudy urine, 366
Clubbing
cardiovascular disease and, 253
gastrointestinal tract disorder and,
341
nail, 63, 64, 90
respiratory disorder and, 211
Coagulation disorders, 104
Coarse crackles, 224
Cochlear nerve, 476
Cognitive disorder, 464
Cogwheel effect, 481
Coin test, 239
Colic
infant and, 513
renal, 372, 373
Collateral ligament, 447–448

Colles' fracture, 569–570
Colon. *See* Gastrointestinal tract
Colonoscope, fiberoptic, 361
Color change of skin. *See* Pigmentation
Coma, 459
Comminuted fracture, 557
Communication skills, 11
Compound dislocation, 559
Compound fracture, 557, 558
Compression
lung and, 233
vertebral body, 562
Computed tomography, 111–112
Concha, 153
Conductive aphasia, 468–469
Conductive hearing loss, 155, 156,
476–477
Condyloma acuminata, 379
Condyle
knee and elbow fracture and, 567–
568
temporomandibular joint and, 179–
180
tibial, 569
Confrontation test, visual, 136–138
neurologic examination and, 470
Congenital disorder
muscle weakness and, 423
palate and, 172
pulmonary regurgitation and, 298,
300
toxoplasmosis and, 150
Congestion, splenic, 352–353
Congestive heart failure, 36
Conjunctiva, 124, 127
redness of eye and, 119
thyroid and, 194
Consciousness
head injury and, 544
neurologic disorder and, 457, 460
Consensual light reaction, 134
Consolidation, 233
Constrictive pericarditis, 276
Continuous murmur, 301–302
Contraction, premature cardiac, 262
Contracture
Dupuytren's, 65, 439
hip and, 443
Contusion
pulmonary, 550
scalp, 545
Conversion reaction, 501
Convulsion
child and, 515–516, 522
neurologic disorder and, 457
Coordination, 517
Cord, spermatic, 380–381
Cornea, 127–128
redness of eye and, 119
scarring and, 141
ulcer and, 129

Corneal reflex
extraocular movement and, 130
neurologic examination and, 472–
473
newborn and, 522–523
Coronary artery
anatomy of, 245
angina pectoris and, 247
Corrigan's sign, 264
Cortical blindness, 134
Costovertebral angle
abdominal palpation and, 348–
349
pain and, 371
Cough, 201–202
abdominal examination and, 347
cardiovascular disease and, 248
Cover test
alternate, 130, 132
child and, 523
Cover-uncover test, 130
Crackle, respiratory, 220, 224–225
elderly patient and, 539
Cradle cap, 519
Cramp, abdominal, 346
Cranial nerve, 469–479
eye and, 133, 134
head examination and, 184
pupillary reflex and, 134
I, 469
II, 470–471
III, IV, and VI, 471–472
V, 472–474
VII, 475–476
VIII, 476–477
IX and X, 477–478
XI, 478
XII, 478–479
Cremasteric reflex, 487, 491
Crepitation, 220
Crown of tooth, 179
Crunch, mediastinal, 228, 549–550
definition of, 225
Crush injury of ribs, 547
Cuff, rotator, 433
Culture, vaginal, 399
Cupping of optic disc, 148, 149
Cushing's syndrome, 70
Cutaneous color change. *See*
Pigmentation
Cyanosis
Chadwick's sign and, 411
finger and, 90
mitral stenosis and, 251
oral mucosa and, 173
types of, 251–252
Cycle, cardiac, 281–282
Cyst
Bartholin's gland, 396
breast and, 322
Gartner's duct, 401

ovarian, 407, 408
  abdominal examination and, 356
pilonidal, 357
retention
  lip and, 170
  mouth and, 176
  nipple and, 316
Cystic fibrosis, 211
Cystitis, 376
  causes of, 377
  male, 365
Cystocele, 395, 396
Cytometry, flow, 112

Dacryocystitis, 125
De Quervain's disease, 437
Deafness, 476–477
Deep tendon reflex, 544
Deformity with fracture, 558
Degeneration, macular, 151
Dehydration, 341
Delirium, 464–465
Deltoid bulge, 566, 567
Deltoid muscle, 420
Delusion, 464
Dementia, 464
Denial, 38
Depersonalization, 463–464
Depression, psychologic, 465
Depressor muscle, 130
Derealization, 463–464
Dermatitis
  seborrheic, 519
  stasis ulcer and, 99
Dermatologic history, 83. See also Skin
Developmental milestones, 508
Diabetes
  pupil and, 131
  retina and, 146
Diaphoresis, 252
Diaphragm
  excursion of, 216
  innervation of, 420
  respiratory failure and, 232
  stethoscope and, 278
Diastole, 281–282
Diastolic extra sound, 286–287
Diastolic murmur, 298, 300–301
Dicrotic pulse, 259
Digital clubbing. See Clubbing
Digital rectal examination, 359–360
Dilation
  pupil and, 139
  ventricular, 275–276
Diplopia, 118
Direct inguinal hernia, 384
Direct light reaction, 134
Disc, optic, 147–148, 470
  cupping of, 148, 149
Discharge
  ear and, 155

eye and, 119
nipple and, 316
vaginal, 392
Disk, vertebral, 431
Dislocation, 558–559
  arterial injury and, 560
  hip and, 564, 565
  olecranon and, 568
  scapulohumeral joint and, 566
  vertebral, 560–563
Distended abdomen, 355–356
  infant and, 513
Disuse atrophy, 422
Diurnal variation in temperature, 72
Diverticulitis, 410
Dizziness, 459–460
Dorsalis pedis, 255
Double vision, 118
Down syndrome, 518
Draping for pelvic examination, 394
Drawer sign, 449
Dribbling incontinence, 365
Drooling, 166
Drug
  ataxia and, 493
  coma and, 459
  perceptual disorder and, 464
  pigmentation and, 89
  pupil and, 131
  sexual dysfunction and, 368
Dry mouth, 166
Duck-billed speculum, 397
Duct
  Gartner's, 401
  parotid, 171
Dullness
  abdominal, 350–351
  chest percussion and, 216
  respiratory, 218
Duodenal pain, 334
Dupuytren's contracture, 65, 439
Dwarfism, intrauterine, 514
Dysarthria, 458
Dysmenorrhea, 391
Dysmetria, 492
Dysphagia, 167, 338
  causes of, 339
Dyspnea
  cardiovascular disease and, 246–247
  child and, 515
  elderly patient and, 537
  patient history and, 35–36
  pulmonary disease and, 203, 206
Dystrophy
  muscular, 482
  nail, 90
  spinal accessory nerve and, 478
Dysuria, 365

Ear, 153–159
  child and, 523–525

cranial nerve and, 476–477
physical examination and, 30
review of systems and, 25
uremia and, 368
Earpiece of stethoscope, 277
Ecchymoses, 95
  flank and, 357
ECG. See Electrocardiogram
Ectopia
  renal, 372, 373
  testes and, 381
Ectropion, 125
Eczematous disease, 83
Edema
  cardiovascular disease and, 264, 265
  cornea and, 128
  eyelid and, 124, 126
  optic disc and, 470
  pulmonary, 236–237, 550
Effusion
  pericardial, 550
  pleural, 231, 233–234, 235
Egophony, 225
Ejection murmur, 288
  aortic systolic, 293–294
  pulmonic ejection, 294
Elasticity of skin, 92
Elbow, 433, 435–437
  fracture and dislocation of, 567–569
  nerve injury and, 560
Elderly patient. See Geriatric examination
Electrocardiogram
  arrhythmias and, 261
  physical examination and, 31
Elevator muscle, 130
Embryoma, 372
Emotional stimuli, skin change and, 91
Empathy, 8
Emphysema, 229–231
  chest and, 211
  mediastinal crunch and, 225
  subcutaneous, 214, 549–550
Endocrine system
  aging and, 536
  short stature and, 514
  sexual maturation and, 391
Endometriosis, 406
Endpiece of stethoscope, 277
Entropion, 125
Epicanthal fold, 125
Epicondylitis, 433
Epidermoid carcinoma, 379, 380
Epididymitis, 380, 381
Epigastric hernia, 343
Epiphora, 124
Epiphysis, 557–558
Epispadias, 379
Epistaxis, 161

Epithelial cell, 395, 397
Epitrochlear lymph nodes, 107
Epitrochlear pulse, 255
Epstein's pearls, 531
Erosion, 95–96
Erythema
  inflammatory versus
      noninflammatory, 88–89
  malignancy and, 84
  of palm, 63, 64
Erythrocytosis, 103
Esophagus
  atresia and, 513
  mediastinal enlargement and, 234
  newborn and, 531
  pain and, 333–334
Esophoria, 130
Esotropia, 134, 523
Essential tremor, 481
Eustachian tube, 167
Eversion
  eyelid and, 124
  foot and, 453
Examination, general, 56–112. See also
      specific organ or system
  general appearance and, 57–70
    face and, 60
    habitus and, 60–61, 67–70
    hands and, 61–65
    history and, 58–59
    patient preparation and, 58
  hematopoietic system and, 101–112
    bone and, 109
    lymph nodes and, 104–108
    optic fundus and, 109
    skin and, 108–109
    special techniques for, 109–112
    spleen and, 108
  skin, 81–99
    anatomy and, 81
    color and, 86–89
    history and, 82–83
    lesions and, 95–99
    nail changes and, 90, 91
    texture and, 91–92
  structure and recording of, 21–33
    history and, 21–26
    impressions and, 32
    laboratory studies and, 31
    oral presentation, 33
    physical examination and, 26–31
    problem-oriented medical record
        system and, 589–595
    progress notes and, 32–33
  vital signs and, 71–79
    blood pressure and, 76–79
    history and, 71
    pulse and, 73–74
    respirations and, 74–76
    temperature and, 72–73
Excoriation, 82, 83

Exercise
  cardiac examination and, 304
  cardiovascular disease and, 246–
      247
Exophoria, 130, 132
Exophthalmos
  causes of, 123
  Graves', 122
Exostosis
  ear and, 157
  hard palate and, 172
  mandible and, 176
Exotropia, 132, 523
Expectoration, 202
Expiratory crackles, 224
Expiratory time, forced, 208
Expressive aphasia, 468
Extensor plantar reflex, 486
External auditory canal, 153
External ear, 157
Extinction, 500–501
Extra heart sound, 286–290
Extradural hematoma, 544
Extraocular muscle, 116
  child and, 523
  motor palsy and, 135
  movement, 130–134
  thyroid and, 194
Extravasation, urinary, 553
Extremities
  cardiovascular system and, 253–272
    arteries and, 253–261
    clubbing and. See Clubbing
    edema and, 264
    veins and, 261, 263–265
  hand and. See Hand
  leg and. See also Foot
    blood pressure and, 78
    fracture and. See Fracture
    straight-leg-raising test and, 428
  neurological examination and, 492–
      493
  muscles of, 421
    innervation of, 420
  physical examination and, 31
Exudate
  pleural effusion and, 235
  retina and, 145–147
Eye, 115–151
  anatomy and, 115–116
  child and, 522–523
  cranial nerves and, 470, 471–472
  elderly patient and, 538
  external examination and, 122–129
    anterior chamber and, 128
    conjunctiva and, 124, 127
    cornea and, 127–128, 129
    eyelid and, 124, 125, 126
    iris and, 128
    lacrimal system and, 124
    sclera and, 127

  extraocular movements and, 130–
      134
  funduscopic examination and, 139–
      150
    blurred visualization and, 141
    chorioretinal scarring and, 149–
        150
    optic nerve and, 147–149
    retinal hemorrhage and, 145–147
    retinal vessels and, 142–145
  hemangioma of, 98
  history and, 117–120
  intraocular pressure and, 150–151
  pain and, 117
  physical examination and, 30
  pupillary testing and, 134
  review of systems and, 25
  thyroid and, 194
  uremia and, 368
  visual acuity and, 120–122
  visual fields testing and, 136–139
Eyelash follicle, 125
Eyelid, 124
  edema of, 126
  lesions of, 125

Face
  cardiovascular disease and, 251
  child and, 522
  erythema and, 84
  gastrointestinal tract disorder and,
      340–341
  general appearance and, 60
  injury and, 546
  weakness and, 474–475, 476
Facet joint, 426
  dislocation and, 562
Facial nerve, 475–476
Fahrenheit scale, 72
Fainting
  cardiovascular disease and, 248, 249
  falls versus, 538
  neurological disorder and, 460
Falls, 538
Familial tremor, 480, 481
Family history, 25
Fasciculation of tongue, 478–479
Fat necrosis, traumatic, 324
Fatigue of inspiratory muscle, 232
Feculent breath, 342
Feculent vomiting, 337
Felon, 411
Female genitourinary system. See
      Genitourinary system, female
Femoral hernia, 385, 386
Femoral lymph node, 103, 107–108
Femoral pulse, 255
Femur, fracture and dislocation of,
      564–565
FET. See Forced expiratory time
Fetid breath, 342

Fetor hepaticus, 342
Fetus, 412
Fever, 72, 73
    child and, 512
    elderly patient and, 537
    gastrointestinal disorder and, 341
    seizure and, 516
FH. *See* Family history
Fiberoptic colonoscope, 361
Fibrillation, atrial, 262
    blood pressure and, 79
Fibroadenoma of breast, 324
Fibrocystic change in breast, 324
Fibroma
    gingival, 168
    ovarian, 407
Fibrosing alveolitis, 230, 231
Fibrosis, pulmonary, 223
Fine crackles, 224
Finger
    clubbing of. *See* Clubbing
    cyanosis of, 90
    hyperpigmentation and, 87
    trigger, 439
Fingernail. *See* Nail
Finkelstein's test, 437–438
First heart sound, 283–284
Fissure, 168
    anal, 360
    mouth and, 170
    palpebral, 124
Fistula, anorectal, 359
Flaccid paralysis, 422
Flail chest, 547
Flank, ecchymoses of, 357
Flatness, percussive, 216
Flexion contracture of hip, 443
Flexion response, triple, 486
Flexor muscles, 420
Floaters in eye, 118
Flow cytometry, 112
Fluid
    ascites and, 356
    intra-abdominal, 356
    knee and, 443, 445
    seromucous, 182
Flush
    malar, 60, 251
    malignancy and, 84
Follicle, eyelash, 125
Fontanel suture, 521, 522
Foot, 451–454
    fracture and, 570–571
    muscles of, 420
    transverse crease of, 531
    vibration and, 497
    vasculitis and, 97
Footdrop, nerve injury and, 560
Footdrop gait, 494, 495
Forced expiratory time, 208
Forearm fracture, 569

Fornix, superior, 124
Fourth heart sound, 287
Fracture, 556–558
    ankle and, 570
    arterial injury and, 560
    Barton's, 569–570
    chest wall trauma and, 547
    clavicle and, 564
    Colles', 569–570
    elbow and, 567–569
    facial, 546
    femur and, 564–565
    foot and, 570–571
    forearm and, 569
    hand and, 570–571
    hip joint and, 564–565
    humerus and, 565–567
    knee and, 567–569
    leg and, 569
    Monteggia's, 569
    pelvic, 563–564
        urinary tract and, 554
    Pott's, 570
    rib and, 211–212
    shoulder and, 565–566
    skull and, 544–545
    Smith's, 569–570
    tibial condyle and, 569
    vertebral, 560–563
    zygoma and, 546
Fremitus, 212–214
    compressed lung and, 233
Frenulum, 170, 176
Friction rub, pericardial, 288–289
Frontal sinus, 162–163
Fundus, ocular, 116
    hematologic disorders and, 109
    examination and, 30, 139–150
        blood vessels and, 142–145
        blurred image of, 141
        chorioretinal scarring and, 149–150
        hemorrhage and, exudates and, 145–147
        mydriatic drop and, 139
        nerve head and, 147–148
        neurologic, 470
Fungal infection of scalp, 93

Gait, 417–418
    child and, 517–518
    general appearance and, 60
    neurologic disorder and, 458
    neurological examination and, 494
    Trendelenburg, 442
Gallbladder, 351–352
    pain and, 334
Gallop rhythm, 288
    atrial, 287
    elderly patient and, 539
    ventricular, 286–287

Ganglion, wrist, 438, 439
Gangrene
    arterial insufficiency and, 254
    Richter's hernia and, 386
Gartner's duct cyst, 401
Gas, arterial blood, 228
    respiratory failure and, 232
Gastric pain, 333–334
Gastritis, 336
Gastrointestinal tract, 331–361
    abdominal examination and, 343–357. *See also* Abdomen
    aging and, 536
    anatomy and, 331–332
    bowel sounds and, 345–346
    general examination and, 340–342
    gynecologic disease and, 392
    laceration and, 553
    male genitourinary tract disorder and, 367
    mouth and, 342
    obstruction and, 336, 337, 346
    pain in, 333–337
    rectum and, 358–361
    review of systems and, 25–26
    rupture of intestine and, 553
    sliding hernia and, 385
    trauma and, 550–553
    uremia and, 368
    vomiting and. *See* Vomiting
General appearance, 57–70
Genetic disease, 514
Genitalia
    child and, 527–528
    female, 394–395, 396
    male, 363, 364, 377–382
    newborn and, 531
    physical examination and, 31
Genitourinary system
    elderly patient and, 539
    child and, 527–528
    female, 389–412
        anatomy and, 389–390
        bimanual examination and, 399, 403, 405
        cervical carcinoma and, 404
        cervix and, 402, 403
        external genitalia and, 394–395, 396
        general examination of, 393–394
        history and, 391–392
        infection and, 408–411
        ovaries and, 406, 407, 408
        pregnancy and, 411–412
        rectovaginal examination and, 406
        special tests and, 399
        speculum examination and, 397–398
        uterus and, 403, 405
        vaginal lesions and, 400–401

Genitourinary system—*Continued*
  male, 363–388
    anatomy and, 363–364
    bladder and, 375–377
    external genitalia and, 377–382
    hernia and, 382–386
    history and, 365–369
    kidney and, 370–373
    prostate gland and, 386–388
    ureter and, 373, 375
    review of systems and, 26
Geographic tongue, 175, 176
Geriatric examination, 533–540
  aging versus disease and, 535–536
  dyspnea and, 537
  falls and, 538
  fever and, 537
  history and, 534–535
  laboratory examination and, 539–540
  memory loss and, 538
  pain and, 536–537
  physical examination and, 538–539
  third heart sound and, 286
  urinary incontinence and, 537
  weight loss and, 537
Gestational age, 531
Gibbus, 210
Gingiva
  lesions of, 168
  leukemia and, 111
  periodontal disease and, 178–179
  signs and symptoms of, 166–167
Gland
  Bartholin's, 394, 396
  prostate, 386–388
  salivary, 165, 178
  skin and, 81
  thyroid, 186–188, 191–194
Glaucoma
  anterior chamber and, 128
  cupping of disc and, 148, 149
  infantile, 128
  mydriatic drops and, 139
  redness and, 119
  test for, 150–151
Globus hystericus, 167
Glossitis
  gastrointestinal disorder and, 342
  rhomboid, 176
Glossopharyngeal nerve, 477–478
Goiter, 191, 193
Gonorrheal infection, 408, 410
Gordon reflex, 486–487, 489
Gouty arthritis, 411
Graham Steell murmur, 298, 300
Granulocytopenia, 102
Graphesthesia, 500
Graves' exophthalmos, 122
Graves speculum, 397
Gray pigmentation, 86

Greenstick fracture, 557
Grey Turner's sign, 357
Grooving of nail, 91
Growth, 505–507
Growth plate trauma, 557–558
Guarding of abdomen, 349
Gum
  lesions of, 168
  leukemia and, 111
  periodontal disease and, 178–179
    signs and symptoms of, 166–167
Gynecomastia, 324–325

Habitus, 60
Hair, 92
  chest auscultation and, 222
  distribution of, 65–66
  loss of, 94
  physical examination and, 30
  sexual, 66
    child and, 527
Hairy leukoplakia, 174
Halitosis, 342
  gastrointestinal tract disorder and, 342–343
Hallucination, 464
Halo, 118
Hamman's sign, 225
Hand, 439–442
  fracture and, 570–571
  general appearance and, 60, 61–65
  muscle atrophy and, 480
  stereognosis and, 500
  thyroid disease and, 194
  vibration and, 497
  vitiligo of, 89
Handgrip exercise, 303
Hard palate, 171–172
Hashimoto's thyroiditis, 194
Head and neck, 113–194
  cranial nerves and. *See* Cranial nerve
  child and, 520–522
  circumference of, 508
  ears and. *See* Ear
  eye and. *See* Eye
  laryngopharynx, 167, 182, 183
  mouth and jaws and, 170–180
  nasopharynx and, 167, 180–182
  neck and, 185–194
  neurological disorder and, 466–467
  nodding and, 251
  nose and, 159–164
  oral cavity and, 164–183. *See also* Oral cavity
  pharynx and, 167
  physical examination and, 30
  review of systems and, 25
  trauma and, 543
  uremia and, 368
Headache
  elderly patient and, 536

eye pain and, 117
  neurologic disorder and, 460
Hearing loss
  elderly and, 534
  infant and, 525
  types of, 155, 156
Heart, 273–310
  anatomy of, 242–244
  child and, 526
  disorders of, 305–308
  failure and
    dyspnea and, 36
    left-sided, 236–237
  heart sounds and. *See* Heart sounds; Murmur, heart
  palpation of precordium and, 272–276
  percussion and, 276–277
  physical examination and, 30
  sternum fracture and, 547
  stethoscope and, 277–278
  thyroid disease and, 194
  uremia and, 368
  valve and. *See* Valve
Heart rate. *See* Pulse
Heart sounds, 280–302
  auscultation technique and, 282–283
  child and, 526
  extra, 286–310
    fourth, 287
    murmurs and, 289–310; *See also* Murmur, heart
    third, 286–287
  first, 283–284
  general, 280–282
  physical maneuvers and, 302–304, 309, 310
  second, 284–286
Heartbeat, palpation of. 248. *See also* Pulse
Heberden's nodes, 442
Heel, 451
Height, 517
Hemangioma
  eye and, 98
  tongue and, 175
Hematemisis, 205
Hematoma
  head injury and, 544
  intrapulmonary, 550
  spleen and, 552
Hematopoietic system, 101–112. *See also* Blood
  anatomy of, 101–103
  bone and, 109
  history and, 102–104
  lymph nodes and, 104–108
  mucous membranes and, 109
  optic fundus and, 109
  skin and, 108–109

special examination techniques and, 109–112
spleen and, 108
Hematoxylin and eosin stain, 111
Hematuria
causes of, 367
male genitourinary tract disorder and, 366
Hemianopsia, homonymous
illustration of, 138
neurologic examination and, 470–471
Hemiballismus, 480
Hemiparetic gait, 495
Hemiplegic gait, 494, 495
Hemodynamics, atrial, 268–271
Hemoglobin, 102
Hemogram, 31
Hemolysis, 110
Hemoptysis, 203
cardiovascular disease and, 248
causes of, 204
Hemorrhage. See also Bleeding
conjunctiva and, 127
intra-abdominal, 551–552
intraperitoneal, 552
preretinal, 147
retina and, 145–147
splinter, of nail, 91
subconjunctival, 119
subdural, 544
subungual splinter, 62
trauma and, 542
urinary tract and, 553
Hemorrhoid, 359
Hemothorax, 548
trauma and, 547
Hemophilia, 104
Hernia
external, 348
illustration of, 381
male patient and, 382–386
types of, 343–344
umbilical, 527
Herpes progenitalis, 379
Hip, 442–443, 444
fracture and dislocation of, 564–565
muscles of, 420
nerve injury and, 560
Hirschberg test, 523
Hirsutism, 66
History, patient, 21–26, 35–53
acute abdomen and, 335
approach to patient and, 44–48
cause and, 43–44
child and, 511–512
dermatologic, 83
experience and, 40
future and, 41–43
general appearance and, 58–59
goals of, 13–19

habitual experience and, 37–38
homeostasis and, denial in, 38
illness as temporal object and, 40–41
pain and, 48–50
patient, 35–53
personal, social, and past, 51–52
of present illness, 23–24
recording of, 22–26
value and, 39–40
vital signs and, 71
Hoarseness, 167
causes of, 169
chest disease and, 206
Hoffmann reflex, 484, 487, 490
Holosystolic murmur, 296–298
Homeostasis, 38
Homonymous hemianopsia, 470–471
Hordeolum, 125
Horizontal rectus muscle, 130
Hormone. See Endocrine system
Horner's syndrome, 131
eye and, 136
Horseshoe kidney, 372
Hum, venous, 269, 270
child and, 526
Humerus
fractures and, 565–567
shoulder and, 432–433
Huntington's chorea, 494
Hutchinson's incisor, 179
Hutchinson's pupil, 137
Hydrocele, 380, 381
canal of Nuck and, 386
Hydrocephalus, 520
Hydronephrosis, 372
Hydropneumothorax, 234
Hygroma, 522
Hyperesthesia, abdominal, 347–348
Hyperinflation, 216
Hyperkeratosis of tongue, 176
Hypermobility of tooth, 179
Hyperpigmentation. See also Pigmentation
adrenal insufficiency and, 69
nipple and, 316
porphyria cutanea tarda and, 87
Hyperplasia, splenic, 352
Hyperresonance, 216, 218
Hypertension, 368
physical findings in, 306
pulmonary
jugular venous pulse and, 269–270
physical findings in, 306
retinal vessels and, 145
retinopathy and, 143
Hyperthyroidism, 193–194
Hypertrophy
asymmetric septal, 296
breast, of newborn, 525

cardiomyopathy and, 259
subaortic murmur and, 296
muscle and, 479, 480
prostatic, 388
subaortic stenosis, 295, 296
physical findings in, 306
tongue and, 176
ventricular, 275–276
Hyphema, 128
Hypocalcemic tetany, 516
Hypoglossal nerve, 478
Hypoperfusion, cerebral, 459
Hypopigmentation, 86, 88
Hypopyon, 128
Hypospadias, 379
Hypotension, 79
abdominal trauma and, 550–551, 552
orthostatic, 538
Hypothermia, 73
Hypothyroidism, 188, 194
Hypoxemia, 206

Iliopectineal bursa, 443
Iliopsoas test, 357
Illumination. See also Transillumination
cornea and, 127–128
fundus and, 139
Illusion, 464
Imbalance, nerve disease and, 460
Immunoperoxidase staining, 111
Impetigo, 98
Implant, endometrial, 409
Incarcerated hernia, 385
Incisional hernia, 343
Incisor, Hutchinson's, 179
Incomplete fracture, 557
Incontinence
elderly patient and, 537
male patient and, 365
Indirect hernia, 382–384
Infant. See also Pediatric examination
history and, 510
premature, 530–531
Infantile glaucoma, 128
Infarction, myocardial
papillary muscle and, 298
physical findings in, 307
"real" disease and, 41
Infection
bone and, 423
chest and, 204
coma and, 459
conjunctiva and, 127
corneal, 128
female genitalia and, 408–411
fever and, 512
hemoptysis and, 203
impetigo and, 98
lymphadenopathy and, 106
muscle weakness and, 423

Infection—*Continued*
  musculoskeletal system and, 418
  nipple and, 316
  respiratory tract and, 206
  scalp and, 93
  urinary tract and, 537
  Vincent's, 179
Infertility, 392
Infiltration
  pulmonary, 218
  splenic, 353
Inflammation
  eye and, 125
  gallbladder and, 352
  gingival, 178
  iris and, 128
  laryngopharynx and, 167
  nasopharynx and, 167
  nipple and, 316
  prostate and, 387–388
  pupil and, 131
Inflammatory carcinoma of breast, 324
Inflammatory thrombosis, 263
Infraspinatus muscle, 420
Inguinal hernia, 382–384
Inguinal ligament, 564
Inguinal lymph node, 103, 107–108
Injured patient, 541–572
  abdomen and, 550–553
  chest wall and, 547–550
  facial examination and, 546
  head and, 543–545
  initial assessment of, 571–572
  musculoskeletal system and, 555–571
    ankle and, 570
    artery and, 560
    dislocation and, 558–559
    elbow and, 567–569
    foot and, 570–571
    forearm and, 569
    fracture and. *See* Fracture
    hand and, 570–571
    hip and femur and, 564–565
    knee and, 567–569
    leg and, 569
    ligaments, tendons, and muscles and, 559–560
    nerve and, 560
    pelvis and, 563–564
    position and, 555–556
    shoulder and, 565–566
    vertebra and, 560–563
  radiologic examination and, 542–543
  spine and, 546–547
  ventilation and, 541–542
Innervation of muscle of extremity, 420
Innocent murmur, 294, 296

Inspiration
  abdominal pain and, 336
  noisy, 218–219
    crackles and, 224
Inspiratory arrest, 351–352
Inspiratory muscle fatigue, 232
Intention tremor, 481
Intercostal space, 294
Interspinous ligament, 562
Intestine. *See* Gastrointestinal tract
Intra-abdominal bruit, 260
Intra-abdominal fluid, 356
Intra-abdominal hemorrhage, 551–552
Intra-abdominal inflammation, 357
Intracondylar fracture, 567–568
Intracranial pressure, 472
Intraductal papilloma, 324
Intranasal examination, 162
Intraocular pressure, 150–151
  mydriatic drops and, 139
  redness of eye and, 119
Intraperitoneal hemorrhage, 552
Intraperitoneal metastasis, 361
Intraperitoneal rupture of bladder, 554
Intrapulmonary hematoma, 550
Intraspinatus muscle, 431
Intrathoracic disease, 357
Intrathoracic pressure, 257
Intrauterine dwarfism, 514
Intussusception, intestinal, 512
Inversion
  eyelid and, 124
  foot and, 453
  nipple and, 316
Iris, 128
  redness of eye and, 119
Irreversible shock, 552
Ischemia
  cardiac papillary muscle and, 298
  pain and, 247
Ischiogluteal bursitis, 443
Ischiopubic junction, 563
Isometric exercise, 303
Isthmus, thyroid, 191
Itching, 82–83
  eyes and, 118

Jaundice
  gastrointestinal disorder and, 341
  infant and, 519
  sclera and, 127
Jaw, 165–166
  examination of, 170
Jaw jerk, 487
Jerk
  ankle, 529
  jaw, 487
Joint, 419. *See also specific joint*
Jugular venous pressure, 266–268

Kayser-Fleischer ring, 129
Keith-Wagener-Baker classification of hypertensive retinopathy, 143
Keratin, mucosal, 173
Keratitis, 129
Keratoconjunctivitis sicca, 129
Keratoconus, 129
Keratopathy, band, 129
Kernig's sign, 467
Kidney, 370–373
  aging and, 536
  pain and, 365–366
  palpation of, 354, 370
  renal stenosis and, 260
  trauma and, 553–554
Kiesselbach's plexus, 161
Kinetic tremor, 481
Knee, 443, 445–449
  fracture and dislocation of, 567–569
  muscles of, 420
  nerve injury and, 560
Knock, pericardial, 287
Knuckle fracture, 570
Koilonychia, 62, 91
Korotkoff sound, 76, 77, 78
  feeble, 79
Kussmaul's respiration, 74
Kyphosis, 210

Laboratory, clinical, 585–586
Laceration
  intestinal, 553
  liver and, 552
  scalp, 545
Lacrimal drainage, 119, 124
Ladin's sign, 411
Laminar flow, 289
Landau reflex, 529
Language, 467–469
Laryngitis, 167
Laryngopharynx, 167, 182, 183
Latissimus dorsi muscle, 420
Leading question, 21
Leg
  blood pressure and, 78
  cardiovascular disease and, 252
  fracture and, 569
  neurological examination and, 492–493
  straight-leg-raising test and, 428
Lens, 128
Leukemia, 103–104
  gums in, 111
Leukoplakia, 174
Levine sign, 247
Lid, 124
  edema and, 126
  lesions of, 125
Ligament
  breast cancer and, 317

broad, 403
collateral, 447–448
interspinous, 562
trauma and, 559–560
Light, photophobia and, 118
Light reflex
corneal, 130
pupillary, 134
neurologic examination and, 471
Light touch test, 500
Limb. *See* Extremities
Limbus, 128
Lindsay's nail, 62
Lingual frenulum, 174, 176
Lingual mucosa, 109
Lip
examination of, 170
gastrointestinal disorder and, 342
Lithotomy position, 394
Liver
laceration of, 552
palpation of, 350, 351–352
portal hypertension and, 343
yellow pigmentation and, 88
Loaded question, 21–22
Lobe, lung, 198
Locking of knee, 447
Lordosis, lumbar, 428–431
Low birth weight infant, 530–531
Lower extremity, 492–493
Lumbar plexus, 554
Lumbar spine, 428–431
Lumbrical muscle, 420
Lung
aging and, 535–536
anatomy of, 197–201
carcinoma and, 211
elderly patient and, 539
hemoptysis and, 203
pain and, 205
percussion and, 216, 218
physical examination and, 30
pulmonary function test and, 238
trauma and, 548–550
Lupus erythematosus, 251
Luschka joint, 426
Lymph node, 101–108
biopsy and, 111
child and, 520, 525
mediastinal enlargement and, 234
neck and, 189
supraclavicular
palpation and, 212
Lymphangiography, 111
Lymphedema, 319
Lymphohematopoietic system, 101–112. *See also* Hematopoietic system
Lymphoma, 103–104

Macroglossia, 176, 177
Macular degeneration, 151
Macule, 92
Malar flush, 60, 251
Male genitourinary system, 363–388. *See also* Genitourinary system, male
Malgaigne fracture, 563
Malignancy
bone and, 423
breast and, 321, 324
detection of, 313
skin retraction and, 317
cervical, 404
cutaneous manifestations of, 84
cystitis and, 376
hemoptysis and, 204
kidney and, 372
lung and, 211
lymph tissues and, 104
mediastinal enlargement and, 234
metastasis and. *See* Metastasis
nasopharynx and, 167
nipple and, 316
ovarian, 407, 408
penis and, 379, 380
prostate and, 388
retinal, 149
testicular, 380, 381
throat and, 167
Malleolus, 450, 451
Mallet finger, 411
Mammogram, 323
Mandible, 179–180
exostosis and, 176
trauma and, 546
Marcus Gunn pupil, 137
Mass
abdominal examination and, 355
bony, 423
breast and, 313
neck and, 186
renal, 366
throat and, 167
Mastitis, 324
Mastoid process, 157
Maxilla, 546
Maxillary sinus, 162–163
McMurray sign, 447
Mean pressure, 76
Meatus, urethral, 379
Meckel's diverticulum, 410
Median nerve, 438–439
Mediastinal crunch, 225, 228, 549–550
Mediastinal lesion
enlargement and, 234
lung and, 233
pain and, 205
Medical records, problem-oriented, 589–596

Mees' lines, 62, 91
Melanin, 86, 88
mucous membrane and, 92
Melanoma, 150
Membrane
mucous. *See* Mucous membrane
buccal, 171
periodontal, 179
tympanic, 153, 155
child and, 523, 525
examination of, 157–158
Memory
amnesia and, 465
elderly patient and, 538
neurologic disorder and, 460, 462
Meningeal signs, 467
Meniscus, torn, 447, 569
Menstruation
abdominal disorder and, 337
menstrual history and, 391–392
review of systems and, 26
temperature and, 72–73
Mental retardation, 515
Mental status, 462
elderly patient and, 538
Metabolic abnormalities
bone and, 423
muscle weakness and, 423
seizure and, 516
Metacarpal fracture, 570
Metaphysis, 557–558
Metastasis
breast cancer and, 320–321
intraperitoneal, 361
retinal, 149
skin and, 84
Microcephalus, 520, 522
Midsystolic murmur, 292–293
Miotic pupil, 131, 136
Mitral valve
anatomy and, 242
disorders of, 305
holosystolic murmur and, 296
prolapse and, 298, 299
prosthetic, 307
regurgitation and, 296, 298
amyl nitrate and, 310
isometric exercise and, 303
stenosis and, 300
cyanosis and, 251
Mixed angina, 247
Mixed hearing loss, 155
Mongolian spots, 519
Monophonic wheezing, paroxysmal, 222
Monteggia's fracture-dislocation, 569
Moro reflex, 529
Motor paralytic bladder, 377
Motor system
cerebral trauma and, 543–544

Motor system—*Continued*
  examination of, 479–481, 497
  extraocular palsy and, 135
  neuron atrophy and, 422
Mouth, 165–166
  breath sounds and, 229
  examination of, 30, 170
  facial nerve and, 476
  gastrointestinal disorder and, 342
  hypoglossal nerve and, 478
  odors and, 342
  review of systems and, 25
Movement
  abnormal, 479–481
  infant's head and, 522
  neurologic examination and, 497
Mucocele, lip, 170
Mucopurulent sputum, 202
Mucous membrane, 342
  lingual, 109
  buccal, 171
  gastrointestinal disease and, 342
  pigmentation and, 92, 173
Mucus
  nasal, 163
  sputum and, 202
Multiple myeloma, 104
Murmur, heart, 289–310
  aortic, 293–294
  child and, 517, 526
  continuous, 301–302
  diastolic, 298, 300–301
  ejection, 288, 293–294
  holosystolic, 296–298
  innocent, 294, 296
  late systolic, 298, 299
  midsystolic, 292–293
  pulmonic, 294
  subaortic, 296
  systolic, 292–298
    thyroid disease and, 194
Murphy's sign, 351–352
Muscle. *See also* Musculoskeletal
    system
  eye, 130, 133–134
    child and, 523
    extraocular, 130
  inspiratory, 232
  laryngeal, 182
  papillary, 298
Muscular dystrophy, 482
  spinal accessory nerve and, 478
Musculoskeletal system, 415–454
  aging and, 536
  anatomy and, 415–416
    history and, 416
  ankle and, 450–451, 570
  arterial injury and, 560
  atrophy and, 422
  bone and, 422, 423

chest auscultation and, 222
cervical spine and, 422–427
child and, 528–529
dislocation and. *See* Dislocation
elbow and, 567–569
examination of, 419, 423
extremity innervation and, 420
foot and, 451–454, 570–571
fracture and. *See* Fracture
hand and, 439–442, 570–571
hip and, 442–443, 444, 564–565
innervation and, 420–421
injury and, 560
joint and, 419
knee and, 443, 445–449, 567–569
leg and. *See* Leg
ligament, tendon, and muscle injury
  and, 559–560
lumbar spine and, 428–431
pain and, 416
pelvic and, 563–564
position of patient and, 555–556
posture and gait and, 417–418
shoulder and, 431–433, 435, 436,
  565–566
spasm and
  abdominal wall and, 348
  cervical, 186, 187
strength and, 481–482
thoracic spine and, 428
trauma and, 555–571. *See also*
  Injured patient
uremia and, 368
vertebra and, 560–563
weakness and, 423
wrist and, 437–439
Myasthenia gravis, 482
Mydriatic drop, 139
Mydriatic pupil, 131
Myeloma, multiple, 104
Myocardial infarction
  papillary muscle and, 298
  physical findings in, 307
  "real" disease and, 41
Myoclonus, 480, 481
Myopericarditis, 251
Myxedema, 67
Myxoma, 287

Nail
  change in, 90, 91
  gastrointestinal disorder and, 341
  hyperpigmentation and, 87
  physical examination and, 30
  pitting of, 90, 91
  systemic disease and, 62–63
Nares, 163
Nasal obstruction, 161
Nasal septum, 161
Nasal speculum, 162

Nasopharynx, 167, 180–182
Nausea
  abdominal disorder and, 337
  central nervous system disorder
    and, 513
Navicular bone, 451
Neck, 185–194
  anatomy and, 185–186
  cardiovascular disease and, 264–271
  cervical spine and, 423–427
  child and, 525
  history and, 186, 188
  neurological disorder and, 466–467
  physical examination and, 30
  thyroid and, 186, 188, 191–194
  vein and, 266–268
Necrosis, fat, 324
Needle paracentesis, 251
Neoplasm. *See* Malignancy
Nerve
  Arnold's, 153
  cranial. *See* Cranial nerve
  muscle of extremity and, 420
  trauma and, 560
  ulnar, 433
    palsy and, 435
  uremia and, 368
Nerve deafness, 476
Nerve head, optic, 147–148
  vessels and, 142
Nervous system, 455–501
  abnormal movement and, 480
  affective disorder and, 465
  aging and, 535
  anatomy and, 455–458
  aphasia and, 467–469
  cerebral function and, 491–494
  cerebral trauma and, 543
  child and, 529–530
  cognitive disorder and, 464–465
  conversion reaction and, 501
  cranial nerves and. *See* Cranial nerve
  esophagus and, 339
  examination and, 31
  fine sensory modalities and, 500–
    501
  head and neck examination and,
    466–467
  history and, 456–460
  mental status and, 462–463
  motor system and, 479–481
  muscle resistance and, 482–483
  pain and, 498
  perception disorder and, 463–464
  psychiatric disorder and, 463
  reflexes and, 483–491
  sensory examination and, 494
  station and gait and, 494, 495, 496
  strength and, 481–482
  temperature and, 498, 500

vibration, motion, and position and, 497
visual field defect and, 136–137, 470
Neurogenic bladder, 377
Neurologic examination. *See* Nervous system
Neuroma, plantar, 453, 454
Neuromuscular system, 26. *See also* Musculoskeletal system; Nervous system
Nevus vasculosus, 519
Newborn, 530–532
  eyes and, 522–523
  jaundice and, 519
Nicotine stomatitis, 172–173
Nipple
  lesions of, 316
  pregnancy and, 411
Nocturia, 366
Nocturnal dyspnea, 246
Node
  hand and, 439
  Heberden's, 442
  lymph. *See* Lymph node
  lymphoma cutis and, 97
  as skin lesion, 95
Nose, 159–164
  child and, 523–525
  fracture of, 546
  newborn and, 531
  physical examination and, 30
  review of systems and, 25
  uremia and, 368
Notes, progress, 32
Nuchal rigidity, 467
Nuck's canal, 386
Numbness
  lip and, 166
  neurologic disorder and, 459
Nutritional status, 341
Nystagmus, 133, 472
  infant and, 523

Obesity, 60–61
  peritoneal irritation and, 357
Obstruction
  airway, 229–231
  apnea and, 206
  arterial, 253–254
  bronchial, 233
    fremitus and, 214
  cardiomyopathy and, 259
  cystitis and, 376
  esophagus and, 339
  eustachian tube, 167
  hydronephrosis and, 372
  intestinal, 337
    bowel sounds and, 346
    vomiting and, 336
  nasal, 161

prostatism and, 368
ureteral, 373
ventricular outflow, 248
Obturator, 564
Occlusion
  aortic bifurcation and, 254
  arterial, 253–254
  dental, 179–180
Occult blood, 337
Ocular fundus. *See* Fundus, ocular
Oculomotor nerve, 471
Oculomotor paralysis, 123, 134
Odontoid fracture, 562
Odor
  breath and, 342
  sputum and, 203
Olecranon, 568
Olfactory nerve, 469
Olfactory organ, 163
Omphalocele, 343
Onycholysis, 62–63, 90
Open dislocation, 559
Open fracture, 558
Open wound of chest, 548
Opening snap, 287
Ophthalmoscopy, 470
Opisthotonus, 517, 518
Oppenheim reflex, 486, 489
Opponens digiti minimi, 420
Optic disc, 147–148
  cupping of, 148, 149
Optic fundus. *See* Fundus, ocular
Optic nerve, 147–148, 470
Oral cavity, 164–183
  gums and, 168, 178–180
  history and, 165–166
  hoarseness and, 169
  laryngopharynx and, 167, 182, 183
  nasopharynx and, 167, 180–182
  newborn and, 531
  oropharynx and, 167
  tongue and, 176–177
  mucosa and, 173, 342
Oral presentation, 33
Orbit
  auscultation and, 466
  pain and, 117
Orchitis, 380, 381
Orchlamydial vaginitis, 400
Orders, standard, 595–596
Orientation, 462
Oropharynx, 167
Orthopnea, 247
Orthostatic hypotension, 78
  elderly patient and, 538
Osteoarthritis
  cervical spine and, 424
  hand and, 440
  knee and, 443
Osteoarthropathy, pulmonary, 211

Otoscope, 157, 524
Ovary, 406, 407
  abscess and, 411
  cyst and, 356
Ovulation, temperature and, 73
Oxygenation, 102, 244, 245

Paget's disease of breast, 315, 324
  nipple and, 316
Pain
  abdomen and, 334–337
    child and, 512–513
  appendiceal, 334
  bladder, 375–377
  cardiovascular disease and, 247–248
  chest
    pulmonary disease and, 203
    sources of, 205
  colonic, 334
  cornea and, 127–128
  duodenal, 334
  elderly patient and, 536–537
  eye and, 117
  fracture and, 558
  gallbladder, 334
  gastrointestinal tract and, 333
  hip bursa and, 443
  intra-abdominal hemorrhage and, 551
  ischemic, 247
  male genitourinary tract and, 365–366
  menstrual, 391
  musculoskeletal, 416
    trauma and, 556
  neurologic disorder and, 460
    examination and, 498, 500
  pancreatic, 334
  patient history and, 48–50
  rectal, 334
  renal, 371
  shoulder and, 433
    causes of, 436
  skin and, 82
  spinal fracture and, 561
Palate, 171–172
  paralysis and, 477–478
Pallor, 108
  gastrointestinal disorder and, 341
Palm, 63, 65
Palpable lesion, skin, 95
Palpation
  abdomen and, 347–357
  blood pressure and, 76
  breast and, 317–323
  carotid pulse and, 189
  fetus and, 412
  foot and, 453
  hip and, 443
  joint and, 419

Palpation—*Continued*
kidney and, 370
precordium and, 272–276
prostate gland and, 387
respiratory disease and, 211–214
rotator cuff and, 433
thyroid gland and, 191
tongue and, 176
Palpebral fissure, 124
Palpitation, 248
Palsy
extraocular motor, 135
trochlear, 134
ulnar nerve, 435
Pancreatic pain, 334
Papanicolaou smear, 399, 403
Papilla, ocular, 109
Papillary muscle dysfunction, 298
Papilledema, 148–149
neurologic examination and, 470
Papilloma, intraductal, 324
Papule, 95
Paradoxical incontinence, 365
Paradoxical pulse, 550
Paradoxical respiration, 232
Paradoxical splitting of second heart
sound, 285–286
Parallelism of eyes, 133
Paralysis
chest wall muscle, 547
cranial nerves and, 477
diaphragmatic, 232
eye muscle and, 130, 134
facial, 522
flaccid, 422
oculomotor, 123
pupil and, 131
vocal cord, 167, 477–478
Paralytic bladder, 377
Paralytic ileus, 346
Paraphimosis, 378, 379
Parenchymal disorder
hemoptysis and, 204
pain and, 205
Parkinsonism, 479, 481
gait of, 494, 496
Paronychia, 411
Parotid duct orifice, 171
Parotid gland, 165, 178
enlargement of, 178
Paroxysmal atrial tachycardia, 262
Paroxysmal monophonicwheezing, 222
Paroxysmal nocturnal dyspnea, 246
Partial pressure of oxygen, 74
Past history, 24–25, 51–52
Patch, 92
white, 173
Patella, 443
dislocation and, 568
reflex and, 483
Pathologic obesity, 60–61

Patient history, 35–53
Patient-physician relationship, 4–13
PCO₂, 74
Pearls, Epstein's, 531
Peau d'orange lesion, 319, 324
Pectoralis major, 420
Pectoriloquy, 225
Pectus carinatum, 208, 210
Pectus excavatum, 208
Pediatric examination, 505–532
abdomen and, 526–527
pain and, 512–513
chest and, 525–526
dyspnea and, 515
ear, nose, and throat and, 523–525
eyes and, 522–523
face and, 522
fever and, 512
fracture and, 556–557
general appearance and, 517–518
genitalia and, 527–528
head and, 520–522
history and, 506–511
innocent murmur and, 294
lymph nodes and, 520
musculoskeletal system and, 528–529
neck and, 525
neurologic, 529–530
newborn and, 530–532
pelvic examination and, 393
rectal, 528
retardation and, 515
seizure and, 515–516
skin and, 519
stridor and, 515
vital signs and, 518–519
vomiting and, 513
weight and
failure to gain, 513–514
growth curves and, 506–507
Pelvis
examination and, 389–412
cervical lesions and, 402, 405–406
competency of examiner and, 393–395
external genitalia and, 394–395, 396
history and, 391–392
infection and, 408–411
saline drop and, 395, 397
special tests and, 399, 403, 405, 406
vaginal lesions and, 400–401
fracture and, 563–564
urinary tract and, 554
nerve injury and, 560
Pelvic inflammatory disease, 408–411
Penetrating wound
chest wall and, 548
head and, 545

Penis, 377–380
child and, 527
Perception disorder, 463–464
Percussion
abdomen and, 347–357
chest and, 214–218
child and, 525–526
heart and, 276–277
kidney and, 370
Percussion wave, 256
Perforation
intra-abdominal hemorrhage and, 551–552
nasal septum and, 161
Pericardial effusion, 550
Pericardial friction rub, 288–289
Pericardial knock, 287
Pericarditis
constrictive, 276
physical findings in, 308
Pericoronitis, 179
Perineal body, 395
Perinephric abscess, 372
Perineum tenderness, 394
Periodontal disease, 178–179
abscess and, 168
Periodontal membrane, 179
Peripheral blood smear, 109–110
Peripheral cyanosis, 252
Peripheral nerve trauma, 554–555
Peripheral vision, 117, 136
Peristalsis, 346
Peritoneal irritation, 357
Peritoneal penetration, 550–551
Peritonitis, 410
Pernicious anemia, 111
Personal history, 51–52
Perthes' test, 263
Petechia, 95
hematologic disorders and, 108–109
Pharyngeal paralysis, 477–478
Pharyngeal tonsil, 181
Phimosis, 378, 379
Phlebothrombosis, 263–264
Phlegm, 202
Phoria, 130
Photophobia, 118
cornea and, 127–128
Physical examination. *See* Examination, general
Physician-patient relationship, 4–13
Physiologic splitting of second heart sound, 284
Pigeon breast, 208, 210
Pigmentation
adrenal insufficiency and, 69
porphyria cutanea tarda and, 87
malignancy and, 84
melanin, 86, 88
nipple and, 316
pregnancy and, 411

oral mucosa and, 173
  yellow, 86, 88
    gastrointestinal tract and, 341
Pilonidal cyst, 357
Pinguecula, 127
Pinprick test, 498
Pitting of nail, 90, 91
Plantar neuroma, 453, 454
Plantar reflex, 484, 486–487
Plaque, 95
Platelets, 103
Pleural effusion, 231, 233–234, 235
Pleural pain, 205
Pleural rub, 225
Plop, tumor, 287
Pneumaturia, 366
Pneumothorax, 234, 237
  bulla versus, 239
  causes of, 237
  hemothorax and, 548
  hyperresonance and, 218
  mediastinal crunch and, 225
  trauma and, 547, 549
Pocket lesions, periodontal, 178–179
Polycystic kidney, 372–373
Polyp, rectum, 360
Popliteal artery, 260
Porphyria cutanea tarda, 87
Portal hypertension, 343
Position
  gastrointestinal disorder and, 341
  heart auscultation and, 281–282
  lithotomy, 394
  Moro reflex and, 529
  neurological examination and, 497
  respiratory examination and, 238
  trauma and, 555–556
Posterior dislocation of hip, 564, 565
Posture, 417–418
  child and, 517
Pott's fracture, 570
Precipitous micturition, 365
Precocious sexual development, 528
Precordium, 272–276
Pregnancy, 411–412
Premature beat
  atrial, 262
  pulse and, 74
  ventricular, 262
Premature infant, 530–531
Prenatal visit, 411–412
Preretinal hemorrhage, 146, 147
Pressure
  intraocular, 139, 150–151
    redness of eye and, 119
  intrathoracic, 257
  pulse, 194
Pulse pressure, 76
  thyroid disease and, 194
  Valsalva maneuver and, 257
  widened, 79

Presystolic extra sound, 287
Problem solving, clinical, 575–583
Problem-oriented medical record,
  589–595
PROM. See Problem-oriented medical
  record
Proctoscopy, 361
Progress notes, 32
Prolapse
  mitral valve, 298, 299, 305
  rectal, 361
Prompt squatting, 310
Pronator digitorum sublimis muscle,
  420
Proptosis, 123
Prostate gland, 365, 368, 386–388
Prosthetic heart valve, 307
Protodiastolic extra sound, 286–287
Pruritus, 82–83
Psoas muscle
  appendicitis and, 336
  transverse process fracture and,
    563
Psoriasis, 90, 91
Psychiatric status, 462, 463
Pterygium, 127
Ptosis, 471
  causes of, 123
Ptyalism, 166
Puberty, abnormal, 528
Pulmonary circulation, 242, 245
Pulmonary disorder
  edema and, 236–237
  trauma and, 548–550
Pulmonary function, 238
Pulmonary hypertension
  jugular venous pulse and, 269–270
  physical findings in, 306
Pulmonary valve
  stenosis, 285
    physical findings in, 306
  murmur and, 294
  regurgitation and, 298, 300
Pulp
  felon and, 411
  tooth, 179
Pulse, 73–74
  arterial, 254–260
  carotid. See Carotid pulse
  child and, 509, 518
  gastrointestinal disorder and, 341–
    342
  orthostatic blood pressure and, 78
  paradoxical, 550
  radial, 73–74, 255
    cervical spine examination and,
      426–427
    palpation of, 75
  thyroid disease and, 194
  venous, 190
    jugular, 268–271

Pulse pressure, 76
  thyroid disease and, 194
  Valsalva maneuver and, 257
  widened, 79
Pulsus alternans, 258, 259
Pulsus bisferiens, 258, 259
Pulsus paradoxus, 259–260
Pulsus parvus, 258, 259
Pulsus tardus, 258, 259
Puncta, 124
Pupil, 128
  abnormalities of, 131, 471–472
  elderly patient and, 538
  redness of eye and, 119
Pupillary reflex, 134
  abnormal, 137
  neurologic examination and, 471
Purpura, 86, 95
  vasculitis and, 97
Purulent sputum, 202
Pus
  corneal infection and, 128
  Skeen's gland and, 395
  sputum and, 202
Pustule, 95
Pyelonephritis, 371
Pyloric stenosis, 513
Pyohydronephrosis, 372
Pyramidal tract disease, 488
Pyrogens, 73

Quadrantanopsia, 138
  neurologic examination and, 471

Radial nerve, 554
Radial periosteal reflex, 485
Radial pulse, 73–74, 255
  cervical spine examination and,
    426–427
  palpation of, 75
Radiography
  chest and, 226–228
  dislocation and, 559
  hematologic disorders and, 111–
    112
  physical examination and, 31
  trauma and, 542–543, 555
Radius, 569
Rale, 224–225
Range of motion
  ankle and, 450, 451
  cervical spine and, 425
  elbow and, 433
  hand and, 439
  hip and, 444
  knee and, 447
  lumbar spine and, 428, 429
Raynaud's phenomenon, 90
Reading, 468–469
Rebound tenderness, 357
Receptive aphasia, 468–469

Record
    history and, 22–26
    problem-oriented, 589–596
Rectal temperature, 73
Rectocele, 395
Rectovaginal examination, 406
Rectum, 358–361
    examination and, 31
        abdominal trauma and, 550–551
        child and, 393, 528
        spinal examination and, 430
    pain and, 334
Rectus muscle, 348
    weakness or paralysis of, 130
Red cell, 103
Red reflex, 522–523
Redness
    erythema and, 88–89
        malignancy and, 84
        palm and, 63, 64
    eye and, 119
Reduction of hernia, 385
Referred pain, 416
Reflex, 483–491
    corneal
        extraocular movement and, 130
        neurologic examination and, 472–473
        newborn and, 522–523
    head injury and, 544
    infant and, 529
    normal, 483
    pathologic, 484–487
    pupillary, 134
        abnormal, 137
        neurologic examination and, 471
    pyramidal tract disease and, 488–489
    superficial skin, 487, 491
Reflex neurogenic bladder, 377
Regurgitation
    aortic. See Aortic valve, regurgitation
        and holosystolic murmur and,
        296–298
    mitral, 298, 300, 305
        amyl nitrate and, 310
        isometric exercise and, 303
    pulmonic, 298, 300
    tricuspid, 307
Relaxation, muscle, 482
Renal artery, 260
Renal disorder. See Kidney
Resistance, muscle, 482–483
Resistance vessel, 242
Resonance, 216
Respiration, 74–76
    abdominal pain and, 336
    cerebral trauma and, 543
    dyspnea and, 515
    gastrointestinal disorder and, 341
Respiratory alternans, 232

Respiratory rate
    child and, 518
    respiratory failure and, 232
    second heart sound and, 284
Respiratory system, 197–239
    aging and, 535–536
    anatomy and, 197–201
    arterial blood gases and, 228
    auscultation and, 218–225
    disorders of, 229–237
    elderly patient and, 537
    failure and, 232
    history and, 201–206
    inspection and, 208–211
    palpation and, 211–214
    percussion and, 214–218
    premature infant and, 531
    roentgenogram and, 226–228
    special maneuvers and, 237–239
    spirometry and, 228
    stridor and, 515
Resting tremor, 479, 480
Retardation, mental, 515
Retention cyst
    lip and, 170
    mouth and, 176
    nipple and, 316
Retinal vessels, 142–145
Retraction, skin, 317
Review of system, 25–26
Rheumatoid arthritis, 440
Rhinitis, 161
Rhomboid glossitis, 176
Rhomboideus muscle, 420
Rhoncus, 220, 223, 224
    child and, 526
    fremitus and, 214
Rhythm, cardiac
    abnormal. See Arrhythmia
    normal, 281–282
Rib fracture, 547
    cough and, 211–212
Richter's hernia, 386
Rigidity
    abdominal, 348
    muscle and, 482–483
    nuchal, 467
    parkinsonism and, 481
Rigor, 73
Ring
    anal, 359–360
    Kayser-Fleischer, 129
    Waldeyer's, 181
Ringworm of scalp, 519
Rinne's test, 159
Roentgenography. See Radiography
Romberg's sign, 494, 496
ROS. See Review of system
Rotator cuff, 433
Roth's spot, 147

Rub
    abdominal sound and, 346
    pericardial friction, 288–289
    pleural, 225
Rubor, 108
Rupture
    bladder and, 554
    intestine and, 553
    splenic, 552–553
    vertebral disk and, 431

Sacroiliac joint, 430–431
    fracture and, 563
    subluxation and, 430
Saddlebag hernia, 386
Saline drop, 395, 397
Saliva, 166
Salivary gland, 165, 178
Saphenous vein, 263
Scalp
    fungal infection of, 93
    hair and, 92
    laceration and, 545
    ringworm of, 519
Scapula, 432
Scapulohumeral joint, 565
Scarring
    chorioretinal, 149–150
    corneal, 128
        funduscopic examination and, 141
Schiotz tonometer, 151
Sciatic nerve, 554
Sciatica, 431
Scissors gait, 496
Sclera, 127
Sclerosis of retinal vessel, 143
Scoliosis, 210
    Perinephric abscess and, 371
Scraping, cervical, 403
Scratching, 83
Scrotum, 380–382
    mass and, 366
Seborrheic dermatitis, 519
Second heart sound, 284–286
Secretion, nasal, 163
Seizure
    child and, 515–516, 522
    neurologic disorder and, 457
Self-examination of breast, 325–327
Senile cataract, 117
Senile tremor, 480, 481
Senile vaginitis, 400
Sensorineural hearing loss, 155, 156
Sensory ataxia, 493, 495
Sensory examination, 494–497
Sensory paralytic bladder, 377
Septum
    cardiac
        asymmetric hypertrophy and, 296
        atrial, 308

holosystolic murmur and, 296
ventricular, 297–298, 308
nasal, 161
Serology, 31
Seromucous fluid, 182
Serratus muscle, 432
Sexual development, 527–528
secondary characteristics and, 509
Sexual dysfunction
female patient and, 392
male, 368
neurologic disorder and, 458
Sexual hair
child and, 527
distribution of, 66
SH. *See* Social history
Shock
abdominal wound and, 552
hypotension and, 79
Shortness of breath. *See* Dyspnea
Shoulder, 431–433, 435, 436
fracture and dislocation of, 565
Shunt, arteriovenous, 242
Sigmoidoscopy, 361
Simple fracture, 557, 558
Sinus
carotid, 264
palpation of, 162
transillumination of, 162–163
Sinus tachycardia, 283–284
Sinusitis, 161
Skeletal system. *See* Bone;
Musculoskeletal system
Skene's glands, 395
Skin, 81–99
adrenal insufficiency and, 69
aging and, 536
anatomy and, 81
breast cancer and, 317, 320
child and, 519
color changes and. *See* Pigmentation
gastrointestinal disorder and, 341
hematologic disorders and, 108–109
lesions of, 92–99
malignancy and, 84
mucous membrane and, 92
peripheral nerve injury and, 554
physical examination and, 30
pruritus and, 82–83
review of systems and, 26
scrotum and, 380
texture of, 89, 91–92
thyroid disease and, 194
uremia and, 368
vasoconstriction and, 253
vasodilation and, 252–253
Skin reflex, 487, 491
Skull
auscultation and, 466
child and, 521

fracture and, 544–545
radiologic examination and, 543
Sleep apnea, 206
Sliding hernia, 385, 386
Sludging, microcirculatory, 103
Small intestine. *See* Gastrointestinal
tract
Smear
Papanicolaou, 399, 403
peripheral blood, 109–110
Smell, sense of, 163
olfactory nerve and, 469
Smith's fracture, 569–570
Snap, opening, 287
Snellen chart, 120–121
child and, 523
Snoring, 206
Social history, 25, 51–52
Soft palate, 171–172
Sole, transverse crease of, 531
Sore throat, 167
Sound
bowel, 345–346
breath. *See* Breath sounds
heart. *See* Heart sounds; Murmur,
heart
Korotkoff's, 79
Spasm, 482–483
abdominal wall and, 348
cervical muscle, 186, 187
tetanic, 480
Speculum
nasal, 162
pelvic, 397–398
Speech
aphasia and, 467–469
child and, 517
cranial nerve and, 477–478
general appearance and, 60
neurologic disorder and, 458
Spermatic cord, 380–381
Spermatocele, 381
Sphygmomanometer, 76
pulsus paradoxus and, 260
Spigelian hernia, 344
Spike-and-dome pulse, 258, 259
Spinal accessory nerve, 478
Spinal injury, 542
Spine
cervical, 422–427
radiologic examination and, 543
injuries of, 546–547
fracture and dislocation and, 560–
563
osteoarthritis of cervical, 424
Spinous process fracture, 562
Spirometry, 228
Splash, succussion, 346
Spleen, 108
palpation of, 352–354

subcapsular hematoma of, 552
trauma and, 552–553
Splinter hemorrhage of nail, 62, 91
Splitting of second heart sound, 284–
286
Spoken voice test, 158
Spondylolisthesis, 428
Spoon nail, 62, 91
Spot
mongolian, 519
Roth's, 147
Spotting of blood, 391
Sprain, 559
Spring sign, 447
Sputum, 202, 203
Squatting, prompt, 310
Stance, 417
Standard orders, 595–596
Stare, Stellwag's, 122
Stasis ulcer, 99
Stellwag's sign, 122
Stenosis
heart sound and, 285
hypertrophic subaortic, 306
mitral, 300, 305
cyanosis and, 251
isometric exercise and, 303
pulmonary, 306
pyloric, 513
renal artery, 260
tricuspid, 301
physical findings in, 307
urethral meatus and, 379
Stensen's duct, 171
Stereognosis, 500
Sternal pectoralis muscle, 420
Sternocleidomastoid muscle
cranial nerve and, 478
innervation of, 420
Sternum, 547
Stethoscope, 277–278
blood pressure and, 76
bruit and, 466
chest auscultation and, 219
Stiff neck, 186, 187
Stokes-Adams attack, 248
Stomach. *See* Abdomen;
Gastrointestinal tract
Stomatitis
angular, 109
gastrointestinal disorder and, 342
nicotine, 172–173
Vincent's, 168
Stone. *See* Calculus
Stool, 337
Strabismus, 523
Straight-leg-raising test, 428
Strain
eye, 120
ligament and, 559

Strangulated hernia, 385, 386
Strength, muscle, 481–482
Stress incontinence, 365
Stricture, ureteral, 373
Stridor, 219
    child and, 515
Stroke, 189
Stroke volume, 79
Stye, 125
Subaortic murmur, 296
Subaortic stenosis, 306
Subcapsular hematoma of spleen, 552
Subcapularis muscle, 420
Subclavian steal syndrome, 466–467
Subconjunctival hemorrhage, 119
Subcostal angle, 209
Subcutaneous emphysema, 214, 549–
    550
Subdural hematoma, 544
Subluxation, 558–559
    sacroiliac joint and, 430
    vertebra and, 562
Submandibular gland, 165, 178
Subungual splinter hemorrhage, 62
Succussion splash, 346
Sucking, 529
Superior fornix, 124
Superior vena cava syndrome, 104
Supraclavicular lymph node, 101, 106
    palpation and, 212
Supraclavicular space, bruit in, 466–
    467
Supracondylar fracture, 567–568
Suprapubic mass, 366
Supraspinatus muscle
    atrophy of, 431
    innervation of, 420
Suspensory ligament of breast, 317
Suture, cranial, 522
Swallowing
    cranial nerves and, 477
    difficulty in, 167
Sweating, 91–92
    cardiovascular disease and, 252
Swelling
    bone and, 423
    foot and, 451
    gingival, 167
    mandible and, 176
    musculoskeletal system and, 418,
        419
    optic nerve head, 148–149
    oral cavity and, 166
        mucosa and, 173
    wrist ganglion and, 439
Swing of gait, 417
Symmetry. See Asymmetry
Symphysis pubis fracture, 563
Syncope
    cardiovascular disease and, 248, 249
    falls versus, 538

Syndactyly, 411
Syphilis
    chancre and, 379
    primary lesion of, 379
    pupil and, 131
Systemic circulation, 242–246
Systole, 281–282
Systolic blood pressure, 259–260
Systolic bruit, 194
Systolic click, 288
    mitral prolapse and, 298
Systolic murmur, 292–298
    thyroid disease and, 194
Systolic wave of pulse, 256

Tabes dorsalis, 494
Tachycardia
    paroxysmal atrial, 262
    pulse and, 74
    sinus, 283–284
    syncope and, 248
    ventricular, 262
Tachypnea, 74, 76
Tactile discrimination, two-point, 500
Tactile fremitus, 212, 214
Tandem walking, 494
Taste, 476
Tattoo, amalgam, 173
Tear
    meniscal, 447, 569
    tendon, 559–560
Tearing of eye, 119, 124
Teeth, 166–167, 179
Telangiectasia, 251
Temperature, 72–73
    child and, 518
    neurological examination and, 498,
        500
    skin, 91
    thyroid disease and, 194
Temporomandibular joint, 179–180
Tenderness
    abdominal, 349
    ankle and, 450
    bladder and, 355
    foot and, 453–454
    fracture and, 558
    hip and, 443
    knee and, 443
    rebound abdominal, 357
    rotator cuff and, 433
Tendon
    Achilles, 450
        newborn and, 529
    reflexes and, 483–491
    trauma and, 559–560
Tendon reflex, deep, 544
Tennis elbow, 433
Tenosynovitis of ankle, 450
Tension pneumothorax, 234, 236, 549
Teres minor, 420

Terry's nail, 62, 91
Testis, 380–382
Tetany
    hypocalcemic, 516
    neurologic examination and, 480
Texture of skin, 89, 91–92
Thermal stimuli, 91. See also
        Temperature
Thinking
    abstract, 462–463
    neurologic disorder and, 460
Third heart sound, 286–287
Thomas test, 443, 445
Thoracic outlet, 426
Thoracic spine, 428
Thorax. See Chest
Thrill
    carotid, 264
    thyroid and, 194
Throat
    child and, 523–525
    pharyngeal paralysis and, 477–478
    physical examination and, 30
    review of systems and, 25
    sore, 167
    uremia and, 368
Thrombocytopenia, 102
Thrombocytosis, 103
Thrombophlebitis, 263
Thrombosis
    hemorrhoids and, 359
    venous, 263–264
Thrush, 531
Thumb
    gouty arthritis of, 411
    muscle weakness and, 438
Thyroid, 186–188, 191–194
    eye signs of, 122
Thyroiditis, 194
Thyrotoxicosis, 187, 188, 193–194
Tibia
    condyle fracture and, 569
    dislocation and, 568
Tidal wave, 256
Tietze's syndrome, 211
Tinea capitis, 93, 519
Tinel's sign, 439
Tinnitus, 155
Toddler, 510. See also Pediatric
        examination
Toe, 451, 453
    muscles of, 420
    vibration and, 497
Tone, muscle, 482–483
    infant and, 529
Tongue, 166, 176
    gastrointestinal disorder and, 342
    lesions of, 174
    macroglossia and, 177
    pernicious anemia and, 111
Tonometer, Schiotz, 151

Tonsil, 171
  child and, 525
  pharyngeal, 181
Torsion of spermatic cord, 380–381
Torticollis, 190
  child and, 525
Torus fracture, 557
Torus mandibularis, 177
Torus palatinus, 172
Touch test, 500
Toxin
  ataxia and, 493
  coma and, 459
  muscle weakness and, 423
Toxoplasmosis, 150
Trachea, 189
  palpation and, 212–213
  tension pneumothorax and, 549
Tracheal breathing, 220, 222
Transillumination
  head of infant and, 522
  hydronephrosis and, 372
  kidney and, 370–371
  scrotum and, 380
  sinus and, 162–163
Transudate, 235
Transverse crease of sole, 531
Transverse groove of nail, 91
Transverse process fracture, 562–563
Trapezius muscle
  cranial nerve and, 478
  innervation of, 420
Trauma. See Injured patient
Traumatic fat necrosis, 324
Tremor, 479–481
  thyroid and, 194
Trendelenburg gait, 442
Trendelenburg's sign, 442
Trendelenburg's test, 263
Triceps tendon reflex, 485
  innervation of, 420
Trichomonas vaginitis, 401
Tricuspid valve
  anatomy and, 242
  holosystolic murmur and, 296
  regurgitation and, 297, 307
  stenosis and, 301, 307
Trigeminal nerve, 472–474
Trigger finger, 439
Triple flexion response, 486
Trisomy 21, 518
Trochanteric bursitis, 443
Trochlear nerve, 471
Trochlear palsy, 134
Tropia, 130
Tubing of stethoscope, 277
Tubo-ovarian abscess, 411
Tumor. See Malignancy
Tumor necrosis factor, 104

Tumor plop, 287
Tuning fork test
  hearing and, 158–159
  vibration and, 497
Turbulent blood flow, 289
Two-point tactile discrimination, 500
Tympanic membrane, 153, 155
  child and, 523, 525
  examination of, 157–158
Tympany
  abdomen and, 355–356
  chest percussion and, 216, 218

Ulcer, 95–96
  anal, 360
  corneal, 127, 129
  lip and, 166
  mucosal, 173
  nipple and, 316
  stasis, 99
Ulna
  dislocation and, 568
  Monteggia's fracture and, 569
Ulnar nerve
  epicondylitis and, 433
  injury and, 554
  palsy and, 435
Umbilicus, 344
  hernia and, 343, 527
Undescended testes, 381–382
Uninhibited neurogenic bladder, 377
Uncovertebral articulation, 426
Unstable angina, 247
Upper extremity. See also Hand
  cardiovascular disease and, 252
  neurological examination and, 491–492
Ureter, 373, 375
Urethra
  inflammation and, 365
  stenosis and, 379
  trauma and, 553–554
Urge incontinence, 365
Urinary bladder. See Bladder
Urinary tract. See also Genitourinary system
  gynecologic disease and, 392
  elderly patient and, 537
  trauma and, 553–554
Urination
  blood in
    causes of, 367
    male patient and, 366
  pain on, 336
Uriniferous breath, 342
Uterus, 403, 405
  palpation of, 355
  pregnancy and, 411
Uvula, 477

V wave, 269, 270
Vagina
  bimanual rectal examination and, 358
  discharge and, 392
  pool sampling and, 403
Vaginitis, 400–401
Vagus nerve, 477–478
Valgus, 449
Valsalva maneuver
  cardiac examination and, 304
  carotid sinus pressure and, 264
  ejection murmur and, 296
  pulse and, 257
Valve
  aortic. See Aortic valve
  mitral. See Mitral valve
  prosthetic, 307
  pulmonary
    stenosis and, 285, 306
    murmur and, 294
    regurgitation and, 298, 300
  relationships of, 242
  tricuspid. See Tricuspid valve
Variant angina, 247
Varicose vein, 261, 263
  hemorrhoid and, 359
Variocele, 381
Varus, 449
Vas deferens, 380
Vascular disorder, 97. See also Cardiovascular system
  abdominal disorder and, 337
  congestion and, 119
  hemoptysis and, 204
  lung and, 205
  mediastinal enlargement and, 234
Vascularity
  conjunctiva and, 124
  cornea and, 128
Vasculitis, 97
Vasoconstriction, 253
Vasodilation, 252
Vein
  abdominal, 343
  extremity and, 261
  neck, 266–268
  respiratory disease and, 211
  retinal, 143, 145
  saphenous, 263
Vena cava syndrome, 104
Venous hum, 526
Venous pressure, jugular, 266–268
Venous pulse, 190
Venous thrombosis, 263–264
Ventilatory function, 207–208. See also Respiratory system
  crush injury and, 547
  pulmonary function test and, 238
Ventricle, 242
  gallop and, 286–287

Ventricle—*Continued*
  hypertrophy and, 275–276
  outflow obstruction and, 248
  premature contraction of, 262
  septal defect and, 297–298
    holosystolic murmur and, 296
  tachycardia and, 262
Vermilion, 170
Vertebral fracture and dislocation, 560–563
Vertigo, 155
Vesical pain, 366
Vesicle, 95
Vesicular breath sound, 219–221
Vestibular nerve, 476
Vibration, 497
Vincent's stomatitis, 168, 179
Vision
  acuity and, 120–122, 470
  child and, 523
  field testing and, 136–139, 470
  loss of, 117–118
  neurologic disorder and, 457, 470
Vital signs, 71–79
  blood pressure and, 76–79
  child and, 509, 518–519
  history and, 71
  physical examination and, 30
  pulse and, 73–74
  respirations and, 74–76
  temperature and, 72–73
  uremia and, 368
Vitiligo, 92
  hand and, 89
Vitreous haziness, 141

Vocal cord paralysis, 167
  neurologic examination and, 477–478
Vocal fremitus, 212, 214
Voice
  chest auscultation and, 221
  cranial nerve and, 477–478
  general appearance and, 60
  nasopharynx and, 167
  respiratory disease and, 225
Voice test, 158
Volvulus, 512
Vomiting, 338
  abdominal pain and, 336–337, 512
  child and, 512, 513
  neurologic disorder and, 457
von Graefe's sign, 122

Waldeyer's ring, 181
Walking, tandem, 494. *See also* Gait
Wasting disease, 422
Water-hammer pulse, 257–258
Wave, fluid, 356
Wave form, jugular venous, 268–271
Weakness
  facial, 474–475, 476
  feigned, 482
  neurologic disorder and, 459
  pulse and, 259
  tongue and, 479
Weaver's bottom, 443
Weber's test, 158–159
Weight
  infant or child and, 513–514, 517

loss of
  elderly patient and, 537
  signs of, 60
Wernicke's aphasia, 468–469
Wheezing, 219, 220, 223–224
Whispered voice test, 158
Whispering pectoriloquy, 225
White arcus, 128
White banding of nail, 91
White noise, 219
White patch, mucosal, 173
White skin, 88
Wilms' tumor, 372
Winging of scapula, 432
Wound
  examination of, 542
  penetrating
    chest wall and, 548
    head and, 545
Wrist, 437–439
  Colles fracture of, 569–570
  nerve injury and, 560
Wryneck, 190

Xanthelasma, 125
Xeromammography, 323
Xerostomia, 166
X-ray. *See* Radiography

Y descent, 271
Yellow pigmentation, 86, 88
  gastrointestinal tract disorder and, 341
Yoked muscle, 131, 133

Zygoma fracture, 546